HEALTH IN ELEMENTARY SCHOOLS

HEALTH IN ELEMENTARY SCHOOLS

Harold J. Cornacchia, Ed.D.

Emeritus Professor of Health Education
San Francisco State University
San Francisco, California

Larry K. Olsen, Dr. P. H., C.H.E.S.

Professor of Health Education
The Pennsylvania State University
University Park, Pennsylvania

Janice M. Ozias, Ph.D., R. N.

Coordinator of Health Services
Austin Independent School District
Austin, Texas

NINTH EDITION

with 116 illustrations

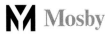

St. Louis Baltimore Boston Carlsbad Chicago Naples New York Philadelphia Portland
London Madrid Mexico City Singapore Sydney Tokyo Toronto Wiesbaden

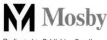

Mosby

Dedicated to Publishing Excellence

A Times Mirror Company

Vice President and Publisher: James M. Smith
Senior Acquisitions Editor: Vicki Malinee
Assistant Editor: Jennifer L. Hartman
Project Manager: John Rogers
Senior Production Editor: Helen Hudlin
Designer: Renée Duenow
Manufacturing Supervisor: Linda Ierardi
Cover photography credits:
 Boy measuring height: Arthur Tilley/FPG International Corp.
 Girl: Steve Dunwell/The Image Bank
 Class with skeleton: Pete Saloutos/The Stock Market
 Boy at keyboard: Paul Barton/The Stock Market

NINTH EDITION

Copyright © 1996 by Mosby–Year Book, Inc.

Previous editions copyrighted 1962, 1966, 1970, 1974, 1979, 1984, 1988, 1991

Printed in the United States of America
Composition by the Clarinda Company
Printing/binding by R.R. Donnelley & Sons Company

Mosby–Year Book, Inc.
11830 Westline Industrial Drive
St. Louis, Missouri 63146

Library of Congress Cataloging in Publication Data

Cornacchia, Harold J.
 Health in elementary schools / Harold J. Cornacchia, Larry K.
Olsen, Janice M. Ozias.—9th ed.
  p. cm.
 Includes bibliographical references and index.
 ISBN 0-8151-1858-9 (alk. paper)
 1. School hygiene—United States. 2. Health education
(Elementary)—United States. I. Olsen, Larry K. II. Ozias, Janice
M. III. Title.
LB3409.U5C63 1995
372.3'7—dc20   95–41874
                                       CIP

95 96 97 98 99 / 9 8 7 6 5 4 3 2 1

About the Authors

HAROLD J. CORNACCHIA, ED.D., is a prominent educator, consultant, administrator, author, and consumer advocate. He is Emeritus Professor of Health Education at San Francisco State University and has been a lecturer with faculty appointments at four other universities. He was chairman of the Department of Health Education for 14 years at the university. He has also had 5 years experience as a school administrator. During his 35-year career, he has developed, promoted, and administered health education programs in elementary and secondary schools throughout the United States. He has conducted many teacher health education in-service seminars and workshops. He was Director of one of the four National Drug Education Training Centers sponsored and financed by the U.S. Office of Education. He was instructor for a series of ten television programs on first aid for the San Francisco Chapter of the American Red Cross. The National Fire Prevention Association Program on Fire Safety that he developed for elementary schools to date has saved hundreds of lives. He has served as a Board Member of the National Council Against Health Fraud. The 17 books in which he has been the primary author include *Health in Elementary Schools, Consumer Health, Drugs in the Classroom: A Conceptual Model,* and *Shopping for Health Care.*

LARRY K. OLSEN, DR. P.H., C.H.E.S., is currently a Professor of Health Education at The Pennsylvania State University. Previously he was a professor of Health Education at Arizona State University and an Associate Professor of Health Education at the University of Illinois and at the School of Public Health at the Chicago Circle Campus of the University of Illinois. He is the author of numerous journal articles and elementary and college level textbooks in the area of health education. As an active member of many prestigious national and international health education organizations, Dr. Olsen has held leadership positions within these organizations at the local and national levels and has served as President of the American School Health Association from 1990-1991. He is a regular presenter at national meetings of professional organizations and has conducted numerous teacher training programs both nationally and internationally. Widely recognized as an expert in the area of school health, Dr. Olsen has also served as a consultant to the Centers for Disease Control and Prevention, the National Center for Health Education, The American Cancer Society, The American Heart Association, and the U.S. Department of Health and Human Services.

JANICE M. OZIAS, PH.D., R.N., is currently Coordinator of Health Services in Austin, Texas, where she oversees a multidisciplinary team including school nurses, the school physician, a vision and hearing screening staff, and a social worker for pregnant youth. Austin School Health Services staff work closely with teachers, parents, and with community resources to protect the health of students in order to promote optimal attendance, participation, and achievement. The Austin Independent School District was the first school nursing program in the United States to promote self-care development of students—prekindergarten through grade 12—using principles of health education. Dr. Ozias is involved in the annual Texas School Health Promotion Conference for teams from school districts throughout the state and is active in the American School Health Association.

Preface

APPROACH

This text provides a unique contribution to school health in the United States for the following reasons:

- Conceptual models for comprehensive school health and health education programs, which must be implemented in schools to affect the well-being of children and to have the greatest impact on learning, are clearly identified.
- The components of school health and health education programs are applied to the concept of health that includes psychological, sociological, physiological, and spiritual phenomena affecting human behavior.
- Critical information needed by teachers and administrators to understand, plan, develop, implement, and evaluate comprehensive school health and health education programs is provided.

Elementary school-age children generally are in good health. However, numerous health and safety conditions that can disturb learning continue to affect these young people, such as respiratory and gastrointestinal disturbances, vision and hearing problems, emotional difficulties, child neglect and abuse, suicide, drug abuse including alcohol and tobacco, dental caries, pregnancies, AIDS, and obesity. Children with problems need to be identified by school personnel in order to assist pupils and parents with information and guidelines for their resolution.

Much of the illness found among school-age children can be prevented or at least reduced in incidence and severity through the avoidance of risk factors and through behavior modification. Because many adult health problems are the result of habit patterns established in the early years of life, programs in schools that provide health education, health services, and a healthful environment, when conducted in cooperation with the home and community, will aid in the establishment of pupil practices of healthful living and contribute to their well-being.

The authors of this text continue to firmly believe that:

- Good health is essential to learning.
- Schools have an important role to play in the well-being of students and must provide comprehensive school health programs.
- Comprehensive school health programs must be planned, developed, and implemented in elementary schools.
- Comprehensive health education programs that impact student behavior must be introduced and expanded in preschool and elementary schools.
- The preventive approach to health problems and the acceptance of responsibility for self-care must be started in children's early years.

It follows, therefore, that teachers and administrators, especially in elementary schools, need to understand the nature and purpose of school health programs and their roles in such programs. The major focus of this text has not changed from previous editions. To this end, this text covers the total school health program, including health education, health services, the healthful school environment, and coordination. However, it has been organized primarily to provide information about health education—curriculum, organizing for teaching, learning principles applied to health education, methods and techniques of teaching, and evaluation procedures. This text will be especially helpful for teachers-in-training and can assist in the professional development of teachers in schools where limited or no health education programs exist.

NEED FOR ELEMENTARY SCHOOL HEALTH EDUCATION

Awareness of the need for health education has greatly increased over the years. It is now widely recognized that individuals must assume more responsibility for their own health. The focus of health education involves not only physiological considerations but also psychological, sociological, and spiritual emphases.

It is recognized that to change health behavior, people need more than an understanding of the parts and functions of body organs. They must be made aware of their own motivations and the peer pressures and other influences that affect their behavior. Health education is needed because of the (1) high cost of medical care, (2) existence of health misconceptions, (3) millions of dollars spent on useless, unnecessary, and harmful products and services, (4) influences on behavior by peers, adults, and the media, (5) confusing and often inaccurate health information disseminated, and (6) desire of people to be healthy.

Health education programs are now supported by the American School Health Association, the Association for the Advancement of Health Education, the National Coalition of Health Education Organizations, The American Public Health Association, The American Association of School Administrators, The National Association of State Boards of Education, The American Medical Association, The American Cancer Society, The American Academy of Pediatrics, and the National Congress of Parents and Teachers. The federal government has established the Division of Adolescent and School Health (DASH) in the Centers for Disease Control and Prevention. Also the U.S. Department of Health and Human Services, Public Health Service, has strongly supported the need for school health education (see Appendix L). It published *Healthy People 2000* that identified the health goals to be reached by the year 2000. These goals support attention to many health conditions as well as the prevention of disease, with much emphasis on school health and health education. As of 1993, one third of these goals have been met or are in the process of being met. In the private sector, the National Center for Health Education has functioned for many years to obtain support for school programs through funds from industry and other sources. Numerous companies and foundations such as the Metropolitan Life Foundation and W.K. Kellog have provided funds for demonstrations of comprehensive school health education programs. Health education is mandated in 19 states (37%) in grades 1 to 6 and is combined with physical education in 3 states (5½%). In grades 7 and 8, health education is mandated in 22 states (43%) and is combined with physical education in 4 states (8%). The Robert Wood Foundation has financed projects to establish health clinics for high-risk youth.

Unfortunately, despite the numbers of elementary schools in the United States that have health education programs, few of these programs are comprehensive. A survey by the National School Boards Association, to which 15% of the 2000 school districts contacted in the United States responded, indicated that only 5% to 14% had some of the components of a comprehensive health education program.

The legal provisions in states often are so loosely written that numerous programs are limited to one or more health topics, such as nutrition, drugs, or safety. The term *comprehensive* has been subject to a variety of interpretations. Its meaning as defined in this text and as accepted by school health experts has not been adequately implemented in U.S. schools. Several problems related to the lack of school finances, the public's demand for a return to teaching the basic subjects, and their basic displeasure with school in general have compounded the difficulty of developing health instruction programs, despite the increased awareness of need and the progress made in the last 5 years.

AUDIENCE

This text has been designed to be a practical guide for prospective and in-service elementary teachers and for health service personnel and school administrators. It can also provide information for school board members. Prospective teachers will obtain a preview of their role in the school health program. In-service teachers may use the text to evaluate and develop health education programs for schools that do not have such programs. School health coordinators, curriculum coordinators, principals, school board members, and health specialists will find this text to be helpful in the development and implementation of curricula and in the preparation of guiding principles and programs. Public health personnel will be able to clarify problems concerning organization, objectives, curriculum development, supervision, and teaching methods and materials related to elementary school health programs.

ORGANIZATION OF THE TEXT

The organization of the text continues to include six parts:

Part I. Identification of the nature and purpose of school health and the role of the classroom teacher.

Parts II and III. Discussion of the healthful environment, covering the physical aspects and emotional climate in the school, and health services, including appraisals, guidance, and emergency care.

Part IV. Discussion of the status of health education today, organizing for health teaching, the learning process in health education, illustrations of popular and effective programs, and principles and procedures of organization.

Part V. Presentation of methods and materials in health education, including an introduction to general methods with over 1200 teacher-tested techniques categorized by subject area and grade level group.

Part VI. Explanation of evaluation with practical suggestions for teacher use in the classroom.

Appendices. Sources of programs and teaching aids, essential updates on AIDS, specific health considerations, evaluation information, listings of children's literature containing health themes with ethnic, cultural, and gender-diverse books noted, and partial health units that may be used to develop units and curricula.

NEW TO THIS EDITION

The ninth edition of *Health in Elementary Schools* has been updated with the latest information in order to provide the most comprehensive book available on school health. Some of the specific new additions that have been made are:

- *Chapter 1: School Health, Its Nature and Purpose* contains the U.S. Surgeon General's Health Goals for the Year 2000 and charts the progress that has been made toward achieving those goals.
- Photos and drawings have been updated throughout the book, with special emphasis on *Chapter 7: Emergency Care,* to provide greater clarity and accuracy.
- *Part III: Health Services* contains increased information about violence, abuse, and homeless children.
- *Chapter 10: Health Education Approaches* provides new examples of successful nationally validated health programs in various states and schools.
- *Chapter 11: Organizing for Health Teaching* includes the Standards for Health Education advocated by The American Cancer Society.
- The difference in organizational pattern for school health as advocated by the American School Health Association is clearly identified.
- Additional and modified "Problems to Solve" have been included at the beginning of many chapters.
- Medical terminology has been updated througout.
- Boxed material, highlighting specific information, has been increased in many chapters.
- References in all chapters have been updated and revised.

- AIDS coverage is expanded and updated throughout. *Appendix A* has been completely rewritten with increased content on HIV/AIDS.
- *Appendix D: A Sample of Health Education Fiction and Nonfiction Books* has been revised to include and highlight books with an ethnic, cultural, and gender-diversity focus.
- *Appendix L* contains the joint statement supporting health education by the U.S. Departments of Education and Health and Human Services.
- *Appendix M: General Criteria for Assessing Health Instruction Software* contains guidelines for the assessment of health instruction materials and software.

PEDAGOGICAL FEATURES

This text is especially useful because of its many pedagogical features:

- Key concepts for each chapter provide a content focus for students.
- Problem(s) to solve have been included to help focus student attention on the practical application of the content.
- Summaries at the end of each chapter contain a brief review of the content and help in the reinforcement of learning.
- Questions at the end of each chapter can be useful for classroom discussions and essay test questions.
- Many subheadings in the text are in the form of questions that can be used as the basis for problem-solving activities.

INSTRUCTOR'S MANUAL

The *Instructor's Manual* provides specific help for teachers when planning course outlines and teacher/learning activities. The manual contains a rating scale using the principles of learning to help in the selection of effective teaching techniques. It contains general and specific student objectives, new suggestions for classroom teaching/learning activities, and audiovisual aids that will enhance classroom presentations. A test bank of true-false, multiple choice, and completion questions for ex-

aminations is included. A computerized test bank for use on IBM and MacIntosh equipment is available for qualified adopters.

Lesson Plan Material

A comprehensive lesson plan manual, *Planning Health Lessons*, a valuable supplement to *Health in Elementary Schools*, can be purchased with the text for an additional nominal fee. This manual contains 120 lesson plans, is organized by health content areas, and contains numerous student handouts and instructor worksheets.

IN CONCLUSION

The philosophical approach to comprehensive school health described in this text provides a *conceptual model* in need of implementation by school districts in the United States.

The authors have made every effort to present the latest and best in research, practice, and the thinking of leading experts in school health in light of what is feasible and practical for elementary schools throughout the nation. We have attempted to provide a synthesis of fundamental principles that are generally accepted by professionals and that in our many years of experience we have found to work best in elementary schools. To be effective, these principles and practices for school health programs must be implemented by teachers, administrators, and school board members.

If this text helps to bring about favorable changes in elementary school health programs, if we lead classroom teachers to recognize the powerful influence they can have on the health of children, if we can motivate teachers to stimulate the inclusion and teaching of health education in their schools, if we can provoke principals to take a critical look at health programs in their schools, if we can touch the conscience of superintendents and school board members to introduce and improve school health programs, if we can pique the curiosity of health department or voluntary agency personnel to lend support for school health programs, if we can motivate private foundations and companies to provide financial aid to add or to improve programs, or if, above all, we can in some way enrich the lives of elementary school children, we will have achieved the goal for which this book was written.

ACKNOWLEDGMENTS

We must express our sincere gratitude to Carl J. Nickerson, Ed.D., for his contributions to this text as a co-author of editions 6, 7, and 8. His expertise and talent provided many valuable improvements to the book that enabled it to continue as an outstanding professional publication. Although we regret his departure as a member of our team, we value the role he played in the successful production of *Health in Elementary Schools*.

Finally, we are grateful to all those people and organizations who have helped us make the ninth edition of *Health in Elementary Schools* a better text. We are especially indebted to those classroom teachers, our friends in the profession, and our students who offered stimulation and useful suggestions.

In addition, we would like to thank the following reviewers for their useful input, which helped in the revision of this edition: Bill Hyman, Ph.D., Sam Houston State University; Karl Salscheider, Ph.D., Bemidji State University; Sherry Salyer, M.A., University of North Carolina—Chapel Hill; and Marion R. Scott, M.S., R.N., Youngstown State University.

Harold J. Cornacchia
Larry K. Olsen
Janice M. Ozias

Contents

HEALTH IN ELEMENTARY SCHOOLS

I

THE ELEMENTARY SCHOOL HEALTH PROGRAM

1

School Health:
Its Nature and Purpose

KEY CONCEPT

Comprehensive school health programs that include instruction, services, and environmental phases play an important role in the promotion, prevention, and maintenance of student health.

For the first time in the history of this country, young people are less healthy and less prepared to take their place in society than were their parents.

CODE BLUE
National School Boards Association and American Medical Association*

Education and health for children are inextricably intertwined. A student who is not healthy . . . is a student who will not profit from the educational process.

MICHAEL MCGINNIS, M.D.
U.S. Office of Disease Prevention and Health Promotion, 1987†

. . . health and fitness are critical to academic performance and need to be improved. . . .

THE CARNEGIE COUNCIL ON ACADEMIC DEVELOPMENT
Report of the Task Force on Education and Young Adults, 1989‡

. . . . 67% of all disease and premature death is preventable . . . prevention should be our first line of defense against medical problems. . . .

JOSEPH A. CALIFANO, JR.
Former U.S. Secretary of Health, Education, and Welfare, 1987§

PROBLEM TO SOLVE

As a sixth grade teacher, a school nurse, or a public health official in a large public school system who believes that a comprehensive school health program would improve the learning capabilities of the students in your school (system), what information would you present to parents, school board members, the superintendent, and others to persuade them to consider the adoption of such a program?

*The National Commission: *Code blue: uniting for healthier youth,* Alexandria, VA, 1990, National School Boards Association and American Medical Association.
†Allensworth DD, Kolbe LJ: The comprehensive school health program: exploring an expanded concept, *J School Health* 57:409-412, 1987.
‡The Carnegie Council on Adolescent Development: *Turning points: preparing American youth for the 21st century: report of the task force on education and young adolescents,* New York, 1989, Carnegie Corporation.
§Stated at US Senate Hearing before Committee on Labor and Human Resources, *National Health Goals,* Jan 12, 1987.

3

SINCE 1900 the death rate in America has been reduced as a result of medical control over such diseases as tuberculosis, diphtheria, poliomyelitis, and gastroenteritis. Infant, child, and maternal mortality have decreased, and the life expectancy of individuals has increased from approximately 50 years in 1900 to 75.5 years in 1994. Improvements in sanitation, housing, nutrition, and immunization have resulted in control over typhoid fever, smallpox, plague, and other diseases. Progress is evident in the control of heart disease, some cancers, and other chronic conditions. Despite these advances, however, many health and safety problems, such as AIDS among young people, especially the poor and minorities, still exist in the United States. Acute illnesses result in an average loss per school year of 5 days for each American child. Numerous children are not completely immunized. Accidents are the primary cause of death. Child abuse and neglect and suicides are of major concern. Students are experiencing learning difficulties related to such problems as attention deficit disorder and dyslexia. Pupils are exposed to a variety of risk factors such as substance abuse, suicide, pregnancy, AIDS, sexual activity, and poor food selection that lead to numerous diseases and conditions. Infants, school-age children, adolescents, and adults are all affected by these risk factors.

The need for preventive actions and services to promote and preserve the health of individuals has now been recognized by Americans who have become increasingly aware and concerned with the preventive aspects of health care. The American Academy of Pediatrics* advocated that children must be healthy to learn effectively and maintains that schools have a responsibility to promote optimal health in pupils. According to the American School Health Association,† a child needs to be healthy to learn. The American Medical Association* believes that many health problems of children and youth are preventable.

The National School Boards Association and the American Medical Association† in a joint statement called on the nation to recognize that adolescent health must be given top priority in schools and in the community. Young people will not reach their potential if social, emotional, and physical health problems interfere with learning. Joycelyn Elders, former U.S. Surgeon General stated, ". . . you don't educate children if they aren't healthy."‡ The importance of school health was emphasized in the National Education Goals established in 1993 when it was stressed that all children in schools must be ready to learn. Attention to life-styles and behavior together with control of environmental factors can reduce the need for medical and hospital care according to Julius B. Richmond, former Surgeon General of the United States. Dr. Richmond indicated the Public Health Service reviewed its priorities for the expenditure of funds in America and decided that the improvement of the health status of citizens could be achieved predominantly through preventive actions rather than through the treatment of disease. However, in 1990 only a fraction of the $660 billion (12% of the Gross National Product [GNP]) went for the prevention of problems.§

In 1979, the first Surgeon General's report on health promotion and disease prevention, *Healthy People,* was published. It stated that good health could be preserved and ill health could be prevented. The report identified 15 priority areas (in three categories: preventive health services, health promotion, and health protection—see Table 1-1) in which, if appropriate actions were

---

*Committee on School Health: *School health: policy and practice,* Elk Grove Village, IL, 1993, American Academy of Pediatrics.
†American School Health Association: *Marketing kit,* Kent, OH, 1985, The Association.

*American Medical Association: *America's adolescents: how healthy are they?* Chicago, 1990, The Association.
†The National Commission: *Code blue: uniting for healthier youth,* Alexandria, VA, 1990, National School Boards Association and American Medical Association.
‡Toch T: Battle plans of a general, *America's agenda,* Winter, 1994, p 13.
§Gibbs N: Shameful bequests to the next generation, *Time* 136:42-48, 1990.

TABLE 1-1 Selected Areas and Objectives From the Surgeon General's Report, *Promoting Health/Preventing Disease,* * Reviewed in *Midcourse Review, 1986* and in *Health United States, 1989*

Areas	Objectives	Midcourse review, 1986†	Health United States, 1989‡
PREVENTIVE HEALTH SERVICES FOR INDIVIDUALS			
High blood pressure	By 1990: At least 50% of adults should be able to state the principal risk factors for coronary heart disease and stroke (i.e., high blood pressure, cigarette smoking, elevated blood cholesterol levels, diabetes).	High blood pressure: est. 92% Cigarettes: est. 91% Cholesterol: est. 86% Diabetes: est. 60%	—
Family planning	There should be no unintended births to girls 14 years old or younger. At least 75% of men and women over the age of 14 should be able to describe accurately the various contraceptive methods, including the relative safety and effectiveness of one method versus the other.	1984: 9965 births 75% knew how 11 of 13 methods used	1987: 10,311 births
Pregnancy and infant health	85% of women of childbearing age should be able to choose foods wisely and understand the hazards of smoking, alcohol, pharmaceutical products, and other drugs during pregnancy and lactation.	No consistent data	—
Immunization	At least 95% of children attending licensed day care facilities and kindergarten through twelfth grade should be fully immunized.	88% or higher	95%
Sexually transmitted diseases	Every junior and senior high school student in the United States should receive accurate, timely education about sexually transmitted diseases.	1982: 66% in metropolitan schools	Some informed: 70%
HEALTH PROTECTION FOR POPULATION GROUPS			
Toxic agent control	At least half of all people aged 15 years and older should be able to identify the major categories of environmental threats to health and note some of the health consequences of those threats.	No data	—
Accident prevention and control	The motor vehicle fatality rate for children under 15 should be reduced to no greater than 5.5 per 100,000 children; the home accident fatality rate should be no greater than 5.0 per 100,000 population.	1983: 6.7 per 100,000 1983: 5.0 per 100,000	1990: 5 per 100,000 1990: 5 per 100,000

Continued.

TABLE 1-1 Selected Areas and Objectives From the Surgeon General's Report, *Promoting Health/Preventing Disease*—cont'd

Areas	Objectives	Midcourse review, 1986†	Health United States, 1989‡
HEALTH PROTECTION FOR POPULATION GROUPS—cont'd			
Fluoridation and dental health	At least 95% of school children and their parents should be able to identify the principal risk factors related to dental diseases and be aware of the importance of fluoridation and other measures in controlling these diseases.	Not available	—
	At least 65% of school children should be proficient in personal oral hygiene practices and should be receiving other needed preventive dental services in addition to fluoridation.	Unknown	—
	No public elementary or secondary school should offer highly cariogenic foods or snacks in vending machines or in breakfast or lunch programs.	Not available	—
	The proportion of 9-year-old children who have experienced dental caries in their permanent teeth should be decreased to 60%.	49%	1986-1987: 34.5%
HEALTH PROMOTION FOR POPULATION GROUPS			
Smoking and health	The proportion of children and youth aged 12 to 18 years old who smoke should be reduced to below 6%.	High school seniors: est. 19.5%	1988: 12%
Misuse of alcohol and drugs	The proportion of adolescents 12 to 17 years old who abstain from using alcohol or other drugs should not fall below the 1977 levels (alcohol, 46%; marijuana, 89%; heroin, 99.9%).	Alcohol: 73.1% Marijuana: 88.5% Heroin: 99.5%	69% 83% Cocaine: 99.2%
	The proportion of adolescents 14 to 17 years old who report acute drinking-related problems during the past year should be reduced to below 17%.	1982: 41%	
	The proportion of adolescents 12 to 17 years old reporting frequent use of other drugs should not exceed 1977 levels (marijuana, 19%; other drugs, 1%).	Marijuana: 9% Other drugs: less than 1%	9% Less than 0.5%
Nutrition	All states should include nutrition education as part of required comprehensive school health education at elementary and secondary schools	12 states	19 states

TABLE 1-1 Selected Areas and Objectives from the Surgeon General's Report, *Promoting Health/Preventing Disease*—**cont'd**

Areas	Objectives	Midcourse review, 1986†	Health United States, 1989‡
HEALTH PROMOTION FOR POPULATION GROUPS—cont'd			
Physical fitness and exercise	The proportion of children and adolescents aged 10 to 17 participating in daily school physical education programs should be greater than 60%.	1984: 36.3%	36%
	The proportion of children and adolescents aged 10 to 17 participating regularly in appropriate physical activities, particularly cardiorespiratory fitness programs, which can be carried into adulthood, should be greater than 90%.	1984: 66%	
Control of stress and violent behavior	Stress identification and control should become integral components of the continuum of health services offered by organized health programs.	Not available	
	Injuries and deaths to children inflicted by abusing parents should be reduced by at least 25%.	40%	1986: 16.3%
	The rate of suicide among people 15 to 24 years should be below 11 per 100,000.	1983: 15-24: 11.9 per 100,000 15-19: 8.7 per 100,000	1990: 11.0 per 100,000

*US Department of Health and Human Services, Public Health Service: *Promoting health/preventing disease: objectives for the nation,* Washington, DC, 1980, US Government Printing Office.
†US Department of Health and Human Services, Public Health Service: *The 1990 health objectives for the nation: a midcourse review,* Washington, DC, 1986, US Government Printing Office.
‡US Department of Health and Human Services, Public Health Service: *Health United States 1989 and prevention profile,* Hyattsville, MD, 1990, National Center for Health Statistics.

taken, further health gains could be expected between the years 1980 and 1990. Broad national goals were established that could lead to the improvement of the health of Americans. These goals were expressed as reductions in overall death rates or days of disability. In 1980, the report, *Promoting Health/Preventing Disease,* was produced. It identified 207 specific objectives necessary to achieve the broad national goals.

Over 65 of these had implications for school programs. Selected objectives that have school implications for most of the areas are listed in Table 1-1.

Progress toward reaching some of the selected goals may be found in the *Midcourse Review, 1986* and the *Health United States, 1989* summarized in Table 1-1. The percentages of objectives by categories to be reached together with the percentages achieved and those "on-track" were:

- Prevention services: 45%, of which 14% have been achieved and 32% are on-track to being achieved
- Health protection: 46%, of which 11% have been achieved and 35% are on-track to being achieved
- Health promotion: 52%, of which 16% have been achieved and 36% are on-track to being achieved

GOALS FOR HEALTHY PEOPLE 2000

The objectives from *Healthy People 2000* (1990) resulted in increased attention to a variety of preventive health problems despite mixed reviews regarding their limited achievement. The effort to set goals for the year 2000 was led by the Office of Disease Prevention and Health Promotion of the U.S. Public Health Service with the assistance of the American Public Health Association and numerous other health organizations in the United States. Table 1-2 provides selected illustrations of some of those objectives that have school significance and their achievement by 1991.

Health United States 1992 presented an overview of the progress toward the year 2000 objectives. This summary provides the percentages to determine progress toward their targets for 300 unduplicated main objectives:

- 3% have been met
- 28% in progress
- 15% show movement
- 4% show mixed results
- 3% no change
- 10% indicated new baselines where none existed
- 28% had no new data to evaluate
- 10% needed baselines

The priority areas that showed the most progress towards their objective targets were heart disease and stroke, 9 of 17 showed progress; unintentional

injuries, 11 of 22 showed progress; alcohol and other drugs, 9 of 19 exceeded the target goal. Those priority areas showing movement away from progress toward their objectives were maternal and infant health, 5 of 16 objectives, and diabetes and chronic disabling conditions, 6 of 20 objectives (Table 1-2).

COMPREHENSIVE SCHOOL HEALTH

The National Commission on the Role of the School in Improving Adolescent Health in the Community concluded that adolescent health must be a top priority in schools and in the community. The Commission recognized that youth health problems are often found in preadolescent and early childhood years.*

Authorities agree that the best time for building foundations for better health is early in life. It follows then that one of society's largest—and potentially most influential—organizations offer vast opportunities for raising the level of health of young people. Obviously we speak here of the approximately 59,000 public and private elementary schools found in the cities, towns, and countrysides of America. There are limitless ways in which elementary teachers and school administrators—with the help of health specialists and the support of parents and the community—can favorably affect the health of 30 million boys and girls (grades K-8) in schools across the land. The provision of a **Comprehensive School Health Program** as identified in Fig. 1-1 will have great impact on children. The basic components of such a program should include **comprehensive health education, health services, provision for a healthful school environment, and coordination** with responsibility for administration, supervision, and integration with the school,

---

*The National Commission: *Code blue: uniting for healthier youth,* Alexandria, VA, 1990, National School Boards Association and American Medical Association.

TABLE 1-2 Selected Examples of the Year 2000 Health Objectives Having School Significance*

Areas	Objectives	Healthy People 2000, Review 1993†
PREVENTIVE SERVICES		
AIDS/HIV infection	Confine the annual incidence to no more than the projected number of new cases in 1992 (baseline: 32,971 cases in 1988; revised in 1989 to 49,000; Target 2000 = 98,000)	87,000
	Reduce the proportion of adolescents who engage in sexual intercourse to no more than 15% by age 15 and no more than 40% by age 17 (baseline: 27% of girls and 33% of boys by age 15; 50% of girls and 66% of boys by age 17; reported in 1988; Target 2000: by 15 years = 15%, by 17 years = 40%)	*Ages* 15 yrs: Boys = 44% Girls = 36% 17 yrs: Boys = 66% Girls = 68%
Family planning	Reduce the proportion of adolescents who engage in sexual intercourse to no more than 15% by age 15 and no more than 40% by age 17 (baseline: 27% of girls and 33% of boys by age 15; 50% of girls and 66% of boys by age 17; reported in 1988; Target 2000: by 15 years = 15%, by 17 years = 40%)	*Ages* 15 yrs: Boys = 44% Girls = 36% 17 yrs: Boys = 66% Girls = 68%
	Reduce pregnancies among girls ages 17 and younger to no more than 50 per 1,000 in adolescents (baseline: 71.1 pregnancies per 1,000 girls ages 15 through 17 in 1985)	10-14 years = 3.3 15-17 years = 74.3
Sexually transmitted diseases	Reduce gonorrhea to an incidence of no more than 225 cases per 100,000 people (baseline: 300 per 100,000 in 1989; Target 2000: 225)	202
	Reduce primary and secondary syphilis to an incidence of no more than 10 cases per 100,000 people (baseline: 18.1 per 100,000 in 1989; Target 2000: 10)	13.7
	Include instruction in sexually transmitted disease transmission prevention in the curricula of all middle and secondary schools, preferably as part of quality school health education (baseline: 95% of schools reported offering at least one class on sexually transmitted diseases as part of their standard curricula in 1988; Target 2000: 100%)	No data
HEALTH PROTECTION		
Oral health	Reduce dental caries so that the proportion of children with one or more caries (in permanent teeth) is no more than 35% among children aged 6 through 8 and no more than 60% among adolescents aged 15 (baseline: 53% of children aged 6 through 8 in 1986-1987; 78% of adolescents aged 15 in 1986-1987)	No data

Continued.

TABLE 1-2 Selected Examples of the Year 2000 Health Objectives Having School Significance—cont'd

Areas	Objectives			Healthy People 2000, Review 1993†
HEALTH PROMOTION				
Alcohol and other drugs	Provide all public and private schools education programs on alcohol and drugs, preferably as part of comprehensive school health education (Target 2000: 100%)			No data
	Reduce proportion of young people who have used alcohol, marijuana, and cocaine in the past month as follows:			
		Baseline 1988	*Target 2000*	
	Alcohol/ages 12-17	25.2%	12.6%	15.7%
	Marijuana/ages 12-17	6.4%	3.2%	4.0%
	Cocaine/ages 12-17	1.1%	0.6%	0.3%
	Cigarettes	No data	12.6%	9.6%
	Average *age* at first use among 12-17 year olds did not change substantially for cigarettes (11.5 years) or marijuana (13.5 years), but declined markedly for alcohol (12.6 years)			
Physical activity and fitness	Increase to at least 75% the proportion of children and adolescents aged 6-17 who engage in vigorous physical activities 3 or more days per week for 20 or more minutes per occasion that promote the development and maintenance of cardiorespiratory fitness (baseline: 66% for youth aged 10-17 in 1985)			Not possible to track
	Increase to at least 50% the proportion of children and adolescents in first through twelfth grade who participate in daily school physical education (baseline: 36% in 1984-1986)			Not possible to track
	Increase to at least 50% the proportion of school physical education class time that students spend being physically active, preferably engaged in lifetime physical activities			Not possible to track
Tobacco	Reduce the initiation of cigarette smoking by children and youth so that no more than 15% have become regular cigarette smokers by age 20 (baseline: 30% of youth had become regular smokers by ages 20-24 in 1987)			28%
	Reduce the use of smokeless tobacco use for males 12-17 years to Target 2000: 4%			4.8%
	Include discussion of tobacco use prevention in 100% of the health curricula of elementary and middle school by 2000			No data

TABLE 1-2 Selected Examples of the Year 2000 Health Objectives Having School Significance—cont'd

Areas	Objectives	Healthy People 2000, Review 1993†
HEALTH PROMOTION—cont'd		
Nutrition	Increase to at least 90% the proportion of school services and child care food services that have menus consistent with the lunch/breakfast nutrition principles in the Dietary Guidelines of America	No data
	Increase to at least 75% the proportion of the nation's schools that provide nutrition education from preschool through twelfth grade, preferably as part of comprehensive school health education	60%
Violent and abusive	Reverse to less than 25.2% per 1000 children the rising incidence of behavior maltreatment of children younger than age 18 (baseline: 25.2 per 1000 in 1986)	No data
	Reduce suicides to no more than 10.5 per 100,000 people (age adjusted baseline: 11.7 per 100,000 in 1987; Target 2000: 8.2)	10.9
	Reduce by 15% the incidence of injurious suicide attempts among adolescents aged 14-19	1.7%
Educational and community-based programs	Increase to at least 75% the proportion of the nation's elementary and secondary schools that provide planned and sequential kindergarten through twelfth-grade quality school health education	No data

*US Department of Health and Human Services, Public Health Service: *Healthy people 2000: national health promotion and disease prevention objectives,* conference edition, Washington, DC, 1990, US Government Printing Office.
†US Department of Health and Human Services: *Healthy people 2000, review 1993,* Washington, DC, 1994, US Government Printing Office.

parents, community agencies, and community organizations. This is a **conceptual model** that has only been partially implemented and whose segments are rarely coordinated or integrated in American schools. In recent years, the American School Health Association* has advocated that an expanded concept of a comprehensive school health program should consist of eight categories: health education, health services, environment, school-community integration, physical education,* food services, counseling, school site health promotion for faculty and staff. Fig. 1-1 includes all of these phases in an integrated pattern

*Allensworth DD, Kolbe LJ: The comprehensive school health program: exploring an expanded concept, *J School Health* 57:409-412, 1987.

*Although physical education makes a significant health contribution to the health of students, especially in the light of its fitness focus, it should be identified as a subject field in its own right. Physical education provides many opportunities for integrated and incidental health teaching rather than direct teaching. Health teachers should integrate and relate learning to and with physical education or vice versa. It differs from health education in terms of teacher preparation, objectives, methods, and activities used in teaching, and procedures for evaluation. Finally, there are aspects of health services and healthful school environment related to physical education directly affecting the health of pupils that should be coordinated with the total school health program.

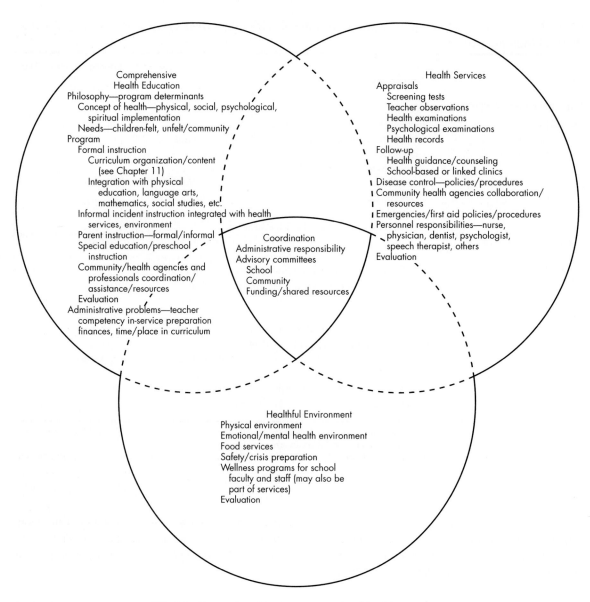

FIG. 1-1 Comprehensive elementary school health program.

and clearly identifies the coordination relationships of the various segments.

In 1993 the United States Secretaries of Education and Health and Human Services issued a joint statement (see Appendix L) in support of the comprehensive school health program concept and established an Interagency Committee on School Health. They also convened the National Coordinating Committee on School Health to bring together major education and health organizations to work with their office for the implementation of comprehensive school health.

Problems With Implementation of Comprehensive School Health Program

There are numerous implementation problems facing schools despite the tremendous advocacy for comprehensive school health promoted by leaders in the field. School superintendents, school boards, and community knowledge and acceptance of the **conceptual model** along with the need for financial assistance are key problems. Achievement of the conceptual model will demand considerable initiative and effort on the part of school leaders and the community plus a massive infusion of funds to become a reality. Few, if any, comprehensive school health programs in the United States today are complete, coordinated, and integrated as outlined in this text.

The Chief School State Officers* identified these things to be missing in health education programs: administrative commitments, adequately prepared teachers, sufficient time in the school day, money, credibility as an academic subject, community/parental support, and the inclusion of controversial subjects in the curriculum.

Health services and provisions for a healthful environment must contend with the loss of nurses; the advent of school-based health clinics; the need for policies regarding AIDS, violence, and emergencies; the tremendous needs of children with special problems; and other issues discussed in later chapters.

To become a reality, the conceptual model for comprehensive school health as described throughout this text needs qualified and identifiable coordinators or administrators to effectively promote, initiate, develop, implement, integrate, and supervise the total school health program.

School problems. But our schools are facing many other troubles. Teachers, prospective teachers, educational administrators, legislators, parents, education faculty in colleges and universities, taxpayers, and the news media have all become increasingly concerned about our schools. As problems continue to mount, cluttering the road to quality education for all children, it is clear that bold measures must be taken if we are to give more than lip service to repeated statements of lofty objectives and high ideals for America's schools.

Our schools and our society are beset with the harsh reality of economic, political, and other social problems that affect the quality of life. The structure of the family has changed dramatically; there are more homes where both parents work and where the number of single parents and minorities have increased. The question of tax sources for the equitable and adequate support of our schools has become critical. Piled atop the money problems are the tangled issues of busing, lowered enrollments, school closings, collective negotiations between teachers and school boards, health and safety conditions for pupils and teachers, conflicts in administrative and learning theories, "accountability" procedures for both pupils and teachers, and, recently, public concern over the quality of education and teachers, and the call for a return to the basic subjects in education.

---

*Butler SC: Chief staff officers rank barriers to implementing comprehensive school health education, *J School Health* 63:130-132, 1993.

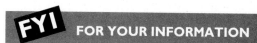

FOR YOUR INFORMATION

> Every 47 seconds a child is abused or neglected.
> Every 67 seconds a teenager has a baby.
> Every 7 minutes a child is arrested for a drug offense.
> Every 36 minutes a child is killed or injured by a gun.
> Every day 135,000 children bring their guns to school.
> The statistics are even worse for poor or minority children.

Modified from Children's Defense Fund: *Children 1990: a report card,* Briefing Book and Action, Washington, DC, 1990, The Fund.

However, because this is a text about elementary schools and their health programs, we cannot properly analyze all those forces that tend to shape our culture and our schools. Nevertheless, the need for *preventive* health care has never been more critical, and its advocacy is increasing substantially each year. Authorities now realize that it is not only necessary but also economically more feasible and desirable to reduce the incidence of health problems. The schools have a vital role to play in such action.

Yet school health does not exist in a vacuum. The school health program is part of the lifeblood of America's better schools, and, like all aspects of good schools, it is sensitive to significant thinking and events in the community in which it thrives. In a very real sense the school reflects the character of its community—local, state, and national. Health instruction must be closely related to day-to-day problems of health and safety; school health services depend in large measure on the community's health resources, and the healthful school environment is in itself part of the community.

It is the basic thesis of education that the thinking and the behavior of people can be changed for the better. It is assumed with the confidence that grows out of research and experience that good teaching in a favorable setting will raise the quality of living for pupils. By enriching the lives of millions of children, elementary education will help contribute to forming a better society.

This "better society" and "the good life" have challenged humans for thousands of years. Along with the family, the church and temple, and the community in general, schools have continuously sought to help people live better individually and in groups. Although there have been shifts in philosophy from time to time, the ultimate purpose of our schools has remained constant.

Teachers and elementary school personnel in the United States are in a unique position to contribute significantly to the preventive concept of health. They can help preserve and promote the well-being of students through the provision of services, programs, and activities that will have great influence on pupil behavior and lifestyles.

WHAT IS PREVENTION?

Prevention has multiple meanings. Literally, to prevent is to keep something from happening. Prevention includes the protection and promotion of health. It involves primary, secondary, and tertiary aspects. Schools generally provide for primary and secondary preventive assistance.

Primary prevention refers to action taken to interfere with something happening or a procedure to stop something before it starts. Specifically, it is an attempt through education and other procedures to help students refrain from the use of or reduce the misuse of drugs, obtain immunizations, and generally make intelligent decisions that will have a positive health impact. This type of prevention may take place in the school or in the community. Within the school the education may be formal or informal and may be provided for students, parents, school personnel, and others.

Secondary prevention relates to procedures taken after an illness or abnormal condition has occurred so that it does not get worse or become more advanced. It includes early detection of conditions and the use of follow-up procedures to obtain the necessary treatment or adjustments. For

 FOR YOUR INFORMATION

Did You Know?

Medical care has only a slight effect on improving health status . . . education appears to have twice the effect and is certainly more cost effective.

S.P. SHELOV, EDITORIAL
American Journal of Public Health
December, 1994

Prevention saves lives, makes people healthier, and is usually inexpensive.

AN OUNCE OF PREVENTION
Newsday, 4/21/1993

example, a teacher who observes a student with a suspicious skin rash sends the child to the school nurse. The nurse concludes that the problem needs medical attention and telephones the child's parent, advising that the student be examined by a physician. The school health program usually provides counseling and guidance that may include referral of children to community resources and follow-up to ensure completion of treatment.

Tertiary prevention is an extension of secondary prevention in which action is taken to interrupt the development of more serious conditions. It refers to treatment and rehabilitation services rendered by physicians, psychiatrists, and other professionals to save lives, restore pupils to high levels of wellness, and prevent serious personality damage. This service is generally not a function of schools and usually takes place outside the school setting. For example, a child with diabetes, epilepsy, heart disease, or hyperactivity needs medical assistance. Communication among the school, parents, and physicians is needed for appropriate adjustments to be made in the school setting.

WHAT IS HEALTH?

Health includes multiple phenomena and cannot be simply or easily defined. Comprehension of the variety of components that comprise health is essential to understanding its nature. These components must receive consideration in the school health program.

Health is a condition of the organism that may be represented on a continuum from so-called good health to so-called bad health, or from "wellness" to "illness," with many variations in between. People desire to find themselves at the positive end of the health scale and not at the negative end. Where any person fits on the continuum at any given time depends on these factors:

- *Health is personal.* Each person is born with a specific constitution or physical body that is provided through the genetic structure inherited from parents. Individuals are the same in many ways (number of arms, legs,

and eyes) and different in many ways (size, shape, and color of skin and eyes). Some children may be tall, obese, have only one kidney, allergies, or perhaps learning disabilities. Some pupils have susceptibilities to certain diseases and conditions. Thus health is individual and variable.
- *Health is frequently changing.* It is the result of the interaction of the individual (genetic, heredity) with many factors and experiences in the environment.
- *Health depends on self-actualization.* It necessitates internalization by the individuals. Children make frequent decisions whether or not to promote and preserve their health.
- *Health is a means to an end.* Good health has an effect on students' learning and living effectively. Children with poor health may have difficulty learning to read, completing math problems, learning to speak correctly, and may have trouble later in life when seeking a job or living independently.

Health is a complex phenomenon that includes a composite of interrelated physiological, psychological, sociological, and spiritual components that have been identified in the modified concept of health (Fig. 1-2). These components must receive consideration in the development of and planning for the comprehensive school health program. They have special significance in helping students make intelligent decisions regarding the environment in which they live and the experiences to which they are exposed. They must receive consideration when establishing curriculum objectives and must be applied when teaching for effective health education.

The isosceles triangle in Fig. 1-2 shows that physiological aspects form the base of the triangle and are fundamental to all learning. Students need to understand the structure and function of the human organism and the nature of good and ill health and diseases and conditions. However, this is of less importance in health instruction than the psychological and sociological aspects represented by the longer, vertical sides of the triangle. The diagram also indicates that emotional and

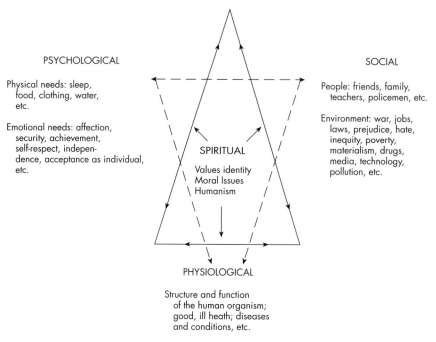

PSYCHOLOGICAL

Physical needs: sleep,
 food, clothing, water,
 etc.

Emotional needs: affection,
 security, achievement,
 self-respect, indepen-
 dence, acceptance as individual,
 etc.

SOCIAL

People: friends, family,
 teachers, policemen, etc.

Environment: war, jobs,
 laws, prejudice, hate,
 inequity, poverty,
 materialism, drugs,
 media, technology,
 pollution, etc.

SPIRITUAL

Values identity
Moral Issues
Humanism

PHYSIOLOGICAL

Structure and function
 of the human organism;
 good, ill heath; diseases
 and conditions, etc.

FIG. 1-2 A modified concept of health.

physical needs are reciprocally related to people—friends, relatives, and others—and to the environment found in the social arena. These interrelating factors influence the structure and function of the human body (see *dashed lines* in Fig. 1-2). Unfortunately, these components are not often stressed in health instruction.

Teachers must understand that student behavior is motivated by psychological needs and the pressure applied by people and other social factors. For example, a pupil may start to smoke cigarettes to satisfy an emotional need for acceptance or affection as part of a school peer group or as a rite of passage to enter into adulthood. Cigarettes are readily available to the public and are widely advertised as an acceptable form of social behavior. Thus the psychological need promotes the demand on the part of the manufacturers to satisfy the need and, reciprocally, the need is satisfied by the availability of the cigarettes and the encouragement of their use. There would be considerably

less lung cancer, bronchitis, and emphysema if students could be directed toward alternative ways of satisfying their psychological needs. Pupils need assistance in this regard as well as help in learning how to cope with societal pressures.

Probably the most important influence on health behavior, yet the one most frequently overlooked or omitted in the classroom, is the spiritual aspect. People's motivations toward health depend on their values regarding health and life, their recognition of moral issues in society, and their concern for the welfare of others. These are the driving forces of human behavior. They provide direction and establish the purpose or meaning of life, helping people determine their life goals. If individuals value their health, they will attempt to satisfy their emotional and physical needs through positive rather than negative behavior. They will learn to cope with the environmental and peer influences previously identified.

They will conclude that their actions can also affect other people.

Unfortunately, few health education curricula in schools (see Chapter 10) have been designed to use the total-person concept of health described in this section. This holistic approach to health education is one that must be widely advocated, promoted, and implemented. There is a need to prepare instructional programs that help students understand their own health motivational factors and make them aware of the influence of the environment on these motivations. In addition, programs must help pupils with the development of values, comprehension of moral issues, and an understanding of their effects. Such emphasis will enable children to *learn to make intelligent health decisions* and *learn to cope;* it will help them make adjustments to the social climate in which they live. Health instruction programs designed to include the total health concept will have more of an effect on the students' lives. The National Commission on the Role of the School and Community in Improving Adolescent Health* stated that youths will not achieve their potential if they have social, emotional, and physical health problems that interfere with learning.

The concept of health described in this chapter, which includes the physiological, psychological, sociological, and spiritual aspects of health, has been used in the development of the illustrative units found in Appendix B. The extent to which the emphasis of these components should be made at various grade levels is also identified in Appendix B.

WHAT FACTORS INFLUENCE PUPIL HEALTH?

A child's health is determined by three basic factors: *heredity, environment,* and *behavior.* Each boy

---

*The National Commission: *Code blue: uniting for healthier youth,* Alexandria, VA, 1990, National School Boards Association and American Medical Association.

and girl, as an individual personality, is a product of these fundamental forces.

As individuals, pupils differ in many ways. Differences in their facial and physical features are readily apparent, even to the casual observer. The teacher discovers that some students learn quickly, others slowly; some show rapid rates of physical growth while others may lag behind. Some learn motor skills easily and quickly; others seem never able to quite "get the hang of it" when a new physical skill is taught. These and more are evidence of biological traits transmitted from parents to children.

It is *heredity* that establishes a child's health endowment fund. What is passed on to the child by genes and their constituent deoxyribonucleic acid (DNA) and ribonucleic acid (RNA) molecules from the parents, grandparents, and more distant ancestors has much to do with the child's basic capacity for good health. Heredity also plays a part in the predisposition to some mental disorders, and chronic conditions such as cancer, heart disease, diabetes, hemophilia, and sickle cell anemia. All experienced teachers have seen the pupil with a strong constitution. This is the boy or girl who is alert, vigorous, seemingly indefatigable, and relatively free from illness. Similarly, teachers are familiar with the opposite—the weak, sickly child who seems always to be perched precariously on the figurative fence dividing health and illness. Often both children are exposed to essentially the same environment and follow much the same daily routine. In the absence of other explanations, such as previous illness or impairment, these health variances must be considered as being significantly influenced by heredity.

Environment has a direct bearing on the health of pupils. Boys and girls must interact with and adjust to an environment that is physical, biological, and social. *Physical* factors, such as weather and climate, housing, soil, water and food supply, medicines, radiation, clean or polluted air, recreational facilities, automobiles, hospitals, school buildings and sites, and many other physical things around us can affect health for better or worse. *Biological* factors include germs, plants, animals, and other people. These, too, may be helpful or harmful to health. For example, a pupil may catch a cold from a parent. At the same time that parent provides shelter, food, clothing, medical care, and other necessities that serve to maintain and improve the child's health. Some "friendly" germs in the intestinal tract manufacture certain vitamins that help prevent deficiencies; other germs are capable of causing disease and death. *Social* or *cultural* factors comprise all the interactions between and among people. These complex human relationships influence and are themselves influenced by patterns of culture at a given time and place. Hence, boys and girls constantly are exposed to the beliefs, attitudes, ideals, values, and customs of family, neighborhood, school, church, peer groups, and the general community (local, state, national, and world) in which they live. In terms of nationwide values, there remains little doubt that the thinking of both children and adults is influenced by vigorous and persuasive advertising through TV and other mass media. These cultural forces can, directly or indirectly, for better or worse, affect the physical, mental, or emotional health of elementary school pupils.

To a far greater extent than either heredity or environment, *behavior*, or *lifestyle* that includes decision making, is generally the most influential factor on pupil health. Behavior undoubtedly is the result of the interaction of the psychological, social, and spiritual factors previously discussed. Young people in elementary schools are at impressionable ages, and teachers and schools can have a great impact on their lifestyles. With proper guidance and motivation from many sources, children can learn to make corrections in their behavior or learn to make adjustments to hereditary limitations and environmental factors. An effective comprehensive health program can guide pupils toward lifestyles that will enable them to live in a healthful manner. It is the fundamental purpose of this text to help teachers and school personnel to assist students in elementary schools to achieve high levels of wellness.

WHAT ARE THE HEALTH PROBLEMS OF CHILDREN?

Despite the apparent good health of many children in the United States, there continues to be a variety of health and safety problems, especially among the poor and homeless, that have a draining effect on their energies, stamina, and capabilities. These problems are of such magnitude and diversity that the quality of education will be affected for students in those schools that fail to give them attention and do not provide a health program of the nature described in this text.

Unintentional injuries are the leading cause of death in children ages 5 to 14, killing 3660 in 1991. In the same age group, cancer is the leading cause of death from illness, killing 1106 children in 1991.

Early elementary school–age pupils have the next-to-lowest mortality and serious morbidity of any age group. Most physical illness in this age group is the result of accidental trauma and respiratory illness, usually of infectious origin. These students also have a variety of problems such as hearing, vision, and speech defects, dental caries, mental retardation, and emotional and educational problems. However, children are facing new major problems, some of which are pre-

 FOR YOUR INFORMATION

Unhealthy teenagers—those who are alienated or depressed, or feel nobody cares, who are distracted by family or emotional problems, who are drinking or using drugs, who are sick or hungry or abused or feel they have no chance to succeed in this world—are unlikely to attain high levels of educational achievement required for success in the 21st century. Thousands of these young people will experience school failure, which for many will be a precursor to an adult life of crime, unemployment, or welfare dependency.

Code Blue: Uniting for Healthier Youth, 1990

ventable, such as cancer, HIV/AIDS, violence, homicide, and suicide.

What Are the Death Rates for Children and Adults?

The average expected lifespan for all Americans in 1992 was 75.7 years.* The average for white males was 73.2 years and for white females 79.7 years. However, the average lifespan in 1991 for black males was 64.6 years and for black females 73.8 years. The average for all racial groups was 75.5: males 72.0 and females 78.9.

The 10 leading causes of death in 1993 are listed in Table 1-3. Almost 1.5 million people die annually from heart disease, cancer, and cerebrovascular diseases and accidents. These conditions may be prevented or reduced in elementary school

children if the students receive attention and develop good lifestyle habits.

The death rates, estimated numbers of deaths, and percentages of deaths from selected causes for young people aged 5 to 14 years are shown in Table 1-4. These rates and numbers are exceedingly low in comparison with other age groups when one considers there are over 30 million children of elementary school age in the United States.

What Are the Safety Hazards for Pupils?

Unintentional injuries from accidents were the leading cause of death among children and youth ages 5 to 14 years; 3660 died. Motor vehicles accounted for 43% of these deaths, drowning for 5%, fires and burns for 4.5%, and firearms for 2%.* Head injury was the primary contributing cause of death in 70% to 80% of all bicycle fatalities; 600

---

*US Department of Health and Human Services, Public Health Service, Centers for Disease Control and Prevention, National Center for Health Statistics: *Health United States 1993*, Washington, DC, 1993, US Government Printing Office.

*National Safety Council: *Accident facts*, Chicago, 1994, The Council.

TABLE 1-3 Death Rates, Percentage of Total Deaths, and Estimated Numbers of Deaths for the 10 Leading Causes of Death in the United States, 1993 (Rates per 100,000 Population)

Rank	Cause of death	Rate	Percent of total deaths	Estimated number of deaths
1	Heart disease	286.9	32.6	739,860
2	Cancer	205.8	23.4	530,870
3	Stroke	58.1	6.6	149,740
4	Chronic obstructive diseases and allied conditions	39.2	4.5	101,090
5	Accidents	34.4	3.9	88,630
	Motor vehicle	15.9	1.8	40,880
	Others	18.5	2.1	47,750
6	Pneumonia and influenza	31.7	3.6	81,730
7	Diabetes mellitus	21.4	2.4	55,110
8	Human immunodeficiency virus (HIV)/AIDS	14.9	1.7	38,500
9	Suicide	12.1	1.4	31,230
10	Homicide	9.9	1.1	25,470
	All causes	879.3	100	2,268,000

From the *World almanac and the book of facts*, New Jersey, 1995, Funk & Wagnalls, as reported by the National Center for Health Statistics, US Department of Health and Human Services.

TABLE 1-4　Death Rates per 100,000 and Estimated Numbers and Percentages for Selected Causes for Children and Youth 5 to 14 Years of Age, United States, 1991

Causes	Estimated rate	Estimated number	Percentage
Unintentional injuries	11.0	3660	43
Motor vehicles	5.6	1680	20
Firearms	2.0	658	7.5
Malignant neoplasms	3.1	1160	13
Homicide and legal intervention	1.4	519	6
Congenital anomalies	1.3	487	5.7
Disease of the heart	.07	281	3.1
Pneumonia and influenza	.04	135	1.7
Chronic pulmonary diseases	.03	122	1.6
Human immunodeficiency virus infection/AIDS*	.025	104	1.2
Cerebrovascular disease	.02	86	1.1
All causes	23.6	8479	100

From US Department of Health and Human Services, Public Health Service, Centers for Disease Control and Prevention, National Center for Health Statistics: *Health United States 1993,* Washington, DC, 1993, US Government Printing Office.
Health United States 1993 reported 744 cases under 13 years in 1992.

were children. More than a half million cyclists suffered injuries that required emergency room attention. Nearly two thirds were children.* In 1991 it was estimated 234,090 head injuries occurred to children requiring emergency room treatment as the result of skateboards and roller skates; over 500 had to be hospitalized.†

Table 1-5 shows the student accident rates and school days lost per injury for 1984-85 and 1985-86. Of the school jurisdiction accidents, 23% were related to playground equipment. One fourth of these were severe—concussions, crush wounds, fractures, and multiple injuries.

What Are the Physical Illnesses and Conditions?

Children's school-loss days from selected causes are shown in Fig. 1-3, and causes of disability

among 10- to 18-year-olds are found in Fig. 1-4. The average number of school days lost per child per year is approximately 5. Children from low-income families, where the mother has less than a high school education, are absent approximately twice that number of days.

Illnesses. Respiratory and gastrointestinal illnesses are the most common physical illnesses among young people. Allergic disease (nasal allergy, asthma, other allergies)* is the number one chronic illness, affecting one in five children. Streptococcal infection ("strep sore throat") has occurred 2 to 3 times in young people by the age of 10 years. Acute rheumatic fever, a serious complication of untreated "strep" throat, may lead to permanent heart disease. Approximately 61% of school days missed by children are because of acute illnesses, primarily respiratory conditions. The common health problems contributing to short-term, self-limiting disability and school absenteeism of elementary pupils may be ranked as follows:

*Dannenberg AL et al: Bicycle helmet laws and educational campaigns: an evaluation of strategies to increase children's helmet use, *Am J Pub Health* 83:667-674, 1993.
†Baker SP et al: Head injuries incurred by children and young adults during informal recreation, *Am J Pub Health* 84:649-652, 1994.

*Richards W: Allergy, asthma, and school problems, *J School Health* 56:151-152, 1986.

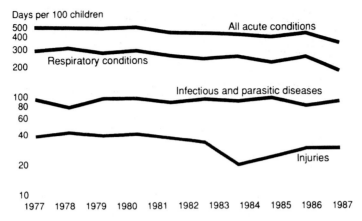

FIG. 1-3 School-loss days from selected causes among children 5 to 17 years of age: United States, 1977-1987. (From National Center for Health Statistics, Division of Health Interview Statistics: National Health Interview Survey. In US Department of Health and Human Services, Public Health Service: *Health United States 1989 and prevention profile,* Hyattsville, MD, 1990, National Center for Health Statistics.)

TABLE 1-5 Student Accident Rates and School Days Lost for Students in Grades K-9 According to Grades and Location of Activity, United States, 1984-1985 and 1985-1986*

	Grades					
Location/activity	K	1-3	4-6	7-9	Total†	Days lost per injury
	(Accidents per 100,000 student days)					
Shops and labs	0.00	0.00	0.01	8.27	.24	1.19
Buildings	1.35	0.85	1.33	2.00	1.26	1.14
Grounds—unorganized activities	1.93	1.99	2.40	0.32	1.16	1.17
Physical education	0.82	0.66	2.28	4.02	2.14	1.12
To and from school (motor vehicles)	0.24	0.10	0.08	0.13	0.11	2.60
To and from school (non-motor vehicles)	0.05	0.07	0.12	0.09	0.07	1.10

From National Safety Council: *Accident facts,* Chicago, 1987, The Council.
*Accidents are those causing (1) the loss of a half day or more of school time, (2) the loss of a half day or more of activity during non-school time, or (3) any property damage as a result of a school jurisdictional accident.
†A rate of 0.10 is equivalent to about 8000 accidents.

1. *Respiratory conditions:* Including the common cold, sore throat, earache, bronchitis, influenza, asthma, and related conditions
2. *Infectious diseases:* Including measles, chicken pox, infectious mononucleosis, and skin infections
3. *Digestive disorders:* Including viral and bacterial intestinal infections, food allergy, constipation, and appendicitis

Although the incidence of measles, rubella, mumps, pertussis, diphtheria, and poliomyelitis has dropped markedly since 1950, only 55% of the

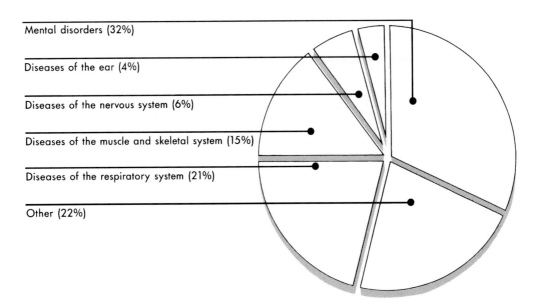

Mental disorders (32%)

Diseases of the ear (4%)

Diseases of the nervous system (6%)

Diseases of the muscle and skeletal system (15%)

Diseases of the respiratory system (21%)

Other (22%)

FIG. 1-4 Causes of disability among 10- to 18-year-olds. (From American Medical Association: *America's adolescents: how healthy are they?* Chicago, 1990, The Association.)

2-year-olds in the United States are fully immunized.* State laws requiring up-to-date immunizations for entry into licensed child care, head start, or school ensure better immunization levels among school-age children.

Approximately one third of 12- to 17-year-olds have skin disorders in need of medical attention. About 8 out of every 1000 children born in the United States each year have one or more congenital heart defects. Until 1993, 4645 cases of AIDS (less than 1% of total) were reported in children under 13 years of age. The numbers of students with chronic illnesses such as cystic fibrosis, leukemia, and spina bifida are on the rise.

Conditions. The two most common dental diseases are caries and periodontal disease. About 60% of pupils also have gingivitis, and 29% of adolescents suffer from severe to very severe malocclusion.† The incidence of these conditions increases as children get older. Decay probably affects more children than any other health problem with the exception of respiratory infections and injuries. *Healthy People 2000* reported that 53% of children 6 to 8 years of age and 78% of 15-year-olds have dental caries. Black and Hispanic children have a higher incidence than the total population.

Dental caries has been on the decline because of dietary changes and the use of fluorides in water, topical applications, and mouthwashes.*

Approximately 1 child in 20 aged 3 to 5 has a vision problem. About 10% of school-age pupils have visual acuity problems, and another 5% to 7% have some form of eye disease. Many of those in need of glasses do not have them. It is estimated that 3% to 6% of students have hearing difficulties, with many of these caused by middle-ear infections. Under 1% of pupils have seizure disorders, and an additional 1% have major speech disorders.

*Children's Defense Fund: *The health of America's children yearbook 1994*, Washington, DC, 1994, The Fund.
†Allukian M: The neglected American epidemic, *The Nation's Health*, May-June, 1990.

*Children's dental caries decreased dramatically, *The Nation's Health*, February, 1982.

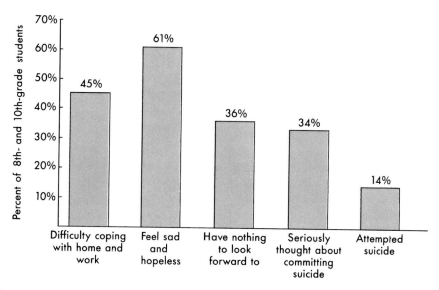

FIG. I-5 Adolescents reporting coping difficulties and depression. (From 1987 NASHS data. In *The National Adolescent Student Health Survey: a report on the health of America's youth,* Oakland, CA, 1989, Third Party Publishing.)

Although almost all adolescents have acne, it is severe in less than 5% of these young people. Boys are affected more severely than girls.

Young people need an understanding of bodily changes during maturation. Almost one half of all female adolescents are affected by dysmenorrhea.

What Are the Psychological/ Emotional Problems?

Psychological problems that may have their onset in adolescence, a period of conflict and crisis, include anxiety, mood disorders, schizophrenia, eating disorders (anorexia nervosa, bulimia), disruptive behavior, personality disorders, and substance abuse, among others. High-risk groups with higher disorder rates are the homeless or abused, those who have mentally ill parents or parents abusing substances, children who live where marital discord or instability exist in the home, those who live in poverty, and those who live where catastrophic events occur. A 1988

Gallup poll* found 85% of young people to be satisfied with their personal lives. Fig. 1-5 identifies a number of problem areas that were revealed when adolescents were asked specific questions about feelings.

The American Academy of Pediatrics and the National Parent-Teachers Association† conducted a survey of 500 teachers who identified these problems as those that interfered with student learning: psychological and emotional (97%), family violence and abuse (78%), and violent behavior (68%).

It is estimated that 12% of pupils (7.5 million) have psychological problems requiring psychiatric help. An additional 2% to 3% have seriously psychotic or prepsychotic conditions. In a class of 30 children, a teacher may expect to recognize emotional difficulties in three children and possi-

---

*American Medical Association: *America's adolescents: how healthy are they?* Chicago, 1990, The Association.
†Conference stresses partnership between learning and health, *The Nation's Health,* Oct, 1992, p. 24.

bly be able to identify one child in need of psychiatric assistance.

Educational failure, or the "failure syndrome," is one of the underlying stress factors related to depression, fears, acting-out in school, and truancy. Stress has a significant correlation to a variety of illnesses, including depression, asthma, high blood pressure, and diabetes. It is also related to skin rashes, children's streptococcal infections, accidents, suicide, and substance abuse.

What Are the Social and Lifestyle-Related Problems?

Approximately 59% of children ages 6 to 17 years have mothers in the workplace or live with single parents and are without supervision for part of the day. About 30% of children are living with only one parent (the mother) or neither. Children in such families have been labeled "latchkey" children. They are alone most afternoons or for longer stretches every weekday. Many of these children have problems that have implications for school health (see Chapter 4). It is estimated there are 10 million latchkey children in the United States.

At least one in five children below the age of 18 years lives in poverty. In 1990 over 5 million (3.1%) adult Americans had experienced homelessness. It is estimated 100,000 children are homeless on any given night.*

Child neglect and abuse. J. Fontana, Medical Director of the New York Foundling Hospital, said child neglect and abuse is increasing in the United States at the yearly rate of 15%.† He adds that these are the children who assault, rob, murder, and commit suicide. Although the incidence is unknown because many occurrences

are never reported, the National Committee for Prevention of Child Abuse stated there were nearly 2.7 million abuse reports in 1991 and 1383 children died.* Many neglect and abuse reports are repeat cases that involve the use of drugs. Abusive parents show poor emotional adjustment and poor parenting skills. The types of child neglect and abuse include physical and emotional neglect (53%) and physical (21%) and sexual abuse (13%). Neglect refers to lack of adequate nutrition, clothing, and shelter, and failure of parents and caretakers to provide an emotionally stable environment. Neglect is more common than physical abuse, which causes bodily harm to children and is manifested by bruises, welts, abrasions, fractures, lacerations, and burns. Sexual abuse includes incest, sodomy, and rape. Many of these children suffer permanent physical and mental impairment.

Suicide. In 1990 over 31,000 people committed suicide, and it is estimated 290,000 to 2,900,000 attempted suicide. White males generally have the highest suicide rate. The rate among teenagers has been increasing steadily over the past three decades. In 1991, the rate for those 5 to 14 years of age was 4.1 per 100,000 with 266 deaths. For those 15 to 24 years of age, there were 4751 suicides with a rate of 13.1 per 100,000.†

It is estimated 60,000 or more of these young people attempt suicide each year. Girls attempt suicide three times more often than boys, but boys succeed more often. The young people with increased risk of committing suicide include those with a history of major psychiatric disorders, drug and alcohol abuse, recent behavioral changes such as depression or truancy, previous suicide attempts, or suicide by another family member. Also involved may be such fac-

---

*Children's Defense Fund: *The health of America's children, 1992,* Washington, DC, 1992, The Fund.
†House of Representatives, Joint Hearing; Subcommittee on Oversight, Committee on Ways and Means, and Select Committee on Children, Youth, and Families: *Child abuse and day care, 1984,* Washington, DC, 1985, US Government Printing Office.

*Adding up early childhood, *America's Agenda,* 4:16, 1994.
†US Department of Health and Human Services, Public Health Services, Centers for Disease Control and Prevention, National Center for Health Statistics: *Health United States 1993,* Washington, DC, 1993, US Government Printing Office.

tors as divorce or separation of parents, loss of a parent or relative, sense of failure, and recent humiliation or punishment. One in five children in need of therapy receive it; the poor and those in minority groups receive the least care.

Homicide. It is estimated that 1 million teenagers yearly are victims of crime. The number of deaths for 5 to 14-year-olds was 519 with a rate of 1.4 per 100,000 population. For 15- to 24-year-olds, the number killed was 8159 with a rate of 22.4 per 100,000 population.

Black youths are six times more likely to be homicide victims. Violent juveniles are likely to be abused children, have alcoholic or criminal parents who divorce or separate, live in poor housing, do poorly in schools, and lack training and the opportunity to work.*

Violence. Teenagers are having to cope with violence inside school buildings as well as on streets. In 1992, the percentage of tenth grade students who were reported to carry a gun, knife, or club to school in the previous month was 10% at least once; 4% for 10 or more days.†

Substance abuse. The percentage of 12- to 17-year-olds who have ever used legal and/or illegal drugs in the United States is shown in Fig. 1-6. Two legal drugs, alcohol and tobacco, are the

*Moyers B: There is so much we can do, *Sunday San Francisco Examiner and Chronicle, Parade Magazine,* Jan 8, 1995, pp 4-6.
†The National Education Goals Report/University of Michigan 1993; Violence in Schools, *America's Agenda* 4:35, 1994.

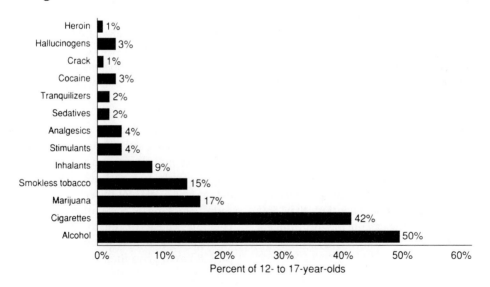

FIG. I-6 Adolescents who have ever used tobacco, alcohol, or other drugs. (From National Institute on Drug Abuse: Highlights of the 1988 National Household Survey on Drug Abuse, Washington, DC, 1989, US Government Printing Office. In American Medical Association: *America's adolescents: how healthy are they?* Chicago, 1990, The Association.)

Grade of First Use Among 1987 High School Seniors Who Ever Used That Substance

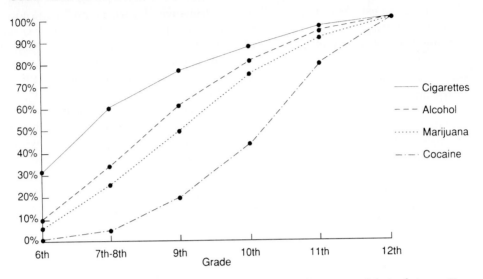

FIG. I-7 Grade of first use among 1987 high school seniors who ever used that substance. (From Johnston LD, O'Malley PM, Bachman JG: Illicit drug use, smoking, and drinking by America's high school students, college students, and young adults, 1975-1987, DHHS Pub No ADM 89-1602, Washington, DC, 1988, US Government Printing Office. In American Medical Association: *America's adolescents: how healthy are they?* Chicago, 1990, The Association.)

drugs of greatest use. Fig. 1-7 shows the grades when selected drugs were first used by high school seniors as reported in 1987. In a national survey conducted by the University of Michigan, marijuana use for eighth graders increased from 6% to 13% and for tenth graders from 16% to 25% between 1991 and 1994; 1993 showed no significant increase in the use of LSD, hallucinogens, stimulants, and cocaine.* More than one half of American youth try an illicit drug before they finish high school.† A Gallup poll of the public's attitude toward public schools revealed that 38% identified the use of drugs as the biggest problem confronting schools.‡

Cigarette smoking. Lung cancer in 1991 caused 30.5% of the cancer deaths or 10% of all deaths in the United States. Over 80% of these cancer deaths (126,000) were caused by cigarette smoking.* Although the evidence shows a decline in adult smoking with the exception of women, the majority of adolescents still experiment with cigarettes. Smokers run a higher risk than nonsmokers of cancer of the larynx, oral cavity, esophagus, and stomach. Smoking is the major cause of emphysema and chronic bronchitis. Smoking is the nation's number one preventable cause of death. Twenty-five percent of high school seniors who ever smoked reported having had their first cigarette by the sixth

*Alexander A: Call to action on teen drugs, *Newsday*, December 13, 1994, p A4.
†National Institute of Drug Abuse: *Overview of selected drug trends*, 1989, Rockville, MD, US Government Printing Office.
‡Twenty-second Annual Gallup poll of the public's attitude towards the public schools, *Phi Delta Kappan*, September, 1990.

*US Department of Health and Human Services, Public Health Service, Centers for Disease Control and Prevention, National Center for Health Statistics: *Health United States 1993*, Washington, DC, 1993, US Government Printing Office.

grade.* By their senior year in high school, 92% of students have tried cigarettes, 11% smoke 10 cigarettes daily, and 20% smoke on a regular basis. There are 4 million teenagers smoking regularly and girls may outnumber boys.†

Smokeless tobacco products, particularly chewing tobacco and snuff, have emerged as popular products among teenagers, especially boys. In 1991, it was estimated that 5.3% of 12- to 17-year-olds were users. Dangers from the use of smokeless tobacco include increased risk of oral cancer, gingival recession (receding gums leading to tooth loss), oral leukoplakia (white patches in the mouth that may become cancerous), and nicotine addiction.

Alcohol. Alcoholic beverages are the primary drug of choice by adults in the United States and have been tried by 92% of all high school seniors. In 1993, 51% of high school seniors reported they used alcohol in the past 2 weeks, and 27.5% claimed to be involved in binge drinking.‡ The National School Health Survey§ revealed that 77% of eighth graders had their first drink while in the sixth grade. In 1993, 26% of eighth graders reported they used alcohol in the past 2 weeks, and 13.5% said they were involved in binge drinking.‖ Sixty-nine percent of tenth graders claimed to have had their first drink while in the eighth grade and 38% have had five or more drinks within the past 2 weeks. The National Institute of Drug Abuse reported that 21% of tenth graders and

13.4% of 8th graders stated they had participated in binge drinking (5 drinks or more, 2 weeks before survey was conducted). The American Academy of Pediatrics* stated there are 500,000 child and adolescent alcoholics. Although the extent of involvement is not known, apparently fourth grade children are being introduced to and trying alcoholic beverages. Early drinking behavior is a predictor of drinking habits later in life. Adolescents who drink alcohol are 10 times more likely than nondrinkers to use marijuana and 11 times more likely to use cocaine.

Other drugs. Other legal drugs identified in Fig. 1-6 such as sedatives, stimulants, analgesics, and inhalants need attention but generally do not pose as great a health threat to most children because of their limited usage. The one exception are the inhalants because they are readily available and are frequently used by some children. Illegal drugs such as cocaine, heroin, and marijuana when used may present serious difficulties. Marijuana, in particular, has become a popular substance among teenagers and may present serious hazards.

The American Medical Association† says current use of cocaine and other illicit drugs among adolescents has declined from 12% in 1985 to 7% in 1988.‡

The most widely used drugs by eighth grade students are inhalants, alcohol, and tobacco. The use of inhalants in 1992 rose from 6.2% to 7.2% but diminished as students got older. Marijuana is a very popular drug among tenth graders (19%) and continues to be the illicit drug most extensively used by high school seniors (26%).§ Marijuana is associated with poor grades, absenteeism, low self-esteem, delinquency, and other problems. In 1988, 14,000 drug abuse episodes were reported in

---

*US Department of Health and Human Services, Public Health Service; *Healthy people 2000: national health promotion and disease prevention objectives,* Washington, DC, 1991, US Government Printing Office.

†Reported in Smoking and Health Reporter, National Interagency on Smoking and Health, 3: April, 1986, in *Health United States and Prevention Profile, 1990.*

‡US Department of Health and Human Services, Public Health Service, Centers for Disease Control and Prevention, National Center for Health Statistics: *Health United States 1993,* Washington, DC, 1993, US Government Printing Office.

§US Department of Health and Human Services, Public Health Service, Alcohol, Drug Abuse, and Mental Health Administration, Office of the National Institute of Drug Abuse: Highlights of national school health survey on drug and alcohol use, *NIDA Capsules,* 1988.

‖*Monitoring the future survey: National high school senior drug use survey, 1975-92,* April, 1993.

---

*Committee on School Health: *School health: policy and practice,* Elk Grove Village, IL, 1993, American Academy of Pediatrics.

†American Medical Association: *America's adolescents: how healthy are they?* Chicago, 1990, The Association.

‡National Institute on Drug Abuse: *Overview of selected drug trends,* Aug, 1989.

§Drug use dips among older teens, rises among younger teens, *Nation's Health,* May/June, 1993, p 7.

hospital emergency rooms involving 10- to 17-year-olds (60% related to suicides) and 88 deaths (51% classified as suicides) occurred.*

We live in a drug-oriented society. We take drugs to wake up, to go to sleep, to keep alert, to escape from reality, to relax, to ease pain, and for many other reasons. People use, misuse, and abuse legal as well as illegal drugs.

Nutrition. Nutrition is generally good among most school-age children but the prevalent problems are overeating, causing obesity and overweight (affecting 27% of children), anorexia nervosa (willful self-starvation) and bulimia (vomiting) in teenage girls, poor food choices that involve excess fat and salt consumption, and under nutrition-hunger (affecting 1 in 5 children in families below the poverty level).

About 5% of adolescents are obese (more than 20% over the maximum recommended weight for their height), and 5% to 25% are overweight. Obesity and overweight can lead to hypertension, increased cholesterol levels, diabetes, and reduced life expectancy. Obese children are significantly more sedentary than thin children. The problem may be one of adjustment and is a precursor to adolescent and adult obesity. Poor food choices result in low intakes of the minerals calcium and copper and the vitamins A, C, and B_2 (riboflavin).

Anorexia can begin at any age and commonly starts in the teens. In 1988 there were 67 deaths.

Exercise and fitness. Sedentary living is one factor that can increase the probability of cardiovascular disease. *Healthy People 2000* reported that regular physical activity can help prevent hypertension, non-insulin dependent diabetes, osteoporosis, obesity, and mental health problems such as depression and anxiety. It can also lower rates of colon cancer, stroke, and may be linked to reduced back injury. In 1984-1986 only 36% of students in grades 1 to 12 participated in daily physical education. The target goal for the year 2000 is to have 75% of American children participating in vigorous activity in physical education. One study of fifth grade students in Texas schools* indicated that on the average 8.5% of class time was spent in vigorous activity.

Sexual activity. Most teenagers begin having sexual intercourse in their mid-to-late teens; 56% of women and 73% of men have intercourse before age 18. Most very young teenagers do not have intercourse.†

One million teenage women—12% of all women aged 15 to 19 (117 per 1000) and 21% of those who had sexual intercourse (207 per 1000)—become pregnant each year. In 1991, about 368,000 unmarried teenagers gave birth. Fifty percent of pregnancies end in birth, one third end in abortions, and the rest are miscarriages.

Teenagers who give birth are much more likely to come from poor or low-income families (83%). Teenage mothers are more likely than older mothers to rely on public assistance to pay for having and raising a child.

Four in 10 teenage pregnancies (excluding miscarriages) end in abortion. There were 364,000 teenage abortions in 1990. Teenage abortions are considerably higher among minorities than among whites (75 versus 36 per 1000 women aged 15 to 19).

Three million teenagers—about 1 in 4—acquire sexually transmitted diseases every year. Infectious syphilis rates have more than doubled among teenagers since the 1980s. The threat of AIDS looms as another problem facing sexually active teenagers. Infertility and cancer can result from a sexually transmitted disease.

A variety of problems complicate pregnancies in young mothers; they include toxemia, anemia, lack of prenatal care, all of which result in such problems as low birth rate, increased infant mor-

---

*US Department of Health and Human Services, Public Health Service, Alcohol, Drug Abuse, and Mental Health Administration, Office of the National Institute of Drug Abuse: Teenagers and drug abuse, *NIDA Capsules*, 1990.

*Simons-Morton BG et al: The physical activity of fifth-grade students during physical education class, *Am J Pub Health* 83:262-264, 1993.
†Alan Guttmacher Institute: *Teenage reproductive health in the United States: facts in brief*, New York, 1994, The Institute.

tality, and mental retardation of the child. Teen parents are often school dropouts and face difficulties obtaining the skills needed to compete in society. Thus they frequently find themselves in low-paying jobs or dependent on welfare.*

Teenage pregnancy is viewed widely as related to poverty. Young black women in the United States are almost seven times more likely than young white women to give birth before age 15.†

AIDS (HIV infection). In 1993 there were 328,392 HIV/AIDS cases. White males constituted more than twice the number of black male cases and four times the number of hispanic cases. Black females were more than twice the number of white female cases and two and a half times the number of hispanic cases. There have been 197,727 deaths in 1993, with the number of white deaths being more than twice the number of minorities.‡

The AIDS epidemic has added a health crisis facing America's children. Adolescent cases have increased 77% in the past 2 years. In 1993 there were 4645 cases in children under 13 years of age and 2501 deaths. Approximately 55% of the children were black, 22% percent were white, and 20% were hispanics.

What Factors Are Related to School Underachievement?

The American Academy of Pediatrics identified a variety of external and internal factors that affect school underachievement of students.

External factors. External factors include (1) improper educational management—curriculum, motivation, resources available to the teacher, teacher attention to emotional needs, class size,

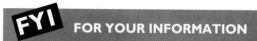

Waldorf DM: *Turning points: preparing American youth for the 21st century*, 1989, New York, Carnegie Council on Adolescent Development.

and school design; (2) family problems—financial, marital discord, anxiety, depression, poverty, and homelessness; (3) unrealistic parental expectations; and (4) lack of motivation—lack of home support, socially and financially successful parents, and peer pressure.

Internal factors. Internal factors include (1) chronic and recurring physical problems—cerebral palsy, activity-limiting chronic illness and disability, overprotection by parents and teacher; (2) sensory defects—defects in vision or hearing, language delays, perceptual disorders; (3) neurological and neuromuscular problems—head injury/traumatic brain injury, epilepsy, and dysphasia; (4) psychiatric and psychosocial problems; (5) developmental disabilities, and (6) undiagnosed conditions—lead poisoning.

Attention deficit disorders. Attention deficit disorders (ADD) describes a group of problems associated with school underachievement. ADD is diagnosed through several behavioral characteristics—hyperactivity, impulsivity, distractibility, and short attention span. It is critical to rule out other problems such as hearing loss or petit mal epilepsy. ADD previously was referred to as minimal brain dysfunction (MBD) or learning disability; the name changed because there was no evidence to show the existence of brain damage.* Students should also be evaluated for learning disabilities such as dyslexia. About

---

*Kenny AM: Teen pregnancy: an issue for schools, *Phi Delta Kappa*, 1987.

†Miller CA et al: *Monitoring children's health: key indicators*, Washington, DC, 1986, American Public Health Association.

‡US Department of Health and Human Services, Public Health Service, Centers for Disease Control and Prevention, National Center for Health Statistics: *Health United States 1993*, Washington, DC, 1993, US Government Printing Office.

---

*Committee on School Health: *School health: policy and practice*, Elk Grove Village, IL, 1993, American Academy of Pediatrics.

2% to 4% of school-age children are affected by ADD, with boys reported affected more often than girls.

Who Are the Children with Special Educational Needs?

There are approximately 5 million (more than 10% of U.S. school children) children with special educational needs, as indicated in Table 1-6. The largest group is the learning disabled, including children with such conditions such as language problems, attention deficit disorders, mental retardation, and emotional problems.

What Are the Special Problems of the Poor?

In recent years the United States population has increased in its diversity. There has been a growing number of racial minority families and children. In 1990, approximately 27% of 5- to 13-year-olds belonged to racial and minority groups. There also has been a sharp increase in the number of homeless families. In 1992, at least one in every five children (13 million) under 17 years of age lived in poverty.

Children from low-income families, especially those families with only one parent, are generally in poorer health than children from high-income families. Poverty increases the chances of chronic disease. Poor children have more sickness and infections as well as other debilitating conditions.

Increasing attention is now being accorded the unusually high rate of illness among the poor and minority groups, such as blacks, hispanics, homeless, and Native Americans. Poverty, homelessness, and ignorance are the common contributory causes of these high disease rates. Poor diet, substance abuse, inadequate medical and dental care, unhealthy housing, teenage pregnancy, health misconceptions and superstitions, high incidence of child abuse and neglect, and lack of adequate childhood immunizations are major reasons for the generally subpar health of low-income families.

Some of the health problems of minority groups are based on genetic variances (such as sickle cell anemia in blacks and Tay-Sachs disease in Jewish and other groups of Middle Eastern origin), whereas others appear to be related to lifestyle and environment (such as alcoholism among Irish Americans, accidents among native Americans, and high blood pressure among black

TABLE 1-6 Number, Percentage, and Percentage of Total School Enrollment of Children and Youth in Educational Programs for the Handicapped in U.S. Elementary and Secondary Schools, 1991-92

Handicapping condition	Number	Percentage	Percentage of total school enrollment
Learning disabilities	2,234,000	45.1	4.96
Speech impairments	997,000	20.1	2.2
Other health impairments	645,000	13.0	1.4
Mental retardation	538,000	10.9	1.2
Serious emotional disturbance	399,000	8.1	.87
Hearing impairments	60,000	1.2	.13
Orthopedic impairments	51,000	1.0	.11
Visual impairments	24,000	.05	.05
Deafness/blindness	1000	.002	.002
	Total = 4,949,000		

From the *World almanac and book of facts,* New Jersey, 1995, Funk & Wagnalls, as reported by US Department of Education, Office of Special Education and Rehabilitation Services.

Americans). Migrant and seasonal farmworkers and their children, most of whom are black or hispanic, suffer severely under the burdens of poverty, poor housing, inadequate diets, discrimination, occupational accidents, emotional problems, and exposure to agricultural pesticides. Among native Americans, a number of conditions are prevalent: tuberculosis, dental decay, alcoholism, drug abuse, diabetes, and a variety of emotional problems.

WHAT IS SCHOOL HEALTH?

Adequate preventive health care for the diverse cultural, racial, and ethnic groups and youth in U.S. schools necessitates the provision of a multiphasic differential program identified as a comprehensive school health program (see Fig. 1-1). The comprehensive school health program is one that includes *health instruction, health services, healthful environment,* and *coordination.* The instructional component should be both formal and informal and for students and parents. The health service phase attempts to identify pupils with problems and provide counseling and guidance where possible and makes adjustments in school programs where necessary. It provides policies and procedures to prevent the spread of communicable diseases and to take care of children who may be injured or become ill while at school. The environmental phase includes a physical plant that is healthful and safe, is staffed by well-adjusted employees, and offers a school climate of friendliness and comfort conducive to learning. No program of this nature can function effectively without coordination.

An understanding of school health is gained through familiarity with the terms that follow:

school health The physiological, psychological, sociological, and spiritual aspects of health as they relate to the school setting.

comprehensive school health program The procedures and activities designed to protect and promote the well-being of students and school personnel, which include four categorical phases: health education/in-struction, health services, healthful school environment, and coordination.

health education A broad term referring to both formal and informal learning about health that will enable individuals to make intelligent, informed decisions affecting their personal, family, and community well-being. It may take place in school, outside school, and through the media.

comprehensive school health education program The planned, sequential, integrative, health instruction program based on student needs for grades K-12 that will enable pupils to live a more healthful life. It should include such content areas as community health, consumer health, dental health, disease control, environmental health, family health, rest, sleep, and fitness, mental health, nutrition, safety, and substance abuse.

health instruction The formal program that takes place in the school. It includes a program of planned activities in a classroom setting that offers understanding and attempts to develop attitudes and practices of healthful living that will enable children to reach high levels of wellness. The formal program is one that is planned, sequential, and includes all grades in a school or school district. It is now considered to be a *comprehensive school health education program.* It should be based on sound principles of curriculum development and include all subject areas necessary to satisfy student health needs and interests. The subject areas must (1) be repeated at several grade levels to ensure reinforcement of learning and (2) increase in depth of content, progressing from simple to complex concepts as pupils move upward in grade.

health services Those activities that involve nurses and other health professionals, through appraisal procedures, in the identification and follow-up of pupil health problems with students and parents, the control of disease, involvement of community health agencies, and pupil emergencies and first aid.

healthful school environment The phase sometimes referred to as healthful school living, relating to those activities that provide a safe and healthful school atmosphere. It includes the physical plant—lighting, heating, ventilation, food services, integration with the health services phase, safety, and health of school personnel—as well as the emotional climate of the school.

coordination Those activities usually carried out by a school administrator in cooperation with school and community health committees or councils. They include the administration and supervision of the school health program with specific responsibilities to integrate the health services and healthful environment phases with health instruction, to develop curriculum, to provide in-service teacher and staff training, to conduct evaluation, and to prepare policies and procedures.

WHY SCHOOL HEALTH?

The health of children and their learning are reciprocally related. Young people must be healthy to obtain optimal benefit from their elementary school experiences. Educational experiences must be provided that will enable pupils to live in a healthful manner.

The curriculum in America's elementary school must include substantially more than the three Rs, despite the trend to return to so-called basic education. Reading, writing, spelling, arithmetic, social studies, and science need not be neglected with the inclusion of health education. Although health should be included as a separate subject area, it also can be integrated easily into all instructional areas. Teachers, with the help of parents, family members, and the community, must aid students to learn how to live and make adjustments to the society in which they find themselves. Health is basic to the basics. Without good health, pupils will have difficulty learning to read, write, add, and perform the necessary activities for learning.

Students who are frequently absent because of illness, uncorrected vision problems, emotional disturbances, malnourishment or undernourishment, or fatigue or other health problems are simply not able to learn most efficiently and effectively even with the best teaching.

Although parents have the primary responsibility for the health of their children, schools must offer supportive and complementary programs to help counsel pupils and parents. However, the extent of poverty and homelessness that occurs in society necessitates the inclusion of school-based or linked health clinics in neighborhoods where families do not have easy access to care.

The role of the school is primarily to educate. Schools are expected to provide education to help students live in and adjust to society. Because society places a high value on human life and health, schools have a responsibility and an opportunity to help protect and promote the health of pupils and to aid in the prevention of ill health.

WHAT IS THE ROLE OF THE SCHOOL AND THE TEACHER IN PREVENTION?

The role of the school in preventive health is identified in the comprehensive school health program (see Fig. 1-1).

Schools have both a legal and a moral responsibility to provide a safe, sanitary, and healthful environment for pupils and school personnel. An atmosphere conducive to learning is one that is friendly and comfortable, offers a curriculum that motivates and meets the needs of students, minimizes stress situations, and includes well-adjusted, competent teachers.

The central purpose of the school health program is to help children learn to be responsible for their own health. Students should be able to acquire scientific understanding and attitudes through the health instruction program, which will enable them to act intelligently. The health habits established in these formative years greatly influence the quality of life that emerges in adulthood. Young people in elementary schools can be exposed to many useful health experiences and activities because they legally must attend school for approximately 6 hours a day, 180 days a year, for 8 or more years.

Children attend school with a variety of illnesses and conditions such as communicable diseases, speech impediments, and dental problems that are in need of identification, or possible correction, or both. The school health services program should provide nurses and access to physicians, dentists, counselors, and other professionals who can assist with these problems to protect other students, to counsel and guide pupils and parents, and to recommend adjustments in school programs for more effective learning.

Teachers are expected to protect and try to improve the health of the children in their charge. Generally they are to be active participants in the comprehensive school health program (see Fig. 1-1). Specifically they need to understand the concept of health previously discussed, to be aware of the factors that influence pupil health, to be enthusiastically involved in the instructional program, and to know how to tell if pupils are in good health. The basic competencies needed for teachers to take part in the school health program are identified in Chapter 2.

HOW CAN YOU TELL IF PUPILS ARE IN GOOD HEALTH?

The classroom teacher is not qualified to dianose illness or make a clinical assessment of pupil health. However, some specific characteristics distinguish healthy children (Fig. 1-8) from those who are not healthy (refer to Appendix J for details). Actually, these attributes help spell out a definition of good health. Generally these behaviors should be looked for in the healthy child:

- Carries out routine learning activities in school and in homework assignments without undue fatigue or emotional upset

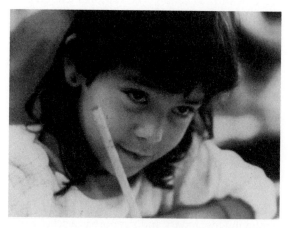

FIG. 1-8 The healthy child. (Courtesy the San Jose Nutrition Project, San Jose, California.)

- Participates regularly in physical education and other physical activities in the school curriculum
- Demonstrates skill in games and body movements appropriate to age, sex, body type, and motor learning experiences
- Shows progressive gains in weight and height without unusually wide deviations
- Has enough energy to do the things that most children of this age and sex want to do
- Has smooth and clear skin, without discoloration, eruptions, or excessive dryness or oiliness
- Has a good appetite
- Has no more illnesses or accidents than are typical of his or her age and sex group
- Is interested in and enthusiastic about most activities that are popular with classmates
- Has confidence in own abilities yet enjoys working and playing with others
- Controls emotions about as well as most of the other children in the class

WHERE DO WE STAND NOW?

Although comprehensive school health programs as described in the text are practically nonexistent, awareness of the concept is being more widely accepted and promoted by governmental authorities, health and educational leaders, agencies, organizations, and some legislators. Undoubtedly such recognition has been stimulated by the Surgeon General's advocacy in *Healthy People 2000.* The statement of cooperation and action by the United States Departments of Health and Human Services and Education in establishing a joint committee to explore cooperative efforts is an encouraging sign. The American Academy of Pediatrics has indicated that such programs have the potential to maximize the health and educational outcomes of children. Senator William S. Cohen (R-Maine)* stated that the importance of relationships between health and education are all too of-

---

*Association for the Advancement of Health Education: *Healthy networks: models for success conference,* Orlando, FL, Oct 22-25, 1991.

ten undervalued and overlooked. Despite this activity, there is no single federal grant program that supports the development and implementation of the concept.

Comprehensive school health education has gained recognition because of the public's increased concern for health and education. Strong and active support in recent years has come from the American Cancer Society, the Association for the Advancement of Health Education, the American Association of School Administrators, the National School Boards Association, the Metropolitan Life Foundation, and the National School Health Education Coalition (60 agencies, corporations, companies, and federal government groups). The American Cancer Society* has made comprehensive school health education development a core priority for the 90s. The Society believes that 50% to 60% of cancer deaths can be prevented, and the positive information acquired by students from such programs can greatly assist in the achievement of this goal.

The advent of school-based health clinics provides an excellent supplement to school health services programs, especially for the poor, the homeless, and those families without health insurance. The introduction of nurse practitioners brings direct health care to children. Efforts directed at removing asbestos in schools and concern about the wellness of teachers and staff demonstrates the intent to improve the school environment.

Support Groups

Some of the many other professional organizations that have helped nurture the growth of school health in the United States include the American School Health Association, the American Public Health Association, the American Medical Association, the American Heart Association, the American Lung Association, the National Educational Association, the American Cancer Society, and the National Congress of Parents and Teachers.

It should be noted that at the federal level, within the Department of Health and Human Services, there is the Center for Health Promotion and Education at the Centers for Disease Control and Prevention and the Division of Adolescent and School Health in the Public Health Service. The Center for Health Promotion and Education, formerly the Bureau of Health, has supported school health education and provided funds for the development of demonstration and model programs. At one time, there was also an Office of Comprehensive School Health within the Department of Education. There is also the Office of Disease Prevention and Health Promotion, (ODPHP), Public Health Service, Department of Health and Human Services. These offices have all cooperated in efforts to advance school health. In 1988 the Centers for Disease Control and Prevention in cooperation with the Education Development Center (EDC) established a Comprehensive School Health Education Network for state departments of education and health and for local school districts to aid in their efforts to develop health education programs.

In the private sector, the National Center for Health Education is an organization supported by funds from industry and other sources that promote health education. The National Congress of Parents and Teachers has for many years conducted a program of support for health education. Several other major curriculum projects are now under way. They have received financial support from several foundations and other sources. The Robert Wood Foundation has financed several health projects for high-risk youths, including programs to establish health clinics as part of the health services programs found in schools.

Health Education in the Curriculum

Health education has made great progress in achieving awareness and support as a school subject in the last 40 years. The number and variety of

*Seffrin JR: America's interest in comprehensive school health education, *J School Health* 64:397-399, 1994.

organizations, agencies, and individuals previously discussed provides the evidence.

Over 90% of teachers believe health education should be a required subject for all students.* The American Academy of Pediatrics believes ". . . schools should teach health education as part of the basic curriculum, giving it the same importance as traditional subjects. They should require comprehensive health education for students from kindergarten through grade 12."†

A Louis Harris survey‡ of students, teachers, and parents in grades 1 to 12 conducted for the Metropolitan Life Foundation in 1988 indicated a growing awareness of the need for comprehensive health education in the public schools. Of the 170 teachers who replied, 67% said they participated in a comprehensive health education program (multitopic, multigrade). However, only 43% of these teachers were very familiar with comprehensive health education. Of the parents polled, 78% said a comprehensive health education program was very important for their children.

In 1993, the American Cancer Society§ funded a study by the Gallup organization that sought opinions and attitudes of adolescents, parents, and school administrators regarding the importance of health education in schools. All three groups believed it was equal or greater in importance than other subjects in the curriculum.

Health Education Today

The present status of school health education and health education and health services in the United States was categorized in a study conducted by Lovato et al.* as follows:

- Health education during grades 1 to 6 is mandated in 19 states (37%) and is combined with physical education in 3 states (5.5). Health education in grade 7 is mandated in 22 states (43%) and is combined with physical education in 4 states (8%). The average number of hours required per year in states with a specific time requirement is 53 or more in grades 1 to 6 and 49 or more in grades 7 and 8.
- In 14 states (26%), there is a network of health educators who are regional coordinators for local school health programs.
- Thirty-one states (58%) have a state information clearinghouse that is available to help local health educators plan school programs.
- Twenty-one states (41%) provide elementary teacher certification in health education. In 10 of these states the certification is solely in health education; 8 states give dual certification in health and physical education; and 1 state offers dual certification in health education and physical education.
- A state curriculum or planning guide for health education is available to school districts in 40 states (75%) to help plan local programs.
- Thirty-four states (65%) have an education code or legislation that provides a legal basis for school health services in public schools.

Twenty-eight of the states (55%) have mandated these services by law. In 20 states (39%), persons responsible for health services are employed by the state department of education, and 13 states (26%) have persons employed by departments of health. In 5 states (10%) these persons are employed by both health and education departments, whereas in 13 states (26%) an agency other than the health or education department employs these persons. Twenty-three (43%) have a state-level school health

*Elam SM; The Twenty Second Annual Gallup Poll of public's attitudes toward public schools, *Phi Delta Kappan* 72:41-55, 1990.
†Committee on School Health: *School health: policy and practice,* Elk Grove Village, IL, 1993, American Academy of Pediatrics.
‡Louis Harris and Associates: *An evaluation of comprehensive health education in American public schools,* conducted for the Metropolitan Life Foundation, 1988.
§American Cancer Society: *Values, opinions of comprehensive school health education in United States public schools: adolescents, parents, and school district administrators,* May, 1994, Gallup Organization.

*Lovato CY et al: *School health in America,* ed 5, Kent, OH, 1989, American School Health Association.

advisory council. Nine states (18%) require a school district to have a school advisory council that includes community representatives.

A survey of school board members' knowledge and attitudes regarding national school health programs in the United States conducted in 1993 by the National School Boards Association* revealed that only 298 (15%) of the almost 2000 school districts contacted had participated.

- Some components of a comprehensive school health program existed in a large majority of districts (86% = 256 districts; 12.8% of 1993 districts).
- One third of the responding districts (99 = 5% of 1993 districts) reported having more complete multi-component programs.
- Closer investigation of reports of districts with programs, however, indicated only a small percentage included some of the components of a comprehensive school health program.

Despite the tremendous increase in awareness and the efforts to support and develop school health education in the United States in recent years, **there are numerous school districts without good programs and others with programs of questionable quality.** Portney and Christenson† stated that 20% of eighth-grade students reported in their survey that they never had a health course.† In addition, the quality of the programs in existence are in need of assessment. Despite the evidence previously reported in the Harris survey, **many of the programs are not comprehensive** and **often are not evaluated in terms of their impact on students.** The effect of learning on pupil health practices in society must be determined. The National Adolescent Student Health Survey‡

of eighth- and tenth-grade students found them somewhat knowledgeable about selected health topics; however, these pupils did not act in a healthful manner. Robert E. Windom, Assistant Secretary for Health, United States Public Health Services, in commenting on the survey findings, said: ". . . many people even when they know better don't always make the right decisions."

State laws requiring health programs, despite their apparent prevalence, are often written in such general terms that schools can comply with the requirements without providing instructional programs such as those outlined in this text.

Although health education exists in some form in most the nation's schools, the majority of districts do not have comprehensive school health education programs. **Few, if any, school systems provide planned, sequential health instruction programs; most are inadequate.** In general, most are categorically focused on these subject areas: substance abuse, nutrition, mental health, and AIDS. This is primarily because of the way federal monies are granted. **The National School Boards Association* estimates that 5% to 14% of school districts have comprehensive school health education programs.** The American Academy of Pediatrics claims that comprehensive school health education is not among the top school priorities.

Health Services

With the exception of some large districts, the health services programs found in schools may not be recognizable as such because they are fragmented, uncoordinated, and poorly planned; in many instances, there may be little or no administrative leadership. In a number of schools and school districts, some of the services may be provided by local health departments. At best a nurse or some administrator may have the responsibility for the supervision and conduct of such programs. In many districts there may be no nurses or

*National School Boards Association: *School board members' knowledge of attitudes regarding school health programs,* Alexandria, VA, 1994, The Association.
†Portney B, Christenson GM: Cancer knowledge and resultant practices, *J School Health,* 59:218-224, 1989.
‡American School Health Association, Association for the Advancement of Health Education, and the Society for Public Health Education: National adolescent student health survey: highlights of the survey, *Health Ed* 19:4-9, 1988.

*National School Boards Association: *School health: helping children learn,* Alexandria, VA, 1991, The Association.

only part-time nurses in schools. Large districts may have specific departments with physicians, nurses, and other health professionals.

In recent years, federal legislation has helped to provide some measure of improvement in health services programs. In 1967 Congress approved a program that required states to provide early and periodic screening, diagnosis, and treatment (EPSDT) as a mandatory Medicaid service to improve the health of children from low-income families through preventive health services. It included identification and preventive care for vision, hearing, and dental problems, among others. The program has been under the supervision of local and state health departments, but it necessitates school involvement and coordination.

In 1975 Congress passed the Education for All Handicapped Children Act (reauthorized as the Individual with Disabilities Education Act [IDEA]), which requires that "free appropriate education" be available to all handicapped children from ages 3 to 21 years regardless of their disabilities and their ability to pay for services. The law requires that provision be made for school health services, speech therapy, medical appraisals, psychological and parent counseling, and other services needed to provide educational benefits.

The patterns of organization for health services vary widely in America's schools. Many schools hire their own nurses and other professionals to conduct programs, some have all services provided by local health departments, and a few schools and school districts coordinate their own activities.

Healthful Environment

School districts in general are attentive to the physical plant, including food services, health services, and to a lesser extent the health of school personnel. The emotional climate may receive consideration to a greater or lesser degree, depending on the nature of the school services rendered and the individual efforts of teachers and personnel.

Coordination

Coordination of the phases of the school health program outlined here does not exist except in some large school districts. In those few districts that have administrative personnel to oversee programs, these individuals may be called supervisors, coordinators, consultants, or directors. In some districts, physicians or other health professionals may serve in this capacity. School health advisory committees can render useful and important aid but such committees are few in number except possibly in large districts. The same probably holds true for community health committees. It should be noted that without administrative supervision, health services or health instruction programs will be hard pressed to develop, and, if in operation, will slowly disappear.

Status today. Despite the progress and advances that have been made in school health, health education does not receive the necessary priority for curriculum inclusion by school, superintendents and school board members to have an impact on student health problems. Additional awareness programs for such individuals, with pressures exerted by parents and community health organizations and professionals, must be initiated. Finances and resources for health instruction are greatly limited. There is no single federal grant program that supports the development and integration of comprehensive school health education. The American Academy of Pediatrics has stated that some school districts provide comprehensive and sequential health education for students from kindergarten through high school. Others provide very little, offering perhaps only brief instruction on dental health, personal hygiene, and other topics in the primary grades, and first aid, mental health, and growth and development instruction in high school.

Perhaps the state of school health programs is best described by these remarks of former Secretary of Health, Education, and Welfare, Joseph A. Califano, when he addressed the American School Health Association annual meeting in Minneapolis several years ago:

Improved school health programs will be a key

element in the comprehensive national child health policy which I will ask the Public Health Service to develop for the Department . . . I believe that the time has come again to forge ahead in expanding and improving these programs.

The school health program outlined in this text may be considered as a conceptual model of the ideal program. It illustrates the pattern for school health that should exist in America's schools and that has been advocated by the American School Health Association and other professional health and governmental organizations. This program identifies the specific components and their organization, which, if implemented, will enable children to achieve high levels of wellness. It will contribute to quality education and help young people to grow into worthwhile and productive adults.

The school health program described herein has emerged as a result of a thorough review of the scientific literature and numerous school health programs, consultation with many school health authorities, discussions with a variety of health professionals, and the authors' years of experience with schools. We have served in numerous capacities in the elementary school at the local and the state level as teachers and administrators. We have participated in professional organizations, conducted many in-service teacher-training activities, and been active in health education projects at the local, state, and national level.

IN SUMMARY WE BELIEVE

- Comprehensive school health programs that include health instruction and health services and provide a healthful environment are necessary to protect and promote the health of America's elementary school children in order to ensure the most effective learning.
- Comprehensive school health programs must continue to develop, expand, and become more readily available to elementary school students.
- Comprehensive school health programs will continue to grow and be supported and imple-

mented because of the public's and community's increasing awareness of their need.
- Comprehensive school health programs need administrative and school board support through the employment of qualified/competent personnel as supervisors and coordinators.
- Comprehensive school health education programs need periodic evaluation to determine their effectiveness on student health and behavior.
- Comprehensive school health programs with an emphasis on health instruction in elementary schools must continue to increase, and their development will require teachers, administrators, school board members, and the community to become more assertive in the support and promotion of these programs.
- Comprehensive school health programs must involve parents as well as professional and community health personnel and organizations in their support, development, and implementation.
- Comprehensive school health programs, to become a reality, must have tremendous financial aid and support by the voluntary and professional health organizations and foundations and companies in the business marketplace.
- Comprehensive school health programs, in order to achieve recognition and implementation, must receive federal funds in large amounts from a single government agency that will not make categorical health instruction grants.
- Comprehensive school health programs are necessary to help resolve and prevent many of the health problems found in children and youth.
- Comprehensive school health programs must give special attention to the health problems of the poor, minority, and homeless children and youth.
- Comprehensive school health programs as described in this text will enable teachers, administrators, and school board members to establish guidelines and programs for their schools and school districts.

QUESTIONS FOR DISCUSSION

1. In the Surgeon General's report, *Promoting Health/Preventing Disease,* what are the three broad categories identified? List five areas that have school implications that were scheduled for achievement in 1990. Give one objective for each area.

2. What are the areas and objectives that the Surgeon General expects will be achieved in the year 2000? (List at least one objective for each area.)

3. What is the nature of a comprehensive school health program? Identify its components and interrelations.

4. What is the meaning of the preventive health concept? Provide illustrations. What are the roles of the school and teachers?

5. What are the components of health as described in the text? Briefly describe their significance to individuals.

6. What is the modified concept of health illustrated in the text? Give examples of its application to health education.

7. What factors influence the health of pupils? Provide illustrations.

8. What are 10 important health problems of children? Identify the extent to which they exist in elementary school pupils.

9. What are five of the social and lifestyle-related health problems of elementary pupils, and what can teachers do about such problems?

10. What are five student health problems in need of special education? What can teachers do to help these children socially and psychologically?

11. What are five special health problems of the poor? Indicate their significance for health education.

12. When covering such topic areas as nutrition, alcohol, tobacco, sex activity, safety, and dental health in a health instruction program for eighth grade students and applying the physical, psychological, social, and spiritual components of the modified concept of health (Fig. 1-2), what content should be included? Provide one illustration for each topic.

13. What is the meaning of the phrase "comprehensive health education"? What is the difference between health education and health instruction?

14. Why do schools have a responsibility to provide a comprehensive school health program?

15. How can a teacher tell whether children are in good health?

16. What is the status of school health programs in the United States today?

SELECTED REFERENCES

Alan Guttmacher Institute: *Sex and the American teenager,* New York, 1994, The Institute.

Alan Guttmacher Institute: *Teenage reproductive health in the United States: facts in brief,* New York, 1994, The Institute.

Allensworth DD: The research for innovative practices in school health education at the secondary level, *J School Health* 64:180-187, 1994.

Allensworth DD, Kolbe LJ: The comprehensive school health program: exploring an expanded concept, *J School Health* 57:409-412, 1987.

Allensworth DD, Wolford CA: *Achieving the 1990 health objectives for the nation: agenda for the nation's schools,* Kent, OH, 1988, American School Health Association.

American Cancer Society: *National action plan for comprehensive school health education,* Atlanta, GA, June, 1992, The Society.

American Cancer Society: *Values, opinions of comprehensive school health education in United States public schools: adolescents, parents, and school district administrators,* May, 1994, Gallup Organization.

American Medical Association: *America's adolescents: how healthy are they?* Chicago, 1990, The Association.

American School Health Association, Association for the Advancement of Health Education, and the Society for Public Health Education: National adolescent student health survey: highlights of the survey, *Health Ed* 19:4-9, 1988.

Association for the Advancement of Health Education: *Healthy networks: models for success conference,* Orlando, FL, Oct 22-25, 1991.

Association for the Advancement of Health Education: *Strengthening health education for the 1990s: summary and suggestions for project replication,* Reston, VA, 1991, The Association.

The Carnegie Council on Adolescent Development: *Turning points: preparing American youth for the 21st century: report of the task force on education and young adolescents,* New York, 1989, Carnegie Corporation.

Children's Defense Fund: *The health of America's children 1992,* Washington, DC, 1992, The Fund.

Comprehensive school health education, *J School Health* 54:312-315, 1984.

Cornacchia HJ, Smith DE, Bentel DJ: *Drugs in the classroom: a conceptual model for school programs,* ed 2, St Louis, 1978, Mosby.

Committee on School Health: *School health: policy and practice,* Elk Grove Village, IL, 1993, American Academy of Pediatrics.

DeGraw C: A community school-based school health system: parameters for developing a comprehensive student health promotion program, *J School Health* 64:192-195, 1994.

Elam SM: The Twenty-Second Annual Gallup Poll of the public's attitudes toward the public schools, *Phi Delta Kappan* 72:41-55, 1990.

English J: Innovative practices in comprehensive health education programs for elementary schools, *J School Health* 66:189-191, 1994.

Gilliam A et al: AIDS education and risk reduction for homeless women and children, *Health Ed* 20:44-47, 1987.

Jackson SA: Comprehensive school health education program: innovative practices and issues in standard setting, *J School Health* 64:177-179, 1994.

The National Commission: *Code blue: uniting for healthier youth,* Alexandria, VA, 1990, National Schools Boards Association and American Medical Association.

National School Boards Association: *School health: helping children learn,* Alexandria, VA, 1991, The Association.

Payne KW, Ugarte CA: The Office of Minority Health Resource Center: impacting on health related disparities among minority populations, *Health Ed* 20:6-8, 1989.

Resnicow K et al: Ten unanswered questions regarding comprehensive school health promotion, *J School Health* 63:171-175, 1993.

Robert Wood Johnson Foundation: *Special report: National School Health Services Program 1985,* No 1, Princeton, NJ, 1985, The Foundation.

US Department of Health and Human Services, Public Health Service: *Healthy people 2000: national health promotion and disease prevention objectives,* Washington, DC, 1991, US Government Printing Office.

US Department of Health and Human Services, Public Health Service, Alcohol, Drug Abuse, and Mental Health Administration, Office of the National Institute of Drug Abuse: Highlights of national school health survey on drug and alcohol use, *NIDA Capsules,* 1988.

US Department of Health and Human Services, Public Health Service, Alcohol, Drug Abuse, and Mental Health Administration, Office of the National Institute of Drug Abuse: Teenagers and drug abuse, *NIDA Capsules,* 1990.

US Department of Health and Human Services, Public Health Service, Centers for Disease Control and Prevention, National Center for Health Statistics: *Health United States 1992,* Washington, DC, 1992, US Government Printing Office.

US Department of Health and Human Services, Public Health Service, Centers for Disease Control and Prevention, National Center for Health Statistics: *Health United States 1993,* Washington, DC, 1993, US Government Printing Office.

US Department of Health and Human Services, Public Health Service, Centers for Disease Control and Prevention, Office of Inspector General: *School-based health centers and managed care,* Washington, DC, 1993, US Government Printing Office.

US Department of Health and Human Services, Public Health Service, National Institute of Drug Abuse: *Monitoring the future survey: national high school senior drug use survey,* Washington, DC, 1993, US Government Printing Office.

US Department of Health and Human Services, Public Health Service, Office of Prevention and Health Promotion, National Coordinating Committee on School Health: *School health findings from evaluation programs,* Washington, DC, 1993, US Government Printing Office.

Waldorff DM: *Turning points: preparing American youth for the 21st century,* New York, 1989, Carnegie Council on Adolescent Development.

World almanac and the book of facts, New Jersey, 1995, Funk & Wagnalls.

2

The Teacher's Role in School Health

KEY CONCEPT

Teachers with appropriate competencies in the comprehensive school health program have a positive effect on student health.

Attainment of the national health priorities will depend substantially on educational and community-based programs to promote health and prevent disease.

HEALTHY PEOPLE 2000

Health education in the school setting is especially important for helping children and youth develop the increasingly complex knowledge and skills they will need to avoid health risks and maintain good health throughout life.

HEALTHY PEOPLE 2000

PROBLEM TO SOLVE

How can teachers prepare plans to develop their competencies, to keep up to date in health education, and to maintain their positive health status in order to provide positive role models for students? How can teachers develop a cultural sensitivity to provide for individual differences within the classroom?

THE elementary classroom teacher has a unique and vital role in the protection and improvement of the health of students through the development of positive health attitudes and behavior. The teacher, one of the most influential factors in the life of young persons, has contact with children during their most formative and sensitive years—a precious time when what they know, what they think, and what they do can be significantly affected. The elementary teacher provides the crucial foundation for the future education of the individual. Often the teacher sees and communicates with a child for more hours each day than do the parents. This reality becomes increasingly important when it is estimated that by the year 2000, as many as 80% of all school-aged children will have mothers in the work force.

Teachers have both a combined opportunity and responsibility to contribute to all facets of the total school health program. By having a good knowledge and understanding of their roles in the total school health program, particularly in health education, health services, and in promoting a healthful school environment (see Fig. 1-1), teachers can contribute in a positive fashion to children's health and safety. The totality of the impact of teachers on child health, however, depends on whether they are ready, willing, and competent to assume a prominent role in school health.

Health instruction, through formally planned and sequentially arranged activities (see Chapters 9 and 11 through 13) and informal counseling and guidance, is designed to promote health knowledge (cognitive), attitudes (affective), and practices (actions) that contribute to the highest levels of individual, family, and community health. Opportunities for both formal and informal instruction occur in health services, as well as in the environmental phase of the school health program. The formal health instruction program provides the greatest responsibility and opportunity for the teacher. Yet, informally, individual health problems often can be given attention through counseling and guidance.

Health services (see Chapters 5 through 7) include activities designed to identify the various health problems of children and to seek possible corrections so that they do not interfere with a child's learning. Adjustments of school programs also must be made to ensure the greatest learning for students. The teacher must be prepared to make classroom arrangements for students with disabilities. The purpose of the school health services program is to protect, maintain, and improve the health of children. This involves nurses, physicians, dentists, and others. Teachers must be prepared to deal with common childhood problems such as colds, stomachaches, fevers, sore throats, toothaches, headaches, and allergies. Teachers must be able to recognize signs and symptoms of student health problems, refer pupils to health personnel, and assist with screening programs. The teacher also may use service activities as teachable moments (see Chapter 12) to provide formal and informal instruction.

A healthful school environment includes the physical aspects (see Chapter 3) and the emotional climate (see Chapter 4) of the school setting. The school must be free of hazards and offer a safe, comfortable, warm atmosphere with stable teachers to enable children to learn most effectively. Although teachers have limited responsibility for the proper lighting, heating, and ventilation of the classroom, they should offer assurance that pupils are free of undue exposure to hazardous conditions. Teachers should be aware of what constitutes a healthful school environment and contribute to keeping the environment a safe and positive one for learning. By teaching students how to maintain a healthful environment, teachers also are contributing to the achievement of community health goals. The emotional climate is a part of the school environment, which includes teacher health, fairness in dealing with pupils, consideration for individual differences, creation of a friendly classroom setting, and avoidance of bias and prejudice.

The elementary classroom teacher often has been called a "specialized generalist," in recognition of the diversity of talents required to be a good teacher. Few people in the entire field of education, or in any of the other professions for that matter, need the diversity of competencies required of the good elementary school teacher. Summarily, that person must be a grammarian, mathematician, psychologist, scientist, computer technologist, nutritionist, editor, art and drama critic, geographer, health educator, sociologist, physical educator, agriculture expert, historian, zoologist, anthropologist, safety specialist, chemist, economist, nurse, counselor, and more.

WHAT COMPETENCIES DOES THE ELEMENTARY TEACHER NEED?

It would be unrealistic to expect each classroom teacher to be a health education specialist. Although an elementary teacher should not be expected to be proficient in the competencies of the specialist, the teacher must have an understanding of the nature and process of health education as well as the total school health program if the program is to be effective. The teacher should be a role model for students. The teacher should be friendly and approachable, a person in whom the students can put their trust. The teacher must be a good communicator—one who is able to present health information that children understand. Specific competencies that will enable the teacher to participate effectively in a comprehensive program are identified on pp. 46 and 47.

In addition to these specific competencies the teacher as a health educator should (1) realize that health education requires the use of a different approach, (2) understand the controversial nature of some health topics, (3) appreciate the special need for the consideration of individual pupil differences, (4) be familiar with a variety of sources of current scientific health information (see Chapter 13 and Appendixes E and F), (5) be able to identify health problems to include in the instructional program (see Chapters 1, 5, and 11), and (6) plan for the orderly conduct of formal educational experiences and use teachable moments for health instruction (see Chapters 8 through 13).

Health Teaching Is Different

Although in many ways health teaching is much like all other teaching, it differs in certain crucial respects.

In the first place, although much of the content of health education is basic to the complete physical, psychological, social, and spiritual development of the child, motivation is often difficult. The normal, healthy child is largely unconcerned about his or her health and safety. In fact, if public apathy toward the value of using auto seat belts and the serious danger of cigarette smoking is any criterion, one may conclude that many youths and adults demonstrate a rather perverse antagonism toward established facts of safe and healthful living. Quite possibly this is because the essential knowledge and favorable attitudes and practices needed to combat this apathy were not developed a decade or more ago when these people were students in elementary school. In any event, the classroom teacher faces special challenges when trying to motivate pupils to make intelligent decisions about health. At the same time, fear psychology, vague exhortation, and the possibility of developing an unhealthy overconcern for health among pupils must be avoided. The balance is often a most delicate one.

Second, health teaching is inextricably bound up in our cultural and social patterns of thinking and doing. Perhaps no other area of learning in the elementary school depends so heavily on positively influencing attitudes and behavior. A person's actions are rooted in feelings, and feelings are colored by experiences and understanding. Health is a very personal thing. It is important that the teacher be aware of cultural differences and diversity within the classroom. Care must be taken to avoid demeaning the cultural beliefs of students and their families. Even though children may come to school without any preconceived notions regarding reading or arithmetic, they often already have begun to develop some false ideas, poor attitudes, and harmful practices in health and safety. Altering these unsound patterns of thinking and behaving is often difficult because of the rigidity of family and community culture and its powerful influence on the child.

Third, health information is constantly changing. What was unknown yesterday will be commonplace tomorrow; what was true last year is false this year; what was an apparently insurmountable problem a decade ago is now relegated to the museum of scientific antiques. Moreover, health science is not a simple listing of pure "blacks and whites." Whereas some concepts are established clearly and unalterably by research, others are supported in varying degrees, given current scientific evidence. The classroom teacher, therefore, must prepare pupils for scientific change without developing a negative skepticism. The teacher must lead children to understand the scientific method to be able to weigh the facts at hand and make choices and decisions that will favorably affect health. This concept of decision making is critical, for unlike most other subject matter areas, health and safety demand that children be participants, not merely spectators.

Health Teaching Can Be Controversial

Because health is such a personal matter, some of the topics in health education may occasionally provoke emotional reactions among pupils, parents, and other concerned persons or groups in the community. Teachers and administrators must be prepared to deal with the issues that arise. Some of the most controversial areas include sex education and human immunodeficiency virus/acquired immunodeficiency syndrome (HIV/AIDS) education; sexually transmissible diseases; tobacco, alcohol, and other drugs; the choice of a health advisor; suicide; violence; and dying and death. These areas are commonly included in comprehensive health instruction programs, and teachers must be thoroughly prepared to present objectively scientific information.

Teachers must be aware that sex education and tobacco and alcohol instruction have certain moral and religious implications. Yet the evidence clearly indicates that despite the hue and cry of small vocal groups, the majority of parents and re-

ligious leaders generally favor school instruction in these areas. Sex education may be the most controversial topic included in a comprehensive health instruction program. When teaching sex education, the teacher should use age-appropriate terminology, and sex-fair language and respect the questions that students might ask. Teachers should keep in mind that the primary responsibility for sex education rests with the home, and that sex education in schools should supplement, not supplant, home instruction. Unfortunately, sex instruction often does not occur at home, or the information that is provided is inaccurate. As a result, it is important that scientifically correct information be provided in the school situation.

School districts should have written guidelines for the teaching of any area that could be considered controversial. Teachers also should be careful not to force their value systems on children. The basic values that should be included in the total education program of the school should be specified in the basic educational philosophy of the school and should reflect community values. Regardless of the topic of instruction, teachers should be aware that personal values that exist within the classroom may come into conflict. The wise teacher will be alert to possible conflicts that may arise and be prepared to manage them effectively.

Fluoridation of water supplies continues to be an emotionally charged topic in some communities, despite the scientific evidence in support of its safety and efficacy in reducing tooth decay. Members of some healing professions may take exception to the generalization that medical diagnosis and treatment are best performed by licensed doctors of medicine and osteopathy. Some persons may urge that an ultraliberal view of medical care—barely short of esponsing acupuncture, homeotherapy, and herbal medicine—be presented in class. Those who oppose this tend to question any approach to medical care that suggests anything other than the traditional fee-for-service agreement between patient and physician.

Because health education is so intimately related to the cultural patterns of any community, teachers can expect that now and then some objections will arise. Neither teachers nor administrators should be intimidated by sporadic criticism of this kind. To be sure of standing on firm ground in these provocative areas, the classroom teacher should follow the recommendations contained in the box on this page.

A variety of teaching techniques should be effectively used in a well-planned health instruction program. However, there are numerous pitfalls to avoid if the program is to be a positive learning experience for children. Some of these pitfalls include the following:

- Using extrinsic rewards—especially "unhealthy" rewards (e.g., candy) for a child who demonstrates positive health behavior

- Inserting personal bias into instruction
- Using students as examples of poor health practices or of health problems
- Creating a "clean plate" club
- Overusing fear tactics or overly graphic portrayals of disease entities or health problems
- Conducting competition between students on health practices such as grooming or posture
- Overly emphasizing perfect attendance at school
- Pushing personal values or interests as fact
- Setting forth unrealistic standards in terms of health knowledge and practices for children
- Ridiculing a child's home situation or using it as an example of a poor health practice or environment

---

Teaching Controversial Topics

When teaching controversial topics the teacher should:
1. Refrain from forcing personal values on students
2. Maintain a scientific, unbiased approach
3. Take care not to ridicule or challenge the personal values of families and allow for cultural differences and student exemptions when subjects or topics interfere with religious or parental beliefs
4. Follow course and unit outlines recommended or approved by local school officials and allow parents to review them
5. Be sure the information being provided is scientifically accurate
6. Wherever possible, use materials that have been prepared by reputable groups and organizations such as those listed in Appendixes E and F
7. Use resources that are up to date and scientifically accurate
8. Keep school administrators informed of classroom activities
9. Inform parents of the intent of the program and the methods to be used (this might be a function of the school administrator)
10. Maintain adequate records of pupil activities, questions, interests, and problems
11. Never have "secret" lessons or admonish students not to discuss lessons at home
12. Be aware of school policy and do not violate that policy
13. Use accurate, nonsexist language and avoid stereotyping
14. Preview all audiovisual materials to be sure that they are scientifically accurate, age-appropriate, and germane to the objectives of the lesson, and allow parents to preview materials
15. Know all guest speakers, and have a preclassroom meeting with them to go over what will be presented in class
16. Invite parents to review materials that will be used
17. Never elicit confidential information from students that will be used in a classroom discussion
18. Be prepared for unexpected occurrences by having a good command of classroom management techniques

- Not being well prepared and organized, particularly in areas that may be controversial
- Challenging the basic beliefs of the children's parents

Teacher-pupil planning of units and including active participation by parents and other citizens in curriculum study and development are procedures that help ensure public understanding and acceptance of what is taught in the schools. Close ties among school, home, and community tend to lessen substantially the possibility of any misunderstandings regarding teaching concepts in controversial areas. This also can help ensure optimal physical, mental, emotional, social, and spiritual development of children.

Ethical Issues

Teachers and all personnel must consider a variety of ethical questions regarding student health that are related to health services and health education. Health records often contain information from a variety of sources including health appraisals, physicians' reports, and parental notes. Such information entrusted to school personnel by parents, medical personnel, and others is for educational purposes and must be considered confidential and not subject to discussion (except possibly with the specific children, parents, physicians, or school nurses). When such information is shared with teachers it is for the purpose of enhancing learning or aiding children to make adjustments. Teachers must value and respect the dignity, worth, and right to privacy of all individuals regardless of their age, gender, socioeconomic or health status, ethnicity, and religion. It is an infringement of student rights for teachers and other school personnel to openly discuss with friends or teachers specific children's conditions or illnesses such as HIV/AIDS, diabetes, epilepsy, mental retardation, or emotional disturbances unless they have specific bearing on the student's educational experiences.

When teaching about health, especially as it applies to the controversial areas previously mentioned, teachers must be aware that students have the right to choose their own styles of living, particularly if the student is fully aware of the risks (informed consent). Since elementary school-aged children may not be able to do this, the wishes of parents or guardians must be honored. All individuals however, have the right to be protected against other individuals if their rights, health, or welfare are endangered. The school, therefore, has the right to prevent illness or injury by imposing restrictions wherever communicable disease or safety is concerned.

Teachers also may become privy to confidential information told to them by students. This information should be held in the strictest confidence. If the information concerns something that could have an adverse effect on the child, however, the teacher must follow district policy and pass the information on to appropriate school personnel for further action. At no time should confidential information be shared with anyone other than designated school personnel. It is quite likely that many parents would be extremely embarrassed if they knew that what their child said in school was discussed openly in a teacher's lounge or elsewhere. Not only is it unprofessional to discuss a child's comments in public forums, it also constitutes unethical practice.

Sources of Current Scientific Information

Elementary education programs in teacher-training institutions have varying school health requirements—from no coursework to one or more courses in personal health, first aid, and perhaps school health. A joint committee of the American School Health Association and the Association for the Advancement of Health Education developed guidelines for the training of elementary teachers in health education. These guidelines should parallel the competencies presented on pp. 47-48. Although a teacher might possess good qualifications for teaching health, because information in the health field changes so rapidly, it is important and frequently necessary that in-service education programs be conducted to assist teach-

Competencies

GENERAL

The teacher understands and appreciates:

1. The meaning of health as a multidimensional state of well-being that includes physical, psychological, social, and spiritual aspects
2. That the health of individuals is influenced by the reciprocal interaction of the growing and developing organism and environmental factors and is necessary for optimal functioning as productive members of society
3. The significance of children's and youth's health problems on learning
4. The importance and the need for the school health program in today's society
5. The nature of the total school health program
6. The role of the teacher in each of the school health program components—services, environment, and instruction
7. The influence of teacher health and teacher health habits on students
8. The need for basic scientific information about a variety of health content areas, including dental health; drugs (alcohol, tobacco, and other drugs); care of eyes, ears, and feet; exercise, fitness, rest, and fatigue; prevention and control of diseases and disorders (communicable and chronic); safety and first aid; family health; consumer health; community health; environmental health; nutrition; mental health; anatomy; and physiology

HEALTH INSTRUCTION

The teacher:

1. Can identify and use a variety of techniques and procedures to determine the health needs and interests of pupils
2. Is able to organize the health instruction program around the needs and interests of students and can develop effective teaching units for the grade being taught
3. Is able to stress the development of attitudes and behaviors for healthful living based on scientific health information
4. Can distinguish between the various patterns of health instruction and attempts to use the direct approach in teaching whenever possible
5. Realizes that health education must receive time in the school program along with other subject areas
6. Possesses current scientific information about a variety of health content areas
7. Can use a variety of stimulating and motivating teaching techniques derived from fundamental principles of learning
8. Is able to identify and use "teachable moments" or incidents that occur in the classroom, in the school, or in the community
9. Uses a variety of teaching aids in the instructional program and is familiar with their sources
10. Is familiar with the sources of scientific information and the procedures necessary to keep up to date with current health information
11. Is able to provide a variety of alternative solutions to health problems to enable students to make wiser decisions
12. Can integrate health into other phases of the curriculum, such as social science, science, and language arts
13. Uses a variety of evaluative procedures periodically to (a) assess the effectiveness of the program on students and (b) determine the quality and usefulness of teaching aids and materials

Continued.

Competencies—cont'd

HEALTH SERVICES

The teacher:

1. Is familiar with the characteristics of the healthy child and can recognize signs and symptoms of unhealthy conditions including child abuse or neglect; refers problems to the school nurse or other appropriate school personnel
2. Is familiar with the variety of health appraisal procedures used in schools and uses them to enrich the health instruction program
3. Acquires limited skill in counseling and guiding students and parents regarding student health problems
4. Understands the value and purposes of teacher-nurse conferences
5. Is familiar with the variety of health personnel found in schools, their functions, responsibilities, and usefulness to the teacher
6. Is able to use information contained on health records
7. Can identify and follow the policies and procedures in schools in regard to such matters as emergency care, accidents, disease control, and referrals, exclusions, and readmittance of pupils
8. Can administer immediate care when accidents or illnesses to pupils occur or can act promptly to obtain sources of help within the school
9. Is able to adjust the school program to the individual health needs of students
10. Is able to relate the health services program to the health instruction program

HEALTHFUL SCHOOL LIVING

The teacher:

1. Is familiar with the standards for hygiene, sanitation, and safety needed in schools to provide a safe and healthful environment
2. Is familiar with the physical and emotional needs of students and adjusts classroom activities to help students satisfy these needs whenever possible
3. Understands the nature and importance of the food services program and is able to relate it to the instructional program
4. Is able to recognize hazardous conditions on the playground, in the classroom, and elsewhere in the school and takes appropriate action to eliminate or correct such conditions
5. Is cognizant of the effect of teacher health, personality, biases, and prejudices on student health and learning and is concerned with the humane treatment of pupils
6. Integrates healthful environmental aspects into the health instruction program

COORDINATION

The teacher:

1. Understands the need for school and community health councils or committees and is willing to participate as a member if requested to do so
2. Realizes the importance of and need for a coordinator, consultant, or a person with administrative responsibility being in charge of the school health program

Modified from Joint Committee of the Association for the Advancement of Health Education and the American School Health Association: Health instruction responsibilities and competencies for elementary (K-6) classroom teachers, *J School Health* 62:77, 1992.

ers and others in keeping up to date with current information. This should be a responsibility of administration, but teachers also should make requests for such training.

Teachers also can supplement the in-service training that they receive by attending local health-related meetings conducted by reputable organizations, by reading professional journals that are available in the school's library, or by taking additional courses at nearby colleges and universities. The advent of computer technology provides opportunities for teachers to obtain new and up-to-date health information through "distance learning."

Unfortunately, the sources of reliable and new information and the methods used to assess such information present problems not readily or easily resolved. There are no simple or definitive ways to discover with certainty whether material contained in publications is truthful and accurate. There are several reasons for this difficulty: (1) data are limited or inconclusive regarding the cause, treatment, or cure of many conditions such as arthritis, cancer, and obesity; (2) published research data are frequently in conflict; and (3) a number of so-called authorities, including scientists, nutritionists, physicians, and others who may disseminate health information may have been motivated to disseminate inaccurate information for purely profit-related reasons—information clearly not in the best interest of the health consumer. Further, the elementary teacher usually does not have access to basic medical literature to double-check the information contained in varied publications. Therefore it is important that teachers attempt to determine the validity of health information they read. The guidelines presented here should be helpful in the evaluation of publications and other printed materials.*

- What is the purpose of the printed material? Is it produced to sell products, make money, or present factual information to the reader?

- Is it presented in an educational or scientific manner, or does it use exaggerated claims and make misleading and inaccurate statements?
- Is the author qualified by way of educational background and professional experience? Even though the author may be qualified, the information may be inaccurate.
- Are the data based on appropriate research and experience of experts in the health field or on the opinions of a few individuals?
- Are the research data acceptable by medical, dental, public health, and other authorities and organizations?
- What evidence exists to support or refute conflicting claims about health information? Has the claimant generalized from a particular incident or from broad research?

Sources of reliable current information and ways for teachers to keep up to date are presented in Chapter 13 and Appendixes E and F.

Providing for Individual Differences

Providing for individual differences, including cultural and ethnic differences, is something we talk about a great deal in education. Doing much about it becomes increasingly difficult. Overcrowded schools and oversized classes make individualization of learning more a theoretical goal than an accomplished fact (Fig. 2-1).

Teachers can learn more about their pupils in several ways. Of course, school records furnish significant information on a child's intellectual capacity, status, and progress. Often these records also contain data about a pupil's social and emotional development. Well-kept cumulative health records should provide information about illnesses, injuries, major surgical operations, allergies, health examination findings, dental health, physical growth, and teacher observations from previous years. These records, combined with notes and recommendations of the school nurse and physician, can be most helpful to the teacher in understanding the health status of each child and the implications such status may have for learning (see Chapter 5).

---

*Modified from Cornacchia H, Barrett S: *Consumer health,* ed 5, St Louis, 1993, Mosby–Year Book.

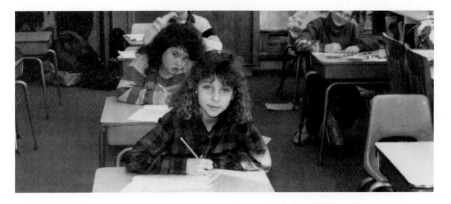

FIG. 2-1 Teachers must provide for individual differences. (Courtesy Galeton Area School District, Galeton, Pennsylvania.)

Intellectually, one must realize that it is not physically possible for a teacher to meet every need of every student within a given classroom. When a teacher must deal with anywhere from 20 to 30 or more students in a classroom and considerably more than that throughout the school day, the chance is quite good that the teacher will come into contact with one or more students with whom it will be difficult to establish rapport. When this occurs, the teacher would be well advised to examine his or her personal biases to determine whether they might be a barrier to the rapport. In like manner, the teacher will have a profound effect on the lives of many other students with whom rapport has been established.

Beyond the variances in the health and growth of pupils (see Chapter 5 and Appendix K), important differences relate to each child's environment. Most important of these is the home background. Economic conditions, cultural level, parental attitude toward the school, social position, marital status, value system, leisure time activities, parents' occupations, and racial or ethnic origins of parents—all these and more tend to leave their mark on the child. The purposes, interests, and values of children will tend to be aligned with those of their parents. Thus whereas one child comes from a home where meals are planned carefully and medical and dental care are readily available, another may leave a home where a full

stomach is the only measure of good nutrition, where breakfast is not served, or where the physician or dentist is seen only for the most extreme conditions, if at all. Surely the needs and interests of these two pupils are different in many respects.

In the same classroom there are pupils whose neighborhoods vary widely. Whereas some live in the town or city, others may be transported to school from outlying rural areas. Some enjoy a pleasant suburban neighborhood, but others live in the shadow of factories, railroad yards, commercial sections, or in the inner city. Home, family, and neighborhood influences shape the pupil's out-of-school experiences. Travel, work, and recreation also play a part in contributing to differences among children.

Attempting to adapt teaching-learning situations and experiences to fit the needs, concerns, and abilities of children, the teacher also must bear in mind that children mature at different rates. What is appealing and important to one fifth grader is, at the moment, beyond the understanding and interest of a classmate. **Children grow and mature according to a general pattern, yet each child sets his or her own unique schedule. This is a most important concept for teachers to recognize.**

Finally, teachers should remember that effective learning also takes place in many situations. A balance must be maintained between individual

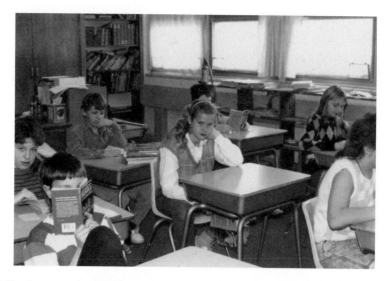

FIG. 2-2 Teachers must be alert for changes in children. (Courtesy Galeton Area School District, Galeton, Pennsylvania.)

guidance and small and large group learning activities. The very nature of these human differences often provides the raw materials with which a good teacher can actually mold a superior setting for health education. Although there are many more similarities than differences among children of the same age and gender, the areas of variance constitute both a stimulating challenge and a rich opportunity for alert teachers to achieve effectiveness in two fundamental functions of good teaching: (1) providing learning experiences suited to individual purposes, needs, concerns, and interests; and (2) providing opportunities for pupil sharing of diversified experiences relating to safe and healthful living.

Teachers Must Choose

Perhaps the most significant function of the classroom teacher is deciding how much time and emphasis to give to various health and safety topics. In general, the teacher designs the curriculum in those districts where none exists. Even with textbooks, courses of study, teaching units, and lesson plans as guides, the classroom teacher usually has considerable latitude in selecting course content at a given grade level. Moreover, the teacher may have to decide just how much emphasis to place on subtopics within a broad unit. More detailed information in this regard is provided in Chapter 11 and Appendix B.

It is important for teachers to remember that their primary responsibility and function is to teach, but they also have a role in all segments of the elementary school's comprehensive school health program (see Fig. 1-1).

THE TEACHER AS COUNSELOR AND GUIDANCE PERSON

The classroom teacher assumes the role of counselor and guidance person mainly in connection with the health services program. The teacher is in a unique position to observe deviances within the student population. The teacher spends a great deal of time with the child and thus is able to see patterns develop within each child. When a deviation from the normal pattern for a given child occurs (Fig. 2-2), the teacher should refer the child to the appropriate school health services personnel.

Once the child has been referred, the conscientious teacher will follow the progress of the child to be sure that the condition for which the child was referred is alleviated. In some cases, all that is needed is to move the child's desk to enable that student to see or hear more easily. In other cases, major alterations may be required. Regardless of what needs to be done, the teacher must maintain contact with the school nurse, the parents, and often the referral source if the school health services component is to reach its full potential.

Another way the teacher serves as counselor and guidance person is through the *informal education approach.* Information, counseling, and guidance that is nondirective, voluntary, and of little if any structure can be provided to children and parents. The teacher must be constantly alert for the child who expresses a need for help.

Naturally, any informal counseling is intended to supplement and complement the formal program. If the school health services program is to be effective, both formal and informal opportunities for counseling must be available to the student. An excellent means of informal counseling is the use of peer groups that can become referral sources for students. By informally discussing the various problems that come to the teacher's attention within the classroom setting, the teacher is enhancing the total school health services program.

The teacher often is sought out or is the first person who becomes aware of student health problems. For this reason, it is critical that children have confidence in the teacher. Young children may be very open in the classroom about things that occur in their homes. Teachers must take care not to discuss specific student situations in class but rather keep discussions on a more general plane. If the teacher suspects child abuse or neglect or other possible home situations that could affect the student adversely, that information must be given to appropriate school administrators. If the student persists in bringing out his or her home situation, the teacher should indicate to the student that some things are better discussed in private and then have a private session, perhaps in conference with appropriate school personnel, and with the student.

HEALTH OF SCHOOL PERSONNEL

The health of school personnel is important when one considers the many daily contact hours these persons have with school-aged children. It is important to know whether they are emotionally well adjusted, have communicable diseases, or are physically able to perform the multitude of required duties.

School districts over the years, however, have not given adequate consideration to personnel health. Varied attention has been given mainly to health insurance, counseling by health professionals, and provisions for sick leave, parenting leave, and leave of absence. In recent years the focus on preventive aspects of health and the need to reduce skyrocketing health care costs have caused some districts and insurance programs to provide monetary rewards at the end of the school year to personnel who stay well. Some insurance companies provide reduced premiums to nonsmokers.

In some 27 states, special conferences are held to assist school districts in developing school-site wellness programs for faculty and staff. These programs are designed specifically to bring teams of educators together in various locations for a week to learn about health and to develop plans for initiating school-site health promotion programs in their respective school districts. The results of these programs have been quite positive, and districts that have had teams of educators participate have reported that teacher morale has improved, teacher absence for health reasons has decreased, and teacher commitment has increased to plan well-developed health programs for the district. These programs need not be expensive, but the benefits they provide are immeasurable.

Teachers and all school personnel have a responsibility not only to protect children's health, but also for their own health. Because they are expected to provide the best physical and emotional climate (see Chapters 3 and 4) for pupils in the classroom, school personnel need to assess their own health needs and problems periodically to maintain a high level of wellness. They also need to use school and community health personnel and services. Teachers are role models for students. A teacher who practices positive health behaviors projects a positive image to students.

Teachers have little opportunity to be completely alone during the school day. Teaching is demanding and time consuming. It is common for teachers to have inadequate sleep, not find the time for proper exercise or relaxation, and feel great stress associated with their responsibilities. The wise teacher periodically engages in introspection to determine whether personal health habits are affecting teaching responsibilities.

The teacher is a role model for the child. As stated in the beginning of this chapter, the teacher exerts a great influence over the child. Thus if the teacher is ill, many additional untoward features may manifest themselves. If the teacher does not feel well, it is quite likely this will show in his or her disposition or in the way classroom problems are handled. How can students gain from the teacher who is chronically tired, is obese, has poor personal hygiene, or constantly complains about one or more physical, psychological, social, or spiritual problems?

Health Standards for School Personnel

When a child is legally mandated to attend school for at least 10 years, it is only right for parents to expect that their child will not be exposed to undue health hazards. Thus having health standards for school personnel benefits children, the school personnel themselves, and the community at large.

The School Health Education and Services Section (formerly the School Health Section) of the American Public Health Association summarized the varied benefits to be derived from having health standards for school personnel. These benefits are presented in the box on p. 54.

COORDINATION OF THE SCHOOL HEALTH PROGRAM

For a school health program to be effective, coordination of all aspects of the program is necessary. In some cases, one individual is given primary responsibility for this administrative function. Thus the likelihood of efficient use of various school resources and facilities is enhanced because the linkage between the instructional, service and environmental aspects of the program can be brought more clearly into focus.

The Teacher and the Health Coordinator

In an ideal situation, each school district or system should have a professionally prepared coordinator or supervisor for the district's school health program. Unfortunately, few districts have employed such a person. In those instances where employment of a health coordinator is possible, the person should be a professionally trained school health educator who works with all of the professional and ancillary school staff, including administrators, to ensure that a well-developed school health program is operating within the district. In those cases where a coordinator is not hired, the classroom teacher may have to assume the role of coordinator for a given building.

Numerous functions have been attributed to the health coordinator. A summary of those most commonly found include the following*:

- Organize and supervise the school health program
- Coordinate the activities of such a program with those in the community—health departments, civic and professional organizations, parents, police safety programs, physicians, dentists, private and voluntary health agencies, and school and community health councils

---

*Modified from Schaller W: *The school health program,* ed 5, New York, 1981, WB Saunders, and Creswell, W, Newman I, Anderson C: *School health practice,* ed 9, St Louis, 1989, Mosby–Year Book.

Benefits Derived from Health Standards for School Personnel

BENEFITS FOR CHILDREN

1. Increased quality of learning experiences when the staff is well
2. Lessening of stress in classrooms and other school areas
3. Greater continuity in the learning experience resulting from fewer absences of teachers and other school staff
4. Lessened exposure to communicable disease
5. Decreased risk of accidents (as from fitness of bus drivers)
6. Increased awareness and value of health when employees are good role models

BENEFITS FOR SCHOOL EMPLOYEES

1. Early detection of conditions that can be corrected or minimized
2. Assistance in locating health resources when needed
3. Financial assistance (for health leaves, sickness disability insurance)
4. Placement in positions or assigned tasks based on consideration of the individual's health status
5. Realization that one's health behavior does relate to his/her fitness and job competency
6. Assistance in coping with stressful situations

BENEFITS FOR THE COMMUNITY

1. Increased cost-effectiveness when staff members have fewer absences
2. Greater competence of personnel when they are well
3. Improved emotional climate in the schools
4. Increased understanding of how teacher and labor negotiations relate to health issues
5. Established and written health policies are available
6. Reduced incidence of communicable diseases
7. Assured compliance with federal regulations for hiring and placement of handicapped persons

From Doster M et al: *Health of school personnel: report of the American Public Health Association, Education and Services School Health Section*, Washington, DC, 1980, The Association.

- Help teach in the instructional program
- Maintain a continuous evaluation program
- Plan for in-service education
- Help develop an articulated health and safety curriculum
- Counsel individual students following referral
- Serve on the community health council
- Chair the school health council
- Establish procedures for purchasing and distributing instructional material
- Furnish the staff with information about the total school health program
- Help prepare policies and procedures for school health services
- Develop a plan for keeping health records
- Provide procedures for student referral
- Prepare and interpret emergency care procedures for faculty and staff
- Provide leadership in the promotion of healthful school living

In-service education. The provision of in-service education programs for teachers is a responsibility of central administration but is often coordinated by the health coordinator. The in-service program provides one way for teachers to keep up to date on health matters that affect the school-aged child. A good program of in-service education can help boost teacher morale and keep the school health program dynamic. Sufficient funds should be allocated for teacher in-service training programs in health areas.

Individual guidance. Through planned conferences and informal talks the supervisor can help teachers analyze and solve the problems that relate to their own classroom situations and teaching. Much of this is concerned with evaluation of the teaching-learning process. The conference may be based on classroom observation by the coordinator. Such observation is concerned with helping the teacher do a better job, *not* with personal criticism of the teacher.

Refer to Chapter 6 for detailed information on health guidance and informal education.

Communication. Helping teachers stay up to date is one of the chief functions of the school health coordinator. Elementary classroom teachers cannot possibly keep up with all the important literature in school health; thus the coordinator has a major function to keep the staff aware of new developments in the field.

Research and curriculum development. An important but often overlooked function of the health coordinator is that of stimulating and guiding teachers in research projects. Of course, most teachers cannot be expected to carry out extensive investigations in addition to their normal teaching load. Yet with help and guidance from the supervisor, significant problems can be selected and delineated for worthwhile study in an elementary school. Important data often can be collected within the framework of routine classroom activities. Policy and procedures based on objective evidence offer far more likelihood of success than those predicated on opinion. By having teachers directly involved in policy making, it is more likely that the policy will be understood and accepted than if the policy were developed externally.

The Teacher and the Administrator

Administrators and school board members who understand the problems and appreciate the values of school health and health education are essential to an effective program. Experience with health programs in elementary schools has shown with vivid clarity that the success of any such program basically depends on the attitude of school administrators and school board members. When administrators favor and support a sound health program, it is more likely to be initiated and carried out successfully. In recent years the leading professional societies of administrators have recommended that school health programs be established for all schools. Teachers should encourage administrators to take active leadership in providing effective school health programs. Teachers may encourage the formation of a school health council and indicate their willingness to serve on such a council.

At the superintendent level this leadership often takes shape through stimulation of school evaluations by professional groups and citizens' advisory committees. Specific criteria for evaluation of the school health program are presented in some detail in Appendix H.

As the official leader in an individual elementary school, the principal has much influence on the health program. Through concern for a sound program, provision of released time for conferences, establishment of in-service programs on health-related topics, encouragement of teachers, efforts to secure textbooks and other learning materials, and consistent interest in the many activities of the school health program, the principal helps classroom teachers assume their responsible roles in school health.

The Teacher and the School Nurse

With the lack of coordinators in the schools, the school nurse commonly may be the individual who promotes and coordinates the health program. The classroom teacher should make every effort to work closely with the school nurse in matters of student health. The nurse should serve as a resource person and can be particularly helpful in allaying the fears of children who may be experiencing screening tests in school for the first time. Although some school nurses are employed directly by the school and others are employed by local or state health departments, it is a fundamental school staff function of the teacher to offer full cooperation to the nurse serving the school.

The teacher and nurse can be of great help to each other in numerous ways. The nurse can help the teacher by letting the teacher know the signs and symptoms of various health problems, establishing referral mechanisms, assisting with the instructional program through securing speakers and material aids, working with the teacher in terms of health guidance (see Chapter 6), and aiding the returning student to readjust to the classroom. The teacher can help the nurse by observing the children daily, assisting in screening, and referring suspected health problems, including child abuse or neglect. Child abuse is not always physically manifested. In fact, mental abuse and neglect may be more devastating to the child in the long run. A child who is "beaten" mentally may become disconsolate, dispirited, and withdrawn. In any case, the basic procedure for reporting any suspected health problem should be part of the written policies (recommended by the National School Boards Association*) and procedures of the school district. The administration should acquaint all employees with these materials.

Once a child has been referred, the teacher is not free of responsibility. It is important that the teacher follow up the referral to see that something is done. Naturally this could and should be done in conjunction with other school personnel. It is usually rather easy to determine if something has been done, as the teacher will have daily contact with the referred child. Further, the teacher can exert some control over the situation through rearrangement of the classroom environment, including seating, and through altering the daily classroom schedule.

The teacher can aid the school nurse through assisting with screening procedures (see Chapter 5). The most common measures include growth and development, vision, hearing, and possibly postural defects (primarily scoliosis). Some schools may offer mental health screening. It must be remembered that these procedures are not diagnostic tools. They are used merely to determine whether a potential problem exists.

The teacher will be able to do some health counseling using the screening procedures as objective evidence. This should be coordinated with the school nurse. Often this counseling occurs on a less formal basis throughout the progress of the average school day.

Screening tests also afford the opportunity for incidental instruction. As the tests are being administered, the teacher has an opportunity to do incidental health teaching on topics directly related to the screening process. Such questions as "Why should this screening be done?", "What might be detected?", and "Will this hurt?" all provide excellent instructional potential.

To ensure close rapport between the teacher and the nurse, teacher-nurse conferences are necessary. Unfortunately, it is often difficult to find the time in the already crowded school day to schedule such meetings, but with the help of the school principal, this problem should not be difficult to resolve. These conferences may be formal or informal, depending on the topics to be considered. Further information concerning teacher-nurse conferences is presented in Chapter 5.

THE TEACHER AS A LINK WITH THE COMMUNITY IN SCHOOL HEALTH

As the school and the community join more closely in their efforts to improve education, many reciprocal advantages accrue. Opportunities that will benefit the school health program are abundantly evident. The teacher has many occasions to work with resource people in the community and should capitalize on these opportunities.

Community organizations and people who are capable of providing cooperative assistance include the following:

- Medical societies and individual physicians
- Dental societies, individual dentists, and dental hygienists
- Local and state health departments
- Local and state voluntary health agencies

---

*National School Boards Association: *School health: helping children learn,* Alexandria, VA, 1991, The Association.

- Parent-teacher associations
- Police and fire departments
- Community health and safety councils
- Child guidance clinics, individual psychiatrists and clinical psychologists
- Red Cross
- Service clubs
- Departments of education
- Departments of welfare
- Youth councils
- Boy Scouts and Girl Scouts
- YMCA, YWCA, CYO, 4-H Clubs, Future Farmers of America, and other youth organizations

These organizations often have speakers' bureaus, among other services, or will provide resource materials to the classroom teacher. For example, the fire department may be willing to present demonstrations of home fire safety hazards or assist the teacher in teaching children techniques of artificial resuscitation. Voluntary, government, and professional organizations and agencies may provide pamphlets, posters, slides, cassettes, or films for classroom use. All the teacher has to do is ask for the material.

The new teacher would be well advised to consult with the school nurse, the school administrator or coordinator, and other teachers in the school to learn the resources available in a given area.

SCHOOL HEALTH COUNCILS

One of the best ways to fully coordinate the personnel resources of the community is through the school health council. Membership of the school health council can include representatives from the following:

- Teachers
- Pupils
- Parents
- Medical society
- Dental society
- Health department
- Voluntary health agencies
- Food service and custodial staffs

- School administrators (principal and school health coordinator)
- School nurses and physicians

The membership of the school health council will vary depending on the size of the school and the nature of the community. Even in small rural elementary schools, however, council membership can include the principal or a delegated representative, parents, pupils, classroom teachers, and custodians. In some communities an advisory health council is established for all schools in the area; in others each school has its own council. Regardless of the size or makeup of the school health council, it has three basic functions: (1) to identify health and safety problems of pupils and school personnel, (2) to study these problems, and (3) to make recommendations to the school administration for solution of the problems. It is important to understand that the council is an advisory body to the superintendent and school board; it is not responsible for taking direct action. The council may, however, conduct evaluation studies; propose changes in the policies for the instructional, service, or environmental aspects of the program; or propose the need for a total curriculum revision. The school health council is also a good forum to receive input from parents and interested citizens on matters related to school health policies and practices.

COMMUNITY HEALTH COUNCILS

The community health council is the community counterpart to the school health council. It has the potential of linking the school health program and the community health program. This council becomes a community voice for the airing of health problems seen by the various groups within the community. By having a close, cooperative link with the community, the school health program can become more responsive to the needs of that community. The membership of the community health council may include representatives from the following:

- School health council
- Voluntary health agencies

- Medical and dental organizations
- Private industry
- Civic or community service clubs
- Religious organizations
- Official health agencies
- Educational organizations
- Parent-teacher groups
- Youth organizations
- Police and fire departments

The community health council can provide a sounding board for the community, particularly when developing curricula related to controversial topics. The council also can assist in mobilizing community resources to assist with the comprehensive school health program.

In cities where the community health council has been successfully established, the school health program has been used as a focal point for community health services. Such things as testing for lead poisoning, school safety (especially crosswalks in the vicinity of the school), drug user referral centers, and many other health problems can be coordinated between the school and community health programs.

THE TEACHER AS A MEMBER OF THE SCHOOL STAFF IN HEALTH MATTERS

As has been discussed, teachers do many things with and for pupils beyond the routine classroom learning activities. The teacher's role as counselor in the various health services, and several ways in which a teacher provides a link between school and community has been presented. In many of these activities the teacher also serves as a member of the school staff.

In the role of the staff member, the elementary classroom teacher also has the responsibility for taking part in committee work and other organized efforts aimed at improvement of the school health program. The teacher may also serve on committees concerned with textbook selection, curriculum development, crisis response, special events planning, safety patrol, school clubs, building and grounds, audiovisual aids, and food ser-

vice. The work of certain committees, particularly the school health council, and the proper concern of all teachers commonly relates to the safety and health of the school environment.

THE TEACHER AS A MEMBER OF THE PROFESSION IN SCHOOL HEALTH

A good teacher tries constantly to improve health instruction by using better methods and keeping abreast of new developments in a variety of fields, including school health. As has been suggested earlier, many teachers will conduct surveys and experiments in connection with their health teaching or other school health work. This, too, is the mark of a professional person. Objective conferences with the health coordinator about teaching methods and materials also help the teacher improve approaches in the classroom.

Through membership in national and state educational associations, the elementary teacher takes part in the profession to a fuller extent. National and state societies generally make provision for school health concerns through member associations, divisions, or sections. Organizations specifically concerned with school health include the American Alliance for Health, Physical Education, Recreation, and Dance; the American School Health Association; the American Public Health Association (School Health Education and Services Section); and regional and state branches of such groups. School administrators should support the efforts of their teachers to become involved in various professional organizations. This can be a positive step in enhancing not only the school health program, but all facets of the school program as well.

All in all, the life of elementary school classroom teachers is diversified in regard to school health. As has been discussed, they must live up to a reputation as "specialized generalists" if they are to make contributions to all phases of the health program. Although many teachers-to-be approach their first positions with some trepidation, all the evidence and experience indicate that the majority of classroom teachers can and do make substantial contributions to school health and health education. All they need is a bit of confidence, a basic understanding of the fundamental concepts of health instruction, health services, and healthful school living and well-planned in-service programs in health. The raw material is America's richest resource; the product is a healthier nation.

SUMMARY

Elementary school teachers have the opportunity to greatly influence the health of students through the instruction, services, and environmental aspects of the school health program. To be effective, these teachers need to be positive role models and acquire the competencies outlined in this chapter. They must be aware that in teaching about health: (1) the approach requires a different emphasis than other subject areas in the curriculum; (2) the inclusion of controversial topics is involved; (3) cultural sensitivity is important; (4) current scientific information must be imparted without bias; (5) ethical issues need consideration; and (6) provision for individual pupil health differences must be made. Teachers must realize that it is important for them to keep up to date with current health information, and that the status of their own health has a considerable effect on student health. They must be ready and willing to coordinate their health efforts with a variety of school and community personnel, organizations, and agencies.

QUESTIONS FOR DISCUSSION

1. Identify the five basic areas of competency for the elementary teacher and list one competency for each area. Is it realistic to expect elementary teachers to possess all these qualities? Why or why not?
2. Why does the teaching of health require a different approach than other subject areas in the school curriculum?
3. What are some of the health areas that may be considered to be controversial and why is this true? How might teachers deal with these areas in the classroom?
4. What are two ethical issues related to the school health program and what can teachers do about them?
5. Why must teachers keep up to date with current scientific information? What evaluation procedures may be used to assess the reliability of sources of health information?
6. Why is it important that the teacher understand the importance of being a role model for students?
7. Why is it important for teachers to provide for individual differences in the classroom?
8. What are two ways teachers may provide health counseling and guidance?
9. How can the health of teachers affect students? What may teachers do to protect student health in this regard?
10. Why is provision of health promotion programs for school faculty and staff important?
11. Identify three ways the school health coordinator may provide services to schools and three ways this person may assist teachers.
12. How can teachers assist the school nurse, and how can the nurse assist teachers in regard to the health of students?
13. Who might become members of a school health council?
14. What might teachers do to start a school health council if none exists in a school or school district?
15. What is the role of the school health council? How do the school health council and community health council complement each other in enhancing the health of communities?

SELECTED REFERENCES

American Public Health Association: *Health of school personnel, report of the School Health Education and Services Section*, Washington, DC, 1980, The Association.

Association for the Advancement of Health Education: Code of ethics for health educators, *J Health Educ* 25:196-200, 1994.

Barnes SE: Ethical issues in health education, *Health Educ* 11:7-9, 1980.

Berryman JC: Health promotion at the school worksite. In Cortese P, Middleton K, editors: *The comprehensive school health challenge,* vol 1, Santa Cruz, 1994, ETR Associates.

Boschee F: Comprehensive health education: directives for development and implementation, *Health Educ* 19(5):136-138, 1988.

Buckner WP Jr: Promoting multicultural sensitivity among educators. In Cortese P, Middleton K: *The comprehensive school health challenge,* vol 2, Santa Cruz, 1994, ETR Associates.

Burks A, Fox E: Why is inservice training essential? In Cortese P, Middleton K: *The comprehensive school health challenge,* vol 2, Santa Cruz, 1994, ETR Associates.

Chen W et al: Impact of a continuing health education inservice program on teacher's competencies, *Health Educ* 21(6):8-11, 1990.

Cleary M, Gobble D: The changing nature of public schools: implications for teacher preparation, *J School Health* 60(2):53-55, 1990.

Cornacchia H, Barrett S: *Consumer health,* ed 5, St Louis, 1993, Mosby–Year Book.

Creswell W, Newman I, Anderson C: *School health practice,* ed 9, St Louis, 1989 Mosby–Year Book.

Davis C et al: Health concerns and teacher training of selected elementary teachers in Michigan, *J School Health* 55:151-153, 1985.

Demian SM, Foulk DF: Characteristics of school health advisory councils, *J School Health* 57(8):337-339, 1987.

Deputat Z, Pavlovich M: School health programs: a comprehensive plan for implementation, *Health Educ* 19(5):47-53, 1988.

Everett SA, Price JH, Telljohann SK: Secondary health educators perceived self-efficacy in teaching mainstreamed mentally disabled students, *J School Health* 64:261-265, 1994.

Furney S: Implementing the nation's health objectives for the 1990s: the role of the secondary and elementary health education specialist, *Health Educ* 20(2):22-25, 1989.

Healthy People 2000: National health promotion and disease prevention objectives and healthy schools, *J School Health* 61:7, 1991.

Hochbaum GM: Ethical dilemmas in health education, *Health Educ* 11:4-6, 1980.

Hosokawa MC: Insurance incentives for health promotion, *Health Educ* 17:9-12, 1984.

Joint Committee of the Association for the Advancement of Health Education and the American Health Association: Health instruction responsibilities and competencies for elementary (K-6) classroom teachers, *J School Health* 62(2):77, 1992.

Kolbe L: Increasing the impact of school health promotion programs: emerging research perspectives, *Health Educ* 16:47-52, 1986.

Kolbe L: Why school health education? an empirical point of view, *Health Educ* 16(2):116-117, 1985.

Mickalide: Children's understanding of health and illness: implications for health promotion, *Health Values* 10(3): 1986.

Miller R: Foreword from the Fourth Delbert Oberteuffer Symposium: administrative aspects of school health education, *Health Educ* 19(5):30, 1988.

Moore RS, Moore D: When education becomes abuse: a different look at the mental health of children, *J School Health* 56(2), 1986.

National Professional School Health Education Organizations: Comprehensive school health education: a definition, *J School Health* 54(8):312-315, 1984.

Rich R: Scheduling and staffing school-based health education, *Health Educ* 19(5):54-55, 1988.

Russo RM et al: The use of community health aids in a school health program, *J School Health* 52:25-27, 1982.

Schaller W: *The school health program,* ed 5, New York, 1981, WB Saunders.

The Comprehensive School Health Program: Exploring an expanded concept, *J School Health* 57(10):409-473, 1987.

Trucano L: *Students speak,* Seattle, 1984, Comprehensive Health Education Foundation.

Valente C, Lumb K: Organization and function of a school council, *J School Health* 51:466-468, 1981.

Wagner DI: Health promotion cooperatives: an alternative delivery system for rural health promotion programs, *J Health Educ* 25:77-82, 1994.

II

HEALTHFUL SCHOOL LIVING

3

Healthful School Environment:
Physical Aspects

KEY CONCEPT

A safe, healthful, and wholesome school environment enhances the quality of student life and learning.

A healthful school environment emphasizes disease prevention and health promotion for both students and staff.

AMERICAN ACADEMY OF PEDIATRICS, 1993

It is difficult to teach a child the value of health if the school environment is not conducive to healthy behavior and if there are no resources with which to practice health skills.

WORLD HEALTH ORGANIZATION*

PROBLEMS TO SOLVE

As a teacher, how might you use the school environment in your classroom instruction in health education? How would you characterize your role as a teacher in promoting a physically healthful school environment?

*World Health Organization: *Education for health: a manual on health education in primary health care*, Geneva, 1988, The Organization, p 136.

When by law we require children to spend so many of their formative years in our schools, we assume a legal and ethical responsibility to provide safe and healthful buildings, equipment, facilities, and services.

Even though this obligation is accepted, tens of thousands of American schools fail to meet minimal health and safety standards for students (Fig. 3-1). Many schools are considered to be firetraps; others maintain overcrowded classrooms; some are unprepared for crisis or violence; still others carry tenured teachers who are emotionally unstable; many are not meeting the emotional needs of students; many are overdue for repairs; some are operating unsafe school buses; and many do not provide nutritious food service.

The physical environment in which students are educated is important to the quality of learning that takes place. A physically and emotionally healthful school environment is essential if the highest quality of education is to be achieved. The quality of life cannot be enriched for students who are forced to learn and grow in schools that fail to provide a safe, orderly, pleasant, healthful, and wholesome atmosphere conducive to learning.

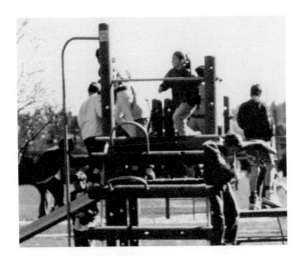

FIG. 3-1 Safe playgrounds contribute to a positive school environment. (Courtesy Health & Welfare, Canada.)

WHAT IS A HEALTHFUL SCHOOL ENVIRONMENT?

A healthful school environment is a dynamic concept that far surpasses consideration solely on the basis of the physical plant. It involves all the internal and external factors that affect the individual during the course of the school day. It is sometimes referred to as *healthful school living*. Healthful school living is the promotion, maintenance, and use of safe and wholesome surroundings and the organization of day-to-day experiences and planned learning procedures to influence favorable emotional, physical, and social health (see also Chapter 4).

Clearly this definition dispels the idea that healthful school living is confined to the mere provision of a safe and sanitary environment in which learning can occur. The overriding purpose for providing a healthful school environment is to establish a climate for children and staff that is supportive of their health and quality of life, enables them to feel good about being in school, and enhances opportunities for student learning.

HOW DO SCHOOL SITE AND BUILDINGS AFFECT STUDENT HEALTH?

Some specific physical components of a healthful school environment include site and building construction and internal organization such as thermal control, lighting and acoustics, water supply, sanitation, food services, school bus safety, and fire prevention and protection. Although teachers do not have control over many aspects of the physical environment of the school, they frequently are invited to participate on committees to consider the construction of new school facilities. A knowledge of basic factors related to school sites and buildings will enable teachers to function more appropriately on such committees.

School Site and Construction

The construction of educational facilities has been a major concern for many decades. In 1829 Alcott

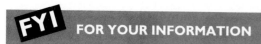

Standards and Frequency of Environmental Inspections of Schools

NUMBER OF STATES WITH ESTABLISHED STANDARDS FOR THE SCHOOL ENVIRONMENT

	Level of standard	
	Standard mandated by law N (%)	Standard recommended N (%)
Lighting	27 (53)	15 (29)
Ventilation	32 (63)	10 (19)
Acoustics	10 (20)	14 (27)
Vermin control	30 (59)	7 (14)
School kitchen	45 (88)	4 (8)
Fire safety	45 (88)	2 (4)
Heating and cooling	29 (57)	13 (25)
Asbestos	32 (63)	6 (12)

NUMBER OF STATES MANDATING INSPECTIONS, ACCORDING TO FREQUENCY OF INSPECTION

	Frequency		
	One per year or less N (%)	More than one per year N (%)	No inspection required N (%)
Cafeteria	27 (53)	19 (37)	4 (8)
Kitchen	26 (51)	20 (39)	3 (6)
Restrooms	23 (45)	6 (12)	20 (39)
Health room/sickroom	20 (39)	5 (10)	24 (47)
Playground/athletic field	17 (33)	6 (12)	27 (53)
Gymnasium	20 (39)	6 (12)	24 (47)
Locker rooms	20 (39)	6 (12)	24 (47)
Laboratories	23 (45)	6 (12)	21 (41)
Waste disposal site	15 (29)	10 (20)	18 (35)
Safety inspection buses	25 (49)	15 (29)	5 (10)
Fire inspection	36 (70)	7 (14)	3 (6)

From Lovato C, Allensworth D, Chan F: *School health in America: an assessment of state policies to protect and improve the health of students,* ed 5, Kent, OH, 1989, American School Health Association, p 25.

wrote an *Essay on the Construction of Schoolhouses,** which emphasized the impact of the environment on the education process. Since that time, many rules, regulations, and standards have been promulgated to help ensure that the school physical plant promotes safety, is sanitary, free of unneces-sary hazards, and is conducive to learning. The critical factor is to plan ahead and not operate on

---

*Means R: *Historical perspectives on school health,* Thorofare, NJ, 1975, Charles B Slack.

a crisis basis. The mere construction of a new building is no assurance that it contributes favorably to the educational experience of the child. A poorly planned facility in terms of location, internal space, color, internal and external traffic patterns, and many environmental considerations may detract from overall learning. The school environment should be developmentally appropriate by age and support the holistic nature of the student.

Numerous innovations in school construction occurred in the early 1960s. Too often, however, these new facilities were based on an architectural idea rather than the effective use of the facility as an institution of learning. Frequently, these new ideas in construction did not adequately facilitate learning. Unfortunately, little research demonstrating what would be best in school facilities has taken place. Now, however, much more consideration is given the interior of the building. Modular construction, open classrooms, learning wings, and central resource libraries as well as the more traditional single-level or multi-level self-contained classrooms may be found in new school building construction.

An expensive problem associated with school construction surfaced in recent years—asbestos removal. Before 1973, asbestos was often used in school construction, primarily as a fire retardant. The Environmental Protection Agency estimates that as many as 35% of the U.S. school buildings involving 15 million children have deteriorating walls and ceilings containing asbestos fibers.* When deterioration occurs, the asbestos fibers are allowed to float free in the buildings. Because exposure to asbestos fibers has been linked with debilitating lung diseases, schools containing asbestos cause a health hazard for the occupants.

In April 1987 the Environmental Protection Agency (EPA) proposed new rules that required school systems that find dangerous asbestos in their buildings to use certified contractors to remove the asbestos. This required school districts to submit a plan for the removal of the asbestos and to begin the work by July 1989. To help school districts pay for the removal, Congress voted to provide $50 million in 1988 to assist in the process. By mid-1993 at a cost of over $3 billion, the EPA reported that an estimated 98% of school districts complied with asbestos removal or abatement. In late 1994, 15,000 school districts participating in a class action lawsuit reached a settlement for $200 million from the 10 largest asbestos manufacturers.

Although there is a great deal of controversy regarding whether the problem of asbestos removal should be a federal, state, or local issue, the fact remains that it has been declared by the EPA to be a hazard that cannot be allowed to remain in the school environment.

Another possible environmental hazard that has surfaced is radon. Radon is a radioactive, colorless, odorless gas that results from the decay of uranium. The gas seeps through soil and rocks and into buildings through openings in the foundation where it can accumulate and attach to dust particles that subsequently are inhaled. The concern with radon is that in a nonsmoking population it constitutes the greatest source of risk for lung cancer,* including cancer caused by exposure to asbestos. In 1988, the EPA projected that indoor radon over 4 picocuries per liter of air posed a risk of lung cancer and advised home testing.† However, researchers at the National Cancer Institute concluded that exposure to the low levels of radon in typical U.S. homes carries little risk.

Specific guidelines for the testing for radon in schools are now available. If testing is completed and high radon levels are noted, the EPA has re-

*Office of Toxic Substances, Environmental Protection Agency: *Evaluation of the asbestos-in-schools identification and notification rule,* Washington, DC, 1984, EPA 560/5-84-005, US Environmental Protection Agency, pp x-xvi; and Lovato C, Allensworth D, Chan F: *School health in America: an assessment of state policies to protect and improve the health of students,* ed 5, Kent, OH, 1989, American School Health Association, p 28.

*Office of Radiation Programs: *Radon measurement in schools,* 1993, EPA 402-R-93-014, Washington DC, 1993, US Environmental Protection Agency.
†US Environmental Protection Agency: *Radon: a physician's guide,* EPA 402-K-93-008, Washington, DC, 1993, The Agency.

leased guidelines relative to school action. Ventilation is important if the radon levels exceed recommended maximum standards.

Schools do not generally receive sufficient local, state, or federal funds to adequately maintain their environments. The U.S. General Accounting Office projected in 1995 that U.S. public schools need $112 billion to repair or upgrade existing facilities. A survey of 10,000 school buildings led to estimates that one third of the 80,000 public schools need considerable repairs or actual replacement. Twenty percent of schools need renovations for basic safety, e.g., sprinkler systems, safer exits.*

Internal organization. It is important when designing a new or refurbishing an existing school building that the architect consider the ages, development, and needs of children and staff. Storage of hats and coats is particularly important because of the possible transmission of head lice through contact between these items (see Chapter 5). Of special concern are the needs of handi-

---

*Lindsay D: Senators say funding to fix schools likely to fall under the budget ax, *Education Week,* XIV (20), February 8, 1995.

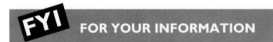

FOR YOUR INFORMATION

Needed School Repairs/Replacements

FEATURE	ESTIMATED NUMBER OF STUDENTS AFFECTED (IN MILLIONS)
Plumbing	12.3
Ventilation	11.6
Security	10.6
Indoor air quality	8.4
Heating	7.9
Safety codes	7.6
Foundation/framing	7.3

From US General Accounting Office: Survey of 10,000 school facilities. Reported in *Education Week*, Feb 8, 1995, p 21.

capped students, staff, and visitors. The Americans with Disabilities Act of 1990 requires programs and services be physically accessible to all persons with disabilities.

In addition, classrooms large enough to permit physical activities of children, areas for quiet study or activity, and internal classroom flexibility such as mobile walls must be planned. The well-being of the faculty and staff must also be provided for with a teacher's lounge and separate restroom facilities that are functional and appealing in appearance. Given the health hazards associated with tobacco use, all campuses should be smoke and tobacco free, including teachers' lounges. Some new constructions contain two teacher/staff lounges, one for smokers and one for nonsmokers. However, only 22 states have a law that restricts smoking in public schools.

Air quality. The teacher often assumes there is adequate heating, ventilation, and air-conditioning in the classroom.

A classroom that is too cold or too warm for children can have an impact on their learning. The recommendation for classroom temperature is between 65° to 70° Fahrenheit, depending on the age of the students and the type of activity that will occur.

The flow of air in a room is important. If the school is not equipped with air conditioning, the teacher should open windows or doors or run fans to improve air movement. These actions will also aid in removal of radon accumulation within the school building.

Concerns about odors or air quality should be investigated by school district staff or local health departments. Frequently, the problems are associated with mold or carbon dioxide caused by poor ventilation design, incomplete duct work, or dirty filters. Air circulation is critical if windows are small or cannot be opened.

Tobacco smoking in schools, whether or not in a restricted area, is an important health matter for children and nonsmoking staff. In a 1988 random sample of public schools, 95% of those who replied had written policy or regulations to control smoking. Most schools restricted smoking by students or adults. Only 17% banned smoking at all times on school property, and only one fourth prohibited staff from smoking within the building. Environmental tobacco smoke can circulate throughout a school that has a common ventilation system; any "smoking room" needs special ventilation to protect children.*

In 1994, as part of the *Goals 2000: Educate America Act,* Congress outlawed smoking in schools that receive federal funding; that includes all public and some private schools. Teachers have a responsibility to support compliance as good role models for children as well as for preservation of their own health.

Lighting. Footcandles of illumination at the work surface and in halls commonly was the determining factor for the number, location, and intensity of lights located in schools. Today, color, natural and artificial lighting, reflection and glare of light, and the type of activity to be performed in the room are factors of greater importance.

Glare is an annoying problem in the classroom setting. Speaking to the class while standing in front of unshaded windows so that the sun is shining brightly into the eyes of students is not conducive to learning. Desks and chairs should be positioned in the classroom to face across or away from windows. Glare can be further reduced by the use of color and placement of student desks or tables. Children should not directly face windows or other sources of illumination. Bulletin board materials need a dull, nonreflecting surface rather than a shiny or highly reflective finish. If the bulletin boards are portable, they should be placed in an area of the classroom where the glare is at a minimum.

Color is another important aspect of the classroom environment. Research has shown that different colors evoke different emotions. Often teachers can suggest a color scheme when a classroom or a building is repainted. Harsh colors such as reds or purples tend to produce anxiety, whereas softer colors, such as blues or mauves tend to exert a more calming effect. Paints should also have a nonglare finish.

Although lead has been removed as a base for paint, some paints still contain a mercury base. Whenever painting of any facility has occurred, the prudent teacher should ensure adequate ventilation of the room until the fumes dissipate and the paint is completely dry. Paint fumes can create headaches among children and staff, so prevention of inhalation of these fumes is important.

Acoustics. For the most part, the teacher will not have much control over the school's acoustics. In newer schools, however, this matter has received attention. By keeping doors and windows closed except when ventilation is needed, the teacher can begin to reduce the amount of outside noise that filters into the classroom. Also, noise control can be maintained by (1) keeping the noise in the classroom at a level not disruptive to others, (2) alerting children to remain quiet or speak softly in hallway travel during class time, (3) carefully planning the location of the school facility, (4) carefully locating areas that have a high level of noise (such as shops, playgrounds, and music rooms), and (5) using carpeting and acoustic tile in construction or remodeling.

Water supply. School authorities have a legal and moral responsibility to provide a safe and sanitary water supply for the schools. Availability of a clean and sufficient water supply is a primary consideration when selecting a site for new school construction.

The best way to ensure a safe water supply is to receive it from the local municipality, which has a civil responsibility to ensure that the water is safe for consumption. In those areas where it is not possible to connect to the municipal water supply, wells can be drilled. Wells must conform to local standards available from the various city, county, and state health departments.

In many classrooms in elementary schools there is a water source within the classroom. If the teacher notices that the water has become turbid

---

*US Department of Health and Human Services: *Preventing tobacco use among young people: a report of the Surgeon General,* Washington, DC, 1994, US Government Printing Office.

or has an odor, the condition should be reported to the school administration for follow-up.

Fountains. In most states, construction standards for schools require that drinking fountains be recessed in the wall, be located in accessible positions, and be operable by those in a wheelchair. Most schools use "arc stream" fountains, but the "bubbler" type fountain may exist in older schools. Use of arc stream fountains is preferable to using the bubbler type fountain because the arc stream is shielded and keeps the person's mouth off the outlet jet. If the individual has a gastrointestinal or respiratory disease, the likelihood of contamination is much greater with the bubbler fountain than with the arc stream fountain. It is also important that the pressure of the water emitted from the fountain be powerful enough that children will not have to put their mouths too close to the outlet jet to drink. If a teacher notes that the water pressure from fountains seems to be low, the condition should be reported to the administrator.

Teachers should educate students about safety and hygienic measures when using water fountains. Horseplay such as pushing a student's head into the fountain should not be tolerated, and students should be told that such behavior might result in dental damage.

Toilet rooms. Although teachers will not have control over the types and placement of toilet facilities in schools, they can make recommendations when problems exist. It is preferable that toilet facilities have an outside exposure to direct, natural lighting because of the effect of sunlight on some disease-causing organisms. It is important that the toilet facilities be accessible; there are supervisory reasons as well as considerations of distance from the classrooms. There should be easy access to toilets for the handicapped, which is another reason for lavatories to be located on the ground level. Both washbasins and commodes should be accessible to the handicapped. At least one commode should have a closable door for privacy for the handicapped.

Washbasins in the restrooms (or in classrooms) should be equipped with hot and cold running water. They should have liquid soap dispensers rather than solid soap. The major problem with bar soap is the possibility of it causing an accident should someone step on it, slip, and be injured.

Paper towel dispensers should be included in restrooms so that children can dry their hands. Although the teacher is not primarily responsible for the physical upkeep of the restroom facilities, he or she should be concerned that the facilities are maintained in a sanitary manner. Maintenance of a clean restroom can also form the basis for incidental health instruction, not only in the area of environmental health but also in the area of disease control. Student behavior is important for maintaining cleanliness and the handwashing supplies in restrooms. Positive peer pressure is necessary to reinforce the desired habits in unsupervised school areas such as restrooms and locker rooms.

Sanitation. Students should not be subjected to an unsanitary environment. Provisions must be made for the safe and effective removal of waste from the school. Where daily pick up of garbage is not possible, refuse should be kept in a secure place where it will not attract animals or vermin. The use of sturdy disposal cans with tight lids for sanitary storage of waste is advisable.

Playgrounds. School playground design, surfacing, and equipment selection and maintenance influences the risk of student injuries. The U.S. Consumer Product Safety Commission issues general guidelines for playground construction.

It is important that students not only have adequate space in which to play but that equipment should be appropriate for the age of the children and be safe for them to use. It is also important that the playground equipment be maintained on a regular basis. The teacher can use the playground as a learning laboratory by having the class periodically report hazardous playground equipment. If unsafe playground equipment is identified, it should be immediately reported to the proper school authorities for repair or removal. Instruction in playground safety may well carry over into the home environment.

SCHOOL FOOD SERVICES: ARE THEY ADEQUATE?

With over 24.8 million lunches and 6 million breakfasts served daily in 1993, feeding children in schools obviously has become big business. It is also big politics, and it certainly is "no small potatoes" when it comes to the nutrition and health of millions of American children.

Yet for millions of America's students the school breakfast, school lunch, or both is their only chance for a nutritious meal during the day. Repeated surveys show that many school-age children and youth, from *all* socioeconomic levels, are subsisting on diets that are nutritionally marginal if not deficient. There is a pressing need for better school lunches and expansion of the school breakfast program. In 1990, over 86,900 schools participated in one or both of these programs.

School Lunch Program

Originating in 1935 under Section 32 of Public Law 74-320 (the Agricultural Adjustment Act) under which the federal government bought farm commodities for distribution to schools as a way to absorb farm surplus and support agricultural incomes, the National School Lunch Act (PL 79-396) was authorized in 1946. The goals of the program were to (1) distribute surplus farm commodities and support farm income and (2) safeguard the health of school children. Today the goals of the school food service program are to provide nutritionally acceptable meals at a fair price and serve as a learning laboratory for health and nutrition education.*

In 1954 the Agricultural Act (PL 83-690), which encouraged fluid milk consumption along with the lunch program, was passed. Because both the National School Lunch Program and the Agricultural Act were basically temporary programs, Congress passed the Child Nutrition Act (PL 89-642) in 1966, giving both prior acts permanent au-

thorization. This act also authorized the school breakfast program. The programs are administered by the U.S. Department of Agriculture.

Participation in the National School Lunch Program has grown from 6.6 million children in 1946 to 24.8 million children in 1990. Over 94% of all schools in the United States participate in the National School Lunch Program.

The cost of school lunches is over $6.8 billion a year. Although the amounts expended in each state differ, about half of the cost is divided between federal and state governments, and the other half comes from "lunch money" from parents. Half of the federal contribution is in the form of food commodities. The federal government contributes to each school meal based on the percentage of students who get free or reduced-price meals.

The basic nutritional goal of the school lunch program is to provide approximately one third of a child's recommended dietary allowances (RDA) of protein, calcium, iron, and vitamins A and C as delineated by the National Academy of Sciences and the National Research Council. An additional goal was proposed by the U.S. Department of Agriculture in the *Dietary Guidelines for Americans:* reducing the dietary intake of sodium, fat, and sugar.

Although the school cafeteria can serve as a learning laboratory for students, only one state has mandated such action. However, 31 states have recommended that the school cafeteria be used as a learning laboratory.*

School Breakfast Program

Because of recognition of the urgent need for many elementary and secondary children to have the opportunity to eat a well-balanced breakfast, breakfast programs have been initiated with the support of the U.S. Department of Agriculture. As

---

*Frank G, Vaden A, Martin J: School health promotion: child nutrition programs, *J School Health* 57(1):451-460, 1987.

*Lovato C, Allensworth D, Chan F: *School health in America: an assessment of state policies to protect and improve the health of students,* ed 5, Kent, OH, 1989, American School Health Association, pp 36-39.

in the school lunch program, all public and non-profit private schools may participate in the breakfast program. In 1993, over 6 million children participated, with 4.6 million enrolled in free or reduced price breakfast.* The federal government paid over $594 million in cash and commodities for the school breakfast program in 1990. In addition, over $19.5 million was spent for the special milk program available in schools.†

Study and experience have shown that, as with the lunch program, when students participate in a school breakfast program, they learn better, have fewer complaints of headache and stomachache, and have fewer behavior problems. School breakfast is intended to provide one fourth of the RDA of protein, calcium, iron, and vitamins A and C.

The Problems

A number of problems have become apparent since the National School Lunch Act was passed during the Truman Administration almost 50 years ago. The program has made a substantial contribution to the health of millions of American students, but critics from the field of nutritional science and the congressional arena continue to point up these problems:

- The *quantity* of food, affected by the changing availability of farm surplus commodities, does not necessarily assure a *quality* diet for growing children and youth.
- Increasing financial burden has fallen on parents because, by implicit Congressional sanction, states can count students' lunch payments as part of the matching formula.
- Economic eligibility guidelines—who pays how much for what students—have contributed to administrative, political, social, and (for the student) psychological problems.

- U.S. Department of Agriculture regulations allow competitive foods to be sold in vending machines in school lunchrooms but not at the time of the regular lunch program. Sharp criticism has been leveled at this modification of the national school lunch program as it opens the door for students to pass up the school lunch for more appealing, but less nutritious, "junk" foods. However, an increasing number of school systems are limiting vending machine sales to milk, fruit juices, and nutritious foods.
- Food and labor costs are causing a financial crisis for schools and parents in providing nutritious school lunches and breakfasts. A U.S. Department of Agriculture study revealed that for every 1-cent increase in cost to the student, there was a 1% drop in participation in the program.

Too Much Too Soon?

Evidence indicates that high serum cholesterol levels are a major risk factor in the development of coronary heart disease and premature fatal heart attack. It has also been clearly established that this buildup of blood cholesterol accelerates during adolescence, especially among boys. We also know that poor dietary habits contribute to 5 of the 10 leading causes of death in the United States: coronary heart disease, high blood pressure, diabetes, atherosclerosis, and some cancers.

Compounding the problem of high cholesterol and coronary heart disease is the fact that obesity continues to be a serious threat to health and a high quality of life for millions of American parents and their children. Obesity and malnutrition often go hand in hand—too many calories with too few essential nutrients.

Most cases of adult obesity have their beginnings in childhood and adolescence. About 40% of obese children become obese adults; over 70% of obese teens will continue to be obese into adult years. Further, obese children may experience psychological problems associated with self-esteem.

*Children's Defense Fund: *The state of America's children yearbook 1994,* Washington, DC, 1994, The Fund.
†Program Information Department, Food and Nutrition Service: *Monthly report,* Alexandria, VA, 1990, US Department of Agriculture.

This may also exacerbate the development of chronic diseases later in life.

Healthy People 2000 goals recommend that 90% of school meals should be consistent with the Dietary Guidelines for Americans. Surveys estimate that school lunches average 38% of the calories from fat, with 15% of all calories from saturated fat.* The Year 2000 goal is no more than 30% of calories from fat and limiting saturated fat content to 10% of the total calories.

The National Heart, Lung, and Blood Institute of National Institutes for Health supported research in four separate U.S. communities to facilitate changes in elementary students' diets through both classroom nutrition education and school food services modifications to reduce fat, saturated fat, and sodium (salt) content.

Too Little Too Late

Early studies showed that many school lunches were deficient in complete proteins, iron, and vitamins A and C. Recent studies indicate that most children's daily vitamin intakes are generally within the RDA regardless of economic status or age differences. This would suggest that school food services have made improvements. However, girls ages 11 and older reported less than the RDA intake of minerals such as calcium, iron, zinc, and magnesium.†

Classroom instruction in nutrition can be effective in imparting knowledge, altering attitudes, and developing skills related to eating practices. Teachers can coordinate nutrition education with events such as National School Lunch Week (October) and School Breakfast Week (March). However, if the meals offered in the school lunch or breakfast program continue to be high in fat,

---

*Perry CL, Parcel GS, Stone E et al: The child and adolescent trial for cardiovascular health (CATCH): overview of the intervention program and evaluation methods, *Cardiovas Risk Factors Inter J* 2(1):36-44, 1992.

†Devaney B, Gordon A, Burghardt J: *The school nutrition dietary assessment study: dietary intakes of program participants and nonparticipants,* Alexandria, VA, 1993, USDA Food and Nutrition Service.

sodium, and cholesterol, students will not have the opportunity to practice concepts learned in the classroom. A goal of the healthful school environment program should be to reinforce healthful behaviors taught in the classroom, not to run contrary to these concepts.

Dispelling the Myths

Although there are still problems with the various school feeding programs, it is important to dispel some of the myths and misconceptions that surround them. Only 20% of the food used in school lunch or breakfast programs is provided by the U.S. Department of Agriculture. The remainder is purchased by local school districts from the same vendors who supply restaurants. Thus the problem of less-than-optimal nutritional value attributed to the government may well be a local problem instead. Improper preparation and storage of the food that is made available through government sources or through local vendors may be responsible for less-than-optimal nutritional value in the school feeding program.

Often teachers grumble about having to pay a higher price for their meals than the students, even though they get the same meal as the students. Federal regulations stipulate that reimbursement, or commodities for the nutrition programs in schools, exclude meals served to adults. As such, no money collected from students, commodities that are either provided or purchased, or money that is reimbursed to the school may be used in serving meals to adults. Thus schools must charge adults an amount for each meal that would pay for the foods that are included in that meal.

Research evidence demonstrates that, if children eat breakfast or lunch at school, they generally show a higher energy level and a better overall nutrient intake than they would if no school feeding program were available. When a school breakfast program exists, more children eat breakfast than would have eaten breakfast if that program did not exist, and students were expected to eat breakfast at home before school.

Streamlining School Food Services

Perhaps like America's railroad dining car—a nostalgic financial failure—our school lunchrooms need to move into the jet age of airline-type central food service. The day of the haphazardly run kitchen must now give way to a more businesslike organization.

Planning and operation of school food services is best done by organizations experienced in large-scale meal delivery systems. Studies show that for the same worker cost, centrally located kitchens can provide three times the number of meals that can be served under the existing unit kitchen system where meals are prepared in each individual school. However, plate wastage (food served but not eaten) may offset any of the advantages that might be attained. Thus careful planning is critical.

The chief drawback to a central kitchen system is the high initial cost. Although such systems usually become economically stable in 1 or 2 years, many school districts cannot afford the initial financial outlay.

Improving School Food Services

Regardless of the merits or limitations of new school food program legislation, teachers, school board members, administrators, and others concerned with student health can get information and assistance from the Child Nutrition Division of the U.S. Department of Agriculture (Washington, D.C. 20250), Advocates for Better Children's Diets coalition members, and the American School Food Service Association (American School Food Service, 1600 Duke Street, 7th Floor, Alexandria, VA 22314). Several available school food nutrition guidelines incorporate the Dietary Guidelines: they include Healthy EDGE (American School Food Service Association), Changing the Course (American Cancer Society), and Health Star: Guidelines for Healthy School Meal Planning (American Heart Association).

At local and state levels there is continuing need to determine the most efficient methods—lowest cost and highest nutrient meals—for sus-

taining the important contribution of the school feeding program to the health of elementary and secondary school children and youth.

At the federal level, the 1994 reauthorization of the Commodity Distribution Program would require improved nutritional quality of the commodities available to schools and better labelling so that food workers can have sufficient information with which to plan balanced meals. Schools would also be able to use 10% of their commodity allocation for fresh vegetables and fruits.*

School Feeding and Nutrition Education

Certainly one of the chief advantages of the school lunch or breakfast program is the opportunity it provides for relating classroom information on healthful diets to school feeding programs. Teachers can have students keep daily records of what they eat, including school meals, and discussions can be a significant part of a unit on nutrition. Of course, any diary records from students must be anonymous if reliable responses are to be obtained.

A news story told about an elementary school principal who was distressed at the food wastage in the lunchroom and had pupils take inventory of what had been thrown in trash cans in 1 day. A pupil-prepared report disclosed that students had discarded sandwiches, milk, bags of potato chips, apples, oranges, and cookies! Obviously, simply offering food to children does not ensure that they will eat it.

Without sound nutrition education, students may discard nutritious foods from the school lunch or breakfast, buy calorie-rich nutritionally poor foods from vending machines, or patronize quick-food commercial establishments in the neighborhood. Again, health education appears as the crucial influence in choices and decisions of students regardless of the environmental situation.

The importance of nutrition education in terms of weight management is exemplified through two

---

*Ford A: Correspondence, June 1, 1994.

of the health goals for the nation for the year 2000. The first of these goals is specifically targeted at obese children age 12 and over; the second is to ensure that nutrition education becomes a part of quality school health education (see the box).

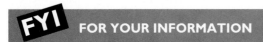

Nutrition-Related Goals for the Year 2000

Increase to at least 50% the proportion of overweight people aged 12 and older who have adopted sound dietary practices combined with regular physical activity to attain an appropriate body weight.

Increase to at least 75% the proportion of the nation's schools that provide nutrition education from preschool through twelfth grade, preferably as a part of quality school health education.

WHAT ABOUT SCHOOL BUS SAFETY?

School buses are part of the school environment because once the child steps aboard the bus he or she is under the jurisdiction and responsibility of the schools. The child's safety on the bus is just as important as when that child is in any other school facility or activity (Fig. 3-2).

Since 1983, an average of 11 school-age passengers have died in school bus-related crashes each year. Another 30 school-age pedestrians were killed in school bus-related crashes yearly; of these, half were between the ages of 5 and 7. Two thirds of these fatalities occurred in or by the school bus, and one third were due to another vehicle.* This is impressively low given that everyday, more than 380,000 school buses carry over 22 million boys and girls to and from school.†

---

*National Center for Statistics and Analysis: *Traffic safety facts 1993: school buses,* Washington, DC, 1994, US Government Printing Office.
†National Safety Council: *Accident facts,* Chicago, 1990, The Council, p 70.

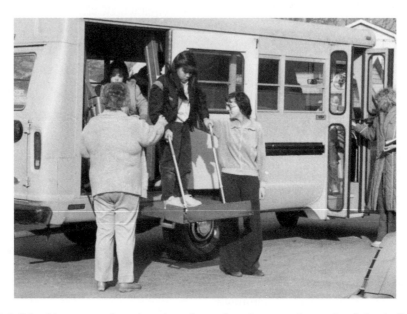

FIG. 3-2 School buses must be safe and can be equipped to meet the needs of physically challenged individuals. (Courtesy Witchita Public Schools, Witchita, Kansas.)

School buses are the safest vehicles on the road and they are 37 times safer than an automobile.* Even so, there is room for improvement. At present, there is continuing effort across the nation to improve the safety of school buses, including the installation of seat belts. Almost all states require children under 5 years to be placed in some sort of car seat or restraint system when they ride in an automobile. However most school buses are not equipped with seat belts. Further, even if seat belts were available, there is no mandate that they must be used.

More school districts are purchasing buses with seat belts factory installed. The estimated cost of these safety devices runs $1,200 to $3,000 for each bus. Only a few states (e.g., New York), however, require seat belts for new school buses. The National Research Council recommended raising the minimum height of school bus seat backs from 20 inches to 24 inches rather than equip the buses with seat belts.† Their rationale was that higher seat backs compartmentalize passengers (i.e., prevent persons from being thrown over another seat) in event of a crash. Only three states have required safety restraints in school buses.‡

The National Highway Traffic Safety Administration proposed tougher requirements for all public transport buses, including school buses. Chief among these is the provision for padded, high-backed seats. The National Standards Conference on School Transportation has developed minimum standards for school buses. This code is available from the National Safety Council in Chicago.

Even when no federal legislation is pending, the National Standards Conference on School Transportation promotes improved safety features. Conference delegates review crash incidents and identify controllable problems. In 1995, the conference will consider upgrading standards for reflectors and stop arms, emergency exits, and the heights of bus bumpers and side skirts. For example, lowering bumper height would prevent an automobile from going under the school bus in a rear-end collision.

Safety experts also recognize the human element in bus safety. Drivers are required to submit to background checks and drug testing. The Omnibus Bill of 1989 requires that, effective January 1995, all public transportation drivers, including school bus drivers, submit to drug testing before employment, after any accident, on a random basis, and for reasonable cause. While every state must have a training course for bus driver certification, the duration varies widely across states (i.e., from 6 hours to 3 weeks). On average, a driver may get 3 to 4 hours first aid training within a 20-hour course. There is no requirement to maintain first aid skills; a local district would do well to update training every 1 to 3 years through a school nurse or the local Red Cross.

Other important factors in bus safety include skilled mechanics who maintain the buses, sufficient bus capacity to prevent passengers from standing, and well-behaved students. The National Highway Traffic Safety Administration promotes bus safety education for students (e.g., School Bus Safety Week [October]).

ARE SCHOOLS FIRETRAPS?

Not too many years ago some fire safety experts stated that many schools in America could be classified as firetraps. Education by the National Safety Council and local and national fire officials have tended to increase public concern for fire prevention and protection. Schools are expected to conform to state and local fire codes. Most school fires are not due to faulty buildings but are caused by behavior such as careless handling of hot materials, pranks by unsupervised students, or deliberate arson—usually when schools are not in session.

---

*Schwartz LG, Klenetsky F: Seat belts in school buses, *J School Health* 55(3):119, 1985.

†Condo, A: Panel recommends against law on school bus seat belts, *Houston Chronicle*, May 9, 1989, p 4A.

‡Lovato C, Allensworth D, Chan F: *School health in America: an assessment of state policies to protect and improve the health of students*, ed 5, Kent, OH, 1989, American School Health Association, p 28.

Still, many schools lack automatic fire alarm systems, and few have automatic sprinkler systems. Such systems should, at least, be installed in shops, chemistry laboratories, boiler rooms, supply rooms, kitchens, and other fire-hazard areas. Local fire inspectors should be consulted by school administrators on regular inspections, and recommendations for eliminating any existing dangerous conditions should be made. The cost of alarm and sprinkler systems is a small price to pay for protecting the lives of children and youth in our schools.

When the American School Health Association conducted its national survey of state policies related to schools, only 43 states required annual school facility fire inspections; of the 43 only 7 required more than one inspection per year. Teachers should be aware of the problems associated with fires and include instruction in fire safety* as a part of the health education program in the school (see the box on p. 65).

The American Insurance Association recommends that the following school fire-hazard conditions be checked and, when necessary, immediately corrected:

- Buildings where the walls or ceilings of exit corridors are surfaced with highly combustible finishes
- Buildings with wood floors and masonry walls, especially if the pupils in the upper floors have no means of exit other than through stairs open to lower stories
- Buildings of wood construction with pupils housed above the second story
- Buildings with unventilated space below them where gas may collect and explode
- Buildings with exit doors to the outside that cannot be readily opened from the inside
- Buildings in which pupils on upper floors have no means of exit except down stairs that are open to lower stories having combustible walls and finishes or contents in storage that are combustible

---

*See the fire safety unit in Appendix B for use in educational programs.

With the increasing use of computers, audiovisual, and other equipment in schools, teachers should ask for new outlets rather than overload outlets.

Monthly fire and disaster drills should be held for students and school personnel, and evacuation plans should be posted in every room. The local fire department can instruct students on crawling to safety when smoke is present. Fire extinguishers should be approved by local fire officials, inspected regularly, and their location and operation understood by teachers and other school personnel. All school personnel and students should be aware of the location of fire extinguishers and manually operated fire alarms in the school and of regular fire alarm boxes near the school.

As with other aspects of a safe and healthful school environment, instruction is essential for optimal fire prevention and protection.

RESPONSIBILITIES FOR HEALTHFUL SCHOOL LIVING

Healthful school living requires shared responsibility among all persons who come into contact with the school. This would extend to those responsible for developing the physical plant (the board of education and the architect), school administrators, students, parents, custodians, and all ancillary staff.

Board of Education

Probably the most critical role in healthful school living falls on the board of education. This group decides if, when, and where a school will be built or if existing facilities will be renovated to meet new standards. The group's authority for these decisions is derived from the voters of the community as their elected representatives. These same voters must ultimately provide the operating or bond funds for any building or renovation programs.

A responsible board will consider carefully any recommendations for the construction of new or the renovation of existing facilities. It will hold meetings with school administrators, teachers, nurses, architects, and community representatives before it makes its decision. The decision to construct a new school is a project of the community. The community will benefit from a well-planned and well-constructed school building that contributes positively to the students who attend the facility or will suffer as the result of a facility that does not meet the needs of the students and the community.

It is the responsibility of the board to retain an architect who is reputable and has experience in school design. Before accepting a school design, the board should implement a process whereby school staff and parents are involved in the overall design and specific features. Support services staff such as the school nurse and counselors need input on floor plans to ensure privacy for their work and to coordinate special programs such as case conferences and school-based health care services. Students may be involved in a survey that explores suggestions for ways to provide a health-promoting environment. All plans must provide accessibility in accord with the Americans with Disabilities Act (1990). By consulting others, the board develops within those individuals a sense of dedication and appreciation of the role they play in maintaining a healthful school environment.

Administrators

School administrators have the major responsibility for keeping the board of education informed of needed changes. They direct and control the daily operation of the school and must be informed of the needed changes in the physical plant that affect safety or the overall quality of education. School population increases or decreases, deterioration of facilities, and other changes must be reported by school personnel to the superintendent, who must then relay this information with proposals for action to the board of education.

Teachers

The teachers are "on the firing line." Although teachers must work with the school facilities pro-

vided, they should maximize the potential for healthful school living and make the school a pleasant place for learning. They must make administrators aware of any special needs they may have. This surpasses the mere physical component of the classroom and extends into all facets of school operation.

New teachers should be oriented to the entire campus to be aware of safety risks and resources in the event of a physical crisis. Teachers should provide a campus or building map with pertinent exits marked for any substitutes or volunteers.

It is important that teachers understand the unique features of a particular building so that those features can be incorporated into Health Education. Teachers can develop a checklist or map for students' use as they investigate the school to identify health and safety features and hazards. By keeping the custodial staff informed of needed repairs and the administrators aware of any special needs, teachers can contribute positively to the overall environment of the school.

Students

The students stand to benefit most from having a healthful school environment. Teachers must help them learn how to assume responsibility for keeping the school safe, sanitary, and clean. Students will greatly assist in keeping a healthful school environment by, among other things, using trash cans rather than throwing paper on the ground or floor, refraining from writing graffiti on the walls, not defacing furniture or equipment, keeping their feet off the walls, using restroom soap and towels responsibly, and wiping their shoes on doormats before entering the building.

Students should take pride in their school surroundings. In the same manner as pride is taken in athletic teams, bands, choirs, and theatrical or forensic groups, pride should be taken in the appearance of the school facilities. Students should learn that the school is their "home away from home" and that each person should assume responsibility for keeping that environment clean, safe, and wholesome.

Custodians

In today's school facility, the custodian must possess a broad range of mechanical and carpentry skills, safety and sanitation habits, and knowledge of disease control. The custodian must also possess the ability to work with both students and staff. The custodian becomes a role model to students and a colleague to teachers. By informing the custodian of problems associated with the school environment, the entire school population serves as a family to protect, promote, and improve the school environment for everyone. In turn, the staff must support the custodian by stressing students' responsibilities to prevent vandalism.

The custodian must constantly be aware of the advantages and hazards of the wide range of cleaning and painting products on today's market and the new equipment available for use in the schools. In many cases the custodian will repair equipment. This person should periodically attend training workshops designed to update custodial knowledge and skills.

The nature of custodians' work puts them at greater risk for cuts and exposure to bodily fluids and bloodborne pathogens. Each school should have a plan to annually review Universal Precautions and ensure that staff have access to latex or vinyl gloves when handling blood or body wastes, disinfectants, and waste disposal materials. All schools need a plan to evaluate staff who have been exposed to blood for hepatitis B and to provide vaccination if indicated. Many, but not all, schools must abide by the federal OSHA (Occupational Safety and Health Administration) regulations.

Secretaries and Clerks

The school secretary is generally an excellent source of information relative to the basic operation of the school. When students, faculty, parents, or other individuals have complaints, it is generally the secretary who first learns of the complaint. The secretarial staff has a responsibility to inform appropriate school personnel about the problem so that preventive or remedial action can take place. Teachers and students should remember that the school secretarial staff are also affected by the school environment. The secretary can enhance the overall school environment, but everyone should remember that secretaries are not personal valets or servants and should be treated with respect and dignity.

Lunchroom Personnel

General sanitation as well as the serving of nutritious, low-fat, and attractive food should be of primary concern to lunchroom personnel. By being aware of and practicing good sanitation and food handling techniques, the lunchroom staff can help control food-borne disease outbreaks.

Most states require all persons who deal with feeding the public to undergo a food handler's sanitation course and a medical examination to show that they are free of any type of communicable disease. The food handler's course generally consists of learning about the need for refrigeration and heating, storage of foods, dishwashing, simple equipment maintenance, and various sanitation standards. Personal health habits and their potential for disease spread are also included.

It is important for teachers to keep the lunchroom personnel informed of nutrition-related projects being conducted in the classroom; thus the lunchroom can become an extension of the classroom. In addition, lunchroom personnel can act in an advisory capacity for the teachers or can assist in the various classroom projects. It is also important for parents to keep school officials informed of special nutrition needs (e.g., diabetes, or diagnosed food allergies of their children). This information must be passed on to teachers, school nurses, and the lunchroom staff so that they can prevent food-related problems. Staff members who monitor students during meals need annual training in choking rescue.

SUMMARY

In general, teachers have no choice in school site selection or construction unless they have the opportunity to serve on a planning committee for renovation or new construction bonds. Hence, they must make the very best of what they inherit. Whatever the age or other problems of the school site, buildings, and facilities, improvements can be affected by concerned administrators, teachers, school nurses, and others involved with the health and safety of students. School and community health councils are especially effective as instruments in bringing about favorable change.

Every school building in America should be maintained in accordance with state and local standards of safety, sanitation, and educational utility. Regular inspections of school buildings and facilities should be made by school administrators, local building inspectors, fire inspectors, health department sanitarians and safety experts, and other qualified personnel. Principals, teachers, students, custodial staff, food service personnel, school nurses, and others in the school should be alert each day for unhealthful or dangerous conditions in the building and on the school grounds.

School boards should assume the responsibility for requiring a nutritious school breakfast and lunch program. Teachers should be aware of the school feeding program and take advantage of the program as a teaching opportunity in cooperation with food service personnel.

School buses should be inspected on a regular basis to ensure that all safety standards are met and that the buses are in perfect mechanical order. Seat belts should be installed, and policies should be developed requiring students who ride the school buses to use seat belts.

School bus drivers should be specifically trained to deal with large numbers of students. They should be particularly safety conscious because the safety of students in their bus is their responsibility. The bus drivers should also be trained in basic first aid and emergency care.

Preventable fire hazards should never be allowed to exist in the school environment. All fire safety equipment such as alarms, fire extinguishers, hoses, and sprinkler systems should be tested regularly and maintained in good working condi-

tion. Regular fire drills should be conducted so that all students and school personnel know how to evacuate the school in a safe and orderly fashion. Finally, all school personnel should know how to use the fire-fighting equipment that is available in the schools.

A healthful school environment contributes to overall student learning and is the responsibility of all persons (who have reason to be) associated with the school. By working together, the health and safety of students and school personnel alike are enhanced.

QUESTIONS FOR DISCUSSION

1. What are the aims of a healthful school environment?
2. What should be included in a good program for healthful school living?
3. How can teachers and other school personnel help make improvements in old school buildings and poor school sites?
4. What can the teacher do to ensure a safe and wholesome internal environment that enhances the learning of students?
5. What responsibility does the teacher have in ensuring that playgrounds are safe? What might be done to minimize the possibility of playground accidents?
6. Why are school food service programs important to student health?
7. What are some of the major problems in developing nutritious school lunch and breakfast meals that students will eat.
8. What are the advantages and disadvantages of centralized food preparation? Campus-site preparation?
9. What organizations can help improve school food and nutrition programs?
10. How can the teacher use the school cafeteria as a "learning laboratory"? What is the role of food service personnel in making this concept become a reality?
11. What changes need to be made in the operation of school buses to make student transportation safer?

12. Do you think seat belts should be made mandatory for all school buses? Why or why not?

13. Should use of seat belts be made mandatory for both students and adults who ride school buses? Justify your response and include how you would suggest implementing any programs to accomplish your ideas.

14. How can school administrators and teachers improve programs for fire prevention and protection?

15. What are Universal Precautions and why are they necessary?

16. Why should the school be obligated to provide a healthful environment for students?

17. What factors have contributed to the school lunch program becoming a national controversy?

18. Discuss how the school physical environment might enhance or detract from the health services program and the health instruction program.

SELECTED REFERENCES

American Academy of Pediatrics: *School health: policy and practice*, ed 5, Elk Grove Village, IL, 1993.

American Cancer Society: *Changing the course: a manual for school food service providers*, 1990, The Society.

American School Food Services Association: Healthy EDGE, *School Food Service J Suppl*, March, 1991.

Behrman RE, editor: *The future of children*, vol 4, no 3, Los Angeles, 1994, Center for the Future of Children.

Children's Defense Fund: *The state of America's children yearbook 1994*, Washington, DC, 1994, The Fund.

Condo A: Panel recommends against law on school bus seat belts, *Houston Chronicle*, May 9, 1989, p 4A.

Devaney B, Gordon A, Burghardt J: *The school nutrition dietary assessment study: dietary intakes of program participants and nonparticipants*, 1993, USDA Food and Nutrition Service.

Dolphin N: Epidemiology on the elementary school playground, *J School Health* 56(3):111-112, 1986.

Ellison R, Capper A, Goldberg R, Witschi J, Stare F: The environmental component: changing school food service to promote cardiovascular health, *Health Ed Quart* 16(2):285-297, 1989.

Environmental Protection Agency: Asbestos containing materials in schools, 40 CFE Part 763, *Fed Register* 52(83):15820-15874, 1987.

Fire Analysis, Division of the National Fire Protection Association: *US school fire trends and patterns*, annual, Quincy, MA, The Association.

Frank GC, Vaden A, Martin J: School health promotion: child nutrition programs, *J School Health* 57(1):451-460, 1987.

Glanz K, Damberg CL: Meeting our nation's health objectives in nutrition, *J Nutrition Ed* 19(5):211-219, 1987.

Hay GH, Harper TB III, Courson FH: Preparing school personnel to assist students with life-threatening food allergies, *J School Health* 64(3):119-121, 1994.

Kansas Department of Transportation: *School bus loading and unloading survey*, Topeka, KA, 1990, The Department.

Kerr D: School bus safety: focus on the danger zone, *J School Health* 57(6):237-239, 1987.

Kolbe L, Green L: Appropriate functions of health education in schools: improving health and cognitive performance. In Krasneor N, Arasten J, Cataldo M, editors: *Child cognitive behavior: a behavioral pediatrics perspective*, New York, 1986, John Wiley.

Lovato C, Allensworth D, Chan F: *School health in America: an assessment of state policies to protect and improve the health of students*, ed 5, Kent, OH, 1989, American School Health Association.

Means R: *Historical perspectives on school health*, Thorofare, NJ, 1975, Charles B. Slack.

National Center for Statistics and Analysis: *Traffic safety facts 1993: school buses*, Washington, DC, 1994, US Government Printing Office.

National Safety Council: *Accident facts*, Chicago, 1990, The Council.

Office of Radiation Programs: *Radon measurement in schools*, EPA 402-R-93-014, Washington, DC, 1993, US Environmental Protection Agency.

Office of Toxic Substances, EPA: *Evaluation of the asbestos-in-schools identification and notification rules*, EPA 560/5-84-005, Washington, DC, 1984, US Environmental Protection Agency.

Olds RS: Promoting child health in a smoke-free school: suggestions for school health personnel, *J School Health* 58(7):269-272, 1988.

Parcel G, Simonds-Morton B, O'Hara N, Baranowski T, Kolbe L, Bee D: School promotion of healthful diet and exercise behavior: an integration of organizational change in social learning theory interventions, *J School Health* 57(4):150-156, 1987.

Perry CL, Parcel GS, Stone E et al: The child and adolescent trial for cardiovascular health (CATCH): overview of the intervention program and evaluation methods, *Cardiovas Risk Factors Inter J* 2(1):36-44, 1992.

Program Information Department: Food and Nutrition Service: *Monthly report,* Alexandria, VA, 1990, US Department of Agriculture.

Riggs S, Woodman K: It's back to basics for school foodservice: refining menus, renovating kitchens, *Restaurants Institutions* 95(2):148-157, 1985.

Roberts SW: Food first, educating our children, *Health Ed* 18(1):17, 1987.

Schwartz LG, Klenetsky F: Seatbelts in school buses, *J School Health* 55(3):119, 1985.

Snyder P, Story M, Trenkner LL: Reducing fat and sodium in school lunch programs: the *LUNCH POWER!* Intervention Study, *J Am Dietetic Assoc* 92:1087-1091, 1992.

Spital M, Spital A, Spital R: The compelling case for seat belts on school buses, *Pediatrics* 78(5):928-932, 1986.

US Consumer Product Safety Commission: *Handbook for public playground safety,* Washington, DC, 1991, US Government Printing Office.

US Department of Health and Human Services; Public Health Service: *Healthy people 2000: national health promotion and disease prevention objectives,* Washington, DC, 1990, US Government Printing Office.

US Department of Health and Human Services: *Preventing tobacco use among young people: a report of the Surgeon General,* Washington, DC, 1994, US Government Printing Office.

US Environmental Protection Agency: *Radon: a physician's guide to radon,* Washington, DC, 1993, The Agency.

World Health Organization: *Education for health: a manual on health education in primary health care,* Chapter 5, Geneva, 1988, The Organization.

4

Emotional Climate and the Teacher

KEY CONCEPT

A positive emotional climate in the classroom depends on adequate provision for the physical and psychological needs of children.

Some teachers are great. . . . They put bandages on my hurts—on my heart, on my mind, on my spirit. Those teachers cared about me, and let me know it. They gave me wings.

THOUGHTS FROM A DROP-OUT*

For every dream, for every aspiration a student holds, there's a teacher who helped turn those ideals into realities.†

PROBLEM TO SOLVE

As a teacher, how will you ensure provision of a classroom atmosphere conducive to the optimal physical, mental, and social development of your students?

---

*McLeod A: *Growing up in America: a background to contemporary drug abuse,* Rockville, MD, 1973, National Institute of Mental Health.
†IBM (in *Educational Leadership,* November, 1990).

WHEN John Locke used the phrase, "mens sana in corpore sano"—a sound mind in a sound body—he expressed the interrelationships between physical and mental health. He envisioned mental health as a condition of the whole personality, not as an entity separate from physical health. He stressed the importance of the total health of children. Current concepts of health also include social and spiritual aspects introduced in Chapter 1.

The mental phase of health today has never had greater meaning. The tremendous anxieties, pressures, and concerns in the world have their effect on children and youth. Young people living in poverty and among bias and prejudice are especially subjected to extensive biological, psychological, sociological, and economic stress. The cultural, ethnic, racial, and economic inequalities; the tensions over world peace; the dichotomy of moral and social values; the stress on materialism; the need for good grades; the conformities to outmoded and antiquated practices and traditions in schools; and the inadequacies of educational opportunities create a social climate conducive to mental illness. The Carnegie Council on Adolescent Development* estimates that about 7 million of the 28 million girls and boys ages 10 to 17 in the United States may be extremely vulnerable to the negative consequences of multiple high-risk behaviors and that another 7 million may be at moderate risk. This means that about one quarter of the nation's 28 million children ages 10 to 17 are in serious jeopardy.

It is imperative that schools recognize these high-risk behaviors and the conditions that promote the behaviors, and that teachers become aware of their roles in the promotion and maintenance of good mental health (see Appendix J).

Teachers can influence students in a positive fashion by creating a classroom atmosphere wherein students can and do achieve, and feel that they have the respect of all individuals in the classroom. The atmosphere should be one of acceptance, appreciation, and sharing. As students recognize their own needs and inherent values and learn skills to interact effectively with other students and adults, they also help shape a positive learning climate.

In Chapter 3 the physical components of the environment as they relate to healthful school living received consideration. However, healthful school living includes the sum of the internal as well as external factors that act on the individual. Therefore the emotional climate in the school is a critical component affecting the mental health of both students and teachers. The *emotional climate* may be defined as a setting that gives consideration to students—their feelings, their beliefs, their physiological and psychological needs—as well as subject matter. It is a setting that treats pupils with kindness and humaneness. The following poem illustrates its meaning:

If a child lives with criticism, he learns to condemn.
If a child lives with hostility, he learns to fight.
If a child lives with fear, he learns to be apprehensive.
If a child lives with pity, he learns to feel sorry for himself.
If a child lives with jealousy, he learns to feel guilty.
If a child lives with encouragement, he learns to be confident.
If a child lives with tolerance, he learns to be patient.
If a child lives with praise, he learns to be appreciative.
If a child lives with acceptance, he learns to love.
If a child lives with approval, he learns to like himself.
If a child lives with recognition, he learns to have a goal.
If a child lives with fairness, he learns what justice is.
If a child lives with honesty, he learns what truth is.
If a child lives with security, he learns to have faith in himself and those about him.
If a child lives with friendliness, he learns the world is a nice place in which to live.

DOROTHY LAW NOLTE

Observations of pupil behaviors may indicate mental health difficulties that may be the result of a poor school atmosphere. They may cause teachers to ask:

"Why is Ann always starting fights?"
"Why does Bill cry easily?"
"Why is Randy so nervous?"

---

*Carnegie Council on Adolescent Development: *Turning points: preparing American youth for the 21st century,* New York, 1989, Carnegie Corporation of New York.

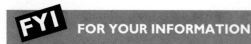

Costs of Preventable Problems

SCHOOL DROPOUT

- Each year's class of dropouts will, over their life-time, cost the nation about $260 billion in lost earnings and foregone taxes.
- In a lifetime, a male high school dropout will earn $260,000 less than a high school graduate, and contribute $78,000 less in taxes. A female who does not finish high school will earn $200,000 less, and contribute $60,000 less in taxes.
- Unemployment rates for high school dropouts are more than twice those of high school graduates. Between 1973 and 1986, young people who did not finish high school suffered a 42% drop in annual earnings in constant 1986 dollars.
- Each added year of secondary education reduces the probability of public welfare dependency in adulthood by 35%.

TEENAGE PREGNANCY

- The United States spent more than $19 billion in 1987 in payments for income maintenance, health care, and nutrition to support families begun by teenagers.
- Babies born to teen mothers are at heightened risk of low birthweight. Initial hospital care for low-birthweight infants averages $20,000. Total lifetime medical costs for low-birthweight infants averages $400,000.
- Of teens who give birth, 46% will go on welfare within 4 years; of unmarried teens who give birth, 73% will be on welfare within 4 years.

ALCOHOL AND DRUG ABUSE

- Alcohol and drug abuse in the United States cost more than $136 billion in 1980 in reduced productivity, treatment, crime, and related costs.

From Carnegie Council on Adolescent Development: *Turning points: preparing American youth for the 21st century,* New York, 1989, Carnegie Corporation of New York.

"Why does Sam use drugs?"

"What can I do to help Laura whose parents are alcoholics?"

"Why is Nancy frequently absent?"

"Why is Robert always so quiet and withdrawn?"

"Why does Michael become frightened so easily?"

"Why is Jane always sullen and unhappy?"

"Why is Marion talking about gangs so much?"

"How can I help and what should I do to best understand children with behavior problems?"

Architects, builders, and school administrators to a large extent control the physical aspects of the school, whereas teachers exert tremendous influence over the emotional climate in the classroom and in the school. The classroom is the teacher's domain. The classroom atmosphere contributes significantly to student learning. The perceptions pupils have of their physical surroundings, their teachers, and their peers all have an impact on learning.

This chapter is designed to provide (1) understanding about mental/emotional health, (2) information about some of the factors that affect mental/emotional health of children, (3) the reasons schools need to be concerned, and (4) ways schools and teachers can improve the emotional atmosphere so children will make worthwhile contributions to the society in which they live by growing into happy, responsible, and productive individuals.

WHAT IS MENTAL/EMOTIONAL HEALTH?

Teachers need to understand the nature of mental/emotional health to be able to have a constructive effect on emotional atmosphere in schools. Although it is difficult to define mental health to the satisfaction of everyone, for the purpose of this chapter it refers to the ability of individuals to make adjustments to self and societal problems in order to face the realities of one's environment with satisfaction, cheerfulness, success, and acceptable behavior.

Mentally healthy persons are able to control their emotions and adequately choose wise responses to environmental problems; they have developed self-esteem, insight, and self-acceptance. The observable features of this adjustment may be identified in what is called *personality* or the *individual's personality*—the sum of the traits and characteristics that make each person unique. Just as children have numerous combinations of traits and characteristics, many types and varieties of personalities exist.

Mental health is affected by the environment in which a person lives and by that person's experiences (Fig. 4-1). It is an outgrowth of one's total life. Teachers and schools can contribute to the mental health of pupils by helping with the satisfactory fulfillment of their physiological and psychological or emotional needs. The physiological needs include food, air, water, warmth, rest and sleep, clothing, and freedom from disease and other health hazards. Psychological or emotional needs include the following:

- Affection—love
- Security—to belong, to have roots, to have protection

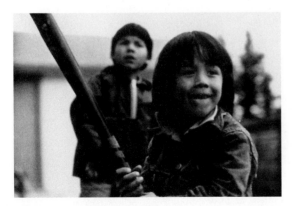

FIG. 4-1 Fun activities contribute to positive mental health. (Courtesy Health & Welfare, Canada.)

- Acceptance as an individual—free of prejudice or bias, respect for the individual differences
- Achievement—success experiences, recognition
- Independence—create and develop things, be on one's own, do things under one's own guidance and direction
- Authority—guidance and direction by adults
- Self-respect—courteous, fair, and just treatment, equating with self-efficacy and self-esteem

Mentally healthy individuals exhibit these characteristics:

- Pursue reasonable goals using their talents and abilities
- Have a sense of self-respect, self-reliance, and achievement; feel worthwhile; have a high level of self-esteem
- Know they are liked, loved, and wanted
- Have a sense of security and are reasonably at peace with themselves and their environment; enjoy life
- Can think and act rationally and realistically when seeking solutions to problems; are able to withstand frustration and anxiety, to persevere despite difficulty, and to ask for help from others without loss of self-esteem
- Can distinguish between feelings and facts
- Can maintain integrity in work and play; exhibit confidence and orderliness
- Have the ability to adapt to change and cope with stressors
- Are able to work in groups; are interested in others
- Respect the rights of others
- Face the realities of life and are able to accept responsibilities; are self-disciplined

The mentally healthy individual has a positive self-concept (Fig. 4-2) and a realistic view of the culture in which that person lives. The individual can accept his or her physical size, looks, talents, and intellectual capacities. The individual gets along with others, obeys fair rules, expresses feelings openly, and behaves in ways that enhance his or her self-esteem and the respect he or she receives from others.

Mental health is usually considered a positive aspect of health. There are varying degrees of positive mental health just as there are varying degrees and kinds of mental illness. Often these variations are difficult to define or identify.

When basic physical and emotional needs are not met or are threatened, a variety of dysfunctional behaviors may result*:

- Overtimidity—withdrawing, crying easily
- Overaggressiveness—bullying, quarreling,
- Excessive daydreaming—persistent inattentiveness
- Excessive showing off or physical risk-taking/"daredevil"

*Modified from Cornacchia H, Smith D, Bentel D: *Drugs in the classroom: a conceptual model for school programs,* ed 2, St Louis, 1978, Mosby–Year Book.

- Poor sportsmanship
- Habit disorders—tics, nail-biting, hair pulling
- Frequent "accidents" or near-accidents
- Abnormal sexual behavior
- Failure to advance in school at rate commensurate with ability
- Disruptive behaviors—nonexperimental/ongoing defiance, temper tantrums, aggression
- Affective (feeling) disorders—depression
- Gradual deterioration or marked drop in educational achievement
- Lack of interest or motivation for previously enjoyed activities
- Constantly seeking attention or popularity
- Anxiety expressions—school phobia (often occurring with depression)
- Conduct disorders—includes multiple types of antisocial behaviors lasting more than 6 months

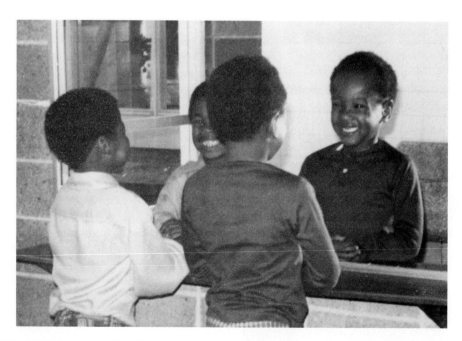

FIG. 4-2 Self-concept identification. (Courtesy Betty Jane Mobley, Tacoma Public Schools, Tacoma, Washington.)

- Soiling or wetting underwear during school day (after toilet trained and if medical conditions have been excluded)*

Depression is of special concern as it is one of the most common mental health disorders of children and interferes with normal psychosocial development. Studies indicate that 3% to 5% of children ages 8 to 12 and attending regular education classes show significant depression. Family history and life experiences are two key factors. Children who are continually exposed to conflict or violence, direct abuse, family disruptions or dysfunction, or homelessness are at considerable risk.

ENVIRONMENTAL IMPACTS ON MENTAL HEALTH

Teachers and students affect and are affected by the overall environment of the school. Thus the emotional climate of the school is a reflection of the various attitudes and behaviors students and staff bring to the school. Teachers and administrators have an ethical responsibility to provide a positive atmosphere for the most effective learning. School personnel should be alert for signs of the deterioration of the school's emotional atmosphere.

The focus of this section is on child abuse, student use of alcohol and other drugs, children of di-

---

*Behrman RE, editor: *Nelson textbook of pediatrics*, ed 14, Philadelphia, 1992, WB Saunders.

vorced or separated parents, and latchkey children. However, many other factors including nutrition, loss of home or loved ones, fear and uncertainty, peer pressure, family standards, and support efforts have an impact on the mental health of students.

Child Abuse

The Child Abuse Prevention, Adoption, and Family Services Act of 1988 defined child abuse and neglect as physical or mental injury, sexual abuse or exploitation, negligent treatment, or maltreatment of a child by a person who is responsible for the child's welfare, under circumstances that indicate that the child's health or welfare is harmed or threatened. Other forms of abuse would include verbal abuse, general neglect, emotional neglect, abandonment, and failure to thrive because of inadequate supervision.*

---

*Lovato C, Allensworth D, Chan F: *School health in America: an assessment of state policies to protect and improve the health of students*, ed 5, Kent, OH, 1989, American School Health Association.

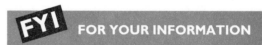
FOR YOUR INFORMATION

Violent and Abusive Behavior–Related Goals for the Year 2000

Increase the number of states to 30 in which at least 50% of children identified as abused or neglected receive physical and mental evaluation with appropriate follow-up as a means to break the intergenerational cycle of abuse.

Reduce by 20% the incidence of physical fighting among adolescents aged 14 to 17.

Increase to at least 50% the proportion of elementary and secondary schools that teach nonviolent conflict resolution skills, preferably as part of quality school health education.

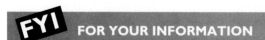
FOR YOUR INFORMATION

Mental Health–Related Goals for the Year 2000

Reduce to less than 10% the prevalence of mental disorders among children and adolescents. (Baseline: estimate 12% in 1989)

A conservative estimate is that over 2.7 million children a year are reported abused or neglected, resulting in the deaths of as many as 1500 children.* In the United States about 43% of substantiated maltreatment is due to neglect, 24% involves physical abuse, and 19% is the result of sexual abuse.† The teacher is in a good position to observe deviations in normal childhood behavior that may be an indication of abuse or neglect (see the box on p. 89). What is generally termed *child abuse* may be physical or sexual in nature, whereas neglect often assumes a more complex nature.

Physical abuse. Physical abuse of the child is often disguised as discipline or punishment of the child. The teacher needs to realize, however, that the distinction between discipline and abuse can be difficult to make. Economic stress and substance abuse are major contributors to overall occurrences of child abuse. The parent or caretaker is usually lonely, unhappy, and angry at a time of family crisis (e.g., loss of job or home, marital strife, birth of another child, or physical exhaustion). The US Department of Health and Human Services has defined physical abuse as "any abuse that results in physical injury, including fractures, burns, welts, cuts and or internal injuries."‡ Whenever the teacher sees any of these physical signs of injury, the child should be gently questioned as to how the injury occurred (see the box on p. 89). Children will often deny that their parents, guardians, or other adults have caused the injury because they fear additional retaliation.

Sexual abuse. Sexual abuse is one of the most difficult forms of child abuse to identify and has been defined as "any contact or interaction between child and adult in which the child is being used *for the sexual* stimulation of the perpetrator or of another person."* Almost all states indicate that any sexual involvement between a child and a parent, guardian, other adult, or an older child is sexual abuse. Girls are not the only targets, but the ratio of girls/boys is more than 2 to 1.†

Another form of sexual abuse is child molestation. Children are the victims of older individuals who manipulate the child into a sexual situation. Molestation does not have to involve only physical contact. Manipulation of the child into a discussion of sexual practices may also be considered molestation. Sometimes older individuals will show pornography to a younger individual; generally the pornography is of a nature that reflects the type of sexual preferences of the molester.

Sexual abuse occurs when there is an imbalance of power between people (e.g., a child abused by an adult or older child). It often is highlighted by an air of secrecy and is reinforced by threats if the action is reported to someone.

Preventive measures should stress that sexual abuse is never the fault of children. Students should learn that it is never proper for an adult or teenager to have sex with a child or to take pictures of the child's genitals.

Neglect. Neglect is the failure of a parent or guardian to care for the basic needs of the child. Neglect includes lack of attention to physical and medical care needs, improper supervision (e.g., leaving a 5-year-old to babysit a toddler), or abandonment.

Emotional abuse or mental neglect denigrates the child so that the child feels that nothing will please the parent. Verbal abuse such as "you'll never get anything right," failure to recognize a child's sincere efforts, or lack of praise for meaningful efforts interferes with development of the child's self-esteem. The child who is mentally abused may suffer emotional deprivation that

---

*National Center on Child Abuse and Neglect, 1992.
†US Department of Health and Human Services: *Child health USA '93,* Washington, DC, 1994, US Government Printing Office.
‡US Department of Health and Human Services: *Child abuse and neglect: curriculum in the schools,* Washington, DC, 1981, PHS Pub #0-81-30312, The Department.

---

*US Department of Health and Human Services: *Child abuse and neglect: curriculum in the schools,* Washington, DC, 1981, PHS Pub #0-81-30312, The Department.
†Coppelleri JC, Eckenrode J, Powers JL: The epidemiology of child abuse: findings from the Second National Incidence and Prevalence Study of Child Abuse and Neglect, *Am J Public Health* 83(11);1622-1624, 1993.

Signs of Possible Child Abuse

TYPE OF ABUSE OR NEGLECT	PHYSICAL INDICATORS	BEHAVIORAL INDICATORS
Physical abuse	Unusual patterns of bruises, including color patterns that might indicate blows over time Loosened or missing teeth, especially if accompanied by swelling around the mouth Black eyes/broken nose Fractures, especially if they are in different stages of healing Burns, especially if they have an unusual appearance Injuries to several body surfaces Unusual skin rashes Ruptured eardrums Cuts on different body surfaces Bite marks, especially if horseshoe shaped Wears long sleeves in warm weather	Complaints of pain when walking, sitting, writing, or using the toilet Story of injury inconsistent with appearance Fear of adults Fear of talking when parent is present Unusual attendance patterns such as arriving early and staying late, reticent to go home Overly aggressive or withdrawn Complaints of earaches Repeated vomiting, abdominal pain
Physical neglect	Usually dirty or dressed inappropiately for the weather Lack of adequate medical or dental care Consistent hunger, brings bad food to school Evidence of poor supervision (e.g., unexplained falls, ingestion of harmful substances)	Complaints of not having anything to eat, begging, or stealing food Delinquency or theft Substance abuse States that parents are not home very much Falls asleep in class
Sexual abuse	Difficulty in walking or sitting or walking with knees bowed in Pain or itching in genital or anal area Torn or bloody underclothing Sexually transmitted diseases Pregnancy Clinging to the teacher or other adult	Fantasy, withdrawal, or infantile behavior Bizarre, sophisticated, or unusual sexual behavior Unwilling to change clothes for physical education or other activities Running away from home Stating, "I would like to live with you."
Emotional neglect	Lags in physical development Repetitive movements Emaciated or lethargic Dirty or torn clothing Verbal assaults on others	Thumbsucking, biting, spitting, throwing items Conduct disorders, e.g., antisocial, destructive Does not accept criticism or compliments well Rigid adherence to instructions

may manifest itself many years later in the various relationships into which the individual enters. When the teacher refers the child suspected of being mentally neglected, often a great deal of time in professional counseling is needed.

The teacher's role. Teachers are in a unique position to notice whenever a student begins to behave or appear markedly different than usual. Teachers also have a responsibility to report suspected abuse or neglect to the proper authorities according to school procedure. All states require school personnel to report any evidence of child abuse to appropriate community authorities. Every teacher should know the specific individual to whom he or she is to report. These procedures should comply with state law and should be expressed as a written policy for all school personnel. It is important to remember that the teacher is not to investigate possible child abuse, only to report to the proper authorities.

Teachers or staff members should document exactly what was seen and what the child said when reporting incidents of abuse. This report should not label the child or interpret personal conclusions. It may be necessary to protect the child from an angry family.

It is important for teachers and staff members to report suspected abuse as soon as it is noticed so action can be taken to help the child and those who are abusing the child. Those who are expected to make reports are generally immune from legal prosecution as long as the report was made in the interest of the child. Failure to report suspected child abuse may result in criminal action being taken against those who fail to make such a report.

Teachers should include instructional programs on abuse and may wish to invite approved community resource personnel to class to discuss ways in which children can try to protect themselves, as well as ways to seek help when in trouble. Students should understand that abuse is not their fault and is unacceptable behavior in society. Pupils need help in the development of skills to be able to say "no" and to learn how to get away from a situation of possible abuse in order to report the incident to a trusted adult.

Violence

Violence has been on the increase in many schools and has become a critical and complex problem in need of attention by school personnel, parents, and community leaders. The introduction by students of guns, knives, and other implements to school buildings and grounds have exposed children to serious dangers of injury and possible death. Those young people at greatest risk of being killed or involved in violent crimes are Hispanic and African-American males in low-income, large, urban, crowded neighborhoods. They grow up witnessing direct or media violence without understanding the painful consequences. They have little hope for a future except one that includes fighting and abuse. Other violence risk factors include:

- *Neighborhood:* High percentage of unemployed men; 40% or more families live below the federal poverty income line; poor organization of networks and institutions to promote safety
- *School-related:* High absenteeism; high drop out rate; lack of central authority; students carrying weapons
- *Peers:* Easy access to weapons, alcohol, and drugs; encouraged to start fights and go to fights
- *Family:* Parents or older siblings involved in crime; lack of supervision; parental abuse or neglect; mother in abusive relationships; condoning of violent TV programs and movies; encouraging children to "fight back"
- *Individual-psychological:* Poor impulse control; low reading and verbal skills
- *Individual-health:* High level of lead in blood (exposure in environment); head injury; prenatal exposure to alcohol; attention deficit hyperactivity disorder; alcohol/drug use*

Schools by themselves cannot solve this complex social problem, but they need to be involved in preventive measures. They can create environments that may cause or increase tensions that can

---

*Earls FJ: Violence and today's youth, *Future of Children* 4(3): 4-23, 1994.

escalate into fights, segregated social groups, and other unpleasant conditions. Some of the actions schools may take to reduce the risks of violent behavior include:

- Establishment of a climate that does not tolerate fights and threats
- Staff training regarding nonviolent crisis intervention
- Building teacher skills and confidence regarding their own safety and ways to diffuse threats of assault on students
- Ensuring weapon-free schools
- Developing and enforcing consistent punishment policies and procedures
- Consider alternatives to corporal punishment
- Providing instruction in health education, health guidance, and in other areas in violence prevention and conflict resolution (see Appendix B)
- Conducting parent education programs in conflict resolution
- Opening the schools after hours for supervised recreation and programs

Alcohol and Other Drug Misuse and Abuse

Alcohol and other drug misuse and abuse can be a personal as well as family problem for a child. Statistical evidence indicates that a teacher will have children in class who come from families where one or more members abuse drugs. Over 7 million children face fear, uncertainty, or other problems daily as a result of parental alcohol abuse. Researchers have shown that children who come from families where alcohol is abused enter school with emotional burdens in addition to the general challenges faced by all children as a result of growing and maturing. Children living in an alcoholic family experience emotional distress often reflected in school behavior problems. Patterns of relationships and rules of "don't talk" about feelings may lead to unacceptable behavior as pupils attempt to deal with the anger caused by matters that cannot be discussed. Such

behaviors have been characterized as (1) the "hero" or successful child who often cares for siblings as well; (2) the "scapegoat" who acts aggressively, gets parent discipline referrals from school, and thereby risks physical abuse by either parent; (3) the "lost" child who withdraws in depression, "never causes trouble," and is unnoticed by teachers; and (4) the "mascot" who clowns around to relieve family tension or is regarded as "hyperactive" in order to mask tremendous anxiety.* This is compounded by the fact that these children often exhibit poor academic and verbal skills. This may be the result of not being able to study at home, talk with their parents, or get assistance with studying.

Evidence indicates that 60% of those who enter an emergency room for an alcohol or drug emergency have their medical symptoms treated and are then released. School officials should be informed when children have been

---

*Behrman RE, editor: *Nelson textbook of pediatrics,* ed 14, Philadelphia, 1992, WB Saunders.

 FOR YOUR INFORMATION

Possible Signs of Drug Misuse and Abuse

PHYSICAL SIGNS

Odor on breath and clothes; mouth and nose irritations; red, watery eyes; fingers with burns from smoking; poor appetite or weight loss; time and place disorientation; needle marks and scars on body; appearance of intoxication

BEHAVIORAL SIGNS

Changes in attendance, discipline and academic performance; unusual degrees of activity and agitation; display of unusual inactivity—moodiness, depression; deterioration of physical appearance and concern for health habits; unpredictable outbreaks of temper and flare-ups.

admitted to emergency rooms for drug-related problems. If these children are to benefit from their educational experience, community and school personnel must help them solve the problems that predisposed them to substance abuse.

According to the National Institute on Drug Abuse, since the formulation of the 1990 Health Goals for the Nation, limited progress has been made in the effort to combat alcohol and other drug problems. Alcohol continues to be the most commonly abused substance among US youth. The 1992 National Household Survey of Drug Abuse found that 3.8% of 12- to 13-year-olds reported alcohol use within the past month.*

For the teacher, the use of alcohol or other drugs may be a symptom of more deeply rooted problems. Use of any of these substances can adversely affect the ability of the child to learn and get the most out of his or her educational experience. In addition, the use of these substances significantly increases the possibility of HIV transmission either through use of shared needles or through unprotected sexual activity. The teacher should be aware

*US Department of Health and Human Services: *Child health USA '93,* Washington, DC, 1994, US Government Printing Office.

TABLE 4-1 Sample—Summary of Drug and Alcohol Administration Guidelines

Situational/category	Immediate action	Investigation
A student is suspected of possible drug or alcohol use. There is no violation or physical evidence.	The student is informed of available help and encouraged to seek assistance.	Limited to the staff member contacting the counselor, nurse, or principal for assistance.
A student volunteers information about personal drug or alcohol use and asks for help.	The student is informed of services available and encouraged to seek assistance.	A staff member may request advice from the crisis intervention counselor, counselor, nurse, or principal.
The student has a drug or alcohol related medical emergency.	The nurse will be summoned immediately. Student will be transported to medical facility.	The principal will investigate the incident. This may include a search of the student, locker, and other possessions.
A student possesses, uses, or is under the influence of drugs or alcohol. First offense—uncooperative behavior.	Principal is summoned. Staff member writes an anecdotal report of the incident.	The student, his/her locker, and other possessions will be searched. Confiscation of substance.
A student is distributing a drug, alcohol, or controlled substance.	Principal is summoned. Staff member writes an anecdotal report of the incident.	The student, his/her locker, and possessions will be searched. Confiscation of substance.

Extrapolated from Pennsylvania Department of Education, Bureau of Basic Education Support Services: *Responding to student drug use: guidelines for school personnel,* Harrisburg, PA, 1987, Division of Student Services, Drug and Alcohol Education Section.

of the possibility of substance abuse when the student begins manifesting signs and behaviors such as those contained in the box on this page.

Young people who may be at high risk for substance abuse include:

- Children of parents with alcohol and drug abuse problems.
- Children seen by health care providers because of abuse, numerous injuries, or psychosomatic disorders
- Children seen by various school personnel because of absenteeism, poor academic motivation, signs of depression, withdrawal, or acting-out behaviors
- Children seen by social service workers because of abuse, neglect, running away, and other home problems
- Children seen by juvenile justice workers for stealing or other delinquent behaviors
- Military dependents
- Youths in institutionalized settings

Telltale evidence such as syringes, pills, solvents, special cigarette papers, and other items found in student possession and around school are additional clues that the student may be involved in substance abuse.

It is critical that schools have specific written guidelines for handling student drug and alcohol use. An example of administrative guidelines is presented in Table 4-1.

Notification of parents	Notification of police	Disposition of substance	Discipline/ rehabilitation
Limited to behavioral problems.	Not applicable.	Not applicable.	None. Referral to the crisis intervention counselor.
Only with the consent of the student, unless there is a clear and imminent danger.	Not applicable.	Not applicable.	None. Referral to the crisis intervention counselor.
Notification of the incident in the case of a health problem or medical emergency.	Only in cases where the safety of the emergency victim or school population is at risk.	Analysis will be made.	Referral to crisis intervention counselor. If there is evidence of further violation, see appropriate situational category.
Yes, parental conference arranged as soon as possible.	At the discretion of the principal.	Analysis will be made.	Informal hearing. 10 days out of school suspension. Required participation in a chemical abuse program.
Yes, requested to come to the school as soon as possible.	Yes.	Analysis will be made for possible use in further proceedings.	Informal hearing. 10 days out of school suspension. Possible formal hearing for expulsion from school. Required participation in a chemical abuse program.

An effective method used by some schools to help students with substance abuse problems is through the use of the Student Assistance Program (SAP) program. This program is a structured way to help students who have personal or chemical use problems that interfere with school performance. It is a strategy to identify, assess, and work with the student and family to ensure evaluation and treatment of serious problems. Key features of SAP include: (1) early recognition of student problems before serious crisis or chronic dysfunction occur and (2) coordinated referrals for assessment and treatment of underlying problems. The strategy is modeled after employee assistance programs that address workers' drug addiction or serious personal problems. A school SAP committee or "core team" is trained to evaluate staff or peer referrals of any student whose behavior suggests emotional distress, family problems, or chemical use; to discuss the concerns directly with the student and parent in an atmosphere of caring; to work jointly with the family to select appropriate community resources for evaluation and treatment to help the student; and to require professional evaluation with a commitment to follow through on recommended treatment as a condition to suspend punishment or to make up missed course work. The success of SAP requires that teachers recognize and take prompt action to seek help when students are showing signs of distress or sudden disinterest in school even though a teacher may not know the reasons.

Children of Separated or Divorced Families

The number of children attending schools from separated and divorced families is growing. Over 1 million divorces occur annually in the United States, and 49% of all second marriages end in divorce as well. Over 12.5 million children are in families where divorce has occurred. In 1992, 26.6% of all young people under 18 years of age

lived with one parent.* Within a 5-year period after a divorce, one third of the children will be unhappy and dissatisfied with their lives, one third will be muddling through, and one third will adjust fairly well.

Children in families going through divorce experience unique problems. These children are preoccupied with the family situation; thus school work and other activities become secondary. They face an inconsistent family life, may spend weekends with the noncustodial parent, and may miss being with friends. These children also may face increased responsibilities at home, especially if there are younger children and the custodial parent must work.

Often these children feel alone or betrayed by parents who no longer are in the household. As a result they may direct their energies at trying to get the parents back together again. Children may feel the need to choose between the parents and also may feel that "unchosen" parents will either be hurt or will not love them as much as before. Children of divorced parents may begin to request more nurse office visits. They also may begin to skip school or look for ways to get suspended from school because they feel they have additional home responsibilities or do not want to be confronted by other children who might ask them about their family situation.

In divorce or separation situations the school may be the only stable element in the life of the child, and these children need a great deal of support, both moral and social. They need to know that divorce is an adult problem, not a child problem, and that even though they live with only one parent, they are still a family unit.

Helping children of divorce. Often the teacher does not know that a child is in a family crisis. However, if the teacher remains alert for behavior changes such as over-aggressiveness or over-

---

*US Department of Health and Human Services: *Child health USA '93*, 1994, Washington, DC, US Government Printing Office.

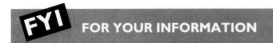

Factors that Influence the Impact of Divorce or Loss on Children

Moving—loss of ties to friends, possibly school change

The types and amount of conflict witnessed before divorce

The parent's inability to provide continuity in lifestyle and routines

The parents' inability to help the child cope while the parent is healing

helpfulness; refusal or reticence to discuss anything related to parents or family; lack of concentration; failure to do homework; constantly seeking adult attention; becoming a "loner"; dropping out of school activities; showing excessive tardiness or absence; or even listlessness, nervousness, or sleepiness; the teacher should certainly suspect that something is awry and refer the child to the school nurse or counselor. The teacher also should discuss the situation with the counselor or parent.

In addition to referring the child, the teacher should be aware of the problems and express a genuine concern to the child that the child was not to blame for an adult decision. The teacher should watch carefully for falling grades, be ready to assist the child whenever needed, and help the child maintain friendships and relationships with other children in the class. The child will eventually realize that the situation is not unique—that there are other children in the same position. Teachers should make sure that when discussions of family arise in the classroom, one-parent families, guardianships, stepfamilies, adoptive families, and foster parents are all included in the discussion.*

Since 1990 the number of children raised by grandparents has increased due to the incapability or death of parents. There has also been an increase in the number of children raised by homosexuals and adoptions by single adults. Teachers should make sure that students from different family structures are included in the discussion. It should be stressed that one type of family is not "better" than another. What is important is the nurturing that occurs within the family, regardless of the type. Children from alternative families may be made to feel inferior if they do not live in a family where the father works and the mother stays at home. Many children come from families where both parents work.

Latchkey Children

Latchkey children is a term used to describe more than 7 million children under the age of 13 whose parent or parents are working; therefore the children must go to school or return home from school without direct adult supervision. They are the result of economic conditions not necessarily divorce. This lifestyle can have an impact on the mental/emotional health of the school-aged child. Often these children come to school without breakfast, and many of them are afraid to return home at the end of the day (Fig. 4-3).*

Several school districts have developed special curricula designed to teach these children skills that enable them to take care of themselves in the absence of parents. They learn how to fix snacks, answer the telephone safely, and to call for help when needed. Other districts have developed after-school supervised recreational activities. However, controversy still exists as to the nature of the school's responsibility to aid these children and their parents. Should programs be provided for those children whose parents cannot supervise them? Should these programs involve the use of

---

*Additional information can be obtained by contacting: Children Facing Divorce, 5136 East Karen, Scottsdale, AZ 85254.

*Seligson M et al: *School-age child care: a policy report,* Wellesley, MA, 1983, School-Age Child Care Project, Wellesley College Center for Research on Women.

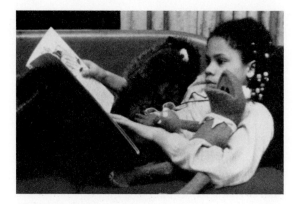

FIG. 4-3 Latchkey children have special needs. (Courtesy Health & Welfare, Canada.)

school facilities? Such action may help to reduce school vandalism and ensure children's safety. However, the additional teacher workloads, costs, and increased facility use create other problems that need to be addressed.

Researchers have shown that latchkey children, especially those in urban areas, face risks. These children must cope with loneliness and the fear of being alone. Faced with general boredom, they may get into trouble just "horsing around," or seek ganglike groups, or they may face academic problems because they do not do their homework, or feel rejected because they have no place to go and cannot invite friends to the house as long as their parents are not there. These children also may experience fear for personal safety either from someone breaking into their homes or from older siblings. Taking all this into consideration, it is clear that latchkey children are expected to assume a great deal of responsibility at an unusually young age.

Some communities have developed telephone "warm" lines for latchkey children. One such program is located in State College, Pennsylvania. This project, called *Project PhoneFriend*, is run by the American Association of University Women. This free line is open from 2:30 to 5:30 PM on weekdays and is staffed by adult volunteers who offer advice, comfort, and general conversation to the school children who call. Other communities have developed recreational programs in cooperation with the parks and recreation departments of the local communities. Increasing emphasis is also being placed on self-reliance activities and programs such as scouting.

The teacher and latchkey children. Teachers should know who the latchkey students are in the classroom. Strother has suggested several ways teachers can help latchkey children*:

- Carefully structure homework assignments as these children do not have adults around to help them complete assignments correctly
- Consider the possibility of establishing a telephone hotline to help students with homework
- During the school day, allow time for children to discuss their personal concerns with the teacher
- Establish streamlined, workable procedures for contacting the parents when emergency situations involving the child arise
- Develop both before-school and after-school day-care programs for these children

Homeless Children

On any given school day, it is estimated 100,000 children are homeless, and many others are temporarily living in another family's home. These children have difficulty attaching to teachers, poor concentration, and poor task completion. Their irregular school attendance, frequent school changes, and limited resources to complete homework often cause them to repeat grades or be assigned to special classes. The U.S. McKinney Homeless Assistance Act of 1987 requires schools to provide appropriate regular educational programs without residency proof or prior school records.

It is critical for homeless children to have teachers help them build self-esteem by providing meaningful, successfully completed schoolwork. These children may need a homework center at

---

*Strother DB: Latchkey children: the fastest growing special interest group in the schools, *J School Health* 56(1):13-16, 1986.

school, adjustment of assignments, and special tutoring.*

McCarty and McCarty† have suggested low-cost, creative ways to help these children and their mental health needs. For example, they identify a "Winner's Pack" as one idea. This includes a picture of the child with his/her classmates, samples of quality work to preserve, and stamped postcards for the child to stay in touch.

WHY SHOULD SCHOOLS BE CONCERNED WITH THE MENTAL/EMOTIONAL HEALTH OF STUDENTS?

The school ranks second to the family as the most important unit in society affecting the mental health of children and must be concerned for these reasons:

- The effectiveness of the educative process will be seriously hampered because approximately 12% of pupils have emotional disturbances.
- Educational failure, or the "failure syndrome," is one of the underlying factors that triggers acting-out in schools, depression, drug abuse, truancy, and other maladjustments. Children who exhibit such behavior have a lower self-concept or self-identity.
- The experiences to which a child is exposed can help prevent serious difficulties or hasten mental problems. Hence, schools play a role in both primary and secondary prevention—before conditions occur and in the control of existing conditions. Early identification of children with emotional difficulties is important because remedial help should be provided at a time when intervention is maximally effective. The increase of problems and limited community mental health services add to the need for emphasis on prevention.

- Behavior is more readily modified and self-esteem can be improved more readily at the elementary level than later in life.
- It is important for children to experience success in school with special attention given to their physical and psychological needs. Many children who enter school are educationally handicapped in terms of readiness to enter school.
- The school is the only agency outside the home that reaches practically all children and youth.

School counseling and psychological services should take a leadership role in developing and implementing a plan to address the physical, intellectual, emotional, and social development of children. These professionals have specific skills that can help enhance all facets of the mental and emotional health of children.

Schools and teachers should promote positive mental health in all students, thus helping prevent mental illness and emotional disturbances and assisting children with mental health problems.

WHAT IS THE TEACHER'S ROLE IN IMPROVING THE EMOTIONAL CLIMATE?

Schools and school personnel can have considerable effect on the emotional health and mental development of children. It has been estimated by some psychologists that the average child is exposed to two emotionally unstable teachers during his school years. This estimate might be considered too conservative.

In any case, the teacher is the person children see day after day during the school year. Next to the parent the teacher probably has more influence on most students than any other person in their young lives. What a challenge this is; yet what an opportunity!

Certified teachers generally have been exposed to information about child development but have received limited preparation in mental health. They find it difficult to deal effectively with emotional problems they face in the classroom and in

---

*Wiley DC, Ballard DJ: How can schools help children from homeless families? *J School Health* 63(7):291-293, 1993.
†McCarty H, McCarty M: Ideas to humanize school and agency settings for homeless children, *Invitational Educ Forum* 13(1): 15-19, 1992.

extracurricular settings. Teachers know that students need to be inherently motivated and have perceivable goals if they are to learn, perform, and develop as individual personalities capable of coping with and contributing to their world. They can reinforce or discourage the joy of learning and the achievement of these goals.

The single most important contribution to student mental health is the development of a wholesome emotional climate in the classroom that contributes to the development of self-esteem in children.

Because self-esteem is learned, children exposed to positive educational experiences presented in an atmosphere of acceptance have a greater chance of developing positive self-esteem than those not exposed to such an environment. When teachers encourage and praise children, they are developing a positive learning atmosphere. Children with positive self-esteem are more likely to perform better in school, be better adjusted both as children and adults, be less defensive, and manifest greater social effectiveness and acceptance of others.* What teachers say, do, and think has a profound and lasting influence on children. The following suggestions should help provide ways to achieve a positive classroom climate:†

- Maximize individual learning through the recognition of individual differences (Fig. 4-4)
- Encourage and increase student involvement in the education process with experiences designed to assist students in learning about self-esteem
- Provide the opportunity for all children to experience success and learn of the various abilities they possess
- Encourage freedom of expression within the classroom without being judgmental, sarcas-

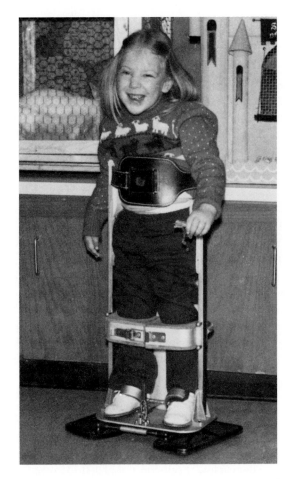

FIG. 4-4 It is important that schools provide for individual differences. (Courtesy Witchita Public Schools, Witchita, Kansas.)

tic, or belittling, and help students do the same, respecting the rights of all
- Provide a meaningful curriculum that satisfies the needs of students and helps them learn how to improve their abilities in coping with a complex world
- Make grades and grading noncompetitive, believing that all children are trying their best
- Help students assess their own value systems, particularly in respecting the rights of others and dealing with cultural diversity

---

*Gurney P: Self-esteem enhancement in children: a review of research findings, *Educ Res* 29(2):130-136, 1987.
†For additional suggestions relative to the role of the school in the physical, intellectual, social, and emotional development of children, see Division of School Programs: *Educating the whole student,* Boston, March 1990, Pub #16,215, Massachusetts Department of Education.

- Accept emotional outbursts from children and utilize the opportunity for incidental instruction related to emotional well-being
- Maintain discipline without becoming overly punitive
- Become a positive role model by practicing tolerance and humanity in dealing with students, teachers, administrators, and staff

Anxieties and tensions can quickly and easily become evident in class. The teacher can help to ease these conditions by being cognizant of the factors previously mentioned and also by providing relaxation outlets through music, art, drama, play, dance, exercise, or creative reading or writing.

Teachers who are self-confident and able to motivate their students will generally realize a greater degree of teaching success by providing a positive emotional climate. The ability of the teacher to handle the daily demands of teaching, as well as the teacher's self-concept, personal appearance, and health status can positively influence the emotional climate of the school.

How Does Teacher Health Affect the School Climate?

Well-adjusted teachers are needed if the most wholesome emotional climate is to be found in the classroom. The teacher who suffers from anxiety and lack of self-confidence will communicate this to children. It is estimated that the percentage of teachers with mental illness is about the same as in the general population—approximately 10%. Teachers therefore need to give attention to their personal needs and make adequate provision for sleep, rest, exercise, appropriate diet, and relaxation to maintain the highest level of health possible.

The teacher's physical health status, diet, sexual activities, and personal health practices, including the use of alcoholic beverages and mood-altering drugs, may impact the emotional climate within the classroom. It is important for teachers to realize that they become role models for students. As such, the way the teacher reacts to varying stressful situations within the school day will have an impact on the students exposed to that teacher. If the teacher cannot handle the daily stresses of the school day, as well as stresses outside of school, how will that teacher be able to transfer good coping skills to students?

Teachers must realize that stress is experienced by everyone. It is a part of living. Individuals vary widely in their ability to adapt to stress. How a person responds to stressful conditions, therefore, is important; it has both positive and negative effects. In the classroom, stress may stimulate and motivate students positively to increase learning, whereas repeated negative reactions may result in adverse behaviors previously identified as occurring when needs remained unmet. When this occurs, a repetitive cycle is initiated wherein the negative behavior evokes negative responses from others, causing more stress.

Stress in the classroom setting, however, is part of the process of education. Any teacher requirement or demand will create differing degrees of stress among pupils. It is important that teachers help children learn how to deal with these as well as other stresses that must be faced as the child grows and matures. It is also important that teachers create among themselves and other school personnel a positive and supportive atmosphere conducive to the optimal physical, mental, and social health of all persons associated with the school. Provision of school-site wellness programs can assist in developing this support. Such programs can contribute to the physical and emotional well-being of staff members. They may include an assessment of needs and activities such as smoking/tobacco use cessation, nutrition education, weight management, and aerobics.*

Health Instruction and Mental Health

The need for health education as part of the curriculum has been mentioned often as a means of promoting positive mental health. Education can

---

*American School Health Association: *Guidelines for the comprehensive school health program*, Kent, OH, 1994, The Association.

help pupils to understand themselves, their drives, their prejudices, their emotions, their ambitions, their growth and personality development, and their values, as well as help them learn how to get along with others, live in society, and be socially acceptable members of the world in which they live. Children need to learn how to resolve conflicts relating to worries, peer pressures, gang threats, fighting, justice, and people differences and interdependence.* Satisfaction that comes with self-esteem and self-concept leads to feelings of confidence, worth, strength, capability, and adequacy. Children who attain such attitudes are able to learn with increased interest, enthusiasm, and efficiency.

Instruction should include both formal and informal programs (see Chapter 1 and Appendix B). The suggested outline of content for mental health, the concepts that should receive consideration, and the objectives to be achieved through grade level groups in the formal phase may be found in Appendix B. They can be integrated into all phases of the curriculum, or specific units can be prepared and taught as part of health education using a variety of techniques (see Chapter 12).

Informally, mental health concepts and understandings of self can be learned and modified indirectly through interpersonal relations between teachers and pupils. The wholesome classroom atmosphere provides numerous opportunities for incidental teaching through informal discussion and counseling and guidance. In addition, support groups can be convened voluntarily to permit students to express opinions and feelings on a variety of topics through verbal and other forms of communication.

Parent education programs are an increasing part of parent involvement in schools. Family understanding of children's needs and the need for communication are extremely important for positive mental health.

---

*Black S: Caught in the middle, *Executive Education* 17:30-34, 1995.

SUMMARY

The teacher plays a primary role in establishing the emotional atmosphere in the school. Teachers therefore must understand the nature of mental/emotional health and its effect on learning. To aid pupils in their development, teachers must help provide for their physical and psychological needs. They must be alert in their observations of changes in students' attitudes and behaviors and understand which ones are in need of attention.

A variety of environmental factors affect the mental/emotional health of children. These include child abuse, alcohol and other drug use, parental separation or divorce, economics, and latchkey and homeless children.

The teacher must be aware of the various stresses that face both student and staff each day. The teacher also must understand that the reaction to these stresses varies for each individual. Knowing how children react to stress, however, is not enough. The teacher also must be aware of how he or she reacts to stress, because the teacher becomes a role model for students. If the teacher constantly reacts in a negative way to stress, it is quite likely that the teacher's students will react in the same way.

Personal health practices are important. If the teacher is constantly slovenly in appearance, or lets mood-altering substances provide substitutes for good judgment and professional pride, then that teacher is not doing much to contribute to the total emotional climate of the school. As Plato stated, "Know thyself." By knowing oneself, the teacher is in a better position to create a positive emotional climate in the classroom and the total school environment.

QUESTIONS FOR DISCUSSION

1. How would you summarize the poem by Dorothy Law Nolte?
2. What is the meaning of the term *mental health*?
3. What is the relationship between mental health and self-esteem?
4. Why do you think child neglect is more prevalent than physical abuse?

5. What are the laws relating to reporting of suspected child abuse in the state where you reside?

6. What provision is made to safeguard the rights of the teacher? In your state, who reports suspected child abuse?

7. Some people feel that alcohol and substance abuse should not be discussed in schools, particularly in elementary schools. State and justify your position on this issue.

8. How can mental neglect or emotional abuse cripple a child?

9. What special problems might confront the child who comes from a family where the parents are separated or divorced?

10. Why should schools have written administration guidelines for dealing with drug and alcohol problems in the school?

11. What do you think the role of the school should be in caring for latchkey or homeless children?

12. Why should teachers be concerned with the mental/emotional health of students?

13. What can the teacher do to provide an emotional climate in the classroom that promotes good mental health?

14. What might teachers do to increase the chances of children in their classrooms developing positive self-esteem?

15. How can health instruction help the mental health of pupils?

16. What impact does the health of the teacher have on the emotional climate of the classroom?

SELECTED REFERENCES

Allegrante J, Michela J: Impact of a school-based workplace health promotion program on the morale of inner-city teachers, *J School Health* 60(1):25-29, 1990.

Behrman RE, editor: *Nelson textbook of pediatrics*, ed 14, Philadelphia, 1992, WB Saunders.

Berne P: Seven secrets for building kids' self-esteem, *Instructor* 11(1):63-65, 1985.

Bickel D, Bickel W: Effective schools, classrooms, and instruction: implications for special education, *Except Child* 52:489-500, 1986.

Blair SN, Tritsch L, Kutsch S: Worksite health promotion for school faculty and staff, *J School Health* 57(10):469-473, 1987.

Bonaguro J, Rhonehouse M, Bonaguro E: Effectiveness of four school health education projects upon substance use, self-esteem, and adolescent stress, *Health Educ Q* 15(1):81-92, 1988.

Bonkowski SE, Bequette SQ, Boonhower S: A group design to help children adjust to parental divorce, *Soc Casework* 65(2);131-137, 1984.

Bryant AL: Hostile hallways: the AAUW survey on sexual harrassment in America's schools, *J School Health* 63(8):125-129, 1993.

Carnegie Council on Adolescent Development: *Turning points: preparing American youth for the 21st century*, New York, 1989, Carnegie Corporation of New York.

Coben JH, Weiss HB, Mulvey EP, Dearwater SR: A primer of school violence prevention, *J School Health* 64(8):309-314, 1994.

Coppelleri JC, Eckenrode J, Powers JL: The epidemiology of child abuse: findings from the Second National Incidence and Prevalence Study of Child Abuse and Neglect, *Am J Public Health* 83(11):1622-1624, 1993.

Cornacchia HJ, Smith DE, Bentel DJ: *Drugs in the classroom: a conceptual model for school programs*, ed 2, St Louis, 1978, Mosby–Year Book.

Dickey J, Henderson PL: What young children say about stress and coping in school, *Health Educ* 20(2):14-17, 1989.

Dunn T: *Educating the whole student*, Boston, March 1990, Division of School Programs, Massachusetts Department of Education, Pub #16,215.

Earls FJ: Violence and today's youth, *The Future of Children* 4(3):4-23, 1994.

Epstein MH, Cullinan D: Depression in children, *J School Health* 56(1):10-12, 1986.

Fisk N: Alcoholism: ineffective family coping, *Am J Nurs* 86:586-587, 1986.

Forte I, Schurr S: Classroom management—the definitive middle school guide: a handbook for success, *Learning* 22:66, 1994.

Frick SB: Diagnosing boredom, confusion and adaptation in school children, *J School Health* 55(7):254-257, 1985.

Glenwick DS, Jason LA, editors: *Promoting mental health in children, youth, and families*, New York, 1993, Springer.

Girvin J, Cottrell R: The impact of the Seaside Health Education Conference on middle school health programs in Oregon, *Health Educ* 18(5):78-82, 1987.

Graham L, Harris-Hart M: Meeting the challenge of child sexual abuse, *J School Health* 58(7):292-294, 1988.

Gray BJ, Pippin GD: Stepfamilies: a concern health education should address, *J School Health* 54(8):292-295, 1984.

Gurney P: Self-esteem enhancement in children: a review of research findings, *Educ Res* 29(2):130-136, 1987.

Hayes D, Fors S: Self-esteem and health instruction: challenge for curriculum development, *J School Health* 60(5):208-211, 1990.

Jones M, Paterson L: *Preventing chaos in times of crisis—a guide for school administrators,* Los Alamitos, CA, 1992, Southwest Regional Laboratory.

Knight S, Vail-Smith K, Barnes AM: Children of alcoholics in the classroom: a survey of teacher perception and training needs, *J School Health* 62(8):367-371, 1992.

Korup UL: Parent and teacher perception of depression in children, *J School Health* 55(9):367-369, 1985.

Laing SL, Bruess CE: *Entering adulthood: connecting health communication and self-esteem,* Santa Cruz, CA, 1989, Network Publications.

Lewis W: Strategic interventions with children of single-parent families, *Sch Counselor* 33(5):375-378, 1986.

Long L: *On my own: the kids' self-care book,* Washington, DC, 1984, Acropolis Books.

Lovato C, Allensworth D, Chan F: *School health in America: an assessment of state policies to protect and improve the health of students,* ed 5, Kent, OH, 1989, American School Health Association.

McCarty H, McCarty M: Ideas to humanize school and agency settings for homeless children, *Invitational Educ Forum* 13(1):15-19, 1992.

Mull S: Help for the children of alcoholics, *Health Educ* 21(5):42-45, 1990.

Myrick RD: *Developmental guidance and counseling,* Minneapolis, 1993, Educational Media Corporation.

Nishioka E: Helping children of alcoholics, *J School Health* 59(9):404-405, 1989.

Olds S: Enhancing self-esteem through mutual self-disclosure, *J School Health* 57(4):160-161, 1987.

Packard V: *Our endangered children: growing up in a changing world,* Boston, 1984, Little, Brown.

Page RM, Allen O, Moore L, Hewitt C: Co-occurrence of substance use and loneliness as a risk factor for adolescent hopelessness, *J School Health* 63(2):106-110, 1993.

Peterson B, Andress P, Schroeder L, Swanson B, Ziff L: The Edina, Minnesota, school crisis response team, *J School Health* 63(4):192-194, 1993.

Redican KJ, Olsen LK, Baffi CR: *Organization of school health programs,* New York, 1986, Macmillan.

Seligson M et al: *School-age child care: a policy report,* Wellesley, MA, 1983, School-Age Child Care Project, Wellesley College Center for Research on Women.

Spirito A, Stark L, Williams C: Coping in children and adolescents, *J Pediatr Psychol* 13:555-574, 1988.

Strother DB: Latchkey children: the fastest growing special interest group in the schools, *J School Health* 56(1):13-16, 1986.

Swan HL, Houston V: Alone after school: a self-care guide for latchkey children and their parents, Englewood Cliffs, NJ, 1985, Prentice-Hall.

Torabi MR, Bailey WJ, Majd-Jabbari M: Cigarette smoking as a predictor of alcohol and other drug use by children and adolescents: evidence of the "gateway drug effect," *J School Health* 63(7):302-306, 1993.

US Department of Health and Human Services: *Child abuse and neglect: curriculum in the schools,* Washington, DC, 1981, PHS Pub No 0-81-30312, The Department.

US Department of Health and Human Services: *Child health USA '93,* Washington, DC, 1994, US Government Printing Office.

Wiley DC, Ballard DJ: How can schools help children from homeless families, *J School Health* 63(7):291-293, 1993.

Zevin D: *Into adolescence: enhancing self-esteem,* Santa Cruz, CA, 1989, Network Publishers.

Zulke J: Among latchkey children problems: insufficient daycare facilities, data on possible harm, *JAMA* 260(23):3399-3400, 1988.

III

HEALTH SERVICES

5

Health Appraisals of School Children

KEY CONCEPT

Systematic observations and appraisals of children by teachers, school nurses and other school personnel can help identify barriers to student attendance, participation, and learning.

. . . early identification of problems can alert school personnel to potential barriers to learning.

SUSAN BRINK AND PHILIP NADER *JOURNAL OF SCHOOL HEALTH,* **1984**

PROBLEM TO SOLVE

As a professional who works in the school, develop a plan to (1) keep up to date with health problems of the elementary child; (2) increase your ability to observe deviations from "normal" health, growth, and development of children; and (3) incorporate the concepts of health appraisal into your daily classroom activities, thus enhancing the ability of children to learn.

TEACHERS frequently ask such questions as the following:

"Why must I be concerned with the health of boys and girls in my class?"

"How can I find out about the health status of children in my room?"

"Is the failure of children to learn related to their health problems?"

"How can the nurse help me protect the health of my pupils?"

"Why must children have periodic vision and hearing tests?"

"What is the teacher's responsibility in preparing children for vision testing, hearing testing, dental inspections, health examinations, and other appraisals?"

"When should I be concerned about a child with a runny nose or a skin infection or one who always seems to be tired?"

"What can I do about inattentive, fidgety, aggressive, or impulsive children in class?"

"Why are health records used in schools?"

"What should I do about children in my class who have diabetes, asthma, seizures, or cancer?"

Although educators and medical specialists generally believe the family has the primary responsibility for the health of children, schools need strong supportive programs because of (1) the relationship of good health to attendance and effective learning, (2) the hazards associated with communicable diseases, and (3) the inability or unwillingness of some parents to accept their responsibilities for maintaining basic health in their children. Students with communicable diseases may transmit these conditions to others. Children who cannot see or hear well may have difficulty benefiting from the usual education. Family crises or personal emotional problems may distract children. Pupils who miss breakfast or regular meals may not have sufficient stamina to endure daily classroom activities. Dental health problems such as cavities, an abscess, or gum disease may cause infection and pain, which adversely affect student's concentration and attention to learning. Children who have asthma, diabetes, seizures, or attention deficit disorders need to be identified so their educational programs can be adjusted as needed.

Unfortunately, many families need help from school staff to recognize and manage their children's health problems. The 1990 Census reported that 28% of US families with children were headed by a single parent.

In some instances parental responsibility has been ignored or has not been recognized. With more mothers working away from the home, communication with parents has become difficult. More than three fourths of all school-aged children have mothers in the work force or living on public assistance. Children continue to be sent to school with physical and emotional conditions that are unknown to parents or are considered less important. The school therefore has found it necessary to help parents recognize children's health problems. The procedures used to identify these children with health problems are called health appraisals.

Health appraisals are part of the comprehensive health services program that should be found in all schools (see Fig. 1-1). Health services are those actions taken to help children with problems. They also include follow-up and guidance (Chapter 6); emergencies and first aid (Chapter 7); health personnel such as registered nurses, nurse practitioners, consulting physicians, and others; and linkages or collaborations with community health agencies and organizations. National, state, and local laws mandate the availability of various service components. However, those services found in schools are uneven in quality and quantity and often barely comply with the law. Except in large school districts, very little money is appropriated for these services, and therefore are generally inadequate. In most schools, nurses or nurse practitioners are responsible for segments of the program. The amount of nursing services provided varies widely and is greatly limited in many school districts.

CHILDREN AT SPECIAL RISK

It was pointed out in Chapter 1 that some children have more severe health problems than others. Children at special risk include those from low-income families, those who are homeless, those who are not covered under any type of health insurance, and those who are victims of violence or who live in families where violence is common.

The American Academy of Pediatrics* has advocated that ensuring students' access to a regular source of primary care is an important goal of every school health program. Where schoolchildren do not receive adequate health care, cooperation from school programs may be necessary to provide screening, preventive, and some treatment services. Since 1967, states have been required by Congress to provide early and periodic health screening, diagnosis, and treatment (EPSDT) for eligible poor children as part of Medicaid. These procedures have included screening tests (vision, hearing, blood pressure, and others), immunizations, dental care, and well-care supervision.

WHAT ARE HEALTH APPRAISALS?

Health appraisals refer to a series of procedures designed to assess the health status of children. Although the nature and frequency of appraisals vary in school districts throughout the United States, they generally include teacher observations, screening tests (vision, hearing, and others), health histories or inventories, dental inspections, medical examinations, and psychological tests (see the box on p. 108).

Appraisals exist for the following reasons:
- To locate pupils needing medical or dental treatment, or child protective services
- To locate pupils who are having problems learning and need special attention at school or assessment by a psychiatrist or child guidance clinic (e.g., concerning behavior problems and emotional disturbances)
- To locate pupils who need modified educational programs (e.g., those with hearing, vi-

sual, or physical problems, or those who are mentally retarded)
- To inform school personnel and parents about the health status of children and to help parents plan how to follow-up
- To make adjustments in school for pupils with health problems
- To serve as learning experiences for children, teachers, and parents

The nature of health appraisals and the responsibilities of teachers are discussed in the pages that follow. The degree to which the teacher participates differs in every school district and depends on the extent of the school program as well as on the availability of special school health personnel.

Three important points related to the teacher's role must be recognized:

1. Teachers, nurses, and nonmedically trained people should not attempt to make medical diagnoses. Registered nurses with training in pediatric physical assessment can

FOR YOUR INFORMATION

America's Children

- Almost 22% of our children lived in poverty in 1992, up from 15% in 1972. Each year the rate increases 1.6%.
- In 1992, over 8 million children had no health insurance all year; another 20 million had no coverage for at least 1 month.
- About 58% of mothers with children under 6 years are working.
- In 1992, 55% of American 2-year-olds were fully immunized; too many wait for day care or school enrollment.
- Every night an estimated 100,000 children are homeless, and in some cities, one in four homeless people is a child.

*Committee on School Health: *School health: policy and practice,* ed 5, Elk Grove Village, IL, 1993, American Academy of Pediatrics.

Modified from Children's Defense Fund: *The state of America's children yearbook, 1994,* Washington, DC, 1994, Children's Defense Fund.

School Health Screening Programs by Grade Level and Frequency

TYPE OF SERVICE	ECE*	K	1	2	3	4	5	6	7	8	9	10	11	12
Vision screening tests†	X	X	X	X	X		X		X		X			
Color vision tests		X												
Hearing screening tests†	X	X	X	X	X		X		X		X			
Dental inspections and education		X			X		X			X				
Dental sealants on first molars				X										
Weight and growth measurements† (often done cooperatively with P.E. program)	X	X	X	X	X	X	X	X						
Nurse interviews with parents of new students	X	X	X	X	X	X	X	X	X	X	X	X	X	X
Medical and/or school nurse practitioner All pupils with suspected health or learning problems without current or complete reports from family or clinic physicians		X	X	X	X	X	X	X	X	X	X	X	X	X
All pupils being considered for placement in special education without current or complete reports		X	X	X	X	X	X	X	X	X	X	X	X	X
Tuberculin skin tests	Recommended for entry if district's prevalence of positive reactors is over 140%													
Scoliosis screening								X	X	X				

*Early childhood education or prekindergarten.
†At certain grades; all new pupils at other grades and referrals.

make judgments about appraisals and plan follow-up action. Observation of runny noses, flushed faces, and fevers does not permit untrained individuals to identify these conditions as colds, influenza, allergies, or other diseases. Signs and symptoms should be reported, and these children should be referred to the school nurse or to a parent.

2. School personnel should not render medical care, and employees should not attempt to provide treatment services; this is the function of physicians, dentists, and other qualified specialists. Some school districts help families enroll in public clinics or gain access to medical care.

3. Health information about pupils should remain confidential. Teachers and others in schools who need this knowledge should have access to school health records, and schools should have written care plans for common or expected health problems.

WHAT ARE TEACHER OBSERVATIONS?

Teachers are in an excellent position to observe the appearance and behavior of children because of daily contact throughout the year. They see children perform a variety of activities under different environmental circumstances. They note pupils with headaches, frequent respiratory infections, recurrent earaches, fatigue, skin rashes, and emotional disturbances. They are capable of becoming skilled observers of the signs and symptoms of ill health. The opportunities to observe boys and girls throughout the day often result in the identification of pupils who are in the early stages of communicable diseases or who need care for physical conditions or emotional disturbances. Prompt attention to behaviors of concern helps maintain and improve the children's health.

The responsibility of observing children for illness indications does not involve responsibility for diagnosing specific conditions. Diagnosis is a matter for individuals with special professional preparation. The more detailed and accurate the teacher's noting of pertinent changes of appearance or activity, however, the more valuable the information can be for diagnosis. A comment such as "George does not seem to feel well today" gives the nurse or parent little specific aid; but a brief account of the signs and symptoms (such as runny nose, frequent fatigue, and constant cough) that led the teacher to believe George was not feeling well is much more helpful.

A pupil's health may change suddenly, and the teacher must constantly be on the alert for such changes. Changes associated with physical, sexual, or emotional abuse are critical indicators; special in-service education programs for school personnel may be necessary to help in these observations. The Colorado Department of Health has prepared a brief list of observations (Table 5-1) that can serve as a guide for referring students to the school nurse or other designated school official. More detailed signs and symptoms of health defects and illnesses may be found in Appendix I.

The teacher must also be aware of the good health characteristics (Appendix J) of children not only to more easily identify problems but also to improve the teacher's competency in making student referrals. This is important, as teachers may have to inform others regarding various conditions that resulted in referral of a student.

Understanding and observing student growth and development characteristics (Appendix K) can have implications for health education, can provide teachable moments, and can be used in the development of curriculum for the instructional program.

Allergies and Asthma

Allergies are one of the common student health problems that confront the teacher. Allergic conditions account for an estimated one third of the chronic conditions seen in children and 130 million lost school days annually. This means that approximately one in five children suffers from some sort of allergy.

Asthma is an allergic condition that accounts for nearly 20% of the school days lost in elementary and secondary schools each year. Students with asthma have significantly more absent days than those without asthma.* When children miss school as a result of any illness, their overall school performance can be affected. However, children who suffer from asthma and other allergic conditions may have to face additional problems even though they remain in school. Some of these problems include fatigue from lack of sleep, discomfort from the various symptoms (e.g., stuffy nose, itchy eyes, and scratchy throat), episodic hearing loss, sleepiness, and other side effects from medications. Additionally, these children affect the concentration of other children in the classroom because they often wheeze, cough, sniff, clear their throats, or blow their noses. They may also leave the classroom to get water or medication or to check respiratory status on a peak flow meter (Fig. 5-1, see p. 112).

Students with allergic rhinitis, or "hay fever," experience eye irritation, itching, congestion, and sneezing. This condition also may cause headaches and numerous ear infections. Obviously, when vision and hearing are impaired, learning may be affected.

The teacher should be aware of children who have allergies, asthma, or other respiratory conditions that may adversely affect school perfor-

---

*Richards W: Allergy, asthma, and school problems, *J School Health* 56(4):4-6, 1986.

TABLE 5-1 Guide for Teacher's Referral to Nurse

It is recommended that the following observations be referred to the nurse:

EYES

a. Sties or crusted eyelids
b. Inflamed eyelids
c. Crossed eyes
d. Repeated headaches
e. Squinting, frowning, or scowl-
    ing
f. Eyes pink or yellow
g. Watery eyes
h. Rubbing of eyes
i. Twitching of the lids
j. Excessive blinking
k. Holding head to one side
l. Complaints of blurry vision

TEETH AND MOUTH

a. State of uncleanliness
b. Gross cavities
c. Crooked teeth
d. Stained teeth
e. Gum boils
f. Offensive breath
g. Mouth habits such as thumb-
    sucking
h. Complaints of toothache
i. Swollen jaw

HEART

a. Excessive breathlessness
b. Tires easily
c. Bluish lips or fingernails
d. Pale color

GROWTH

a. Failure to gain regularly over 6-
    month period
b. Unexplained weight loss
c. Unexplained rapid weight gain

EARS

a. Drainage from ears
b. Earache
c. Failure to hear questions
d. Picking at the ears
e. Turning head to hear
f. Talking loudly or in a monotone
g. Inattention
h. Anxious expression
i. Ringing in ears
j. Dizziness

GLANDS

a. Enlarged glands at side of neck
b. Enlarged thyroid

GENERAL APPEARANCE AND CONDITION

a. Underweight—very thin
b. Overweight—very obese
c. Does not appear well
d. Tires easily
e. Chronic fatigue
f. Vomiting or diarrhea
g. Faintness or dizziness
h. Chronic menstrual discomfort

POSTURE AND MUSCULATURE

a. Alignment of shoulders
b. Walks or runs with unusual gait
c. Obvious deformities of any type
d. Alignment of spine on "stand-
    ing tall"
e. Muscular development lacking
f. Coordination problems
g. Muscle tone

RESPIRATORY

a. Persistent mouth or noisy
    breathing
b. Frequent sore throats
c. Recurrent colds
d. Chronic nasal discharge
e. Frequent nose bleeding
f. Nasal speech
g. Frequent tonsillitis
h. Chronic coughing

ANY CHRONIC ILLNESS (KNOWN OR SUSPECTED DIAGNOSIS), FOR EXAMPLE

a. Diabetes
b. Epilepsy/seizures
c. Arthritis
d. Cystic fibrosis
e. Orthopedic condition
f. Severe hearing loss
g. Unremedial visual loss

OTHER

a. Students who lack medical care
b. Known or suspected social, fam-
    ily, financial situations affect-
    ing the health of the student
c. Prolonged or frequent absen-
    teeism
d. Homebound students
e. Suspected or known pregnan-
    cies
f. Suspected abuse
g. Children receiving medications
    for a prolonged time and for
    chronic conditions
h. Frequent injuries

TABLE 5-1   Guide for Teacher's Referral to Nurse—cont'd

SKIN AND SCALP	BEHAVIOR	
a. Tatoos/ink or cut marks	a. Overstudious, docile, withdrawing; unusually afraid	g. Lying (imaginative or defensive)
b. Eruptions or rashes		h. Intentionally breaks known rules
c. Habitual scratching of scalp or skin	b. Bullying, overaggressiveness, domineering; starts fights	i. Scratching or rubbing genital or rectal area
d. Nits or lice on the hair	c. Unhappy and depressed	j. Antagonistic, negativistic, continual quarreling
e. State of uncleanliness/odor	d. Impulsive, low tolerance for frustration	
f. Excessive redness or yellowness of face		k. Excessive use of toilet
	e. Stuttering or other forms of speech difficulty; speech hard to understand for age	l. Wetting or defecation in clothing
g. Bruises or burns		m. Doesn't want to go home
	f. Poor accomplishment in comparison with ability	n. Unusual hunger and/or thirst
		o. Refuses to do assignments

Modified from Colorado Department of Education and Colorado Department of Health: *Colorado school health guidelines,* ed 2, Denver, 1986, The Departments.

mance. Certain sustained physical activities, especially if done in cold, dry, or dusty environments, can trigger the symptoms of asthma.* Swimming and activity done in spurts such as running/walking are least likely to evoke problems (Fig. 5-2, p. 113).

Learning Disabilities or Perceptual Problems

Approximately 7% of all school-aged children exhibit one or more learning disabilities. Learning disabilities may be characterized as problems in understanding or using spoken or written language. The use of language involves complex psychological processes, and failure of these processes to function properly may result in a learning problem.

Teachers also may observe a variety of children's problems called attention deficit disorders with or without hyperactivity or specific learning

disabilities. Learning disabilities include such conditions as dyslexia (inability to read more than a few lines with understanding), autism (disturbances of language, cognition, and human relations), and developmental aphasia (inability to transmit ideas by language, including writing and speaking, and through reading). These central nervous system disorders are not clearly defined but generally refer to those pupils with near above-average general intelligence with learning or behavioral abnormalities ranging from mild to severe that are associated with subtle dysfunctions of the central nervous system. Difficulties in listening, thinking, talking, reading, writing, spelling, or arithmetic occur. They involve memory and control of attention, impulse, or motor function. Testing reveals a significant difference between children's achievement level and their capabilities based on their mental abilities. These conditions are independent of errors of refraction, muscle imbalance, and imperfect binocular vision, including problems caused primarily by hearing or motor handicaps, mental retardation, emotional disturbance, or environmental disadvantage.

Children with learning problems or attention

*National Asthma Education Program: *Managing asthma: a guide for schools,* Bethesda, MD, 1991, The National Asthma Education Program Information Center.

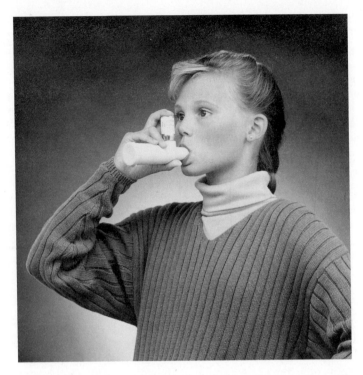

FIG. 5-1 Peak flow meters, such as Personal Best, help students monitor asthma. (Courtesy HealthScan Products Inc, Cedar Grove, New Jersey.)

deficit disorders may exhibit the following behavior:

- Hyperactivity—constantly moving, poor concentration, short attention span, talkativeness
- Impulsiveness—act without planning
- Variability and unpredictability—may cry or laugh easily; explosive irritability
- Emotional instability—overreaction to trips, parties, and such activities; delay and failure may produce tears and temper tantrums; not accepted by peers; gullible and trusting; low tolerance for failure and frustration
- Perseveration—inordinant focus on irrelevant stimuli or tasks,* continuous repetition of an action or response after a successful performance; may write a letter over and over, or talk incessantly about a subject for months
- Poor sleep habits—easily awakened; difficulty falling asleep
- Poor muscle coordination—cannot function in sports; exceptionally clumsy; difficulty with buttoning, writing, speaking, reading (dyslexia)
- Narrow, poorly transferred variety of strategies for task demands

The diagnosis of students with perceptual problems is difficult and complex. It may involve a team of individuals including school personnel. The procedure involves a complete prenatal and medical history, a thorough physical examination including a neurological survey, and a psychological examination.

Treatment for learning disabilities may include

---

*Levine MD: Attention and memory: progression and variation during the elementary school years, *Pediatr Ann* 18(6):366-372, 1989.

Date: _____, 19____

Dear Physical Education Instructor:

_____ is under my care for ASTHMA.

(Name of student)

Because exercise is important for the asthmatic child, both physically and psychologically, I am providing information and instructions concerning this child's participation in physicial education.

1 He/she should be permitted to remain in regular PE classes and should be able to engage in *regular* physical education activities most of the time. However, during asthma episodes (characterized by cough, wheeze, shortness of breath), activities may have to be *temporarily* curtailed.

2 Each asthmatic child has a different limit of tolerance to exercise. *Please permit the youngster to set his/her own pace on a daily basis.* In particular, asthmatics may have difficulty "running laps" and playing competitive soccer and basketball; please do not "force" the child, but let the student participate at his/her own level. Swimming is usually well-tolerated and an excellent activity for asthmatics.

3 Warmup exercises are often useful in warding off wheezing episodes.

4 We do not wish the student with asthma to feel "different." Please do what is necessary toward accomplishing this end.

5 If this student does have some problem with "endurance" sports, please permit him/her to take the following medication★: _____ *before* participating to *prevent* symptoms.

6 In case of breathing difficulty, talk to the child reassuringly and calmly; have child take prescribed medication (_____).★
If the treatment is ineffective or symptoms severe, notify school nurse or parent immediately.

We welcome your help.

★The student's parent has been given a "school medication request" form to transmit to the school. Where indicated, permit the child to self-medicate her/himself if authorized by physician and parent.

Sincerely,

_____   _____
Physician's Signature   Parent's Signature

_____   _____
Address   Address

_____   _____
City, State, Zip Code   City, State, Zip Code

_____   _____
Telephone   Telephone

Recommendations developed by
American College of Allergy and Immunology
The American College of Allergy and Immunology
800 East Northwest Highway
Suite 1080
Palatine, IL 60067
(312) 359-2800

Endorsed by the Asthma & Allergy Foundation of America, the
American Academy of Allergy & Immunology and the American Academy of Pediatrics

FIG. 5-2 Letters from physicians/parents to school personnel.

helping students recognize sensory information (perception), improve memory, understand oral and written language, or increase cognitive skills. It may also include the trial use of such drugs as stimulants (Ritalin, pemoline [Cylert]) or antidepressants. Anticonvulsants are used for seizure control and are beneficial to some children. The teacher's responsibility to record behavioral and learning changes should be clearly defined (see Prescribed Medications at School, Chapter 6).

Medical research has not demonstrated value for the following interventions: restrictive diets, motor patterning, decrease of the child's sugar intake, or increase of the child's intake of vitamins. Eye-tracking exercises for reading disability (dyslexia) do not help because the brain learns to read, not the eyes.*

Control of Communicable Diseases

Although state and local health departments have the legal responsibility for the control of contagious disease, all school personnel have important roles in the control of communicable diseases because of the hazards they present. A variety of microorganisms including bacteria, viruses, protozoa, and fungi can enter the body and cause infectious disease. If the diseases these organisms cause are transmissible from person to person, they are called *communicable diseases.*

Teachers must be alert for symptoms (Table 5-1 and Appendix I) of suspected disease conditions in pupils. They need to isolate those children and send them to the nurse, principal, or appropriate school authority for possible exclusion from school. Schools need written policies developed with the counsel of local health departments. If such policies do not exist, however, registered school nurses or pediatricians can provide information when needed, and local or state health departments can render school assistance when necessary. When pupils who had been excluded from

school as a result of communicable disease return to school, teachers should be familiar with the readmission procedures to be certain that the pupils have sufficiently recovered to permit their return.

It is possible to prevent and control many diseases through immunizations: diphtheria, whooping cough, tetanus, poliomyelitis, measles, mumps, German measles, and *Haemophilus influenzae* type B (Fig. 5-3). Most states have laws requiring immunizations for school enrollment. These laws should be known by school personnel, and evidence of completion of the required immunizations should be provided by the parents of students entering school.

Vaccine for hepatitis B is recommended for infants and sexually active youth but is not required by schools.* Chickenpox vaccine will soon be widely available; it has been used for children with limited resistance (e.g., during cancer treatment).

AIDS† was first reported in the United States in May, 1981.‡ It is estimated that 1 million Americans may be infected with the virus. The U.S. Centers for Disease Control stated that there were 361,509 cases, and 38,500 persons had died from the disease through 1993.§

The *San Francisco Chronicle*‖ reported 5734 children under 13 years had AIDS. *The World Almanac*¶ stated 629 children had died as of 1993

---

*Committee on School Health: *School health: policy and practice,* Elk Grove Village, Ill, 1993, American Academy of Pediatrics.

*Massachusetts will require hepatitis B vaccination for children entering kindergarten, September 1996. New York, in the summer of 1994, enacted a law requiring the vaccine for entry into day care or preschool.

†For a more detailed discussion of AIDS, see Appendix A and the January 1994 (vol 64, no 1) issue of *The Journal of School Health.*

‡Toolief MS et al: *Pneumocystic carinii* pneumonia and mucosal candidiasis in previously healthy homosexual men: evidence of a new acquired cellular immunodeficiency, *N Engl J Med* 305:1425-1431, 1981.

§US Department of Health and Human Services: *Healthy people 2000, review 1993,* Washington DC, 1994, US Government Printing Office.

‖Study reveals AIDS case total: *San Francisco Chronicle,* Aug 8, 1994, p A3.

¶*The World Almanac,* Funk & Wagnalls, 1995, p 971.

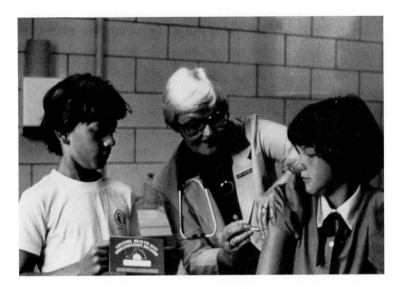

FIG. 5-3 Control of communicable disease is part of the school health services program.

and officials estimated up to 20,000 children would be infected by 1995.*

The majority (estimates range as high as 80%) of cases of AIDS among children are the result of the human immunodeficiency virus (HIV) passing through the placenta of an infected mother and infecting the unborn child. Although a mother may be infected, there is evidence that HIV is not transmitted to the fetus in all cases. Current research indicates that 20% to 50% of infected mothers will not infect their unborn children.†

AIDS is caused by a virus that invades many cells of the body but particularly those vital to the immune defense system and central nervous system. It reproduces rapidly and destroys T-helper cells that are crucial to resisting some kinds of disease. Thus many diseases like chickenpox, measles, and thrush, ordinarily would not be harmful with a normal immune system, can pro-

duce devastating and ultimately lethal diseases in persons with HIV. Specific blood tests can identify people with HIV antibodies. Once the infection is established, it is probably a lifelong infection and those people who carry the virus are potentially infectious to others. No cure has been found.

Treatment is limited to fighting the opportunistic infections and giving antiviral drugs to bolster the immune system. Because treatment reverses nervous system damage, the best result may be prolonged life.

Controlling the spread of HIV and the impact of infection has many research fronts. Education about behavior is one of the school's primary responsibilities. Teacher/staff in-service programs conducted by the school nurse, consulting pediatricians, or local health department personnel must address several aspects of the disease. First, schools should instruct and model universal precautions for handling any bodily fluid that can transmit disease-carrying organisms. For example, blood can carry hepatitis B virus from an infected person, as well as carrying HIV. Second, schools have to abide by federal and state laws that govern confidentiality for any person—child

*Cohen HJ, Papola P, Alvarez M: Neurodevelopmental abnormalities in school-age children with HIV infection, *J School Health Suppl* 64(1):11-13, 1994.
†Arpadi S, Caspe WB: Diagnosis and classification of HIV infection in children, *Pediatr Ann* 19(7):409-420, 1990.

or adult—who has HIV infection. Third, schools need to implement appropriate educational or work adjustments for students or staff with HIV or AIDS. Federal law prohibits discrimination or exclusion based on the diagnosis of an illness, including HIV infection.

Although HIV has been found in body fluids such as blood, semen, saliva, and tears, there are no documented cases showing that anyone has become infected with HIV as a result of contact with saliva or tears. Also, there is no documented evidence that HIV is transmitted person-to-person through the air or by casual contact.

Clearly this provides documented evidence that an exclusionary policy for students or staff in schools is not warranted. There has not been a single case of HIV infection acquired through casual contact in settings such as school or day care.*

The American Academy of Pediatrics and Centers for Disease Control and Prevention have set guidelines for school and day-care attendance for those children with HIV. The guidelines indicate that HIV-infected children can attend school and daycare without restriction and should not be isolated from others, either for their own or anyone else's protection. Their education ought to be developmentally appropriate, and activity participation is altered only as their health status changes, as for any child.†

Philip Nader, MD, Professor of Pediatrics at the University of California, San Diego, and former President of the American School Health Association, stated:‡

No greater public health urgency exists today than to inform students frankly and explicitly how to avoid AIDS infection. The education needs to be directed to all students, regardless of their developing sexual preferences and behaviors. To fail to do so may sentence unknown numbers of children and adolescents to contract not just

a sexually transmitted disease (STD) but one with potential mortality.

The National Association of State Boards of Education reported that as of January 1990, only 29 states had HIV/AIDS education policies. The Association stated that the majority of the policies indicated that it was preferable to begin HIV/AIDS education before children reach the age of puberty. In 1990 a survey of 2150 school districts in the United States by the National Center for Chronic Disease Prevention and Health Promotion, with 78% reporting, HIV education increased from 29.7% in kindergarten to 82.3% in seventh grade and declined to 37.3% by 12th grade.* However, as of 1989, only 66% of school districts in the United States required HIV education of any sort, and only 5% required this education each year from grade 7 through grade 12.

When planning HIV/AIDS education, it is important that the education be developmentally appropriate for the students. To assist school districts who were starting HIV/AIDS education programs, the Centers for Disease Control and Prevention developed guidelines that could be used (see references at end of chapter). It is integral to these guidelines that HIV/AIDS education should not be an isolated program but should be part of quality school health education. The importance of this type of education is exemplified in one of the health goals for the nation for the year 2000†:

Increase to at least 95% the proportion of schools that have age-appropriate HIV education curricula for students in 4th through 12th grade, preferably as a part of quality school health education.

Pediculosis (head lice). Lice are tiny crawling insects that require an animal host and that lay eggs on hair shafts. The most common louse that

---

*Rogers MF et al: Acquired immunodeficiency syndrome in children: report of the Centers for Disease Control: National Surveillance, 1982 to 1985, *Pediatrics* 79:1008-1014, 1987.
†Committee on School Health: *School health: policy and practice,* Elk Grove Village, IL, 1993, American Academy of Pediatrics.
‡Nader P: AIDS: a commentary, *J School Health* 56(3):107-108, 1986.

*Holtzman DS: HIV education and health education in the United States: a national survey and local school district policies and practices, *J School Health* 62:421-427, 1992.
†US Department of Health and Human Services: *Healthy people 2000: National health promotion and disease prevention objectives,* Washington DC, 1990, US Government Printing Office.

FYI   FOR YOUR INFORMATION

Checklist for Classroom Lice Control

_____ Play items (hats, wigs, sweaters, shirts, dresses, etc.) cleaned after each child's use

_____ Headphones sprayed after each child's use

_____ Sweaters and coats hung separately (on backs of chairs or on racks) and not touching

_____ Children's personal items (combs, brushes, hats, scarves, sweaters, coats) not shared

_____ Carpet vacuumed daily

_____ Frequent observations of children for:
  • Nits/lice in hair (on nape of neck, over ears and within ¼ inch of scalp)
  • Scratching of head and neck

Courtesy Austin Independent School District Health Service, Austin, Texas.

needs a human host is the head louse. It is important to understand that pediculosis is not a disease but an infestation that is spread directly between people when the hair of one person, or an object that has been in contact with the hair of an infected person, comes into contact with the hair of an uninfected person.

It is important for teachers to stress with children that they should not share combs, brushes, hats, or other headgear or clothing because this type of contact is another way head lice are transmitted. In classrooms, teachers should be aware that sharing costumes or play items, especially wigs, can result in the spread of head lice. In addition, headphones should be sprayed with a pediculicide to stop head lice spreading from person to person. Coats, hats, and sweaters should be hung separately, as contact between these items can also promote the spread of head lice. Contact with the bed linen of an infested individual, such as a friend invited to spend the night, also can result in spread of lice (see the box).

Itching seems to be the major complaint of students infested with head lice. Infections can result from the open wounds that may result from the scratching that accompanies itching. When teachers observe a student continually scratching his or her head, or if children complain of an itchy scalp, pediculosis should be suspected. The nurse can train teachers and office staff to recognize lice and the whitish oval egg cases (nits) attached to the hair shafts. If the teacher notes these nits, the child should be referred to the school nurse or parent.

Teachers must observe students unobtrusively on a daily basis. The school nurse will prepare instructions so parents can treat any infestation and the child can return to school. Effective shampoos are available without prescription. Nit removal and re-shampooing in about 7 days are important. Some families will need ongoing follow-up to control lice at home to prevent reinfestation of the child.

Scabies. Like head lice, scabies is highly contagious. Scabies is caused by a mite that burrows under the skin, and the individual who has scabies will scratch a lot or will complain of severe itching, especially at the finger webs, wrists, elbows, beltline, armpits, thighs, or buttocks. Once the mite has burrowed into the skin, small lesions will appear. Because of the intense itching and subsequent scratching, secondary infections are common.

The major means of transmission of scabies is by direct person-to-person contact. However, the fabric of undergarments or bed linens of an infected person can also carry the mite. Once the mite has moved to a new individual, it can burrow beneath the skin in less than 3 minutes.

Any student suspected of having scabies should be referred to the school nurse or parent. Specific prescription external lotions to kill mites must be used. Once a child has been referred, the teacher should watch the class closely for other children who may have become infected.

Tuberculosis. Tuberculosis in school-aged children in the United States is more likely if they were born in a country with high rates of infection or have been homeless or living in crowded quarters with an infected adult. A procedure used to detect the disease through the identification of positive reactors is tuberculin testing. In the preferred Mantoux test, a fluid containing proteins extracted from tubercle bacilli is injected intradermally (between the layers of the skin). If the test is positive, a reaction, a raised, inflamed, or red area, appears in 48 to 72 hours where the injection was made.

A positive reaction to the test (inflammation, redness) does not necessarily mean that a person has active tuberculosis. It simply indicates that the person has been exposed to tubercle or similar bacilli and there has been an allergic reaction to these germs. In most communities less than 2% of elementary children have positive reactions. Some children who receive a BCG vaccine in other countries may have a positive skin test. Children with positive reactions to tuberculin tests should receive medical examinations, including chest radiographs to determine the source of exposure and whether active tuberculosis exists. Preventive medicine may be prescribed for daily use for 6 to 12 months when no disease is detected.

Tuberculosis testing should be concentrated in areas where the prevalence of infection is constantly high over a period of time. Therefore routine or periodic testing of schoolchildren should be required only in those schools where the reactor rate is 1% or more* and should take place in other schools on a selective basis only. Local health departments can determine whether the incidence of tuberculin sensitivity exceeds 1% by requiring tests for all those starting school for the first time and children in target grade(s) or by testing randomly selected subsamples annually.

WHAT ARE SCREENING TESTS?

Screening tests are preliminary health evaluations used to identify signs of possible health problems. They are not diagnostic tests. The primary goal of conducting selected screenings in schools is to identify those health conditions among students that may adversely affect the child's ability to learn. Secondary goals include serving as a referral and resource mechanism and making recommendations for adjustments in the school program to accommodate children found to have educationally limiting health problems. Screening may include tests for vision and hearing problems, growth and development, tuberculosis, dental problems, spinal curve deviation, nutrition, lead poisoning, anemia, and others. They should be low cost to provide but not lead to over-referral. They are likely to be administered by trained teachers, nurses, technicians, and other school personnel. They are specific procedures that, in addition to teacher observations and regular checkups, are used to determine the health of students. Proper screenings include criteria by which children should be referred to their health care provider for diagnostic tests.

Vision

Vision screening is usually concerned with problems of central visual acuity, direct vision of near and far objects, and ability to perceive the shape and form of objects in the direct line of vision. However, alertness for signs of eye diseases and other abnormalities must also be maintained. Children with acuity defects may have difficulty perceiving and discriminating details of objects or printed symbols. Thus they are at risk for learning difficulties.

School vision screening usually attempts to reveal the following eye problems:

1. Errors of refraction—eye defects in which images are focused improperly on the retina.
   a. Hyperopia—farsightedness; light rays focus behind the retina, common in those under 10 to 12 years and may change as the eye matures.
   b. Myopia—nearsightedness; light rays focus in front of the retina.

---

*Starke J: *Screening for tuberculosis in school children: what priority should it have?* Austin, TX, 1994, Migrant Clinicians Network.

c. Astigmatism—irregular curvature of the cornea or lens.

d. Anisometropia—difference in refraction of the two eyes.

2. Strabismus—crossed eyes caused by muscle imbalance; the muscles of the two eyes do not work in coordination, resulting in failure of the alignment of the eyes. About 1.5% of children are so afflicted. One eye may not be used, resulting in deterioration of visual acuity, a condition known as amblyopia, which usually can be prevented if treated early.

a. Tropia—constant unequal alignment of the eyes due to muscle imbalance; easily observable.

b. Phoria—a tendency for one eye to turn out of line, especially under visual fatigue or general stress; cover-uncover test can identify.*

3. Color blindness—inability to perceive colors; this condition is usually congenital. Total color blindness is rare and when it occurs, all colors appear as grays. The partial type is more common and is primarily inherited through the mother who carries the recessive gene and is generally not affected. Red and green colors are usually confused in most cases. Approximately 3.8%† of children 6 to 11 years of age have color vision deficiencies; 6.95% of boys and 0.53% of girls are affected; the problem among young white males is about twice as great as among young black males.

The American Academy of Pediatrics states that every child should have a test for visual acuity and strabismus by the age of 4 years.‡

Minimum recommended procedure. The minimum recommended vision screening program varies in schools throughout the United States. The National Society to Prevent Blindness* claims that where a professional eye examination is not possible a child should have an *annual* test for distance visual acuity. However, realizing that time and personnel may not permit such screenings, the minimum for using the Snellen charts or the (H:O:T:V) Matching Symbol Chart should be:

- Prekindergarten—H:O:T:V or Snellen "E"
- Kindergarten or first grade (5 to 6 years)—use Snellen "E" chart
- Third grade (8 years), fifth grade (10 to 11 years), eighth grade (13 years), tenth or eleventh grade (15 to 17 years)—use Snellen letter chart
- All new students as well as teacher and self-referrals—use age or developmentally appropriate test
- All children who exhibit a change in behavior or signs of learning disability

Continuous observation by the teacher and the tester for symptoms related to eye problems should be combined with the screening procedure. Several research studies have indicated a high correlation of this approach with clinical findings by ophthalmologists.

Preschool vision screening is also recommended. Identification of defects such as cross-eye and amblyopia or so-called lazy eye is important. These conditions can lead to unnecessary loss of vision unless detected and treated before the age of 6 years. For nonreaders and hard-to-test children, the H:O:T:V, LH Symbol test,† or Snellen "E" chart is recommended.

Snellen. The most reliable distance vision screening test is the Snellen, using charts that are designed to discover those children with

---

*Texas Department of Health: *Vision screening manual,* Austin, TX, 1992, The Department.

†US Department of Health, Education and Welfare, Public Health Service, National Center for Health Statistics: *Color vision deficiencies in children, United States,* Washington, DC, 1972, US Government Printing Office.

‡Committee on Practice and Ambulatory Medicine, American Academy of Pediatrics: Vision screening and eye examination in children, *Pediatrics* 77:918-919, 1986.

---

*National Society to Prevent Blindness: *Vision screening for children,* New York, 1980, The Society.

†The Lighthouse Inc: *The LH symbol tests,* Addison, IL, 1992, School Health Supply.

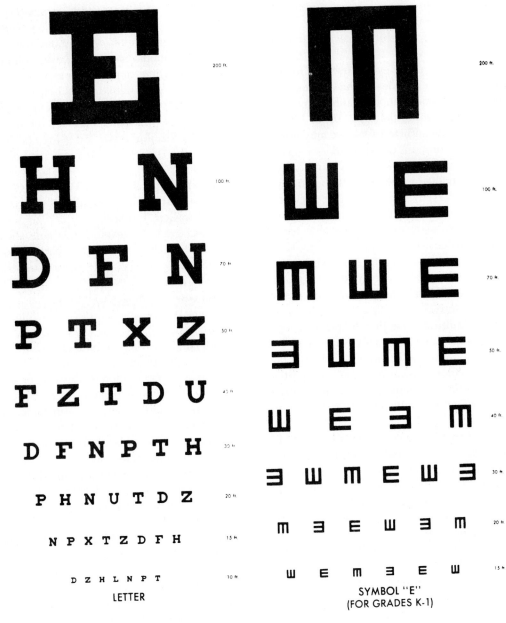

FIG. 5-4 Snellen charts. (Courtesy National Society to Prevent Blindness, New York.)

myopia, although other difficulties may also be found. The Snellen test has been widely used in schools because the charts (Fig. 5-4) are simple, economical, and practical. The test is considered by the National Society to Prevent Blind-

ness as the best single measurement for vision screening.

The Snellen tumbling "E" chart has square-shaped letters or symbols resembling the letter E. These are in specific sizes and in printed rows. The symbol at the top line of the chart is of such a size that a person with normal vision is able to recognize it from a distance of 200 feet, whereas the person with a vision problem may recognize it only from 20 or fewer feet. In each succeeding row, from the top downward, the size of the symbols is reduced to a point that a person with normal vision can see them at distances of 100, 70, 50, 40, 30, and 20 feet, respectively.

To determine visual acuity, the student stands at a distance of 20 feet from the chart and, with one eye covered, reads the smallest letter that can be seen. The student's acuity is recorded as the distance at which the test has been completed and the line at which the student identifies one symbol greater than half the total number of symbols. These numbers are recorded as fractions: 20/20, 20/40, 20/70. They are not actually fractions, but represent a simple method of estimating visual acuity. Thus an acuity of 20/70 means that the student was tested at 20 feet and could identify more than half the letters on line 70. The student was unable to identify more than half the symbols on line 50. The vision of each eye is tested separately. To properly administer the test, the chart should be placed at eye height and be well lit. Frosted light from a 60-watt bulb to reduce glare from other sources should be used.

Criteria for recommending students for a retest may be the following*:

- Through 4 years of age—20/50 or worse in either eye (i.e., cannot read one more than half the symbols on 20/40 line; or two or more line difference between the eyes, e.g., 20/20 in one eye and 20/40 in the other).
- Five years or older—20/40 or worse in either eye (i.e., cannot read over half the symbols on 20/30 line).

Individuals are considered legally blind if their vision is not correctable beyond 20/200 or if

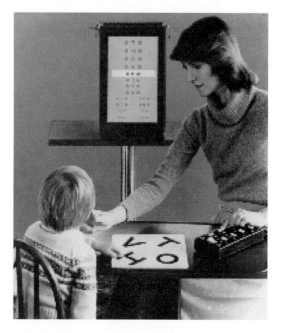

FIG. 5-5 Children must be taught how to respond to vision screening. (Courtesy Good-Lite Co.)

they have a loss of 80% or more of their field of vision.

H:O:T:V test. The H:O:T:V test was developed for use specifically with very young children, children who are developmentally delayed, or children who are unable to read. This would include children from other countries who have not yet developed English language skills. The basic procedures for administration of the test (Fig. 5-5) and the bases for referral are the same as for the Snellen "E" test. The test uses the letters H, O, T, and V (Fig. 5-6). Children are given cards that contain these letters and are asked to match letters on the screen with a letter on the card that they are given.

For any test, within about 2 weeks after being retested, children, for whom the second findings are the same as the first and provided that the teacher's observations indicate an abnormality, should be referred for examination by a professionally qualified person (Fig. 5-7).

---

*Texas Department of Health: *Vision screening manual,* Austin, TX, 1992, The Department.

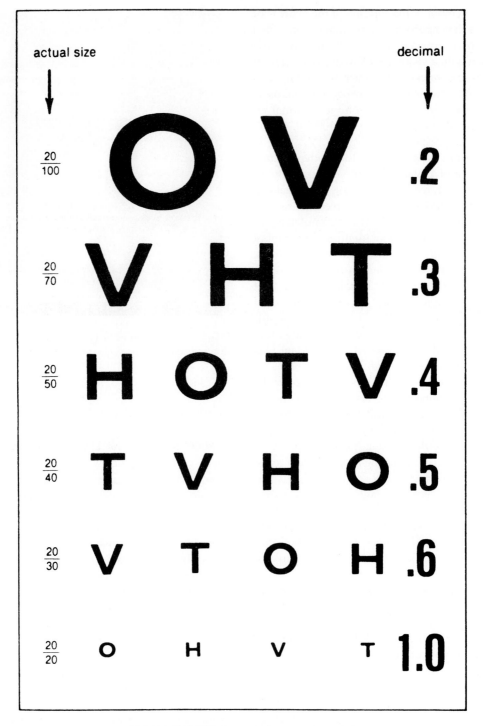

FIG. 5-6 H:O:T:V chart. (Courtesy Good-Lite Co.)

V10 (Parent) Rev. 01/94

Austin Independent School District
Vision referral

Dear Parent:

Your child did not pass the school vision screening. The results of the vision screening indicate the need for a professional eye examination by an eye doctor of your choice. **If your child is currently under treatment by an eye doctor or has had an eye examination within the past year, please call the vision and hearing office (450-1604).** If you have any other questions about the vision screening or think you may qualify for financial assistance for eye care, the screening specialist will be able to help you. Please take this form with you to the examination. The doctor will complete it and return it to the AISD Vision and Hearing Office so that your child's health record can be kept current.

Remember: How well your child sees may determine how well your child learns.

Estimado padre/madre de familia:

Su hijo(a) no pasó la prueba de visión de la escuela. Los resultados de la prueba selectiva de los ojos indican la necesidad de un examen profesional de los ojos con un oculista elegido por usted. Si su hijo(a) está ya recibiendo atención médica de un oculista, o se le ha hecho un examen de los ojos durante el último año, haga el favor de llamar a la Oficina de Visión y Audición (450-1604). Si tiene alguna pregunta que hacer con respecto de la prueba de visión, o cree llenar las condiciones para ayuda financiera para el cuidado de los ojos, el técnico de las pruebas podrá ayudarle. Haga el favor de llevar esta forma al examen. El doctor la llenará y la devolverá a la Oficina de Visión y Audición del AISD

Recuerde: La Medida en que su hijo(a) vea bien puede determinar la medida en que aprenda bien.

Student's name _____   Date of birth _____   Grade _____

School _____   Teacher or counselor _____

Date of test _____   Screening specialist _____

Report of school vision screening

Reason for test: ☐ Routine screening   ☐ Retest of known case   ☐ Referred by _____

Results:

Distance acuity	Near acuity	Muscle function
Right eye 20/ Left eye 20/	Right eye 20/ Left eye 20/	Far: Pass Fail Near: Pass Fail

Student was tested with/without glasses

Test used: HOTV   Titmus E   Titmus letters   Sloan
(20/30 is considered passing for school screening)

Comments: _____

Eye specialists report

Diagnosis: ☐ Myopia   ☐ Hyperopia   ☐ Amblyopia   ☐ Strabismus   ☐ Astigmatism   ☐ Phoria

☐ Other: (Please explain) _____

Acuity:

Without correction	With correction
Right eye 20/ Left eye 20/	Right eye 20/ Left eye 20/

Treatment: ☐ Glasses   ☐ Medical   ☐ Surgery   ☐ Patching   ☐ Observation
☐ Constant wear
☐ Near vision only   ☐ Other _____
☐ May remove for P.E.   ☐ Treatment not needed at this time

Re-examination recommended in: _____ Weeks _____ Months _____ Years _____ Not required

Comments: _____

This referral was: ☐ Valid   ☐ Invalid   Doctor: Please return this form completed to:

Dates of examination _____

Doctor's name _____ M.D./O.D.

Address _____

City _____ State _____ Zip _____

FIG. 5-7 Vision Screening Record.

Additional tests. The National Society to Prevent Blindness recommends several other tests that may be added to the minimal procedure. These include the plus sphere lens, muscle imbalance, and color vision tests. Training is specifically needed to administer any of these screening tests.

Plus sphere lens. The plus sphere lens is used to detect hyperopia. The test is administered by having children wear a pair of glasses with convex (hyperopic) lenses of specified strength (+2.25 diopters* for the first three grades and +1.75 diopters from fourth grade on) and requiring them to read the 20-foot line of the Snellen chart. Each eye is tested separately. If they read the line, they have failed the test. The convex lens blurs the vision of the children with no refractive error and makes correction for the hyperopic youngsters enabling them to read the chart. Pupils who fail the test should be retested. If the results are the same or there are other signs noted through teacher observations, these children should be referred for professional diagnosis. The plus sphere test should be given only to those pupils who do not wear glasses and who satisfactorily pass the Snellen distance acuity test.

Muscle imbalance. Muscle imbalance refers to the inability of the two eyes to work together. There are a number of tests to measure this condition. The cover-uncover test is a simple way to detect latent strabismus (crossed eye not readily noticed) or phoria. In some children this condition reveals itself when they are very tired or under emotional stress. Latent strabismus may manifest itself in only one eye, or it may alternate between the eyes.

The cover-uncover test determines whether eye alignment is maintained when one eye is covered while the other is fixed on an object. The alignment of each eye should be determined for both distant and near points.

The procedure for testing should be as follows:

---
*Diopter, unit of measurement of strength or refractive power of lenses.

- Have the pupil look at a small light or object 20 feet away.
- Place a cover card in front of one of the pupil's eyes so that the light or object cannot be seen with that eye. Watch to see if the alignment of the covered eye is maintained; note whether the eye turns in, out, up, or down or holds its fixed position.
- After a few seconds, move the cover card to the other eye. The previously covered eye is watched for a shift in the direction of its fixation.
- Repeat the test, having the pupil look at a small light or object 8 to 10 inches in front of the nose. If the muscle balance of the eye is essentially normal, there should be no marked change in its fixation on covering or when the cover is removed.

Pupils who show marked deviation from normal should be retested by a different screener if possible, and if the same results are discovered, they should be referred for professional diagnosis.

Color vision test. The color vision test is a procedure to determine whether a person is color blind, or unable to discriminate between certain colors, usually red and green and sometimes blue and yellow. Two satisfactory tests for school use are the Hardy-Rand-Ritter test and the Ishihara test.

Color blindness is inherited, affects more boys than girls, and cannot be corrected. Adjustments to the abnormality are important, and students should be aware of this limitation, especially when making vocational choices or when learning to recognize traffic lights. It is desirable to test young people once before they complete elementary school.

Other devices and procedures. Numerous other instruments and procedures are available for vision screening and testing. Adequate screener training and awareness of language or developmental characteristics of the child are critical to avoid unnecessary referrals. Some of these instruments and procedures include the Telebinocular (a stereoscopic instrument to measure muscle imbalance, visual acuity, and color vi-

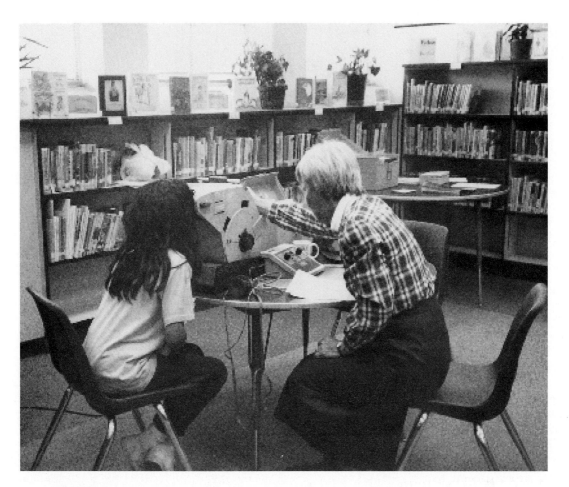

FIG. 5-8 Titmus vision tester aids mass screening in any school location. (Courtesy Austin Independent School District Health Services, Austin, Texas.)

sion), the Ortho-Rater (similar to the Telebinocular), the Titmus vision tester (for near- and far-sightedness) (Fig. 5-8), and the Massachusetts vision kit (visual acuity, plus sphere, and muscle balance test).

Several modified clinic techniques have been used. The procedures used to test vision include visual acuity (Snellen "E" chart), binocular coordination (cover test for muscle imbalance), refractive error (retinoscope for myopia, hyperopia, and astigmatism), and use of ophthalmoscope to inspect the internal eye.

Photoscreening devices are now available and

hold promise for effective screening of very young children or special populations who are difficult to screen.* Use of photography-based tools such as the MTI Photoscreener† or VisiScreen OSS-C‡ can identify children whose eye conditions may lead to amblyopia (Fig. 5-9). All screening programs

---

*Freedman HL, Preston KL: Polaroid photo screening for amblyogenic factors, *Ophthalmology* 99(12):1785-1795, 1992.
†MTI Photoscreener, Medical Technology, Inc, Cedar Falls, IA.
‡Cogen MS, Ottemiller DE: Photorefractor for detection of treatable eye disorders in preverbal children, *Ala Med* 62(3):16-20,1992.

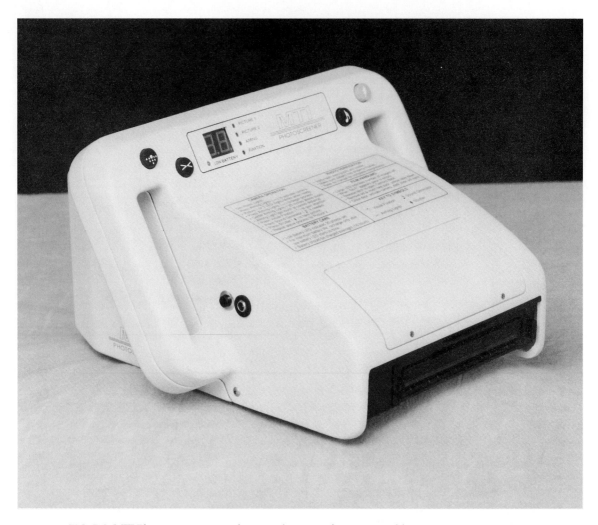

FIG. 5-9 MTI Photoscreener uses photography to test for vision problems (Courtesy Medical Technology, Inc.)

and instruments should be planned in coordination with local eye care professionals.

Teacher involvement. The individual who conducts and manages screening differs among schools and school districts. Often a health professional or administrator is responsible for the program, but trained teachers or volunteers can perform mass screenings. Although the nurse is often involved in the screening of vision, teachers' involvement in vision testing is important because:

- They better understand the children with vision problems in their classes
- They become more sensitive through continually observing children who may have vision problems
- They can make the vision screening program a part of the health instruction program
- They can describe to parents the impact of a vision problem on the child's academic progress and stress the importance of fol-

lowing prescribed treatment (e.g., patch, glasses).

Hearing

Approximately 3% to 6% of all children are affected with some type of hearing impairment.* This impairment can affect the child's speech development, attentiveness, behavior, and learning. Early detection of hearing impairment can lead to possible remediation of the problem before it becomes a handicapping condition.

Hearing loss may be classified in three ways; however, the most serious losses are conductive loss, sensorineural loss, and mixed (conductive/ sensorineural) loss. Conductive loss is the most common among children and is usually correctable. This means that the sound waves are being blocked from reaching the inner ear. Such things as a buildup of earwax, foreign objects in the auditory canal, colds that cause a stuffiness in the eustachian tubes, and congenital malformations are some of the causes of conductive disorders. Sensorineural disorders are more serious, as they may not be remediable. This type of disorder may be caused by damage to the auditory nerve as a result of viral infections, constant exposure to loud noises such as gunfire or loud music, or head trauma.

The procedure generally used to test the hearing of children is performed with the puretone audiometer. It requires special training to administer and interpret.

Puretone audiometer. The puretone audiometer (Fig. 5-10) is an individual testing device that measures the ability to hear sounds of varying frequencies† or hertz (Hz) at different intensities of sound called decibels.‡

A procedure known as the sweep-check test

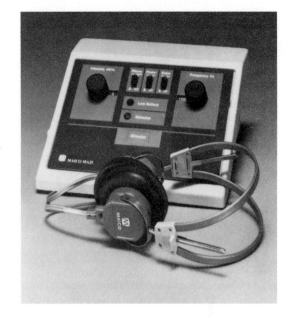

FIG. 5-10 Puretone audiometer. (Courtesy Maico Hearing Instruments, Inc.)

method has been used in schools to expedite the hearing screening process. It is best if a sound-proof booth is available. Each ear is tested separately with the intensity dial set at 10 decibels. The tone dial is changed rather quickly through 1000, 2000, 4000, and 6000 frequencies (CPS; cycles/second) and reset at 20 decibels for 4000 frequencies. The extremely low and high tones may be omitted. Many sweep-check methods involve the 500, 1000, 2000, and 4000 frequencies at 20 decibels. From 5% to 10% of the students fail this test. Those students who fail to hear one tone or more in either ear in this sweep-check method should be given a second screening test. Failure to pass the repeated screening should be followed by a threshold test. In this test, pupils listen to all the intensities of sound of each frequency, with the results plotted on audiograms. The findings are then interpreted by the trained screener administering the test, and decisions are made whether to refer these children for specialized examinations (Fig. 5-11). The criteria for referral include hearing losses of 20 decibels or more at any two fre-

---

*Wold S: *School nursing: a framework for practice,* North Branch, MN, 1981, Sunrise River Press.
†Frequencies, qualities of sound caused by the number of vibrations per second of an object resulting in high and low tones, for example, strings on a piano.
‡Decibels, units of sound intensity.

H10 (Parent) Rev. 01/94 .... Austin Independent School District
.... **Hearing referral**

Dear Parent:

Your child did not pass the school hearing screening. The results of the screening indicate the need for a thorough ear examination and hearing evaluation by an ear specialist (otologist) or doctor of your choice. If your child is currently under medical care for an **ear infection, allergies,** etc. please call the Vision and Hearing office (450-1604). If you have any questions about the screening or if you think you may qualify for financial assistance, the screening specialist will be able to help you.

Please take this form with you to the examination. The doctor will complete it and return it to the AISD Vision and Hearing Office so that your child's health record can be kept current.

Remember: How well your child hears may determine how well your child learns.

Muy estimado Padres de familia:

Su hijo(a) no pasó la prueba del oído de la escuela. Los resultados de la prueba indican la necesidad de un examen completo y de una evaluación de su facultad auditiva por un especialista (otólogo), o un doctor que ustedes escojan. Si su hijo(a) está actualmente bajo cuidado médico por alguna infección del oído, alergias, etc., tengan la bondad de llamar a la oficina de VISION AND HEARING (Visión y audición), al 450-1604. Si tienen preguntas sobre la prueba o creen que reúnen las condiciones para ayuda financiera, la especialista en las pruebas podrá ayudarles. Haga el favor de llevar esta forma al examen. El doctor la llenará y la devolverá a la Oficina de Visión y Audición del AISD

Recuerde: La Medida en que su hijo(a) oiga bien puede determinar la medida en que aprenda bien.

Report of school hearing screening

Student's name _____   Date of birth _____   Grade _____

School _____   Teacher or counselor _____

Date of test _____   Testing technician _____

Reason for test: ☐ Routine screening   ☐ Retest of known case   ☐ Referred by _____

Results:

Hearing screening performed at 20 dB

Frequency (cps)	250	500	1000	2000	4000	6000
Right ear:						
Left ear:						

(✓=pass   X=did not pass)

Comments:

Report of otologist or examining physician

Diagnosis: ☐ Otitis   ☐ Cerumen   ☐ Sensorineural loss   ☐ Conductive loss   ☐ Perforated TM

☐ Other: (Please explain) _____

Patient was: ☐ Examined and treated

☐ Examined, no treatment prescribed due to: ☐ Permanent neurosensory loss .... ☐ Right ear ☐ Left ear

☐ Congenital disorder .... ☐ Right ear ☐ Left ear

☐ Examined, no problem found   ☐ Other _____

Treatment or recommendations prescribed: _____

I expect that on completion of treatment there will be: ☐ No significant hearing handicap that may interfere with learning.

☐ A handicap that may interfere with learning.

Comments: _____

This referral was: ☐ Valid ☐ Invalid   Doctor: Please return this form completed to:

Dates of examination _____

Doctor's name _____ M.D.

Address _____

City _____ State _____ Zip _____

FIG. 5-11 Audiogram.

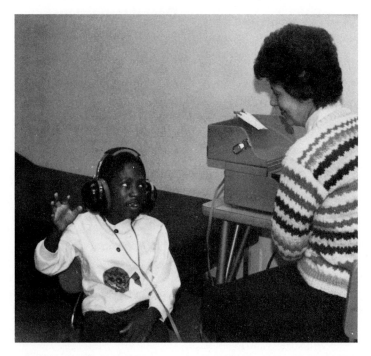

FIG. 5-12 Hearing screening is used to identify sporadic or constant hearing losses. (Courtesy Wichita Public Schools, Wichita, Kansas.)

quencies in either ear, or a loss of 30 decibels or more at any single frequency in either ear.

Audiometers are usually calibrated in round-numbered frequencies such as 125, 250, 500, 1000, 2000, on up to 8000—the range of sounds that are normally heard by human beings. The machines are also calibrated by sound intensities, with the step intervals being from 5 or 10 decibels to a maximum of 100 decibels.

The American Academy of Pediatrics* recommends that every child have a hearing test by the age of 4 years (Fig. 5-12). Children with ear disease, language or speech problems, or other indications of possible hearing abnormality should be tested when conditions are first recognized regardless of age. Hearing testing in schools should be done annually in preschool, kindergarten, and grade 1 and then in grades 3, 6, 9, and 12. Children with persistent hearing impairments or frequent middle ear infections should be tested annually.

Growth and Development

Periodic measurements of the heights and weights of children will aid in understanding the growth and development (see Appendix K) of boys and girls in terms of: (1) normal progression, (2) extent of overweight, and (3) extent of underweight. Growth monitoring as a part of health supervision through accurate measures made at school or during medical office visits is a more responsible approach than infrequent public mass screenings.* Routine measurement of children's

---

*Committee on School Health: *School health: a guide for health professionals,* Evanston, IL, 1987, American Academy of Pediatrics.

*Rosenbloom AL: Height screening in the community, *Clin Pediatr* 29(5):288-292, 1990.

height and weight is useful if it is part of a health education program, is used as a follow-up or evaluation of a nutrition program (e.g., weight control), is part of a battery of tests to monitor growth and development, or is used as a screening test to detect growth problems in areas where there is a treatable condition that produces growth retardation. Mere observation of weight and height increases, or the failure of children to gain weight, may not in themselves be significant in the growth process. Children's growth patterns are individual, and unless an instrument is used to show this, school personnel may be led to erroneous conclusions about overweight, underweight, or abnormal growth conditions. Weighing and measuring can be valuable in the appraisal process if the information is recorded and plotted on growth charts for interpretation, as illustrated in the height-weight records shown in Figs. 5-13 and 5-14.

Measures of body fat composition or percentages are being introduced to measure fitness. A teacher, nurse, or volunteer can be trained to accurately use a quality set of skin-fold calipers. Data on young people collected during the National Children and Youth Fitness Study II* are currently being analyzed. At this point, one can measure skinfolds for changes over time.

Height and weight should be measured at the beginning, middle, and end of the school year. It is important that measurements be accurately taken and recorded (Fig. 5-15).

Children in grade 3 and up can be taught to take these measurements. Teachers or volunteers can record data on the growth charts. This activity provides an excellent teachable moment for health instruction about growth patterns and fitness.

The school or public health nurse should review the charts and follow-up on students whose growth change or inadequate growth is of concern.

---

*Ross JG, Pate RR: The national children and youth fitness study. II. A summary of findings, *J Phys Educ Recreation Dance* 58(9):51-56, 1987.

Dental Inspections

Dental inspections refer to procedures generally performed by dentists or dental hygienists using mouth mirrors and explorers to locate decayed teeth, as well as to check for diseases of tissue surrounding the teeth and for malocclusion. These inspections are not complete examinations because they do not include radiographic examinations.

Ideally, children should visit their family dentists twice yearly for appraisal and necessary treatment. There is evidence to indicate that only 20% of the population is following this practice.

Opinions differ regarding whether periodic dental inspections should be conducted in schools. Several reasons causing this dilemma include the following:

- There is little need to locate cases because dental decay is the most common health defect found in school-aged children.
- There may be a poor geographic distribution of affordable dentists and dental hygienists. Access to dental care is also limited by financial resources.
- Most families do not have dental insurance through private or public-funded plans.

Dental inspections and preventive care in schools vary widely as to their inclusion and frequency. In Pennsylvania, dental examinations by a dentist must be conducted by schools on the original entry of children, as well as in the third and seventh grades. In elementary schools, dental hygienists may provide a screening, prophylactic care, and an educational program. Some schools coordinate with the local health department or dental society to administer flouride treatment (rinses) and/or surface sealants on the first molars of children with high caries risk.

Sickle Cell Anemia

Sickle cell anemia is a rare disorder of red blood cells caused by abnormal hemoglobin that affects the cells' ability to carry oxygen. The normal red blood cells that usually appear disk shaped are crescent or sickle shaped. The condition is found among the Black population and to a lesser degree

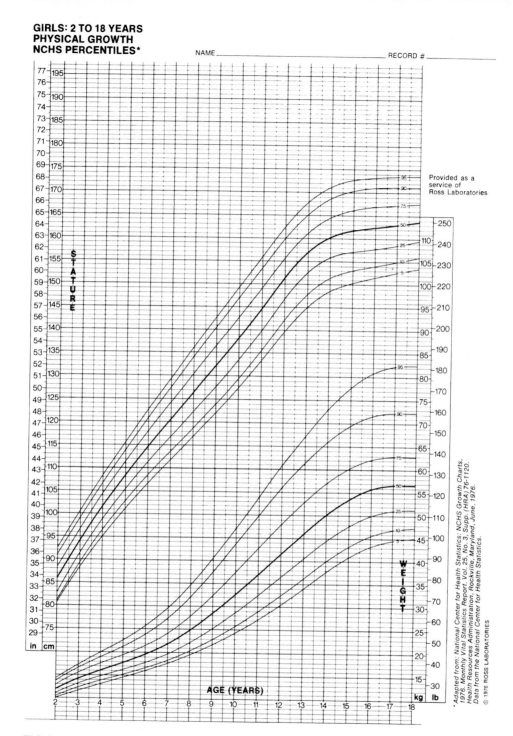

FIG. 5-13 NCHS growth chart for girls. (Modified from Hamill PVV, Drizd TA, Johnson CL, Reed RB, Roche AF, Moore WM: Physical growth: National Center for Health Statistics percentiles, *Am J Clin Nutr* 32:607-629, 1979; data from the National Center for Health Statistics (NCHS), Hyattsville, Maryland; courtesy Ross Products Division, Abbott Laboratories, Columbus, Ohio.)

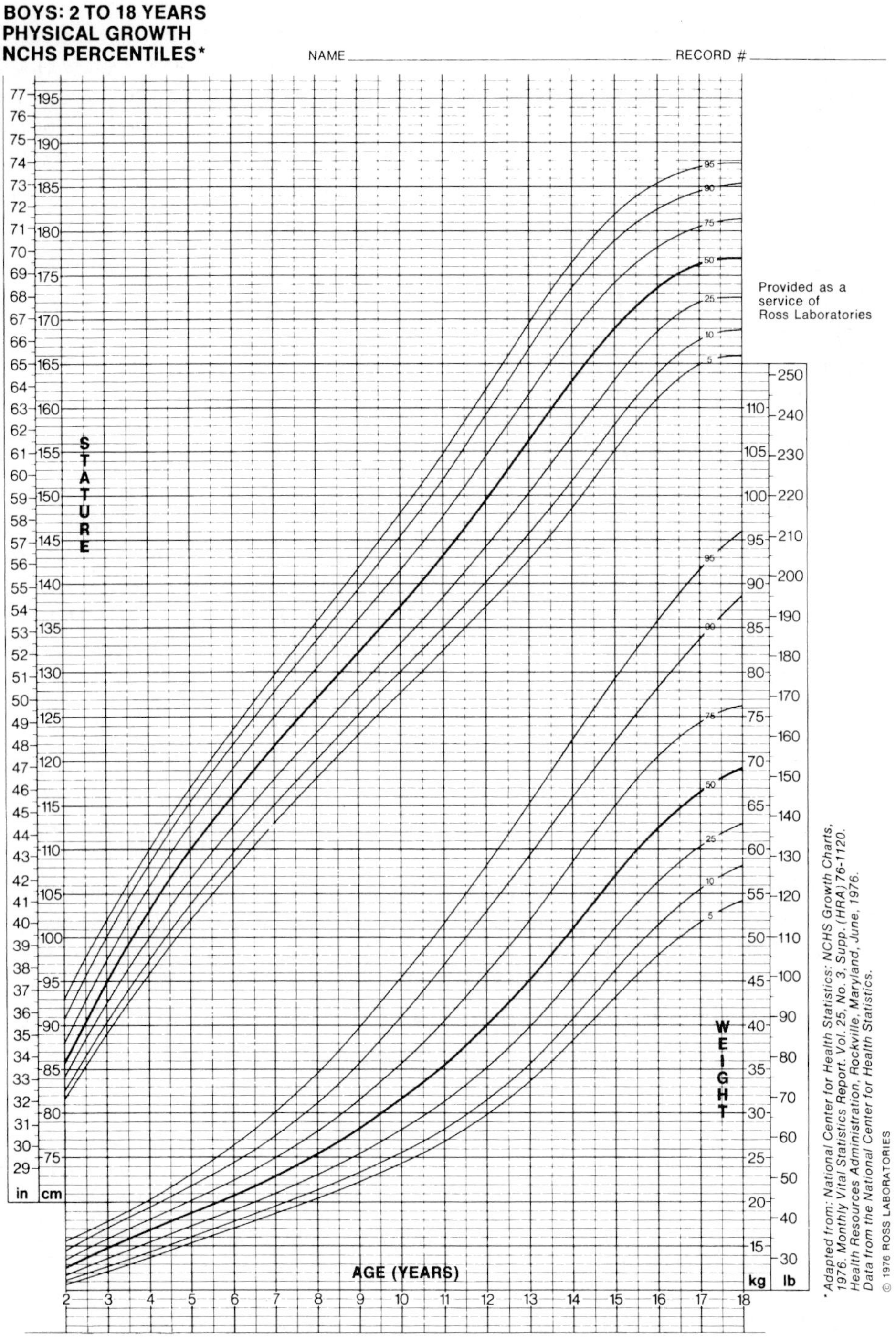

FIG. 5-14 NCHS growth chart for boys. (Modified from Hamill PVV, Drizd TA, Johnson CL, Reed RB, Roche AF, Moore WM: Physical growth: National Center for Health Statistics percentiles, *Am J Clin Nutr* 32:607-629, 1979; data from the National Center for Health Statistics (NCHS), Hyattsville, Maryland; courtesy Ross Products Division, Abbott Laboratories, Columbus, Ohio.)

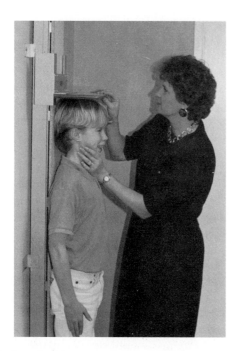

FIG. 5-15 Height assessment. (Courtesy Austin Independent School District, Austin, Texas.)

in individuals with Mediterranean ancestry (Greek, Italian), in Caribbean islanders, and in people in South and Central America. The sickle cell trait is a genetic factor found in an estimated 8% of the Black population,* whereas the disease itself, sickle cell anemia, is found in approximately 1 in 400 to 500 Blacks. The condition results in the swelling of joints; pain in the abdomen, legs, and arms; poor appetite; and weakness. The anemia cannot be cured, but the "crisis" situation, which is usually triggered by a bacterial infection, can be treated. The school nurse should be sought for advice about first aid for "crisis situations." Sometimes a crisis condition can be prevented by ensuring adequate water intake and avoiding infections, chilling, and contact sports.

Some community programs provide screening in conjunction with health education. The purpose of the screening is to identify sickle cell trait. Most children with the disease will be identified and diagnosed before school age. Venous blood is tested by direct hemoglobin electrophoresis to determine if the blood cells differ from normal ones. Only one test is needed to determine an individual's status. The American Academy of Pediatrics* states that screening of well school-aged children is not indicated.

Diabetes

Diabetes is the most common chronic endocrine disease of individuals 10 to 69 years of age. The prevalence among school-aged children is 1.9 per 1,000.† Diabetes is not an infectious disease. It can be detected by blood test to determine the level of sugar and ketones (acids) in the blood. Although schools do not conduct such tests, every effort should be made to identify diabetic children in order to provide needed help. When students first enter school, parent completion of health histories or visits should be used to identify diabetic pupils.

Diabetes results from failure of the pancreas to make a sufficient amount of insulin. Without insulin, food cannot be used properly. Diabetes currently cannot be cured but can be controlled by daily injections of insulin and a prescribed food plan.

There are two types of diabetes: type I and type II. Type II, or noninsulin dependent diabetes, usually develops in individuals over 40 years of age. Thus the teacher will generally see the child who has type I, or insulin-dependent diabetes. In general, students with type I diabetes will already be under the care of a physician, but the teacher should be aware of which children in class have this disorder in case one of them begins to show symptoms of insulin shock or diabetic acidosis. Schools should have a written plan of action to respond to these signs. If a child with diabetes seems to show uncharacteristic sleepiness or com-

*Behrman RE, editor: *Nelson textbook of pediatrics*, ed 14, Philadelphia, 1992, WB Saunders.

*Committee on School Health: *School health: a guide for health professionals*, Evanston, IL, 1987, American Academy of Pediatrics.
†Behrman RE, editor: *Nelson textbook of pediatrics*, ed 14, Philadelphia, 1992, WB Saunders.

plains of stomach pain and begins vomiting, the care plan should be initiated immediately and the office notified.

Children with diabetes can participate in all school activities but should wear a medical identification tag and be observed during unusual schedule changes. Physical education should not be scheduled just before lunch, nor should a child be assigned a late lunch period. Most will check their blood sugar level once or twice during the school day using a small lancet and device called a glucometer. The care plan indicates what actions to take depending on the reading.* Most will need midmorning and midafternoon snacks. Teachers should have sugar packets or cubes readily available in the event of insulin shock (a condition in which too much insulin is circulating in the bloodstream). The sugar or sugared drink should be referred to as "medicine" or "treatment," not as "candy" or "treat."

Epilepsy and Seizures

Epilepsy is a disruption of the electrical impulses to the brain that causes nerves to send out erratic impulses through the body, resulting in a seizure, or sudden alteration of consciousness, or spastic movements known as convulsions. Teachers should be aware of seizure disorders among children, because to an uninformed teacher who encounters a child undergoing a seizure, the experience can be traumatic. Epilepsy occurs in approximately 6 children/1000,* with 75% of the cases beginning before the eighteenth birthday. Four of five cases of epilepsy, where known, can be controlled with medication; 50% can be totally controlled and 30% partially controlled. Excessive fatigue, overexposure to heat or sunlight, and situations that cause stress can affect the seizure threshold in children and increase the incidence of attacks.

*From Graff JC, Ault MM, Guess D, Taylor M, Thompson B: *Health care for students with disabilities*, Baltimore, 1990, Paul H Brookes.

Schools must identify students with epilepsy to be able to best provide for their safety and to enable classmates to understand and not tease these pupils. Identification is best when students first enter school through parent interviews and the completion of health histories, or through a review of health records. Teachers may be asked to record seizure events, as well as students' cognitive and behavior development. The doctor needs this information to prescribe the medication dosage that will adequately limit seizures and minimize side effects (see Chapter 7 for ways to handle seizures at school).

Spinal Curves

Scoliosis is a condition in which there is a lateral curvature and rotation of the spine. It is found in 0.5% to 2.0% of young people. It is most commonly observed in children aged 12 through 16 years and progresses until skeletal maturity is attained. Serious curves needing bracing or surgery occur more often in girls than boys. Spinal curves may also include severe roundback or be a result of other conditions such as unequal leg length during adolescence.

The purpose of scoliosis screening is to detect abnormal curvature of the spine at an early stage so that corrective procedures can be instituted. Screening should occur when skeletal growth is rapid—in girls at 9 to 14 years of age and boys at 11 to 15 years of age. As of 1989, 21 states required spinal screening for students. Schools commonly conduct the screening in grades 5 through 9 or 10. The number and frequency of these procedures depend on the resources available and local school district policy. The procedure can be completed by nurses and others with special training. Health department personnel or local orthopedic specialists can help develop program guidelines.

The screening procedure for scoliosis should be performed after pupils have removed their shirts or blouses. Girls may wear brassieres or swim tops. Pupils should be observed from the back and should stand erect with the shoulders back, head up and looking forward, hands hanging at sides, knees straight, and feet together. The screener should note whether the shoulders, scapulae, arm hang, and hips are in a level plane; one should not be higher or lower than the other. Also, the straightness of the spine should be checked; it should not bend right or left. The pupil should then bend forward at the waist, head hanging relaxed, arms dangling from the shoulders, and knees straight (Fig. 5-16). The screener should observe the surface of the back at eye level to detect prominence of the thoracic ribs and the area around the vertebral column. The chest should be symmetrical, and an imaginary line drawn from scapula to scapula should be parallel to the floor. As the student resumes an upright position, the back movement should be checked to note prominences or spinal curvatures. Abnormalities detected should be referred to a physician for examination and treatment.

Scoliosis screening may be controversial because the testing procedure (the bending test) produces a large number of false-positive results and marginal cases that may not need attention. Nevertheless, it has been suggested that this screening

become a part of the child's physician examination at every visit.*

Other Screening Procedures

A variety of additional types of screening appraisals for such problems as speech difficulties, hypertension, and learning disabilities also can occur in schools. Their frequency and extent vary widely throughout the United States.

WHAT ARE HEALTH HISTORIES AND INVENTORIES?

Histories and brief inventories (Fig. 5-17) are informational accounts of the health practices and behavior of children that take the form of written questionnaires or checklists. They are often neglected, yet they are one of the most important parts of periodic health appraisals. In-depth nursing reviews should include information about past health problems (physical and emotional)

---

*Morais T, Bernier M, Turcotte F: Age- and sex-specific prevalence of scoliosis and the value of school screening programs, *Am J Public Health* 75(12):1377-1380, 1985.

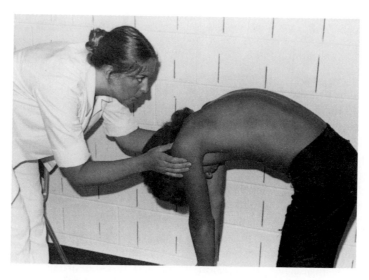

FIG. 5-16 Scoliosis screening. (Photo by L.K. Olsen.)

Medical Alert Card

(1) The information on this card is to alert the school nurse to any health problem which may need attention or limit the student's activities.

STUDENT _____ SCHOOL _____

(2) STUDENT'S BIRTHDATE: _____ / _____ / _____ GRADE _____

TEACHER _____ DATE _____
TELEPHONE NUMBERS WHERE PARENTS MAY BE REACHED DURING THE DAY:

(3)

_____	_____	_____	[ ]	[ ]
Parent/Guardian Last Name	First Name	Initial	Phone # during school	Home phone #
_____	_____	_____	[ ]	[ ]
Parent/Guardian Last Name	First Name	Initial	Phone # during school	Home phone #

Health Problem or other information for the nurse _____

(4) _____

_____

_____

List any medicines the student takes regularly:

A. At home _____

B. At school _____

FIG. 5-17 Annual medical alert card. (Courtesy Austin Independent School District Health Service, Austin, Texas.)

and their treatment, an orderly review of body systems, relevant information about current and past special problems of other members of the family, and information about the student's academic achievement and school adjustments. This information provides background data about the health of children not usually revealed by other procedures but are useful in the health appraisals of pupils. The teacher needs to know that a child with asthma carries an inhaler. A periodic health examination may not reveal that a student has migraine headaches or occasional seizures. These inventories help in understanding the health status of boys and girls and may be particularly useful if medical examinations are conducted for school-related purposes. The forms should be completed during enrollment. The data become a part of the child's health record.

WHAT ARE MEDICAL EXAMINATIONS?

Medical examinations refer to those appraisals completed by physicians. Examinations conducted at school are usually for specific purposes such as appraisal for special education eligibility or athletic participation (Fig. 5-18).

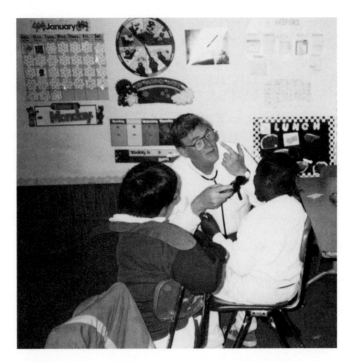

FIG. 5-18 School physicians can perform appraisals in the school where the student is comfortable. (Courtesy Austin Independent School District Health Services, Austin, Texas.)

The health examination includes a comprehensive review of the health history and body systems:

- Growth measures
- Vital signs: pulse, blood pressure, respiration
- Appearance: skin, hair/nails
- Head to toes: eyes, ears, nose, throat, lymph nodes

  Chest, lungs, heart

  Abdomen

  Genitalia

  Back: spine and limbs

  Neurological system: reflexes
- Urine

The American Academy of Pediatrics believes an ongoing health care provider or family physician is the most appropriate source for a health appraisal to ensure proper treatment for identified problems. Therefore it generally should be performed outside the school setting. Circumstances such as legal requirements, poverty, and lack of health care resources, however, may require such examinations to be conducted in some schools.

The Academy states that routine, periodic, health examinations in schools have low effectiveness in the identification of serious, uncared for medical problems. They do not recommend such appraisals.

The frequency of health examinations for children in school is set by law in some states. Where there are no legal directives, local school and medical officials must make these decisions. Appraisals probably should be performed when pupils start school, again in grades 6 or 7, and before leaving school in grades 11 or 12. In addition, they should be conducted for those who have been identified as having particular problems. The Academy states that priority for school examinations should be given to high-risk children: those who may be homeless or have low socioeconomic status, poor school performance, existing handicaps, frequent absence, and disciplinary problems.

WHAT ARE PSYCHOLOGICAL EXAMINATIONS AND TESTS?

Psychological examinations and tests include a variety of procedures to test personality, behavior, and social acceptance of pupils as well as intelligence, achievements, and aptitudes. They are usually administered by psychologists and psychometrists who are members of a child guidance or pupil personnel services program. School counselors and school psychologists have the expertise to train teachers to recognize signs of chronic emotional distress or crisis responses. The findings from formal appraisals, together with teacher observations, help determine the necessary action. Pupils with suspected emotional difficulties who are identified through these evaluations may need to be referred for medical or psychiatric consultation. Parent conferences and sometimes additional testing at school facilitate referral for proper medical attention.

Recognizing Emotional Problems

An estimated 12% of young people under age 18 years suffer from mental disorders serious enough to require treatment. These disorders include attention deficit, depression, alcohol or drug use, and severe conduct disorders.* Children who are emotionally disturbed or who exhibit behavior that causes one to suspect mental illness or crisis reactions need to be identified early to receive the greatest help. Elementary schools with a Student Assistance Program or other multidisciplinary "case conference" process frequently can provide attention to students with behavior problems. The teacher is the main contact person with pupils and is in a strategic position to render valuable service. The importance of teacher observations was previously stressed; however, the specific signs of concern that the teacher must recognize are found in Table 5-1 and Appendix I. It has been estimated that teachers can identify

70% of the emotionally disturbed children, and with a clinic team, 90% of their problems can be discovered. Dysfunctional behaviors result from an array of causes: biochemical, family changes, school or learning problems to name a few. Depression in children is not well recognized by many teachers. Teachers must be alert in their informal contacts, conferences, and interviews with pupils and parents for clues that will help to identify unmet needs and problems of their pupils.

Some procedures teachers may use with discretion to help identify indicators that children may have problems include the following:

- Sociometric technique—the teacher may ask pupils to list the three classmates they would like to have sit next to them in order of preference. This information can then be plotted on paper, and those pupils with few, if any, friends in class can be readily identified.
- Examination of school records including health records—these contain reports of children's performances and health status. Children who move or change schools often are at greater risk.
- Assignments—the teacher may have pupils draw pictures or write compositions on topics such as the following:

    "What I criticize about myself"
    "What others criticize about me"
    "What makes me mad"
    "The person I would like to be"
    "My life 10 years from now"
    "My family"

Finding children in distress is not easy and is the responsibility of many school personnel, including teachers, nurses, and counselors. Their specific responsibilities vary in schools; but they should be observant of pupil behavior, assess attendance, achievement, and discipline records, and use a variety of formal procedures.

---

*US Department of Health and Human Services: *Healthy people 2000: national health promotion and disease prevention objectives*, Washington, DC, 1990, US Government Printing Office.

Numerous personality and adjustment inventories and tests used by school or private psychologists can be used to help identify emotionally disturbed children.*

Counselors, nurses, social workers, psychologists, psychiatrists, and parents may be involved individually or collectively in case studies of pupils. Teachers, parents, and other school personnel need to report their observations. In this technique, the conclusions of a variety of people are brought together to help identify and understand children and families, determine needed action to help children, and suggest school adjustments.

The assessment of the mental health status of pupils is both difficult and complex. Accurate, objective observations of behavior together with the pooling of information obtained from many sources are necessary.

Teacher feeling, emotions, and expressions affect pupil emotions. Teacher attitudes are reflected in the attitudes of pupils. The teacher who is kind but firm, sympathetic but exacting, and friendly but reserved exerts a beneficial influence on emotional health. The nagging, scolding, domineering, sarcastic, or emotionally unstable teacher may cause serious stress in pupils.

WHAT ARE HEALTH RECORDS?

Health records (Fig. 5-19) refer to those materials that contain pertinent data about the health status of pupils. Cumulative records should be maintained for all pupils in school and not merely for those with known health problems. They should be managed by health professionals and interpreted to those persons who need information. They should follow students from grade to grade, from school to school, and from school district to school district.

There is no common health record used in schools. The American School Health Association and other school nurse leaders are trying to develop one. Regardless, record information should be kept confidential and should not be available without permission of school health personnel. They should not contain personal observations by the teacher that label children as slow learners, mentally retarded, and the like. By law, parents or guardians have access to contents and must give written consent to release the records to anyone outside the school.

Records usually contain the following information:

- Teacher observations and pupil attendance
- Results of screening tests
- Findings of medical, dental, and psychological examinations
- Notes on health counseling and follow-up procedures
- Known health conditions, care plan, and names of medications

Despite the amount of information found in health records, the records are not used with any degree of consistency by teachers and others. This is probably because of any, or all, of the following reasons: (1) there is no central, master file on every student, and retrieval of information is difficult; (2) it takes a great deal of time to transcribe the data by hand; (3) information is often lost or misinterpreted, and records may be incomplete; (4) little anecdotal information can be included; (5) if a record is lost, a new one must be reconstructed; and (6) an adequate study of the total student population is virtually impossible.

In an effort to solve problems related to health records, including recording and having access to data, school districts are beginning to computerize these records. The technology exists today to do this on a wide scale.*

Teachers can better understand the health status of students by having conferences with the parent or school nurse at the beginning of the semester. They may be expected to record their observations and other essential information about the health of children.

---

*For a discussion of various tests that may be used in mental health evaluation of children, see Reinert, HR: *Children in conflict*, ed 2, St Louis, 1980, Mosby–Year Book.

---

*One example is Healthmaster Computerized Student Medical Record, Walled Lake, Michigan.

NAME ___ Last, ___ First, ___ Middle ___ **Birthdate** ___ **Sex** ___

Father's Name ___ **Mother's Name** ___

GROWTH AND SCREENING RECORD

SCHOOL							
YEAR							
LEVEL							
Height							
Weight							
Vision—With glasses R.							
Vision—With glasses L.							
Vision—Without glasses R.							
Vision—Without glasses L.							
Vision referral							
Near vision							
Stereo test							
Color vision							
Hearing, R.							
Hearing, L.							
Hearing referral							
Dental screening							
Dental referral							
Scoliosis							
Scoliosis referral							
Physical Examination							
Health Assessment							
Special ed Staffing							

HISTORY OF IMMUNIZATION
Code: Date of immunization D for disease

	DATE	DATE	DATE	DATE	BOOSTERS	
DPT						
DT						
Tetanus						
Polio (Trivalent)						
Measles (Rubeola)						
Measles (Rubella)						
Mumps						
Other						

MAJOR HEALTH CONCERNS

KINDS	DATE	KINDS	DATE
Allergies:		Hospitalizations	
Animal		Operations	
Drug		Serious injury	
Food		Seizures	
Insect stings		Skin infections	
Chickenpox		Prone to colds	
Dental		Prone to strep	
Diabetes		Pneumonia	
Ear infections		On medications	
Eye concerns		Other:	

If yes to any of these, please remark:

FIG. 5-19 Cumulative school health record. (Colorado Department of Education and Colorado Department of Health: *Colorado school health guidelines,* ed 2, Denver, 1986, The Departments.)

THE NURSE AND APPRAISALS

Employed professional registered nurses who work as school nurses have an important role in school health (Fig. 5-20). They are an integral part of the professional health team within the school and community. Their responsibilities vary depending on the size of the school district, whether physician or dental services are available, and the amount of time they serve in schools. Generally, they: (1) supervise and conduct screening programs, (2) train teachers to conduct certain appraisal procedures; (3) coordinate examinations conducted by physicians and other health professionals; (4) aid teachers with pupil observations and referrals; (5) interpret appraisal findings to pupils, teachers, and parents; (6) counsel pupils and parents; (7) recheck students and initiate referrals with parents; (8) assist parents to follow through on examinations and treatments; and (9) maintain health records.

Referral of students to private and public resources for the remediation of health problems is an important part of the school health service program. Unless follow-up activities including telephone calls, health counseling, and health education are conducted, however, the value of the referral may be lost.*

In some communities, registered nurses may be assigned to more than one school. They need to have clerical support for tasks such as immunization records; they can train campus teachers and clerks in special care orders such as urinary catheterizations and basic first aid, so students' emergencies are safely managed until parents or the nurse is summoned.

In recent years school nurses have assumed expanded duties in the assessment of school-aged children. Some have acquired additional specialized training to become *nurse practitioners.* They are especially useful in schools with limited physician services in the community. In addition, they provide a close relationship with physicians and community health professionals. They are competent to conduct a comprehensive assessment including neurological examinations to screen for

---

*Oda D: Cost documentation of school nursing follow-up services, *J School Health* 561:20-23, 1986; and Oda D, Fine JT, Heilbran DC: Impact and cost of public health nurse telephone follow-up of school dental referrals, *Am J Public Health* 76:1348-1349, 1986.

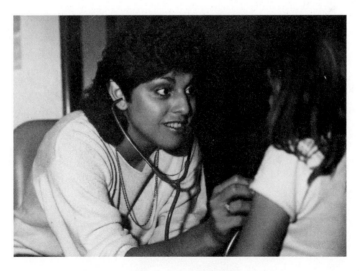

FIG. 5-20 A school nurse plays a vital role in elementary schools. (Courtesy Austin Independent School District Health Service, Austin, Texas.)

learning difficulties. Their functions include completing health histories, performing developmental and physical examinations (Fig. 5-21), conducting laboratory tests, initiating preordered medications within written protocols, and health teaching and counseling.

The expanded role of the school nurse practitioner has met with controversy. A 5-year study supported by the Robert Wood Johnson Foundation found that use of nurse practitioners in schools could improve the health care and status for children. However, not only is the cost considerably greater than is generally spent by school districts for nursing services,* but also questions have been raised as to whether schools should provide such services.

School-Based Health Care

Because of the failure to take care of the needs of poor children and youth, four school districts

(Cambridge, Mass.; Hartford, Conn.; Galveston, Tex.; and Chicago, Ill.) made an attempt to provide primary health care in the school settings several years ago.* The emergence of the school nurse practitioner made this possible. Later, the Robert Wood Johnson Foundation funded a 5-year demonstration project in medically underserved areas in 18 school districts in New York, Colorado, Utah, and North Dakota. The purpose of the project was to establish primary health care centers in the schools and determine whether school nurse practitioners supported by community physicians could improve student health.† The findings revealed that nurse practitioners could correctly diagnose and treat many health problems of the school-aged child.

---

*American Public Health Association: School nurse practitioners: effective, but expensive, *Nation's Health*, July, 1985.

*Cronin GE, Young W: *400 navels, the future of school health in America,* Bloomington, IN, 1970, Phi Delta Kappan.
†Robert Wood Johnson Foundation: *National school health service program,* Princeton, NJ, 1985, Special Report No 1, The Foundation; and Kort M: The delivery of primary health care in American public schools, 1890-1980, *J School Health* 54(11):453-457, 1984.

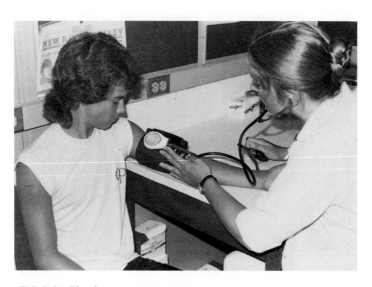

FIG. 5-21 Blood pressure screening is important. (Photo by L.K. Olsen.)

Primary care via school-based health clinics is increasing in the United States. By 1992, 418 school-based or community-linked health centers had been established. The majority of the clinics service secondary students in urban areas, but some are geared toward families in low-income areas who lack access to primary health care.*

The school-based clinic concept is controversial for some of the following reasons: (1) concern that schools are being asked to bear too much responsibility for health care, thereby permitting parents and community agencies to reduce the care they are expected to provide; (2) failure to provide continuity of emergency medical care outside of school hours and during school holidays; federal funding for Medicaid requires continuity; (3) high cost per client; and (4) distrust that mental health or reproductive health care will be given without or contrary to parental approval.

TEACHER-NURSE CONFERENCES

The purposes of periodic teacher-nurse conferences are coordination of services and education and referral of students. In districts where the nurse serves more than one building, these conferences are particularly important. Often the nurse first sees a child when the child is referred for service; thus the teacher may know more about the child's basic health status and appearance and the effect of the health status on the child's learning. This information must be communicated to the nurse.

In like manner, the nurse can interpret medical findings to the teacher. The teacher is then in a much better position to make alterations in the school program for the student, thus enhancing the ability of the student to learn. Despite the significance and recognition of the need for teacher-nurse conferences, however, they are not often held because of time constraints. In general, the following are some reasons for these conferences to be a priority for teachers and nurses alike:

- To discuss teacher observations
- To understand known health problems, such as diabetes, epilepsy, and heart conditions and to plan for individual pupil needs
- To help teachers know what action to take in emergencies to help pupils with known health problems, such as epilepsy and diabetes
- To help teachers make appropriate adjustments in their classrooms and in school, such as having children sit in the front of the room or having them participate in limited activities
- To make decisions about referrals to parents for diagnosis, information, or other action
- To help teachers with the techniques of discussing health problems with parents
- To inform teachers about future examinations and screenings
- To help teachers identify ways to integrate health instruction into the health services program

Teacher observations supplement screening procedures and examinations. They help identify pupils with health problems in the interval between medical examinations and identify children with problems who need special examinations. In schools that do not conduct or require periodic medical and dental examinations, teacher observations combined with screening tests and health inventories or histories, together with teacher-nurse conferences, may provide the "safety net" to identify the health problems that affect learning.

SUMMARY

A review of the various procedures for assessing the health of pupils indicates that the teacher should:

- Become aware of the characteristics of good health and growth and development of students
- Observe children for signs and symptoms of health deviations and be familiar with the

---

*McKinney DH, Peak GR: *School-based and school-linked health centers: update 1993,* Washington, DC, 1994, The Center for Population Options.

school's procedures for handling pupils with problems; especially those with HIV

- Understand the meaning and importance of medical and psychological examinations and observations, dental inspections, and other assessment procedures
- Be familiar with a variety of screening tests and be prepared to help conduct several, such as growth measurement and vision and hearing tests
- Know the type of information required and importance of health records to better understand the pupil
- Be prepared, when appropriate or where nurse services may be limited or nonexistent, to discuss or counsel students and parents regarding pupil health problems
- Periodically meet with the school nurse to exchange information about pupils, learn about school adjustments for students, and obtain help with the health instruction program
- Encourage parents to consent to and participate in health appraisals

The teacher should also realize that health appraisals offer numerous opportunities for health education:

- Teaching about care of the eyes and ears is appropriate when pupils are taking vision and hearing tests.
- Health examinations and dental inspections can have their greatest impact when the instruction period coincides with the examinations or the inspections.
- The control of communicable disease should be discussed when tuberculin tests are being administered.
- Student understanding about growth can be achieved more easily by integrating the periodic measures and graphs of heights and weights with the teaching of math.

The more the teacher knows about the health status of pupils, the better that teacher will understand them, make necessary classroom and school adjustments, provide functional health teaching, and increase the effectiveness of the total educational program.

QUESTIONS FOR DISCUSSION

1. Why must schools be concerned with the health status of students?
2. What is the meaning of the term *health appraisals?*
3. What are the purposes of health appraisals?
4. What is the role of the teacher when observing children?
5. What are some of the signs and symptoms of pupils' health problems that teachers can observe?
6. What is the meaning of the term *learning disabilities?* How can a teacher identify such conditions, and what can be done to help children with these problems?
7. What are some communicable conditions, and how are they prevented or controlled?
8. Why are teacher-nurse conferences necessary?
9. What are the general categories of health screening tests used in schools, and why are they necessary?
10. What types of vision screening tests may be used in schools?
11. How is hearing tested, and who can do it in schools?
12. What are the values, problems, and frequency of periodic height and weight measurements?
13. What is meant by tuberculin testing, and under what conditions should it be completed in schools?
14. What are dental inspections, and why are they valuable?
15. What is sickle cell anemia? What are its signs and symptoms, and how can it be identified?
16. What is diabetes and what can schools and teachers do to help children with diabetes?
17. Why is it important for schools to have a written policy for dealing with HIV-positive individuals? Should there be a policy for every disease?
18. What are the purposes of medical examinations?
19. What are psychological examinations and tests, and what can schools and teachers do to help discover children's problems?

20. What procedure is used to screen for scoliosis and why is it important?

21. Why is scoliosis screening controversial?

22. What is the meaning of the term *nurse practitioner,* and how may they help children with health problems?

23. What is the role of the nurse in health appraisals?

24. How would you characterize the role of the teacher in health appraisals?

SELECTED REFERENCES

American Academy of Pediatrics: *School health: a guide for health professionals,* Evanston, IL, 1987, The Academy.

American Academy of Pediatrics: *School health: policy and practice,* Elk Grove Village, IL, 1993, The Academy.

American Foundation for AIDS Research: AIDS and children: a growing crisis, Am*FAR Reports Winter* 1-2, 1989.

Arpadi S, Caspe WB: Diagnosis and classification of HIV infection in children, *Pediatr Ann* 19(7):409-420, 1990.

Ballard D, White D, Glascoff M: AIDS/HIV education for preservice elementary teachers, *J School Health* 60(6):262-265, 1990.

Balzer M: *Scoliosis: an annotated bibliography: articles on scoliosis screening in the schools.* II. Supplement, Raleigh, NC, 1988, The Scoliosis Association.

Behrman RE, editor: *Nelson textbook of pediatrics,* ed 14, Philadelphia, 1992, WB Saunders.

Behrman RE, editor: School-linked services, *Future of Children* 2(1):Spring, 1992.

Benenson A, editor: *Control of communicable diseases in man,* ed 15, Washington, DC, 1990, American Public Health Association.

Black J, Jones L: HIV infection: educational programs and policies for school personnel, *J School Health* 58(8):317-321, 1988.

Block CE: Scoliosis: school screening specifics, *School Nurse* 2:7-10, 1988.

Brown L, Nassau J, Barone V: Differences in AIDS knowledge and attitudes by grade level, *J School Health* 60(6):270-276, 1990.

Carvey A, Kittell S, Hadeke M: A method for documentation in school health services, *J School Health* 57(9):390-391, 1987.

Centers for Disease Control: Guidelines for effective school health education to prevent the spread of AIDS, *MMWR* 37(S-2):1-4, 1988.

Children's Defense Fund: *The status of America's children: yearbook 1994,* Washington, DC, 1994, Children's Defense Fund.

Coalition of National Health Education Organizations: Instruction about AIDS within the school curriculum, *J School Health* 58(8):323, 1988.

Cogen MS, Ottelmiller DE: Photorefractor for detection of treatable eye disorders in preverbal children, *Ala Med* 62(3):16, 1992.

Cohen HJ, Papola P, Alvarez M: Neurodevelopmental abnormalities in school-age children with HIV infection, *J School Health Suppl* 64(1):11-13, 1994.

Committee on Practice and Ambulatory Medicine, American Academy of Pediatrics: Vision screening and eye examination in children, *Pediatrics* 77:918-919, 1986.

Committee on School Health, Academy of Pediatrics: Acquired immunodeficiency syndrome education in schools, *Pediatrics* 82:278-280, 1988.

Council on Scientific Affairs: Providing medical services through school-based health programs, *J School Health* 60(3):87-92, 1990.

Copeland L: *The lice-buster book,* Mill Valley, CA, 1994, Authentic Pictures.

Cronin GE, Young W: *400 navels, the future of school health in America,* Bloomington, IN, 1970, Phi Delta Kappan.

Division of HIV/AIDS: *HIV/AIDS surveillance: US AIDS cases reported through August 1990,* Atlanta, September, 1990, Center for Infectious Diseases, Centers for Disease Control.

Dryfoos JG: *Full-service schools,* San Francisco, 1994, Jossey-Bass.

Education Funding Research Council: *Federal funding for school health programs,* Arlington, VA, 1994, The Council.

Edwards L: The school nurse's role in school-based clinics, *J School Health* 57(4):157-159, 1987.

Falick HL: A standard health form for all children, *J School Health* 64(7):302-303, 1994.

Frager A: Toward improved instruction in hearing health at the elementary level, *J School Health* 56(5):166-169, 1986.

Freedman HL, Preston KL: Polaroid photoscreening for amblyogenic factors, *Ophthalmology* 99(12):1785-1795, 1992.

Futrell M: AIDS education through schools, *J School Health* 58(8):324-326, 1988.

Graff JC, Ault MM, Guess D, Taylor M, Thompson B: *Health care for students with disabilities,* Baltimore, 1990, Paul H. Brookes.

Guidelines: school-based clinics, *American Academy of Pediatrics News* 3(4):7, 1987.

Harbit M, Willis D: Lyme disease: implications for health educators, *Health Educ* 21(2):41-43, 1990.

Hertel V, Doyen H: *Colorado school health guidelines,* ed 2, Denver, 1986, Colorado Department of Education and Colorado Department of Education.

Holtzhauer FJ et al: Reye's syndrome, *Am J Dis Child* 140(12):1231-1236, 1986.

Joint Statement of ANA, ASHA, NAPNAP, NASSNC: *Recommendations for delivery of comprehensive primary health care to children and youth in the school setting,* Kent, Ohio, 1988, American School Health Association.

Kornguth ML: Preventing school absences due to illness, *J School Health* 61(6):272-274, 1991.

Kort M: The delivery of primary health care in American public schools, 1890-1980, *J School Health* 54(1):453-457, 1984.

Levine MD: Attention and memory, progression and variation during the elementary school years, *Pediatr Ann* 18(6):366-372, 1989.

McCormick K: Bringing health care to the kids, *Governing* 56-61, 1989.

McKinney DH, Peak GR: *School-based and school-linked health centers: update 1993,* Washington, DC, 1994, The Center for Population Options.

Miller CA, Fine A, Adams-Taylor S: *Monitoring children's health: key indicators,* Washington, DC, 1989, American Public Health Association.

Monheit BM, Norris MM: Is combing the answer to headlice? *J School Health* 56(9):158-159, 1986.

Morais T, Bernier M, Turcotte F: Age- and sex-specific prevalence of scoliosis and the value of school screening programs, *Am J Public Health* 75(12):1377-1380, 1985.

Nader P: AIDS: a commentary, *J School Health* 56(3):107-108, 1986.

National Asthma Education Program: *Managing asthma: a guide for schools,* Bethesda, MD, 1991, The Program Information Center.

National Education Association: Recommended guidelines for dealing with AIDS in the school, *J School Health* 56(4):129-130, 1986.

National Heart, Lung and Blood Institute: Expert panel report to provide clinical guidelines for diagnosis and treatment of asthma, *J School Health* 61(6):249-250, 1991.

National Reye's Syndrome Foundation: *Facts . . . you really need to know,* Bryan, OH, 1990, The Foundation.

National Society to Prevent Blindness: *Vision screening for children,* New York, 1980, The Society.

Newacheck P, Jameson WJ, Halfon N: Health status and income: the impact of poverty on child health, *J School Health* 64(6):229-233, 1994.

Newcorn JH, Halperin JM, Schwartz S et al: Parent and teacher ratings of attention-deficit hyperactivity disorder symptoms: implications for case identification, *J Dev Behav Pediatr* 15(2):86-91, 1994.

Oda D: Cost documentation of school nursing follow-up services, *J School Health* 56(1):20-23, 1986.

Oda D, DeAngelis C, Meeker R, Berman B: Nurse practitioners and primary care in schools, *Matern Child Nursing* 19(2):127-130, 1985.

Oda D, Fine JT, Heilbran DC: Impact and cost of public health nurse telephone follow-up of school dental referrals, *Am J Public Health* 76(11):1348-1349, 1986.

Price J: AIDS, the schools and policy issues, *J School Health* 56(4):137-140, 1986.

Reinert HR: *Children in conflict,* ed 2, St Louis, 1980, Mosby–Year Book.

Richards W: Allergy, asthma, and school problems, *J School Health* 56(4):4-6, 1986.

Robert Wood Johnson Foundation: *National school health services program,* Spec. Rep. No. 1, Princeton, NJ, 1985, The Foundation.

Rogers MF et al: Acquired immunodeficiency syndrome in children: report of the Centers for Disease Control: National Surveillance, 1982 to 1985, *Pediatrics* 79:1008-1014, 1987.

Rosenbloom AL: Height screening in the community, *Clin Pediatr* 29(5):288-292, 1990.

Ross JG, Pate RR: The national children and youth fitness study. II. A summary of findings, *J Phys Educ Recreation Dance* 58(9):51-56, 1987.

School-based clinic policy initiatives around the country, Washington, DC, 1986, Center for Population Options.

Schumacher M: *HIV/AIDS education survey: profiles of state policy actions,* report of the National Association of State Boards of Education, Washington, DC, 1989, The Association.

Starke J: *Screening for tuberculosis in school children: what priority should it have,* Austin, TX, 1994, Migrant Clinicians Network.

Sullivan L: How   effective is preschool vision, hearing and developmental screening? *Pediatr Nurs* 14(3):181-183, 1988.

Supports for children with HIV infection in school, *J School Health Suppl* 64(1), 1994.

Terwillinger SH: Early access to health care services through a rural school-based health center, *J School Health* 64(7):284-289, 1994.

Texas Department of Health: *Vision screening manual*, Austin, TX, 1992, The Department.

The Lighthouse Inc.: *The LH symbol tests*, Addison, IL, 1992, School Health Supply Co.

Toolief MS et al: Pneumocystic carinii pneumonia and mucosal candidiasis in previously healthy homosexual men, evidence of a new acquired cellular immunodeficiency, *N Engl J Med* 305:1425-1431, 1981.

US Department of Health and Human Services: *AIDS prevention guide*, Rockville, Md, 1993, US Government Printing Office.

US Department of Health and Human Services: *Healthy people 2000: national health promotion and disease prevention objectives*, Washington, DC, 1990, US Government Printing Office.

US Department of Health and Human Services: *Healthy people 2000, review 1993*, Washington, DC, 1994, US Government Printing Office.

US Department of Health, Education, and Welfare, Public Health Service, National Center for Health Statistics: *Color vision deficiencies in children, United States,* Washington, DC, 1972, US Government Printing Office.

Walsh M, Bibace R: Guidelines for HIV and AIDS student support services, *J School Health* 60(6):249-256, 1990.

Wasserman RC, Croft CA, Brotherton SE: Preschool vision screening in pediatric practice: a study from the pediatric research in office settings network, *Pediatrics* 89(5):834-838, 1992.

Wold S: *School nursing: a framework for practice*, North Branch, MN, 1981, Sunrise River Press.

Wood SP, Walker DK, Gardner J: School health practices for children with complex medical needs, *J School Health* 56(6):215-217, 1986.

Zanga JR, Oda DS: School health services, *J School Health* 57(10):413-416, 1988.

6

Health Guidance

Parents or guardians have primary responsibility for the health care of their children.

AMERICAN ACADEMY OF PEDIATRICS

PROBLEMS TO SOLVE

As a teacher you have noted a considerable change in the attendance habits and quality of work of one of your students. Develop a health guidance plan to deal with this problem.

The school district in which you are employed as an administrator has decided to include a guidance component as part of its total school health program. What guidelines would you develop, and how would you present these guidelines to the Board of Education?

THE developmental needs and health problems of school-aged children involve a broad spectrum of social, emotional, behavioral, and technological issues that require a complex range of services delivered by various individuals and systems in a flexible, coordinated manner.* Identification of health problems such as vision and hearing deficiencies, attention deficit disorder, malnutrition, dental decay, emotional disturbances, or skin infections, all have an impact on student learning and clearly indicate that schools should become involved in providing assistance for children with these problems. The decision by schools to aid in the improvement of students' wellness should be considered because many parents are not informed, nor are able, or even refuse to give adequate attention to their children's needs or health. Failure to attend to pupil conditions may interfere with attendance or educational experiences and thus adversely affect learning. Many schools therefore have shown leadership in collaborating with community, private, and public agencies to help parents and students.* The methods used are part of the school health services program and are referred to as *follow-up* or *guidance procedures.* They include guidance and counseling, use of community health resources, and adjustment of school programs. The emphasis in this chapter is on the guidance and counseling aspects.

The most important part of the health services program, and the one given least attention, is the follow-up phase. Many public and private schools lack full-time nurses to obtain the needed corrective action by students and parents. By way of illustration, Oda identified a 10% increase in dental referral completion when additional nurse time was used to add telephone contact to the written referral.†

WHAT IS HEALTH GUIDANCE?

Health guidance in schools is a broad term that refers to a variety of processes involving the interaction of school and community health personnel, students, and parents to aid in the discovery, understanding, and resolution of mental or physical health concerns through self-effort and self-direction. Health guidance includes those activities in which individuals participate voluntarily in incidental, individual, or small-group counseling or in support group sessions to obtain information regarding health concerns or to seek solutions to health problems. It involves communication with parents to help them identify and have access to resources or community services and to encourage and persuade them to take action. The general aim of health guidance is to enable pupils to acquire the highest levels of wellness in accordance with their individual needs. Guidance plays an important role in *primary prevention* (before a condition arises such as immunization, smoking, inability to cope with crisis situations) and in *secondary prevention* (after a condition such as diabetes, hearing loss, or learning disabilities has been discovered) (see Chapter 1).

Health guidance involves the use of health appraisals and health records; more specifically, it involves counseling to provide information and aid in regard to health problems, immunizations, reports of health examinations, program adjustments, identification of community health resources, and relations between pupils and parents with medical, dental, and other health specialists. Its objective is not to give advice but to encourage, motivate, help, and empower individuals to achieve good health through their own efforts. It is purposeful action and organized effort directed toward intelligent decision making regarding corrections, care, service, treatment, and assistance.

What Are the Purposes of Health Guidance?

Health guidance seeks to achieve the following:

- Provide information about and interpretations of pupils' health status, concerns, or problems
- Provide information to parents of the nature of the health conditions that exist in their

---

*Melaville AI, Blank MJ: *Together we can: a guide for crafting a pro-family system of education and human services,* Washington, DC, 1993, US Government Printing Office.
†Oda DS: Cost documentation of school nursing follow-up services, *J School Health* 56(1):21-22, 1986.

children and to encourage needed care (Fig. 6-1)

- Support pupils' self-care skills and appropriate responsibility for the promotion of their own health
- Motivate parents and pupils to seek care and treatment when needed for existing health conditions and to accept needed modifications in the school program
- Enable pupils and parents to use available medical, dental, and other health resources to the best advantage
- Contribute to the health education of pupils and parents in both formal and informal settings
- Assist in adapting school programs to the individual needs and abilities of students with health problems; to train and inform teachers
- Inform teachers of pupils' health problems and to identify responsibilities

- Work with community groups to ensure availability of treatment services, especially those with minimal access barriers.
- Encourage and promote, where necessary, the establishment or expansion of school and community health services and facilities, especially for needy and homeless children and families

Following health appraisals, the procedures used in guidance are frequently referred to as *health counseling*. Health counseling focuses on helping an individual promote his or her own well-being. This counseling is the direct personal contact between students or parents and counselors (nurses, teachers, physicians, and others) for the purpose of interpreting the nature and significance of a student's health problem. The focus of the discussion should be to provide information and skill training so the student or the parents can formulate a plan of action that will lead to a solution of the problem.

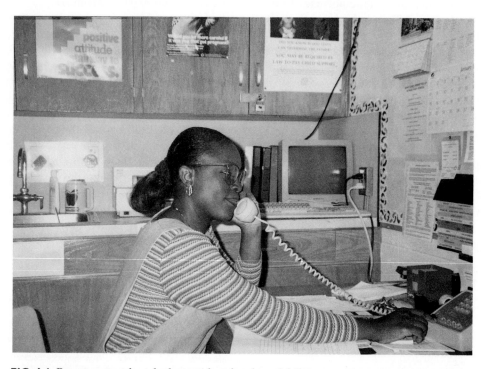

FIG. 6-1 Parent contact by telephone aids referrals and follow-up. (Courtesy Austin Independent School District Health Services, Austin, Texas.)

The results of screening procedures or medical examinations are often reported to parents on preprinted forms that may read something like:

Dear parent: On February 14, your child, John, was screened for possible visual problems. This screening revealed a visual problem that could interfere with John's health and school work. We recommend that you take John to an eye specialist for further diagnosis and recommendations for treatment.

This message by itself has several major shortcomings:

- It may not be given to the parents by the student.
- If it is given to the parents, they may not read it.
- If it is read, it may be misunderstood.
- There is no explanation or interpretation of what was found during the screening.
- The importance of the message may not be clear and thus may not motivate the parents to take additional action.
- There is no provision for knowing what help was needed or if additional action was taken by the parents.

Although making referrals is an important aspect of a school nurse's role, follow-up is also critical. However, referral alone is not enough. It is important that the nurse counsel and consult with teachers, parents, and pupils, both in groups and individually. Nurses, teachers, or other school personnel should always use "teachable moments" to guide students facing health problems or emotional crises. This process may be identified as the *informal school health education program.*

Informal Health Education

Informal health education must receive greater emphasis in schools if educational programs are to adequately address the differing health needs of children and youth. It is a phase of the school health education program that has been neglected and has generally been thought to be the responsibility of the nurse. A great deal of such education has occurred "accidentally."

Although the nurse is an important contact person, the nurse's time in school is often limited. There are others who can learn to provide assistance. On occasion, students require special, individual attention that cannot be obtained from a formal health education program. These young people need and often desire someone, some group, or some way in schools to be able to discuss concerns and interests about sex, drugs, adolescent development, stress and pressure, self-care, family problems, and other health matters. Most young people talk to their peers about their problems or ask where to obtain help in solving problems. The school nurse, a teacher, a counselor, the school psychologist, or someone who will listen in a nonjudgmental fashion and have empathy for student concerns might also help. Informal health education needs to be recognized as valuable and integrated in schools. It would be helpful in secondary prevention of health problems and also could serve a useful purpose in primary prevention.

Informal education is unplanned, unstructured, but purposeful learning. It may occur in the classroom, nurse's office, or other school locations. It may take place in a meeting with a parent or pupil, or by telephone, note, letter sent home, newsletter, or other procedure. It may take place outside the school, in the home, watching TV, talking with a parent, friend, or neighbor, reading a magazine or newspaper, or through a variety of activities. It usually occurs on a one-to-one basis or in small groups. It can also occur as the result of hallway or library displays and staff members engaging in wellness activities. It is a communication procedure that provides information, models, counseling, and guidance that is nonthreatening but relevant to students and voluntary in terms of participation.

Implementation of informal health education may occur in a variety of ways. A student may ask a teacher a question about health or about what action to take because of the sudden appearance of a skin rash. A pupil visits the nurse for information and guidance about losing excess weight, a severe cough, or fear of being beaten by an aggressive student. The nurse, counselor, or other staff member should encourage children and youth to visit them to discuss health problems or concerns whenever they are free, during lunch time, or in after-school group sessions. The school newspaper prints articles written by students on student health problems. The nurse makes pamphlets and publications available to students or coordinates a Health Fair with invited community agencies. Special voluntary educational programs on drugs, sexually transmitted diseases, teenage pregnancies, and emotional problems may be held as needs arise. Parent-teacher-nurse conferences also should be planned.

Opportunities for health guidance also exist in the *formal school health education program*, but they are not discussed in this chapter. The procedures used in the formal program may be considered to be group guidance methods. Pupils' requests for informal assistance often arise from the formal program. Chapters 9 through 13 and Appendix B on organizing, learning, and teaching techniques provide numerous suggestions for helping students in the classroom in a group or formal setting.

What Are the Kinds of General Problems for Which Children Need Health Guidance?

The health problems of children that require guidance may be categorized in the following manner:

In some situations *more detailed examination* of the child is needed to establish a diagnosis. Observations of signs and symptoms might necessitate tests for attention deficit disorder, or auditory or visual problems; a medical examination when chronic fatigue, serious menstrual cramps, frequent headaches, frequent colds, or blackouts are noted; or a dental examination for decay or periodontal (gum) disease.

There are some conditions for which the child needs *treatment services*, such as obesity, depression, vision refractive errors, epilepsy, dental decay, ear infections/hearing difficulties, skin infections, and asthma.

Other conditions need *home care improvement.* These may include the need for breakfast, lice control, bathing, first aid for minor wounds, cleanliness, dental care, nonprescription medicines for simple allergies and "colds," or better sleeping facilities.

Problems of emotional and social adjustment may make *special counseling* mandatory. Opportunities to talk with understanding people may be most helpful to students. Teachers, nurses, and counselors who have success communicating with pupils may be able to assist them with their problems regarding coping with change such as moving, death, or parent's job loss, family disruption, or use of drugs. It also may be necessary to interpret the emotional problem to parents to encourage their seeking additional help. These problems often are difficult to present to parents in ways that will not cause them to scold the child.

For some problems, *assistance regarding health practices and behavior* is advisable. This might call for confidential discussions with students regarding bathing, unusual body odor, obesity, the importance of washing the hands before eating and after using the toilet, safe use of medicines, the abuse of drugs, remaining home when ill, eating breakfast, and what to do about sexually transmitted diseases. Some of these matters also may involve parental communication and should be handled discreetly.

ORGANIZATION FOR SCHOOL HEALTH GUIDANCE

Although schools try to provide health guidance, in most cases it is done on an incidental basis. Schools in general do not have well-organized health guidance programs, as presented in this chapter. In elementary schools the nurse is usually the key person in the health counseling program. Where health guidance does exist on an organized basis, the best results accrue when the program is carried out collaboratively; all departments and personnel of a school concerned with any phase of mental, emotional, and physical health of children should cooperate and participate in the formulation of health guidance policies. Objectives, responsibilities, and communication methods need clear definition.

Organized health guidance programs may be considered a relatively new development; therefore it may be well to consider some of the fundamental factors that are basic to sound organization. It is essential to consider factors such as (1) desirable principles of operation, (2) role and skills of the individual who counsels, (3) responsibilities of various school personnel, (4) nurse-teacher/nurse-teacher-parent conferences, and (5) techniques for counseling.

Principles of Operation

As in other functions of the school, health guidance should be based on certain fundamental principles for effective operation. The following generalized list may serve as a guide for the establishment of such principles in local school situations:

- The health guidance program should complement and supplement the total educational program within the school.
- The health program should be tailored to serve individual pupil needs.
- The health guidance program should have visible support of the school administrators.
- Written policies and procedures identifying purposes and responsibilities of personnel should be provided.
- School staff responsible for health guidance services should know community agencies and specialists available for referral.
- The objectives of the health guidance program should be communicated to students, parents, teachers, and others.
- Regular in-service training to identify best practices in health guidance should be provided for teachers, administrators, nurses, and counselors.
- All school departments concerned with the health of pupils should be well coordinated.
- The purposes and scope of each school department concerned with child health should

be clearly defined to ensure efficient service delivery to pupils.
- Responsibility for leadership in the health guidance program should be assigned to individuals who possess interest, ability, and preparation for such service.
- Procedures for effective school and community coordination in health guidance should be developed.
- The health guidance program should be subjected to continuous evaluation so that constructive improvements may take place (see Appendix G).
- All health guidance personnel should keep abreast of the latest research and changing conditions as they relate to their specific health area.

Role of Individuals Who Counsel

The responsibility for counseling involves a variety of school personnel including teachers, nurses, physicians, psychologists, principals, counselors, and even students. Although there is no single correct philosophy or way to counsel, the person who functions as a counselor and is involved in human relations should know how to: (1) gather data to identify an individual in need of assistance, (2) be competent to interpret findings to pupils and parents, and (3) encourage and motivate them to make realistic plans for action. Because parents have the primary responsibility for the health of their children, school personnel should not try to tell them how their children should be raised. School personnel should attempt to describe the health conditions of pupils that warrant attention, interpret the importance of care especially as it relates to attendance and learning, and inform parents about community health services and parenting support, and make any necessary adjustments of the school program.

School personnel should understand the cultural heritage and customs of people of all ethnic backgrounds. Some personnel should be conversant in the different languages for effective communication.

Responsibilities of Various School Personnel

One of the principles previously mentioned suggested that the responsibilities of all concerned with the health of pupils should be clearly defined and designated. This should perhaps be amplified to the extent that *every* person in the school system should accept responsibility for the health guidance of the school population. In other words, every person associated with the school should have the physical, spiritual, mental, and social well-being of pupils as a major concern. The fact that pupils' academic and nonacademic interests relate to their physical and mental health cannot be overstressed. For example, the child who is fatigued, hungry, hurting, anxious, or unable to understand why people do not seem to want him or her around is likely to have difficulty concentrating on learning.

Although all school personnel rightfully should take an interest in health guidance of pupils, the extent of responsibilities naturally must vary. Someone should be available in schools with whom students are able to communicate when necessary about health matters, but especially regarding sexually transmitted diseases, use of drugs and tobacco, human sexuality, pregnancies, violence, and home and school problems. This might be the school counselor, nurse, teacher, or some other capable individual. Following are some of the specific counseling responsibilities of various school personnel who participate in health guidance programs.

School administrators and officers. The responsibilities of the school board, superintendent, and principal of the school must focus on the leadership necessary to set goals, parameters, and plans to carry out a successful health guidance program. These individuals actually have the final approval concerning the budget, the acquisition of new equipment, in-service training, and the hiring of personnel. The health services program needs cooperative leadership in which the administrator plans with school staff members on decisions pertaining to the scope of the program. The combined competencies of health professionals and educators are needed to achieve the related goals of better health and effective learning for more schoolchildren.

School administrators need to be acquainted with the objectives of the program, because they are usually the liaisons between the school and the community who are expected to interpret program objectives. In addition, administrators should initiate plans for the coordination of school and community relationships and strive to maintain high standards for total school health. Principals, with input from staff, should establish committees to address student needs (e.g., student assistance programs). They also may need to initiate community action to help ensure the provision of comprehensive health care services, especially for children who lack access to care.

Health service personnel. The main responsibilities of the school physician, school nurse, and others in health services involve helping youths who exhibit health needs that may affect their school attendance, activities participation, and focus on learning. Regular follow-up is necessary. For example, certain pertinent information derived from examinations of students by the school physician can be relayed to teachers and guidance counselors. More use is being made of the case study or student assistance methods whereby those people directly working with a child meet and discuss their findings, progress, and barriers. The reports add to the separate impressions, and the goal of assisting in the development of the whole child is more fully realized. In other cases either the school nurse or school social worker serves as a case manager or direct link between the home and school. The nurse or social worker routes vital information to guidance counselors and teachers that may reveal physical, mental, and emotional health problems that arise out of home situations.

School physician. The practice of medicine in schools is a special interest area requiring expertise in identifying, observing, advising, and preventing children's health problems in the school setting. School physicians must be familiar with the total school health program, not just the services component. Unlike clinical practice wherein the physician-patient relationship is the focus, the school physician is a member of a team and must work in a physician-group relationship.

A physician has specialized knowledge of diseases, chronic conditions, and human development. Although a variety of job descriptions may exist for part-time, full-time, or consulting physicians, in general, the school physician may volunteer or be employed by the school district for any of the following:

- Administrative and advisory activities including consulting and developing health policies, procedures, and forms
- Liaison activities between the school and the medical community, parents, and other child- or health-oriented groups
- Consultation with school nurses regarding their health service activities, including controlling communicable diseases and special care plans for uncommon conditions
- Consultation with teachers regarding health concerns and health education activities
- Involvement in special education programs, including medical appraisal of students, interpretation of the findings for other staff professionals regarding school placement, referral for detailed examinations, and in-service training of staff
- Involvement in employee health programs such as mental health, physical examinations, control of communicable disease, and employee assistance
- Attention to environmental health in the school setting for both students and employees
- Participation in school programs such as drug and alcohol abuse prevention and crisis response planning

School nurse. The work of the professional school nurse (i.e., registered nurse) continues to gain importance in the school health program. The committee on School Health Service of the World Health Organization states that nurses, like physicians, have a different type of task when they work within the framework of the school, for it is not the clinical situation to which most have been accustomed. School nursing combines the prevention agendas of public health, emotional support skills of psychiatric practice, and acute care needs of ambulatory pediatric care. Nurses must direct their energies to the educational goals of the school and remember they are not in a hospital or clinic setting. To the teacher, the nurse must be a source of information and guidance. To the parent the nurse must be a skilled health counselor cognizant of community resources, and family problem solving, and an interpreter par excellence of the child's needs as revealed by medical examination and school behavior. They also must help guide parents and school staff to recognize the impact of health problems on learning.

Although the responsibilities and duties of school nurses are numerous and varied, special emphasis should be placed on their part in health guidance. The following list summarizes some of the ways the school nurse contributes to the health guidance program:

- Conducting assessments and assisting with medical examinations that may reveal a need for counseling, especially for students in high-risk situations
- Interpreting the results of health appraisals to pupils, teachers, and parents (Fig. 6-2)
- Providing information and direction concerning community resources available for health promotion and the care of physical, mental, and emotional problems of children
- Helping pupils to develop skills and habits to maintain optimal health
- Helping children to find solutions to their personal problems, particularly those involving or likely to involve physical, mental, and emotional health
- Assisting in the identification of pupils needing modified education programs and designing care plans
- Counseling pupils with health problems
- Counseling parents concerning the health problems of children
- Serving as a liaison between home, school, and community organizations and agencies

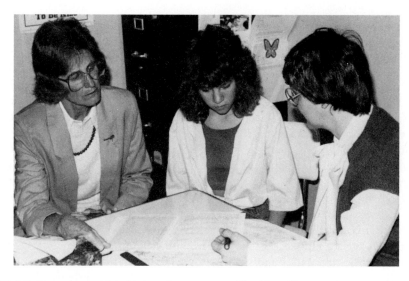

FIG. 6-2 Nurse/parent/student conference: part of health guidance. (Photo by L.K. Olsen.)

- Providing student and staff training and direct care in emergencies, injuries and specific health procedures
- Participating in formal and informal health education
- Keeping individual health records for descriptive reports and for specific use when health counseling is indicated

As early as 1974, Oda identified expanding school nurse duties that included the following*:

- Greater stress on health education, counseling, and consultation
- Emergence of school nurse practitioners who complete additional preparation for competency to conduct in-depth assessment of physical, psychomedical, and psychoeducational behavior and learning disorders of children
- Involvement in the development, implementation, and evaluation of health care plans and programs
- Use of increased technologies for health assessment and care

The expectations expressed by Oda are now a central part of the school nurse's duties. These roles have been expanded to include advocacy for children and parents; support for staff wellness; implementation of "mainstreaming;" coordination with community agencies; and coordinating medically ordered care (e.g., tube feeding, catheterizations, and administration of medications at school).*

The number of registered nurses including school nurse practitioners in schools varies because standards are not uniform or consistent throughout the United States. Ideally it is advisable to have a full-time nurse in every elementary school, but at the present time most districts do not budget for this. It is generally believed there should be one nurse for every 800 to 1200 pupils depending on the number of medically fragile or special need students; however, common practices differ widely. Some schools have no nurse services, and in others nurses are limited to one-half day weekly. Because there are so few school nurse

*Oda DS: Increasing role effectiveness of school nurses, *Am J Public Health* 64:591-595, 1974.

*Snyder A, editor: *Implementation guide for the standards of school nursing practice,* Kent, OH, 1991, American School Health Association.

practitioners and their usage is so limited, no standard has been established regarding how many should be found in schools. In recent years nurse services have been eliminated in some districts because of budget limitations. The quality of the health services programs in these districts undoubtedly has been lowered because of this action.

Some school districts are using nonprofessional *clerks, screeners,* or *aides* to assist school nurses. These hired staff members or volunteers may perform a variety of clerical or routine, technical skills that do not require any professional judgment. Helping with tasks such as scheduling home visits, recording screening data, ordering supplies, or coordinating a health fair frees the nurse's from non-nursing, but important, activities. Volunteers and student aides are not permitted to read students' records. With training and supervision by the school nurse, employed aides may conduct routine vision or hearing screening or perform a special health care procedure for assigned students who need help with eating, bladder or bowel elimination, or diabetic blood sugar checks. The nurse is legally responsible for preparing the care plan and procedures and judging that the assigned person can safely provide care.*

Health coordinator. A joint committee of the National Association of State Boards of Education (NASBE) and the American Medical Association (AMA)† recommended that all schools should employ a health coordinator to serve as a link between students and individuals in and out of schools who can provide students with needed services. The joint committee also recommended that schools could assign a current employee to be the health coordinator, create a new position and hire someone, or house a coordinator who works for a different agency. Regardless of the employment pattern

utilized, the job of health coordinator should be a full-time position. The person assuming the responsibilities of school health coordinator should direct, supervise, and coordinate all activities concerning the health of students. The success or failure of health guidance programs may depend on the extent to which proper use of information is made. For example, many schools have excellent health appraisal programs, yet do not have adequate organization or means of following up the findings of appraisals. The school health coordinator should fill gaps that may exist by coordinating all information that might be used to guide the pupil in health matters. This person should be well informed about the total school health program as presented in Chapter 1.

Another important function of the school health coordinator is that of conducting needed research. All too often records are kept, and up-to-date entries made so that the pupils growth and development are charted, but little if any attempt made to use the data for study purposes. The analysis of records could certainly aid in identifying trends; changes in physical, social, and emotional patterns of boys and girls; and the limitations of the school's health program.

Health coordinators are responsible for managing formal linkages with community resources. The coordinator may represent the school health department in community projects or in the creation of school-based health and social services centers or clinics. Many centers started with a single focus on preventive health care (such as described in Chapter 5), but have evolved into multiple-services or "one-stop" centers where families can even apply for social assistance or take literacy or parenting classes. Some centers also offer before- and after-school recreation programs for students to ensure safety while parents are at work.*

Unfortunately, health coordinators per se are not commonly employed in school districts. Where they are found, these individuals may be

---

*Snyder A, editor: *Implementation guide for the standards of school nursing practice,* Kent, OH, 1991, American School Health Association.
†The National Commission on the Role of the School and Community in Improving Adolescent Health: *Code blue: uniting for healthier youth,* Alexandria, VA, 1989, National Association of State Boards of Education.

---

*Winerip M: Public school offers a social-service model, *The New York Times,* December 8, 1993, p A1, B7.

the nurse, physician, health educator, or general administrator.

Guidance personnel. The school guidance and counseling program includes guidance counselors, school psychologists, associate psychologists, educational diagnosticians, and sometimes social workers or drug counselors. Among their diverse responsibilities, many have skills to help pupils handle health problems.

The school counselor's guidance program should focus on student development, not just crisis management or problem prevention. The purpose of a developmental guidance program is to help students gain knowledge, understanding, and skills through activities that address students' developmental stages, self-concept, and interpersonal relationships within the school and families. Some of the goals of a developmental approach to school guidance that is consistent

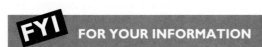

Developmental Guidance for Elementary and Middle Schools

The goals of such a program should be to help students:

- Understand their abilities and develop skills for relationships with others as well as recognize the value of differences among people
- Recognize the effects of their habits and thoughts on behavior; they also recognize how they can choose behaviors, considering goals and consequences
- Gain skills for decision making and problem solving with increasing emphasis on age-appropriate personal responsibility
- Develop interpersonal and communication skills for positive relationships with others
- Experience community involvement (e.g., service projects) and identify helping resources.

From Myrick RD: *Developmental guidance and counseling,* Minneapolis, 1993, Educational Media Corporation.

with the promotion of mental health are identified in the box below.

If counselors expect to have pupils referred to them for individual help, knowledge of the objectives of health guidance is essential. They should have a good background in the psychodynamics of behavior and an understanding of health education, as most of the behavior or learning problems found among children involve, either directly or indirectly, physical, mental, social, or emotional health. Counselors can contribute to the health guidance program by offering in-service education to teachers and other school personnel with respect to counseling methods that would be most effective for pupils with specific needs. School counselors also coordinate student and family referrals for special mental health evaluation and crisis support to community resources.

Because guidance personnel are generally involved in a helping relationship, children, parents, teachers, and others often share with them various types of personal concerns, some of which may relate to the school environment. It is possible, without breaking confidence, for guidance personnel to assist in calling attention to health problems that are not receiving care.

School psychologist. A comprehensive program includes mental health evaluations and services to help students cope with problems. School psychologists have advanced degrees and may represent the schools as liaison to community mental health professionals to identify gaps in needed services for students or their families. Psychologists may supervise mental health counseling provided by social workers or associate psychologists. These staff and educational diagnosticians also are often involved in the assessment of children with learning difficulties. They have a key role in explaining assessments to parents and preparing an Individual Education Plan required for students who need special education services.

School psychologist time should be available to the school administrator, school physician, school nurse, school social worker, teachers, and family physicians and psychiatrists who may be in a position to act on recommendations regarding school services or adaptations for children with emotional or mental health problems. Although most school professionals have taken course work in behavioral sciences, the school psychologist can provide staff development in the understanding of unusual behavioral patterns. Often the school psychologist will administer various types of tests and submit a report of these findings for the school. Because these reports are psychologically descriptive, care must be taken in their use and circulation.

Drug counselor. Certified alcohol and drug counselors are hired in some junior and senior high schools or placed there by a community agency at the principal's request. These counselors should be trained in special skills related to drugs and drug use. The duties of the drug counselor may include referral and aftercare for students needing drug-treatment support; establishing student assistance programs and peer support groups; liaison with community resources, including the police and the courts; and the preparation of policies and procedures for the school or school district. This individual should be approachable by students, readily available and accessible, willing to talk and not preach, honest and trustful in approach, willing to discuss any topic of interest to pupils, and knowledgeable about the drug scene.

Elementary school teachers. Classroom teachers are actually the heart of a successful health guidance program at the elementary school level. Elementary school teachers are expected to observe pupils daily. It becomes their responsibility to detect physical, social, and emotional behavior patterns that are unusual and refer students to the nurse, parents, counselor, or administrators. Elementary teachers are the most important people, outside of the family, for cultivation of health attitudes and values through the health instruction program. The student will seek out the teacher for information in individual and informal settings if communication has been established.

The elementary teacher contributes to health guidance by*:

---

*King LS, Dodd N: The health educator as counselor: what does it take? *Health Educ* 17(2):17-22, 1986.

- Participating in school health appraisals, orienting students about the appraisals, and using the findings to discuss health with children
- Providing descriptive classroom observation information to medical and guidance personnel
- Listening to students and trying to assist them in clarifying and understanding their health problems
- Observing for sudden or gradual changes in child appearance or behavior and referring children suspected of having health problems (see Table 5-1 and Appendix I).
- Contributing to the child's school records
- Developing a good emotional climate for learning
- Respecting students' needs and helping them develop a sense of their own well-being
- Aiding in adapting the school program to meet the needs of the physically challenged or emotionally distressed student
- Aiding in the follow-up of students
- Assisting in interpreting the significance and results of health appraisals to parents
- Providing reports to parents about their child's positive growth

As a counselor, the following must be avoided:

- Trying to diagnose or prescribe treatment; this includes labeling children or insisting the parent secure medication for hyperactivity.
- Taking the decision making away from the students and parents relative to what to do about a health problem
- Suggesting only one way or personal remedies to resolve a health problem
- Embarrassing or ridiculing the child
- Arguing basic values such as religion and culture as they relate to health care
- Conveying a judgmental or condescending attitude

Special teachers. Teachers dealing with special groups, such as new immigrants, special education students, and special subjects (physical education, home economics, and health education), have considerable responsibility in all matters of pupil health, including health guidance, because of their close contact with situations that deal with health. For instance, the physical education teacher has an opportunity to observe the growth and development of pupils as well as peer relationships. Whether physical educators are aware of their responsibility for health guidance has been questioned, but physical development should not be their only concern.

Students. Many schools prepare student peers to try to help pupils with problems. Upper elementary school youths make dramatic or formal presentations to younger students in their own schools. They also have been available for informal individual and group meetings. The value of such activities has not been defined clearly, but indications reveal they create interest and enthusiasm. The use of students in a variety of health counseling situations therefore should receive greater consideration and experimentation in schools. Success with this type of program depends on extensive training of peer educators and careful planning by program developers.

Nurse-Teacher/Nurse-Teacher-Parent Conferences

Casefinding and follow-up in the interest of the child requires a three-cornered arrangement—nurse or medical professional, teacher, and parent. The absence of participation of any one of these members makes effective action on behalf of the child much less likely.

GEORGE A. SILVER, MD*
Professor of Public Health,
Yale University School
of Medicine

The need for communication within as well as between the school and the home is clearly identified in Dr. Silver's remarks. Conferences are indi-

cated when student needs are dealt with by a team or case manager, with key staff serving as school liaisons with parents and community resources. Limited nurse time in many schools, extensive teacher responsibilities, and parents' difficulty leaving work or obtaining transportation to the school are factors that make problem management more complicated (see Chapter 4). Effective guidance of pupils will not take place without effective communication procedures. Perhaps teachers need to take more initiative to arrange conferences if the health needs of their pupils are to receive adequate attention.

Conferences may be planned or spontaneous. In planned nurse-teacher conferences, the nurse should:

- Review each student's record in conjunction with teacher observations, and interpret recommendations and adjustments for school environment and/or instructional program
- Plan for those students needing follow-up care; the teacher can be a valuable ally in contact with parents, especially through observation of the students and knowledge of each student's behavior in the class situation
- Stimulate interest in health teaching utilizing upcoming screenings or the known needs of the student as learning opportunities
- Help the teacher plan and evaluate classroom health programs and discuss availability of quality health education material
- Adopt a plan for notifying the teacher of nurse follow-up on individual cases.*

The nurse or teacher who knows that a student, parent, or other staff member has a special health condition such as HIV infection must respect the confidentiality of the information. Most states have public health laws or rules that make it illegal for anyone to reveal the HIV or AIDS diagnosis of another person without written consent. This law pertains to minor students; their parents

---

*Silver GA: Redefining school work health services: comprehensive child health care as the framework, *J School Health* 51:157-162, 1981.

*Hertel V, Doyen M: *Colorado school health guidelines,* ed 2, Denver, 1986, Colorado Department of Education and Colorado Department of Health.

must document the names or positions of persons who can be told.*

These basic procedures for planned teacher conferences also apply to parent meetings, but the focus must be on the individual student. The nurse or teacher also should be prepared to deal with the student or parent who drops in to talk about health-related matters.

Techniques for Counseling

Although there is no best way to counsel, the specific procedures for communicating with students and parents include informal and formal talks, notes home, home and school visits with parents, and telephone calls.

These are the basic principles to be followed when counseling†:

- Start where counselees are and accept them as they are
- Treat each individual with respect and recognize the individual's potential for growth
- Do not moralize, preach, or impose personal values or other values
- The key to successful or effective counseling is attentive and nonjudgmental listening

When teachers counsel parents or students, or both, the following suggestions will facilitate problem solving:

- Try to develop rapport to improve the effectiveness of the communication. Attempt to be friendly and nonofficious in approach. Demonstrate sincerity in wanting to be helpful. Clarify the information and indicate that aid, if desired, is the intent of the meeting. Refrain from telling the parent or student what action to take; ideally a request for help will be forthcoming. Be familiar with differences in cultural and family values without being judgmental. Permit cultural identification to emerge as a strength and resource.

- Help parents and pupils analyze or recognize the problem. A child's inattentiveness may be annoying to the teacher. Although a condition may be serious, it may not be significant for learning for that particular child. Only medical diagnosis can determine the cause of the behavior.
- Help parents and pupils understand the nature and significance of the problem by encouraging questions and by supplying information. Be certain understanding occurs.
- Help parents and pupils determine the courses of action to be taken and discuss the consequences. The solution may be relatively simple if parents have a family physician. However, if parents do not know where to go or do not have a physician or the funds, the next step may be a referral.
- Encourage parents and students to choose a particular course of action, but indicate that the decision will rest with them.

Cormier and others* suggest the following behavior:

- Speak in a soft, soothing voice
- Maintain interest and focus; do not allow telephone calls or other interruptions
- Lean toward the student, keeping a relaxed posture
- Look directly into the student's eyes if this is culturally appropriate
- Make sure gestures are open and welcoming
- Keep a physical proximity that is comfortable for the other person (Fig. 6-3)

When contacting parents about student health problems that are common, such as vision or hearing difficulties, the school nurse may send home a form notice because it is the quickest and easiest way to communicate with a large number of parents. The limitations of this procedure have been previously discussed and suggest that the procedures used to get in touch with parents must receive careful consideration, especially if the health

*Majer LS: HIV-infected students in school: who really "needs to know?" *J School Health* 62(6):243-245, 1992.

†Litwack L, Litwack J, Ballou M: *Health counseling,* New York, 1980, Appleton-Century-Crofts.

*Cormier L, Cormier W, Weisser R: *Interviewing and helping skills for health professionals,* Monterey, CA, 1984, Wadsworth.

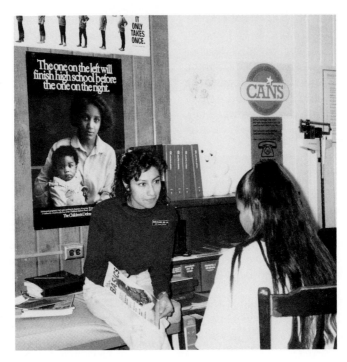

FIG. 6-3 Effective communication skills are important for counseling. (Courtesy Austin Independent School District Health Services, Austin, Texas.)

problem is other than a routine matter (see pp. 150-151).

Studies on effective ways of communicating with parents to get action found that children of parents at high socioeconomic levels are more likely to receive attention than those at low socioeconomic levels; children whose parents give defects a high urgency rating are more likely to receive attention; notification about a child's defect by more than one contact technique (written notice, telephone call, home or school visit, and others) is more likely to prompt action than if parents are notified by one contact only. Those contacts involving personal interaction by telephone or visitation are more productive than those using a written medium. Also, parents who receive two notifications of children's defects are more likely to pay attention than parents who receive only one notification. Three notifications do not appear to be worth the extra effort.

The most effective techniques of communication for parent action are notices written by a physician and telephone calls by school nurses. However, Ozias found that face-to-face contact by a home call or a nurse-parent conference at school or at the parent's place of work resulted in over 70% of the referrals being completed by the parents.*

WHICH COMMUNITY HEALTH RESOURCES ARE ESSENTIAL?

School personnel should be familiar with and use local community health resources that can help meet the health guidance needs of pupils. Schools must take the initiative to learn about the services

---

*Ozias J: *Influence of parental health beliefs on follow-through on school nurses' spinal screening referrals,* unpublished doctoral dissertation, University of Texas at Austin, 1990.

available and establish referral arrangements with physicians, dentists, psychiatrists, and other health specialists in private practice, health clinics, and hospitals, as well as the voluntary health agencies, health departments, child guidance clinics, social service agencies, family service agencies, civic and service organizations, welfare agencies, and religious services located in the community.

For example, resources in the community for emotionally disturbed children may include privately practicing psychologists and psychiatrists, child guidance clinics, general and mental hospitals with inpatient and outpatient care, youth agencies, associations for the physically handicapped, special schools, family service agencies, welfare agencies, and a variety of professional and voluntary organizations.* They offer services including diagnosis, treatment, transition, rehabilitation, education, information, and consultation. In several states, public health departments make available some or many of these services. The extent of community mental health services differs in school districts, with many of them being in short supply. Services for the poor are frequently inadequate. The cost for help may be partial or full payment, depending on the need of the patient. Some organizations provide free services.

At least one person in the school must be familiar with the kinds and variety of resources available so the best guidance can be provided to students and parents. The school nurse often assumes this responsibility and is the best-informed person. Where nurses or counselors are not available, teachers may have to: (1) try to locate someone in the school or school district who knows the resources, or (2) contact the local health department for assistance. A school administrator or committee should prepare a print or computer

*Professional organizations include American Academy of Child Psychiatry, American Association for Mental Deficiency, American Association of Psychiatry Services for Children, American Orthopsychiatric Association, American Psychiatric Association, American Psychological Association. Voluntary organizations include National Association for Mental Health, Child Study Association of America, Council for Exceptional Children, National Society for Autistic Children, Inc., Al-Anon Family Group Headquarters, and Alateen.

database directory of local resources indicating services and how to apply for them.

HOW DO SCHOOLS ADJUST PROGRAMS?

Teachers who recognize symptoms of physical, mental, emotional, or social disturbances in children should initially examine their own activities in class or their relationship with the pupil to determine whether they may be the cause of, or a factor contributing to, the behavior exhibited. Sometimes student difficulties may be prevented by teachers modifying their activities or relationships with pupils. The teacher may provide additional help to a child who is having difficulty in reading or to motivate the gifted student with appropriate new challenges. They may have to help pupils who have trouble with emotions or behavior. Teachers need to arrange successful experiences for all students. They may need to be friendlier with a pupil. They may have to try to gain the trust of a child rejected by parents or peers. These are some of the considerations that teachers must make before determining whether the problem needs to be referred to others.

Although attention deficit hyperactivity disorder (ADHD) has no known specific cause, children with ADHD appear to have different responses to mental stimuli. Careful professional evaluation is needed because this condition is easily confused with behavior (conduct) disorders, learning disabilities, petit mal seizures, or high levels of anxiety. Teachers are not qualified to label a student with an ADHD diagnosis, nor is it ethical to pressure parents to ask their physician for medication. Often, the student with hyperactivity also experiences depression and family conflict. Stimulant medication is useful for ADHD, but only as part of a comprehensive health guidance plan including behavior management and counseling with students, their teachers, and parents.*

*Behrman RE: *Nelson textbook of pediatrics,* Philadelphia, 1992, WB Saunders; and from Schnaiberg L: Experts, educators question ADD diagnoses, *Education Week* 14(22):1,8,1995.

After appropriate care or treatment has been started, it may not always mean that the child has been cured or that the child's health problem has been corrected. A child with a severe vision problem may wear corrective lenses, but still not be able to read the type in a textbook. A student with epilepsy may be receiving medication to control seizures, but may still have seizures at school. It becomes necessary therefore for schools to adjust programs to reasonably fit the needs of students with health problems.

Many but not all modifications occur in special education. Among the numerous ways schools have modified and adjusted educational programs are the following:

- Special consideration for students in the regular classroom. The visually handicapped or hard-of-hearing child may need to be placed near the front of the room. Special rest periods during the day may have to be provided for some pupils. For children with diabetes, midmorning snacks and blood sugar testing may be necessary.

- Special education teachers assist assigned children in the regular school. The partially sighted child may need to have special large-print textbooks and other materials provided. The pupil with speech difficulties may need special attention. Children with learning disabilities may need special guidance. Students go to special teachers for individualized instruction to help them master content in such areas as arithmetic and English.

- Special classes in the regular school. Those who are mentally handicapped, blind, or deaf may be grouped into special classes with specially prepared teachers. Greater attention to a curriculum to satisfy the needs of these children may therefore take place.

- Special day schools. Severely physically challenged children, those who are emotionally disturbed or deaf or severely developmentally delayed may be educated in a school separate from the regular school. These schools are designed for highly structured skill and behavior training.

- Special residential care facilities and schools. Some severely emotionally or mentally handicapped students live for extended periods of time in these schools to receive appropriate care and behavior management. Schools are responsible for education; they may place a teacher in the facility or bus the children to a public day school.

- Home and hospital teachers. Those children who are ill or injured and who must remain at home or in hospitals for long periods of time may have teachers go to their homes or hospital rooms.

Schools differ in the nature and extent of the educational services provided for handicapped pupils. The larger school districts and those with more funds are usually able to provide greater services. Federal and state funds subsidize local costs.

With the passage of Public Law 94-142, the Education for All Handicapped Children Act of 1975, amended to the Individuals with Disabilities Education Act (IDEA), more students who previously stayed home or attended separate schools are attending classes in regular schools. Guidelines expect schools to provide an "appropriate education" in "the least restrictive environment." The process of educating students in regular schools with meaningful interactions with other students is called *mainstreaming*. Placing students in classes in their "home school" with their age-peers and bringing special services as needed into the class is called *inclusion*.

Some students have health conditions such as diabetes or HIV infection, but they are not handicapped as defined by special education if the condition does not interfere with learning. However, they may qualify for certain protection under Section 504 of the federal Rehabilitation Act of 1973. This law prohibits discrimination against persons with disabilities in schools or other programs receiving federal funds. It is intended to ensure that all children have equal access to educational programs. This may mean that schools provide individual services, such as ensuring that a student takes a daily medication or adapting the school food for a medically prescribed special diet so that the student can participate fully in the school day. This law is reinforced by the Americans with Disabilities Act of 1990, Public Law 101-336, which requires that all schools and public places be physically accessible to any persons with disabilities as described in Chapter 3.*

It is important to realize that the problem is not mainstreaming per se, but rather mainstreaming effectively. Teachers must realize that traditional methods may not be effective with these students. According to the IDEA, individualized educational plans (IEPs) must be developed by an established committee (to include parents) so each student can benefit from the educational experience. Individual appraisals and creative teamwork facilitate the planning of a teacher's assignment, instruction, and related services (occupational therapy, physical therapy, speech, extra nursing care) for meeting students' unique educational needs. Clearly these students face problems beyond those of the regular student, and all school personnel should be alert for any additional problems that may emerge. Positive adjustments must be made.

Prescribed Medications at School

Many students with chronic health problems need to take physician-prescribed or nonprescription medications during school hours. Because school personnel must oversee the administration of medication to students, concerns about liability arise. Errors in judgment, including use of the wrong drug, a wrong dosage, or not keeping an exact schedule and record of the administration of the medications to various students contribute to the problem. It is necessary therefore for schools to establish written policies and procedures. According to Lovato, Allensworth, and Chan,† fewer

than 55% of states have written policies that deal with the administration of medications at school.

The purposes of a written policy concerning prescription and nonprescription medications are: (1) to ensure that exact instructions are followed (right drug, right student, correct amount, and proper time), (2) to keep from embarrassing students who have to take the medication, and (3) to minimize the amount of disruption in the school day for the student who must take medication. In developing a set of regulations, The American Academy of Pediatrics* recommends that the following should be included:

- A physician or parent should provide written orders with the name of the drug, dose, time when the medication is to be taken, and diagnosis or reason (unless it should be confidential) the medicine is needed.
- The parent or guardian should provide a written request that the school district comply with the physician's order (Fig. 6-4).
- Medication should be brought to school in a container appropriately labeled by the pharmacist or the physician. Nonprescription drugs must be in the original package.
- When the student does not regularly take his or her own medication, or if the parent or physician requests that school personnel administer the medication, the medication must be kept in a locked cabinet. Designated personnel must be available to administer the medication at agreed-upon times, and arrangements should be made for alternate personnel to perform the task in case of absence. The person administering the medication must keep a written record (Fig. 6-5).
- When the child is responsible for carrying and taking his/her own medication safely, he/she may do so in school without supervision by school personnel, provided the physician and parent have provided the required written authorizations. The school

*Oberg CN, Bryant NA, Bach ML: Ethics, values, and policy decisions for children with disabilities: what are the costs of political correctness? *J School Health* 64(6):223-228, 1994.

†Lovato C, Allensworth D, Chan J: *School health in America: an assessment of state policies to protect and improve the health of students* ed 5, Kent, OH, 1989, The American School Health Association.

*American Academy of Pediatrics: *School health: policy and practice,* Elk Grove Village, IL, 1993, The Academy.

Permit to Administer Medicine

According to AISD policy and state law, school personnel, including the nurse, can administer medicine to your child only as prescribed by the doctor, if prescription, or not more than directed on the label if non-prescription (over-the-counter), and only with your written permission. You must also supply the medicine in what appears to be the original container. If it is a prescription medicine, the child's name must appear on the label. If it is not prescription, we suggest you put your child's name on the container.

Prescription suggestion: When you take the doctor's prescription to the pharmacist, ask her/him to prepare two labeled bottles—one for home and one for school. This method may prevent missed doses because the medicine was left at school.

Any change in the amount of medicine to be given or the time medicine is to be given must be accompanied by another written note or permit.

If you have any questions or comments, please call the school nurse.

- -

Student's name _____ **Teacher** _____

Medicine _____ **Purpose** _____

Amount _____ **When** _____

Form of medicine to be given (please circle one):

Tablet   Pill   Capsule   Liquid   Inhalant

Drops   Cream   Other _____

Any special instructions or side effects:

Parent's signature _____ Date _____

Telephone number (home) _____ work _____

Medicine	Dose	Time	Wk of	M	T	W	Th	F	Wk of	M	T	W	Th	F

The person giving the medicine signs his/her initials in the box under the corresponding day.   School Year: _____

FIG. 6-4 Parental request and physician's order for medication. (Courtesy Austin Independent School District, Health Services, Austin, Texas.)

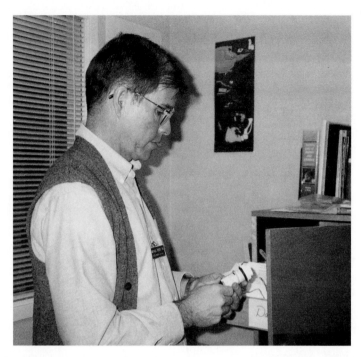

FIG. 6-5 School nurses set campus procedures to prevent medication errors. (Courtesy Austin Independent School District Health Services, Austin, Texas.)

administration should cooperate with the physician, parent, and child. In such instances, it is understood that the school bears no responsibility for safeguarding the medication or ensuring that it is taken, and the parent should provide a written statement relieving the school of such responsibility.

- Individual school districts should seek the advice of counsel as they assume the responsibility for giving medication during school hours. Liability coverage should be provided for the staff including registered nurses, teachers, athletic staff, principals, superintendents, and members of the school board.

- Opportunities should be provided for communication between the parent, school personnel, and physician regarding the efficacy of the medication administered during school hours.

Certain types of medication merit special attention. **Stimulants** such as those for attention deficit–hyperactivity are legally controlled drugs; the tablets should *always* be kept in a locked cabinet and regularly counted. **Inhalers** for asthma may be carried by responsible students; teachers should not insist on keeping these in the school office or locked in the classroom when the students are in other areas, especially physical education or field trips. Only the school's registered nurse should consider administering **injected** medications; the only exception is a student's prescribed injection kit for sudden, life-threatening allergies caused by bee or other insect sting. The school nurse may train the principal or other staff to use an automatic injection kit. Finally, **aspirin** use by children during viral illnesses such as chickenpox or influenza has been connected with Reye's syndrome, a serious disease that attacks the brain and liver. For this reason, school staff should not give aspirin sent by the parent if they have any concern about the child's illness and should ask the parent to get a physician's advice.

SUMMARY

Health guidance is an important and essential part of the school health services program. It should receive adequate consideration in schools. Without follow-up procedures to obtain corrections, treatment, and care including the adjustment of school programs, health appraisals by themselves are not important to the educational process. Assistance in guidance should be forthcoming from a variety of school personnel. School nurses spend a considerable portion of their time in health guidance and are important resources not only for teachers, but also for parents, students, and others. Teachers should clearly understand their responsibilities in health guidance.

For effective results when counseling, it is necessary to follow fundamental principles and techniques. School personnel should be familiar with the community resources available to help children with health problems. Schools use a variety of procedures when adjustments of programs for children with special needs are necessary.

QUESTIONS FOR DISCUSSION

1. What procedures are necessary when children with health problems have been discovered in schools?
2. What is meant by the term *health guidance*, and what is its relationship to informal health education?
3. In your own words, define health counseling.
4. Why is informal health education an important part of the total school health program?
5. What are some pupil health problems needing health guidance?
6. What are the major purposes of health guidance in schools?
7. What organizational factors must receive consideration when a school health guidance program is being introduced?
8. What guiding principles are necessary for an effective school health guidance program?
9. What should be the role of the individual who counsels in the health guidance program?
10. How would you characterize the role of a physician in the school health program?

11. What are the responsibilities of a school drug counselor, and how can such a position be justified?
12. What are some of the duties of the school nurse as the nurse's responsibilities expand?
13. What are the responsibilities of the various school personnel in health guidance?
14. What are some effective techniques for health counseling?
15. What guidelines should be used when students or parents are being counseled?
16. What health resources may be available in the community to help with student health problems?
17. What federal laws or regulations influence school adaptations for children's special needs?
18. What ways have schools tried to adjust programs to help pupils with health problems?
19. What policy regulations should be established in schools in regard to the use of physician-prescribed medications?
20. It has been said that "students do not care what you know until they know that you care." What does this mean for elementary school teachers, counselors, and nurses?

SELECTED REFERENCES

American Academy of Pediatrics: *School health: policy and practice,* Elk Grove Village, IL, 1993, The Academy.

American Academy of Pediatrics, Committee on School Health: *Guidelines for the administration of medication in school,* in press.

American School Health Association: *Guidelines for the comprehensive school health program,* Kent, OH, 1994, The Association.

Cormier L, Cormier W, Weisser R: *Interviewing and helping skills for health professionals,* Monterey, CA, 1984, Wadsworth.

Creswell WH Jr, Newman I: *School health practice,* ed 10, St Louis, 1993, Mosby–Year Book.

Curran D: Adolescent suicidal behavior, *Issues Ment Health Nurs* 8(4):175, 1986.

Davis TM, Allensworth KK: Program management: a necessary component for the comprehensive school health program, *J School Health* 64(2):80-82, 1994.

Dryfoos JG: *Full service schools,* San Francisco, CA, 1994, Jossey-Bass.

Evans D: A school health education program for children with asthma aged 8-11 years, *Health Educ Q* 14:267, 1987.

Evans D: Explaining suicide among the young: an analytical review of the literature, *J Psychosoc Nurse Manage Health Serv* 20(8):9-16, 1986.

Fagan TK: School psychology's dilemma: reappraising solutions and directing attention to the future, *Am Psychol* 41(8):851-861, 1986.

Gibson RL, Mitchell MH: *Introduction to counseling and guidance,* ed 2, New York, 1986, Macmillan.

Hertel V, Doyen M: *Colorado school health guidelines,* ed 2, Denver, 1986, Colorado Department of Education and Colorado Department of Health.

Joachim G: The school nurse as case manager for chronically ill children, *J School Health* 59(9):406-407, 1989.

King LS, Dodd N: The health educator as counselor: what does it take? *Health Educ* 17(2):17-22, 1986.

Klingman A: Health-related school guidance: practical applications in primary prevention, *Pers Guidance J* 62(6):576-580, 1984.

Litwack L, Litwack J, Ballou M: *Health counseling,* New York, 1980, Appleton-Century-Crofts.

Lovato C, Allensworth D, Chan F: *School health in America: an assessment of state policies to protect and improve the health of students,* ed 5, Kent, OH, 1989, American School Health Association.

Majer LS: HIV-infected students in school: who really "needs to know?" *J School Health* 62(6):243-245, 1992.

Melaville AI, Blank MJ: *Together we can: a guide for crafting a profamily system of education and human services,* Washington, DC, 1993, US Government Printing Office.

Myrick RD: *Developmental guidance and counseling,* Minneapolis, MN, 1993, Educational Media Corporation.

National School Board Association: *School board member knowledge of and attitudes regarding school health programs,* Alexandria, VA, 1994, The Association.

Nelson S: *How healthy is your school: guidelines for evaluating school health promotion,* New York, 1986, National Center for Health Education Press.

Niebuhr VN, Smith LR: The school nurse's role in attention deficit hyperactivity disorder, *J School Health* 63(2):114-117, 1993.

Oberg CN, Bryant NA, Bach ML: Ethics, values, and policy decisions for children with disabilities: what are the costs of political correctness? *J School Health* 64(6):223-228, 1994.

Oda DS: Cost documentation of school nursing follow-up services, *J School Health* 56(1):20-22, 1986.

Oda DS: Increasing role effectiveness of school nurses, *Am J Public Health* 64:591-595, 1974.

Ojanlatva A, Hammer AM, Mohr MG: The ultimate rejection: helping the survivors of teen suicide victims, *J School Health* 57(5):181, 1987.

Ozias J: *Influence of parental health beliefs on follow-through on school nurses' spinal screening referrals,* unpublished doctoral dissertation, Austin, TX, 1990, University of Texas at Austin.

Palfrey JS, Haynie M, Porter S, Bierle T, Cooperman P, Lowcock J: Project School Care: integrating children assisted by medical technology into educational settings, *J School Health* 62(2):50-54, 1992.

Passarelli C: School nursing: trends for the future, *J School Health* 64(4):141-149, 1994.

Reed-McKay K: Role transition for school nurses in Spokane Public Schools, *J School Health* 59(10):444-445, 1989.

Silver, GA: Redefining school work health services: comprehensive child health care as the framework, *J School Health* 51(3):157-162, 1981.

Snyder A, editor: *Implementation guide for the standards of school nursing practice,* Kent, OH, 1991, American School Health Association.

The National Commission on the Role of the School and Community in Improving Adolescent Health: *Code blue: uniting for healthier youth,* Alexandria, VA, 1989, National Association of State Boards of Education.

Thomas A: School psychologist: an integral member of the school health team, *J School Health* 37(10):466-468, 1987.

Thomas PS, Texidor MS: The school counselor and holistic health, *J School Health* 57(10):461-464, 1987.

Turner-Henson A, Holaday B, Corser N, Ogletree G, Swan JH: The experiences of discrimination: challenges for chronically ill children, *Pediatr Nurs* 20(6):571-577, 1994.

Wallace H, Parcel GS, Igoe JB, Patrick K, editors: *Principles and practices of student health,* Oakland, CA, 1992, Third Party Publishing.

Walsh M, Ryan-Wenger NM: Sources of stress in children with asthma, *J School Health* 62(10):459-463, 1992.

White DH: A study of current school nurse practice activities, *J School Health* 55(2):52-56, 1985.

Williams RA, Horn S, Daley SP, Nader PR: Evaluation of access to care and medical and behavior outcomes in a school-based intervention program for attention-deficit hyperactivity disorder, *J School Health* 63(7):294-297, 1993.

7

Emergency Care

Every school administrator should develop a systematic procedure for handling any accident or emergency illness that occurs while children are under the school's jurisdiction.

A.E. FLORIO AND WES ALLES*

KEY CONCEPT

Pupil and staff safety can be enhanced when school personnel are prepared in the basic elements of emergency care.

PROBLEM TO SOLVE

You are a fifth grade teacher and one of your students, while on the playground and under your supervision, is injured from a fall. What action must you take to provide emergency care that will protect the injured student?

*Florio AE, Alles W: *Safety education,* ed 4, 1979, McGraw-Hill.

BECAUSE children are required to attend school, all school personnel have an ethical and legal responsibility to ensure that pupils have a safe and hazard-free environment and are provided care in emergencies when injuries or illnesses occur.

Sudden illness and injuries are unplanned occurrences at school or on sponsored trips that all employees should be prepared to handle with skill, promptness, and efficiency. Regardless of the care with which a school facility is constructed, and regardless of diligent care to prevent accidents it is not possible to provide a completely safe environment. In any situation in which relatively large numbers of young people are assembled, emergencies occur, despite precautions that might be taken.* Consequently, all school personnel should know and understand basic first-aid and emergency care procedures.

This chapter contains basic elements of emergency care including first-aid procedures that will enable both the teacher and staff to assist children. All teachers, however, are encouraged to take a course in emergency care and first aid, as well as cardiopulmonary resuscitation (CPR). It is preferable that at least one person certified in emergency care procedures be present at all times when children are in the school. This is also important when after-school activities take place. All school personnel should be adequately trained in current emergency care procedures and CPR whether provided by the American Red Cross, National Safety Council, American Heart Association, or through a program provided by a college or local organization that certifies the individual to render first aid.

Unintentional injury is the leading cause of death and disability for all persons in the United States aged 1 to 34. The financial cost of injury in 1991 was (estimated) over $224 billion—including medical and rehabilitation costs, lost wages, and reduced productivity.†

Elementary teachers are critical people in safety education. Over the past half century the death rate due to injuries for children in the 5- to 14-year age range has continued to drop, mostly from use of seat belts and other improvements in motor vehicle safety. Yet there is room for improvement when some 4000 elementary schoolchildren die each year from injuries. More tragic is the fact that half of these unintentional injuries could have been prevented.

WHAT CAN TEACHERS DO?

Because health and safety are so closely related to the optimal welfare of the school child, teachers need to understand the importance of health and safety in the school program.

Teachers, parents, and others responsible for the optimal growth and development of children should be cognizant not only of the problems in health education, but also of those in safety education. Historically, the schools have accepted responsibility in health education to help each child develop to his or her greatest possible capacity not only academically, but also emotionally and physically. Teachers also have a responsibility to help children know and understand that the potential for injury exists at all times. Children should be taught to be always alert for possible hazardous situations and to avoid those situations whenever possible. The way teachers handle fire and tornado drills with a swift, calm, matter of fact attitude stresses the importance of following emergency procedures to students.

Training in first aid at appropriate levels should be an integral part of the school's health education program. One of the health goals of the nation for the year 2000 is to "provide academic instruction on injury prevention and control, preferably as a part of quality health education, in at least 50% of public school systems (grades K-12)."*

---

*Creswell W, Newman I: *School health practice,* ed 10, St Louis, 1993, Mosby–Year Book.
†Data from National Center for Injury Prevention and Control, Centers for Disease Control and Prevention (CDC), 1991.

---

*Public Health Service: *Healthy people 2000,* Washington DC, 1990, US Department of Health and Human Services, p 283.

WHAT PROVISIONS SHOULD BE MADE FOR EMERGENCY CARE OF INJURED AND ILL PUPILS?

Every school, regardless of size, should have carefully organized, written plans and procedures for the proper care of injured and ill pupils. These plans should be made for emergency care of both mass and individual injuries and illnesses. It is important that emergency care plans be well organized and accessible to all.

Organization and administration of the school emergency care program are the responsibility of the board of education. This responsibility, however, is usually delegated to the superintendent, principal, and other school administrators.

A school district should establish a uniform policy for the emergency care of the injured and ill, and that policy should be available to all school personnel and parents. Plans based on recognized first-aid practices should be used for the general student body. Any student with an identified health condition such as seizures or serious bee sting allergy needs an individualized, written care plan (updated or reviewed yearly). The school nurse or the student's doctor/clinic is responsible for the care plan and teacher training. Explanation of the emergency care policy should be an integral part of the orientation for all new teachers and staff members, regardless of when they enter the school district.

The policy established by a particular school depends on a number of factors, including the size of the community and school; availability of nurses, physicians, hospitals, and ambulances; effective communications; and trained first-aid personnel. In formulating the emergency care policy, school administrators should seek the advice and cooperation of local emergency medical services, school and community safety councils, parents, local medical and public health groups, and community organizations or agencies, such as the police department, fire department, and ambulance and auxiliary services, which may be able to lend assistance when necessary.

The main responsibilities of the school in emergency care are to (1) *give immediate and proper first aid, (2) notify the parents, (3) not increase the severity of the injury, and (4) be certain that the injured or ill are placed under the care of parents or a physician designated by the parents.* Policies should address emergencies that result from such situations as natural disasters (e.g., earthquake, fire, floods, hurricanes, tornadoes), as well as problems such as drug overdoses and injuries resulting from violence. A teacher might encounter a violent situation, for it seems that violence has become more common in many cases of emotional and mental distress and interpersonal conflict.* Teachers also should be aware that some students take weapons to school on a daily basis, usually reportedly for self-defense, and that these weapons may be utilized in conflict situations (see box on p. 173).

The majority of emergency situations that the elementary teacher encounters are rather minor. Regardless, all teachers should have basic first-aid and emergency care training. It is critical that at least one specially trained person also be available to respond to emergency situations and be able to get to the scene of an emergency within 3 to 5 minutes. This person can render basic emergency care until the services of more qualified personnel can be obtained.

In violent situations, school personnel might be exposed to blood. Specific precautions used when dealing with students who are bleeding are called *Universal Precautions.* This is a method of infection control in which blood and all body fluids visibly containing blood are considered to be infected by hepatitis B virus, HIV, or other blood-borne pathogen. The key strategies are:

- Using latex gloves when aiding a person
- Handwashing
- Using disinfectants

---

*Public Health Service: *Healthy people 2000,* Washington DC, 1990, US Department of Health and Human Services, p 226.

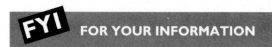

FOR YOUR INFORMATION

What American Children Face

Each day 135,000 children bring a gun to school.

Each day 30 children are wounded by guns.

Each day 13 children die from guns.

Each day, over 1 million latchkey children go into a home where there is a gun.

In 1987, 4% of eighth-grade students were involved in a physical fight.

In a survey of eighth- and tenth-grade students, almost 7% of the boys and 2% of the girls carried knives to school every day.

In 1992, almost 2 million students were suspended from public school.

In 1992, 614,000 students were corporally punished.

Every year almost 3 million children and adolescents are reported abused or neglected; more go unreported.

From Children's Defense Fund: *The state of America's children yearbook 1994,* Washington, DC, 1994, The Fund; Public Health Service: *Healthy people 2000,* Washington DC, 1990, US Department of Health and Human Services; American School Health Association, Association for the Advancement of Health Education, and Society for Public Health Education: *The national student health survey: a report on the health of America's youth,* Oakland, CA, 1989, Third Party Publishing; The National Commission on the Role of the School and the Community in Improving Adolescent Health: *Code blue: uniting for healthier youth,* Alexandria, VA, 1990, National Association of State Boards of Education, and American Medical Association.

• Disposing blood-containing trash properly into plastic bags

"Fanny packs" can be handy for carrying latex gloves, disinfectant, hand wipes, and simple bandages on the playground or field trips. Each staff member should be aware of the danger in dealing with blood and should be instructed in the universal precautions described by the school.

Appendix A contains guidelines that could be utilized by schools in developing policies to deal with blood-related injuries.

Plans for Emergency Care

Every school district needs detailed written procedures that cover emergency situations. Although it is impractical to list the detailed plans that may be necessary for every district, there are many common procedures that should be used in all schools.

For any student with a condition that may lead to an emergency, an individual health care plan, prepared by the school's registered nurse or the child's own physician or clinic must be used.

Emergency transportation. Every school should have written plans for transporting injured or ill children to their homes, hospital, or physicians' or dentists' offices. Previous arrangements should be made with the community emergency medical service system. School buses, ambulances, or other suitable transportation should be available. Often the school nurse or other school personnel needs to transport children in private vehicles, but only in the absence of other alternatives. When injured children are transported in private vehicles, proper insurance coverage should be carried on those vehicles. Staff's own automobile liability insurance may be claimed by an injured student. Regardless of the means, some acceptable type of emergency transportation should be available to the school at all times when children are in attendance, especially during contact sports events. It is important to remember, however, that it is always best not to move seriously injured persons unless the individual is in immediate danger of further injury. Competent medical assistance should be brought *to* a victim.

Facilities and equipment. Proper first aid and emergency care imply that there will be sufficient facilities and equipment in every school. There should be an emergency area containing cots, blankets, lavatories, towels, chairs, and a table. The emergency room should be equipped with adequate first-aid supplies for any type of injury or sudden illness. The first-aid supplies should be maintained in accordance with recognized standards for first-aid care. The kinds and amounts of first-aid material depends on the size of the school and the availability of community resources for emergency medical care. In addition to the first-aid supplies found in the emergency room, classroom teachers should have such supplies as latex gloves, soap, and small dressings for minor wounds. A heavy-weight, zipper-closure plastic bag provides waterproof storage and visibility for classrooms. Students can be assigned to keep them stocked from the school office.

Every elementary school should have adequate first-aid supplies, depending on the enrollment, location, and availability of medical assistance. In most elementary schools the first-aid supplies should be kept in central places, such as the health service room, gyms, science laboratories, kitchens, and the school office. The following list shows usual first-aid supplies needed by the school:

- Adhesive bandages (assorted sizes), flexible fabric type
- Adhesive and paper tape
- Sterile gauze sponges ($3 \times 3''$, $4 \times 4''$)
- "Steri-strip" skin closure, $\frac{1}{8} \times 3''$
- Roller bandages, 1 inch
- Triangular bandages (for slings)
- Cotton swabs, sterile and nonsterile
- Scissors
- Sterile eye wash
- Oval eye pads
- Alcohol, 70% isopropyl, pads
- Liquid soap or skin cleanser (antibacterial)
- Tongue depressors
- Hand brushes
- Elastic bandages, 2 and 3 inches wide
- Blankets
- Thermometers
- Splints
- Pillows (thin)
- Paper cups (5 oz)
- Finger ring cutter
- Safety pins
- Tweezers/splinter forceps
- Hot-water bottle
- Ice bag or zipper-closure freezer bags
- CPR mask with one-way valve (for rescue breathing)
- Latex gloves (vinyl gloves for persons allergic to latex)

No medicines of any kind should be part of a first-aid supply! Periodic inventory and restocking should ensure that first-aid kits are complete and up to date.

Reports and records. An accurate report of each emergency injury or illness should be made. The National Safety Council standard accident report form is shown in Fig. 7-1. Ordinarily the principal delegates the responsibility of making this report to the person who witnessed the event, or the school nurse, or teacher. In any case, teachers are likely to initiate reports, particularly when children under their supervision are injured or become ill. The report should contain such information as the name of the pupil; time, location, and nature of the injury or illness; witnesses, teachers, or other persons present; possible causes of the illness or injury; description of the illness or injury including the part of the body seemingly injured; first aid given; notification of parents; and disposition of the case.

School policy on emergency care. When caring for any injury or emergency situation, the classroom teacher must follow the policy of the school. If an illness is mild, the child should be kept warm and on a cot and be under constant or regular supervision. If the illness progresses, the parent should be called and the usual procedure invoked for caring for more serious illness. The teacher should remember that no medication should be given. The only medicine that can be given is what is noted on the child's existing care plan and furnished by the parent in an original prescription container.

First aid for injuries such as minor cuts and scratches usually can be safely cared for by the teacher. The teacher should be cognizant of any bleeding and take precautions such as wearing latex gloves. The importance of cleanliness for wounds should be stressed, and sterile dressings should be applied. Whenever possible, students should clean and apply pressure to their own minor cuts.

For seemingly major illnesses, the school policy concerning the notifying of parents and taking whatever steps necessary must be put into opera-

STANDARD STUDENT ACCIDENT REPORT FORM
Part A. Information on ALL Accidents

1. Name: _____ Home Address: _____
2. School: _____ Sex: M ☐; F ☐. Age: _____ Grade or classification: _____
3. Time accident occurred: Hour _____ A.M.; _____ P.M. Date: _____
4. Place of Accident: School Building ☐   School Grounds ☐   To or from School ☐   Home ☐   Elsewhere ☐

5. NATURE OF INJURY

Abrasion	_____	Fracture	_____
Amputation	_____	Laceration	_____
Asphyxiation	_____	Poisoning	_____
Bite	_____	Puncture	_____
Bruise	_____	Scalds	_____
Burn	_____	Scratches	_____
Concussion	_____	Shock (el.)	_____
Cut	_____	Sprain	_____
Dislocation	_____		
Other (specify)	_____		

DESCRIPTION OF THE ACCIDENT

How did accident happen? What was student doing? Where was student? List specifically unsafe acts and unsafe conditions existing. Specify any tool, machine or equipment involved. _____

_____
_____
_____
_____

PART OF BODY INJURED

Abdomen	_____	Foot	_____
Ankle	_____	Hand	_____
Arm	_____	Head	_____
Back	_____	Knee	_____
Chest	_____	Leg	_____
Ear	_____	Mouth	_____
Elbow	_____	Nose	_____
Eye	_____	Scalp	_____
Face	_____	Tooth	_____
Finger	_____	Wrist	_____
Other (specify)	_____		

6. Degree of Injury: Death ☐ Permanent Impairment ☐ Temporary Disability ☐ Nondisabling ☐
7. Total number of days lost from school: _____ (To be filled in when student returns to school)

Part B. Additional Information on School Jurisdiction Accidents

8. Teacher in charge when accident occurred (Enter name): _____
Present at scene of accident: No: _____ Yes: _____

9. IMMEDIATE ACTION TAKEN

First-aid treatment	_____	By (Name): _____
Sent to school nurse	_____	By (Name): _____
Sent home	_____	By (Name): _____
Sent to physician	_____	By (Name): _____
		Physician's Name: _____
Sent to hospital	_____	By (Name): _____
		Name of hospital: _____

10. Was a parent or other individual notified? No:___ Yes:___ When:_____ How: _____
Name of individual notified: _____
By whom? (Enter name): _____
11. Witnesses: 1. Name: _____ Address: _____
             2. Name: _____ Address: _____

12. LOCATION

Specify Activity		Specify Activity		Remarks
Athletic field	_____	Locker	_____	What recommendations do you have for pre-venting other accidents of this type? _____
Auditorium	_____	Pool	_____	
Cafeteria	_____	Sch. grounds	_____	_____
Classroom	_____	_____ shop	_____	_____
Corridor	_____	Showers	_____	_____
Dressing room	_____	Stairs	_____	_____
Gymnasium	_____	Toilets and		_____
Home Econ.	_____	washrooms	_____	_____
Laboratories	_____	Other (specify)	_____	

Signed: Principal: _____ Teacher: _____

(National Safety Council- Form School 1)   Printed in U.S.A.   Stock No. 429-21
Rep. 100M106002

FIG. 7-1 National Safety Council accident report form. (Courtesy National Safety Council, Inc., Chicago, Illinois.)

tion immediately. The child should rest and body temperature should be maintained. Someone should stay with the child until the school has carried out the parents' instructions or, if parents cannot be contacted, call the family physician for instructions or take the child to a hospital. In cases of major injuries the school policy for rendering first aid under such circumstances should be put into effect. Specific policies for dealing with emergency cases during lunch or after-school hours when offices are closed should also be established.

Information for Emergencies

Certain information must be readily available to facilitate the rapid and proper handling of emergency cases. The following kinds of information should be carefully listed, organized, and placed near a telephone in the principal's office where it is accessible to the school nurse, all teachers, or other school personnel who may be expected to assist in any way with emergency care:

- A list of all pupils with full and correct names
- The names of both parents or guardians, if available
- Home address
- Home telephone number
- Work telephone, address, and name of business of each parent/guardian
- Name and telephone number of child's physician and alternate physician of family's choice
- Names and telephone numbers of relatives to be called in case parents cannot be reached
- Hospital of choice and the telephone number
- Any special directions from parents concerning the handling of emergency injury or illness
- Homeroom teacher
- List of pupil's daily class schedule

In a central location, and on every telephone should be numbers of local ambulance services, fire department, police department, and poison control center.

An increasing number of communities are centralizing their emergency communication sys-

tems. More towns and cities are using 911 as the all-purpose number. School administrators, teachers, other school personnel, and students should know how to use the local emergency communication system.

Notification of parents. Schools often request parents to sign a permit authorizing school staff to contact emergency care for their children in case of injury and certain illnesses. This is helpful in situations in which parents or guardians cannot be contacted promptly. The school can call the designated physician or hospital or take any other action necessary for the child's safety. The school permit is *not* an authorization for emergency room treatment other than life support.

When notifying parents by telephone, the person making the call should speak in a calm, reassuring voice to allay fear. A full description of the child's injury or illness should be given so far as it is evident. Parents should be told whether immediate medical attention seems needed. The school nurse or principal may need to insist that parents come for their child and secure medical care. The person making the call should learn from the parents how soon they will come to school or who they will send for the child. Parents should be encouraged to come whenever possible. Occasionally, parents may want to call the physician for instructions or to arrange to take the child to the office, clinic, or hospital. If an ambulance is needed, parents should be told before the school takes this action. The school is not financially responsible.

In the event of ambulance transport, the school may send staff to accompany the child. Usually the nurse or principal arranges assistance.

As most physicians are not prepared to provide emergency care in their offices in critical situations, it is usually most advisable to call 911 or another emergency phone number for quick transport to the emergency unit of the nearest hospital. It is important to call the hospital and inform them of the nature of the injury or illness while the child is en route to the emergency room. This gives hospital personnel time to set up whatever may be required. It also alerts them to possible need to call a surgeon or other specialists.

Sick or injured children should never be sent home unless accompanied by a responsible adult *and* unless the parents or some responsible person designated by the parents is there to care for them. In cases in which parents or guardians cannot be immediately contacted, school authorities must use their best judgment. It may be necessary to call a physician or dentist directly, or in some cases it may be necessary to call an ambulance and take the child to a hospital. In every case school personnel should give the parents every possible aid in caring for a sick or injured child. Often if specialized medical attention is indicated, the parents may be at a loss concerning the selection of a physician. In this case the school nurse or other authorities should be prepared with the names of available medical specialists such as pediatricians, orthopedists, ophthalmologists, and dentists from which parents can make a selection.

It is advisable that the school follow up emergency cases. Parents or guardians should be called within 24 hours to learn the condition of the child. If the condition is serious, periodic telephone calls from the school might be made until the child is improving. Follow-up of emergency cases costs little and brings goodwill to the school. It is also important that school officials know the recovery period needed for any injury or illness so that the child's schedule can be altered appropriately. All follow-up actions should be noted in the student's record.

TEACHER'S ROLE IN EMERGENCY CARE

All teachers need sufficient training to manage basic emergency situations, particularly those involving breathing and bleeding. The teacher should be able to assess an emergency situation and carry out appropriate care procedures. Teachers and other school staff also should be totally familiar with the school's emergency care program, including emergency assistance numbers to call. The teacher must be prepared to accept certain responsibilities, such as the following:

- Survey the scene for safety

- Assist with any emergency in which large numbers of pupils are injured or become suddenly ill
- Render first aid or contact those who are officially designated to give first aid when a pupil is injured or becomes ill
- Assist those who are giving first aid, when necessary, by doing such things as calling parents or physician
- Give first aid for minor injuries such as small wounds that do not require the attention of a physician, nurse, or others who give first aid

The legal duty of school personnel falls into four categories:

- To foresee possible hazards and take reasonable steps to correct the hazard
- To provide warnings about hazards that are not immediately remediable
- To render proper first aid to the injured
- Not to increase the severity of the injury

The teacher should be prepared to assume full responsibility for those few times when there is no immediate help. Providing first aid does not involve medication of any kind, even such a seemingly harmless thing as aspirin, unless directed on the student's written care plan and provided by the family. The teacher should use *only* those supplies and soaps indicated in the written policy of the school. All first-aid supplies in the schools should have the approval of those responsible for formulating the policy for emergency and first-aid care.

Teachers must provide emotional support for students who witness accidents, particularly if the accident was severe or the result of violence. Such support is a type of informal health education; it is also an example of a teachable moment in schools. The counselor would provide or coordinate support in dealing with student adjustments as the result of witnessing an unintentional injury. Cooperatively, the teachers and counselors assist students in dealing with the situation in such a fashion to help them cope with loss or fear and return to normal school routines as soon as possible.

WHO IS LIABLE AND RESPONSIBLE FOR SCHOOL ACCIDENTS?

Although teachers have always been concerned about injuries involving schoolchildren, some teachers have not understood their responsibility in such circumstances.

Fear of being sued often dissuades teachers from rendering first aid to students. State policies differ in regard to teacher responsibilities and although in some states there may be no legal obligation, *there is a moral obligation* for teachers to provide care for students in need. Teachers who act in a reasonable and prudent manner when providing emergency care are generally protected from tort liabilities (monetary compensation). Good Samaritan laws protect persons who act in good faith to give first aid according to their training and without gross negligence.

Legal Responsibility

The question is often asked, "Why is there a greater tendency today to attempt to hold the teacher financially liable for injuries to pupils?" The answer to this question in part is that today most people have come to expect injuries to be paid for. When an action or object causes injury, usually the first question asked is, "Who is to pay?"

Because the teacher is acting *in loco parentis* (in the place of a parent), any time a student is injured at school, the teacher runs the risk of being sued for negligence. Negligence is generally based on failure to act as a reasonably prudent and careful individual would act given the same or similar circumstances. In general, negligence may take three forms: (1) failing to perform an expected duty (nonfeasance or an act of omission), (2) performing a duty incorrectly (misfeasance or an act of commission), or (3) performing an illegal procedure or performing a procedure without consent (malfeasance or an act of commission).

In case of *negligence,* a teacher or a school board, or both, may be held responsible and financially liable for injury to a pupil. Increasing numbers of court procedures and damage suits for accidental injuries to school children are being recorded. States laws define and control the liability of public schools.

The teacher would be well advised to carry a personal liability insurance policy. This policy may be purchased through private insurance companies, or, often at less cost, through a professional organization to which the teacher belongs.

Teachers should familiarize themselves with not only local school emergency care procedures, but also with the school law in their own state regarding negligence and personal liability to civil suit.

The law of negligence is partly based on the theory that everyone has the right to live safely and must be protected from the negligence of others in this right. In the school situation the teacher owes a duty to the school child. In many cases the failure to act to prevent an accident to a school child would be considered negligence on the part of the teacher.

The law of negligence implies, so far as the duty of the teacher to the pupil is concerned, that there must be *foreseeability*. The teacher acting as a reasonably careful and prudent person should anticipate danger or an accident.

For negligence to be established, the court must determine that[*]:

- The student was injured as a result of a school-related incident
- The action or inaction of the school official resulted in additional injury or caused the severity of the injury to increase
- The school official acted in a manner different from the way a reasonable and prudent person would have acted under the same or similar circumstances

---

[*]Modified from Hafen B: *First aid for health emergencies,* ed 3, St Paul, 1985, West.

- The school official did, in fact, have a duty to act

Some conditions that may make teachers liable to legal action include:

- Permitting pupils to play unsafe, unorganized games
- Maintaining attractive nuisances (conditions of school environment, apparatus, equipment, machinery)
- Permitting pupils to use dangerous devices
- Planning and organizing inadequately for field trips
- Permitting use of defective equipment, particularly on playgrounds, in physical education activities, shops or laboratories
- Failing to provide adequate supervision or instruction for pupil activities
- Use of "excessive force" in corporal punishment
- Transportation in a motor vehicle

Although these points may seem rather obvious, the basic laws associated with liability were developed to protect and compensate innocent victims of accidents that might have been prevented through prudent action. The laws were also enacted to protect the school or staff from frivolous lawsuits.

In some cases the injured student may be partially or wholly at fault. If the teacher gives specific directions or warnings and the student ignores them, depending on the age of the student, it is possible that the student, not the teacher, could be held liable for the injury. This is called "contributory negligence," and means that the child failed to exercise care, follow directions, or heed specific warnings. In comparative or shared negligence, both the teacher and the student contribute to the situation that results in an accident or injury. In this case, damage recovery is proportional to the amount of negligence contributed by each party to the circumstances that led to the injury.

In addition to the possibility of the teacher's being held financially liable for the injury of a child, especially in a case of negligence, there is another factor that should be taken into consideration. In many cases the teacher may not be financially responsible. The teacher may be quite vulnerable, however, from the viewpoint of failing to take proper responsibility in case of an accident to a child. That is, the superintendent of schools or the board of education could hold the teacher negligent, perhaps resulting in discipline or even discharge for failing to use reasonable care in providing safe conditions.

Legal Defense

Fortunately, teachers generally exercise caution in their dealings with students. Further, the courts have realized the difficulty of controlling or keeping under close supervision as many as 35 to 40 students. Also, there has not been a successful prosecution for negligence against any person who has followed established first-aid procedures when providing aid to an injured individual. The low cost of personal liability insurance is also mute testimony to this low incidence of successful prosecutions.

Several defenses are generally used in lawsuits against teachers. These are as follows:

assumption of risk The person injured failed to heed warnings or voluntarily and with full knowledge of the possible consequences entered a hazardous situation (e.g., climbed over a fence surrounding a hazard)

contributory negligence The failure of the injured person to use due care for his or her own personal safety

proximate cause The injury was not the result of teacher negligence and would have occurred regardless of safety precautions that were taken

vis major A natural cause that could not be guarded against or anticipated by a person acting in a reasonable and prudent fashion (e.g., an earthquake or other act of God)

Obviously the best defense is not to become involved in litigation initially. This means that a well-planned safety program should be functioning within the school and that the teacher and other school staff should be prepared to handle emergency situations as they arise.

EMERGENCY CARE PROCEDURES IN SCHOOLS*

The emergency care given at the time a person is injured or becomes suddenly ill is known as first aid. It is the care given before medical aid is available. The duties of the person giving first aid end immediately when medical assistance is obtained. Actions such as repeated bandaging of wounds or attempting to care for extended illnesses is not a responsibility of the teacher.

Every elementary school classroom teacher should have a knowledge of first aid to provide care and to teach students basics in care for themselves or others. Some states require elementary teachers to complete a course in first aid or have comparable American Red Cross instruction. Every person employed by the school district, every parent, and every student needs basic first-aid skills.

The following points should be kept in mind when giving first aid:

- First aid is given to an injured person to prevent further harm and reduce suffering and discomfort.
- Always call for emergency medical assistance in serious cases.
- Haste is seldom necessary as most schools are in relative proximity to emergency medical services.
- The person giving first aid should know what not to do as well as what to do in an emergency.
- Improper emergency care may result in permanent injury or even death.
- An injured person should not be moved unless it is absolutely necessary, until the exact nature of the injury is known, and until provisions have been made to prevent further damage.

The teacher or person responsible for giving first aid should remember that the three emergency situations requiring immediate and instant action to save life (hurry cases) are serious bleeding, suspended breathing, and poisoning.

Calling Emergency Medical Services

Many communities have centralized emergency communication systems. These systems are generally activated by calling 911. Regardless of the emergency system used, the following information should be told to whomever answers the emergency number:

- The location of the emergency, including the specific address, if known, and key landmarks such as names of buildings or statues.
- The exact telephone number being used to make the emergency call. This number can be traced and can assist emergency medical services.
- The name of the individual initiating the call.
- The exact nature of what happened.
- The number of victims involved.
- The condition of each of the victims, including approximate age of each.
- What is currently being done to aid each victim.

Whoever initiates the call to the emergency service waits until the dispatcher hangs up. If the caller hangs up first, the dispatcher may need additional information and will have no way to recontact the caller.

Evaluate the Scene

Before rendering care to an injured child, it is important to assess the situation. The purpose of surveying the scene is threefold. First, the teacher must determine whether it is safe to enter the scene. A teacher cannot help an injured child if the teacher also becomes a victim. For example, a teacher should not attempt to provide care in

---

*Modified in part from Airhihenbuwa CO: *First aid and emergency care: procedure and practice,* Dubuque, IA, 1986, Kendall/Hunt; American Red Cross: *Community first aid and safety,* St Louis, 1993, Mosby–Year Book; Hafen BQ: *First aid for health emergencies,* ed 3, St. Paul, 1985, West; Heimlich HJ, Uhley MH: The Heimlich maneuver, *Clinical Symposium, CIBA* 31(3): 1979; National Safety Council: *First aid and CPR,* 1991, Boston, Jones and Bartlett; Rinke CM, editor: Standards and guidelines for cardiopulmonary resuscitation (CPR) and emergency cardiac care (ECC), *JAMA* 255(21):2905-2984, 1986; Parcel GS, Rinear CE: *Basic emergency care of the sick and injured,* ed 3, St Louis, 1986, Mosby–Year Book.

which there are environmental dangers such as exposure to electrical currents, toxic gases, or explosions, or in situations where there is violence, such as in knife fights or where firearms are involved. Second, the teacher may gather clues as to what happened. Finally, during this time, the teacher may identify witnesses and bystanders who may assist in rendering care.

CARDIOPULMONARY EMERGENCIES

Every year more than 400 children die of respiratory or cardiac emergencies. Children are much less likely to have heart conditions or cardiac emergencies than older adults. There are two types of cardiopulmonary emergencies: respiratory arrest and cardiac arrest. Respiratory arrest occurs when a person stops breathing. Cardiac arrest occurs when a person's heart stops beating. A person may go into respiratory arrest without going into cardiac arrest, but the situation requires swift and proper first aid.

ABCs of Life Support

In emergency situations, people use the ABC of emergency care (Airway, Breathing, and Circulation). The ABC begins with a primary survey of the situation. The purpose of the primary survey is to assess the most life-threatening conditions and treat those first. Thus the primary survey consists of an assessment and a subsequent action. The ABC of life support is a first-aid procedure that consists of recognizing cessation of breathing and heartbeat and then applying cardiopulmonary resuscitation (CPR), which involves (A) opening and maintaining a victim's *Airway*, (B) giving rescue *Breathing*, and (C) providing artificial *Circulation* by external cardiac compression (heart massage). CPR should be performed only by people with special training. Local Heart Associations or the American Red Cross can provide certified training. Schools can sponsor training for staff, parents, and students over 12 years old. These are the essential points of the ABCs:

A, airway open. Roll the victim over (Fig. 7-2) and check for responsiveness by gently tapping the person and asking if he or she is all right. If the victim is unconscious, open the airway. The airway is opened by placing your hand on the victim's chin and lifting while tilting the head as far as possible with the other hand (Fig. 7-3). Doing this moves the base of the victim's tongue away from the back of the throat and provides a clear airway.

B, breathing restored. The next step is to assess whether a victim is breathing. The rescuer should check for breathing by looking for the rise

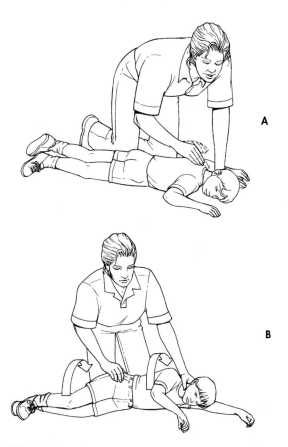

FIG. 7-2 Initial stages of cardiopulmonary resuscitation. **A,** Determine unresponsiveness and call for help. **B,** While supporting the head and neck, position the victim for resuscitation. (Courtesy the American Red Cross. All rights reserved in all countries.)

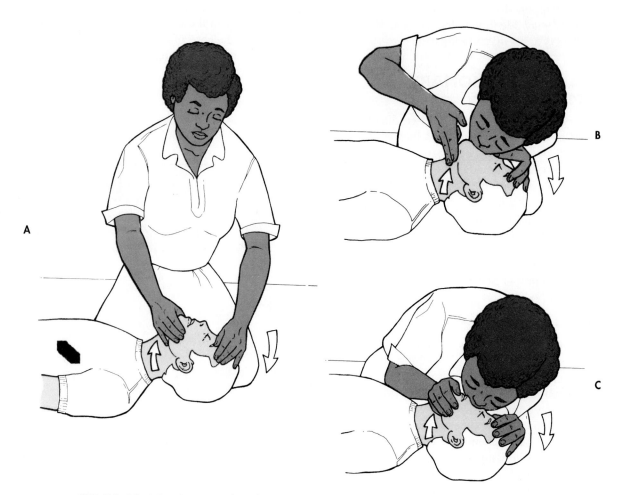

FIG. 7-3 Administering rescue breathing. **A,** Move the child's head so that the chin is pointing upward. **B,** Close the child's nostrils and place your mouth tightly over the child's mouth. **C,** If the mouth-to-nose method is used, close the child's mouth and place your mouth over the child's nose.

and fall of the chest, listening for breaths, and feeling for breaths against the rescuer's cheek. If the victim is not breathing, place your mouth tightly over the victim's mouth, pinch the nostrils, and give two slow, deep, and separate breaths with enough air to make the victim's chest rise. After giving two breaths, check for a carotid pulse located in the neck artery under the side angle of the lower jaw near the "Adam's apple." To do this, keep the victim's head tilted with one hand and use the index and middle fingers of the other hand to feel the carotid pulse (Fig. 7-3, *B*). For children (1 to 8 years) the pulse should be checked at the brachial artery located on the inside of the upper arm.

C, circulation maintained. If no carotid or brachial pulse is identified, cardiopulmonary resuscitation must be initiated.

Cardiopulmonary Resuscitation

The purpose of CPR is to act as a life-support system for victims in either respiratory or cardiac arrest. CPR involves two important procedures: rescue breathing and external chest compressions. Victims of respiratory and cardiac arrest risk brain damage if they do not receive CPR within 4 to 6 minutes. If CPR is given within 4 minutes after the victim goes into cardiac arrest, the chances for survival and full recovery are four times greater than if the victim did not receive CPR.

Rescue Breathing

Artificial respiration, now called *rescue breathing,* is given to a victim in respiratory arrest. During rescue breathing, the rescuer is breathing for the victim because a person cannot live without oxygen. It is extremely important when administering first aid to begin rescue breathing immediately after the cessation of breathing because the heart will stop a short time after breathing has stopped.

Rescue breathing can be administered in several ways. However, the mouth-to-mouth or mouth-to-nose method is recommended as the most efficient and usually the most practical.

The following directions briefly explain how to give mouth-to-mouth and mouth-to-nose rescue breathing.

As stated previously, the person is gently tapped and asked loudly whether he/she is alright. If you get no response, open the airway, call out for help, and place your ear near the mouth to listen for breathing. To open the airway, the head is tilted back and the chin lifted to ensure an open airway. Breathing is rechecked. If there is still no breathing, rescue breathing is initiated.

In the most effective, mouth-to-mouth technique, close the person's nostrils with your fingers or cheek. Place your mouth tightly over the person's mouth as shown in Fig. 7-3, *B*. Some do not wish to come in contact with the person if there is blood on or near the mouth, so they place a pocket mask or handkerchief over the nose and mouth of the victim. If you use the mouth-to-nose technique, close the person's mouth and place your mouth over the person's nose as shown in Fig. 7-3, *C*. Blow two slow, full breaths into the person's mouth until the chest gently rises. Remove your mouth and turn your head toward the chest while you inhale. Check for a pulse at the side of the neck, just below the chin. Feel for a pulse for 5 to 10 seconds. If you feel a pulse, maintain rescue breathing. If there is no pulse, CPR is required. To continue rescue breathing only, repeat the blowing of air into the person's mouth and remove your mouth to inhale and check for breathing. The rate of breathing in this way should be about *1 breath every 5 seconds* for adults, 1 breath every 3 seconds for a child. Blow deeply for an adult or older child; use your diaphgram muscles, not your cheeks. Continue until the victim starts breathing on his or her own, the airway becomes obstructed, or qualified help arrives. Recheck for pulse and spontaneous breathing about every minute.

There are a few differences in using the mouth-to-mouth method of artificial respiration on small children under 8 years of age.

Place a small child on his/her back with chin pointed upward and lower jaw in a jutting position. The child's chin is lifted and the forehead tilted back. Place your mouth over *both* the child's nose and mouth tightly enough so that air cannot escape. Breathe gently and smoothly into the child's nose and mouth until the chest rises. When you have breathed enough air into the child's lungs, as indicated by the rising of the chest, turn your head toward the chest and allow the air to pass from the child's lungs. Remember to *repeat this cycle about once every 3 seconds.*

Airway Obstructions

At times, breathing cessation is caused by an obstructed airway. At other times, the cause of complete or partial cessation of breathing is electric shock, drowning, inhaling certain gases, choking, strangling, inhaling certain chemical fumes or glue, and consuming drugs such as morphine,

barbiturates, and alcohol. In the school, mechanical obstruction is likely to be the most common cause of suspended breathing. The causes of breathing interference include foreign bodies in the throat and windpipe, drowning, and strangulation.

If you come upon a person who is not breathing, you should again remember the ABC of life support. Sometimes merely opening the airway will suffice and the victim will resume breathing. However, if the victim is unconscious and you have unsuccessfully tried tilting the head back to open the airway, with the victim lying on his or her back, straddle the victim's legs at the thighs or move to the victim's side and deliver 6 to 10 upward and inward, quick, forceful, abdominal thrusts (Fig. 7-4). The rescuer's hands are placed

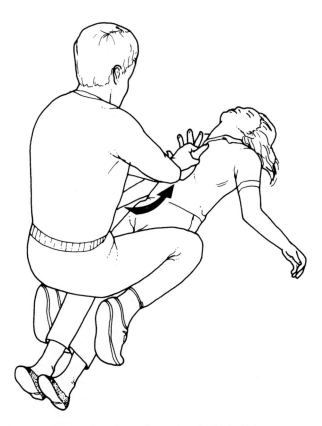

FIG. 7-4 Rescuer kneeling when using the Heimlich maneuver.

in the same location as in the Heimlich maneuver. After giving 6 to 10 abdominal thrusts, move to the victim's head to sweep the mouth and remove any foreign bodies that may be obstructing the airway. This procedure is repeated until the victim begins breathing. Once the obstructing body is removed, give rescue breathing until the victim begins breathing or qualified medical help arrives.

Choking. Occasionally students, infants, and adults will experience severe choking. About 3000 people died (40 in the 5- to 14-year age group) in 1994 as a result of a foreign body obstructing the airway.* In 1974 Dr. Henry Heimlich developed a technique to deal with foreign-body airway obstruction. Heimlich's technique consists of external compression of the air in the lungs in order to create an "artificial cough" strong enough to dislodge a foreign body blocking the airway. In 1985 a National Conference on Cardiopulmonary Resuscitation (CPR) and Emergency Cardiac Care (ECC) recommended the Heimlich maneuver be the procedure for dealing with victims of an obstructed airway unless the victim is younger than 1 year of age. For infants, a combination of back blows and chest thrusts was recommended.

Identifying a choking victim. In more than 90% of the instances of choking, the victim chokes on food or an object. Over 98% of persons dying suddenly in eating establishments have choked on food. The choking victim cannot breathe or speak, becomes cyanotic, and collapses. This is obviously a life-threatening situation.

When an individual is choking, there is a universal signal that has come to be known as the *Heimlich sign,* which indicates, "I am choking." Victims grasp their neck between their thumb and index finger to indicate the choking situation (Fig. 7-5). It should be noted, however, that not every victim of choking will show this signal. The rescuer should ask "Are you choking?" and let a person who is coughing try to cough out the object first.

Heimlich maneuver. To be safe and effective, the Heimlich maneuver should be performed in one of the following ways:

1. When you as rescuer are standing or slightly kneeling and the victim is standing or sitting, you should do the following:
   a. Stand behind the person, slide your arms under the person's arms, and wrap your arms around the victim's waist. Point your elbows outward to avoid injuring the victim's ribs. Position your feet to support the victim in case the victim falls.
   b. Make a fist and place it thumb side against the victim's abdomen slightly above the navel and below the ribcage (Fig. 7-6).
   c. Grasp your fist with the other hand and press into the victim's abdomen with firm, quick inward, and upward thrusts (Fig. 7-7).
   d. This process may need to be repeated several times.
2. If the victim is sitting, you should stand behind the victim's chair and perform the maneuver in the same manner as for a standing victim.

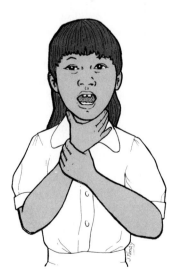

FIG. 7-5 Universal signal used to indicate choking.

---

*National Safety Council: *Accident facts,* Itasca, IL, 1994, The Council.

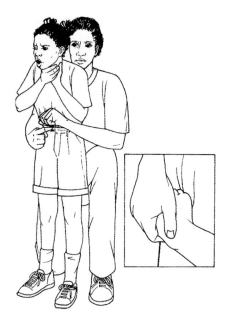

FIG. 7-6 Heimlich maneuver with child upright. (Courtesy the American Red Cross. All rights reserved in all countries.)

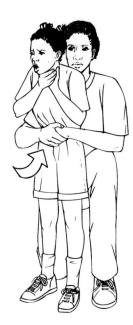

FIG. 7-7 Give quick upward thrusts in the Heimlich maneuver. (Courtesy the American Red Cross. All rights reserved in all countries.)

3. However, when the victim is lying face up and you are kneeling, you should take the following steps:
   a. With the victim lying on his or her back, face the victim and kneel alongside the hips.
   b. With one hand on the top of the other, place your hands on the victim's abdomen slightly above the navel and below the ribcage.
   c. Press into the victim's abdomen with quick upward thrusts.
   d. Repeat several times if necessary.

The standing and sitting positions are used most often; however, it is extremely important that rescuers learn the supine position (victim lying face upward). Only in that position can a small person—one who cannot reach around the victim's waist or who is not strong enough to press a fist upward under the diaphragm with sufficient force—save a heavy victim. In the supine position,

the rescuer uses weight, not strength, to press upward on the diaphragm.

It is important to remember that the Heimlich maneuver is to be used only in emergency situations. Training mannequins are available for practice. The maneuver should *not* be practiced on people because damage to internal organs could occur.

External chest compressions. External chest compressions are performed only on a victim who is in cardiac arrest. Any person giving CPR needs prior training. The following description of key steps illustrates CPR, but is not a substitute for proper training. If no pulse is detected, compressions should be administered as follows. First, place the victim on his or her back on a firm surface such as the floor. Place the heel of your hand on the center of the lower half of the sternum, or sternum breastbone, with your fingers off the person's chest. Place your other hand on top (Fig. 7-8). Apply a forceful, downward thrust, pressing 1

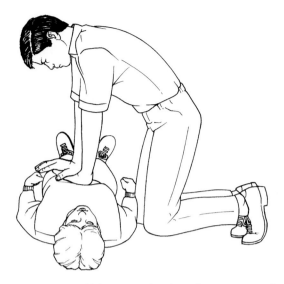

FIG. 7-8 ABC of life support (cardiopulmonary resuscitation, CPR). (Courtesy the American Red Cross. All rights reserved in all countries.)

to 2 inches, with your hand to force blood out of the heart. Repeat this procedure 15 times, then administer two full breaths, following the procedure indicated in the section dealing with rescue breathing. The rate of administration of chest compressions to adults and children over 8 years of age should be about 80 to 100 times a minute. Repeat this cycle of 15 compressions to 2 breaths four times, then reassess breathing and pulse. If you do not detect either breathing or a pulse, you must continue to repeat this procedure until the victim is revived, you are too tired to continue, or qualified help arrives.

For small children (1 to 8 years old). Locate the center of the breastbone. Using *only* the heel of one hand, pressing 1 to 1½ inches, deliver chest compressions at a rate of 100 a minute. The ratio of breaths to compressions in a child is 1:5.

Bleeding

Severe bleeding must be stopped immediately. In addition to danger from the loss of blood, it is likely to cause shock. Furthermore, children are usually frightened by the sight of their own blood if the bleeding is serious. If a large blood vessel is severed, a quart of blood can be lost from the body within 1 minute. Consequently, in an emergency of this kind, the teacher must act instantly. Direct pressure with elevation is recommended to stop most bleeding. Latex gloves should be worn and sterile gauze pads obtained. In most cases, hand pressure with a sterile dressing, towel, or cloth is the accepted procedure. A compress directly on the wound with a tight bandage and elevation will control the blood flow in most cases. Blood flow from the head and face usually can be controlled in this way. If bleeding cannot be controlled using direct pressure and elevation, the rescuer should apply pressure on a main artery that supplies the wound area with blood. Pressure is applied on the artery against an underlying bone.

If a large artery of the upper arm or thigh is cut, *it may be necessary, under rare circumstances, to apply a tourniquet. Because a tourniquet is an extremely dangerous piece of equipment, its use is highly restricted and should be viewed in the light that a limb may be sacrificed to save a life.* Improper use of a tourniquet may cause the following:

- The artery may be permanently damaged through crushing by too much pressure.
- Keeping the supply of blood from a part of the body too long may cause loss of the limb.
- Additional bleeding resulting from removing the tourniquet too soon.
- Removing the tourniquet after an extended period of application may increase the possibility of shock.

If a tourniquet is needed anywhere on an upper arm or thigh, it should be applied between the heart and as close to the wound as possible, on the nearest uninjured tissue, and only tight enough to stop or slow bleeding so that direct pressure on the wound will be effective. Any material fairly thick and soft that can be tied around the arm or leg and twisted tight enough to stop the bleeding can be used as a tourniquet. *It must not cut or bruise the flesh.* Materials such as wire or rope should *never be used as a tourniquet.*

A tourniquet should be used *only in case of serious bleeding that threatens life* and cannot be stopped by other means. If a tourniquet is applied, it should not be released other than by a physician or medical personnel. The time of application should be attached to or, if possible, written on the forehead of the victim.

Wounds

Any injury to the skin or tissue is classed as a wound. Any break in the skin or mucous membrane is considered a wound if germs are allowed to enter.

Wounds may be classified according to the way the injury occurs, the type of wound made, and the kind of first aid required. The general types of wounds with which the person giving first aid is likely to be concerned are cuts or lacerations, abrasions or scraping, or rubbing types of wounds made by the body sliding on the floor or on a rough surface. Puncture or stab wounds are made by objects such as knives, needles, and nails.

Puncture and stab wounds are ordinarily more serious than other types of minor wounds for the following reasons:

- Tetanus, or "lockjaw" germs, may grow when there is a lack of air, such as in a puncture wound.
- Punctures do not bleed freely; consequently, dirt and germs are not washed out as in an open wound.
- It is difficult to clean the wound, and germs may have been deposited in the bottom of it by the instrument making the wound.

A physician needs to treat a puncture wound with antibiotics and/or tetanus immunization.

Infection is a risk of wounds. Although thousands of organisms may enter even a tiny wound, not all wounds become infected. The body resists and overcomes organisms, depending on a number of factors.

Clean-cut wounds usually bleed freely and are less likely to become infected. Wounds made by machines or other rough objects, however, are more likely to become infected. They may not bleed freely, and often there may be dirt and grease in the wound.

In giving first aid for wounds in which serious bleeding is not a factor, a main purpose is to control bleeding, prevent infection, and keep germs from entering the wound. If the cut gapes and stitches (sutures) are probably needed, the student needs medical attention within 2 to 4 hours. If a physician is available, the person giving first aid is only required to apply direct pressure using a sterile dressing, elevate the wound area above the level of the heart if possible, and apply pressure to the nearest pressure point. Never try to clean a wound or apply an antiseptic if a physician is needed. If it is necessary to cleanse a wound, use antibacterial soap and running tap water adjusted to room temperature. The first-aid care of small wounds requires only skin cleansing, a sterile compress and bandage to keep dirt from entering the wound.

Nosebleed

A nosebleed frequently results from a blow on the nose, although there may be other causes. Low humidity or a coldlike infection can irritate the mucous membrane of the nose. Most nosebleeds in children will stop without emergency care. For minor cases, have the person sit, lean forward, and breathe through the mouth. The student or person giving first aid presses the side of the nose that is bleeding with the thumb for 5 to 10 minutes (Fig. 7-9). This technique keeps the blood from flowing back into the throat. Cold packs may be applied to the nose. After a nosebleed ends, the person should not blow his or her nose for about 12 hours. If a nosebleed cannot be stopped after 10 minutes, medical care is needed.

Dental Emergencies*

In the event a permanent tooth is knocked out, the teacher needs to calm the student and find the

---

*American Academy of Pediatric Dentistry: *First aid for dental emergencies,* Chicago, 1986, The Academy.

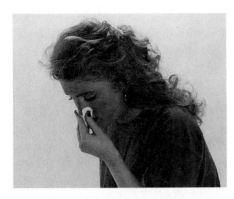

FIG. 7-9 To control a nosebleed, have the victim lean forward and pinch the nostrils together until the bleeding stops. (Courtesy the American Red Cross. All rights reserved in all countries.)

tooth. Handle it only by the top (crown), not the root. A helper can rinse dirt from the tooth, but never clean it. Try to replace it immediately in the socket and have the child hold it in place by biting down on a clean gauze pad or cloth. If the tooth cannot be reinserted, keep it moist in a zip-top bag of water or milk. A dentist *must* be seen immediately to increase the chances of saving the tooth. Likewise, if part of a tooth breaks, try to find the broken pieces. A dentist should evaluate the child's tooth as soon as possible.

Shock

Broken bones, poisoning, severe burns, hemorrhage, perforation or inflammation of internal organs, or reactions to drugs or proteins may cause *shock*. Intense pain, loss of blood, tissue destruction, and sometimes strong emotions may affect the nervous system's control of the circulatory system. Blood pressure may fall so low that circulation is inadequate. The brain fails to get enough blood to supply sufficient oxygen and nutrition, and, as a result, consciousness may be lost.

Shock may not be clearly noticeable following most minor injuries. However, some degree of shock may follow any injury, particularly if it is accompanied by strong emotional reactions.

An injury that causes only slight or moderate shock in one person may cause serious shock in another. Severe shock usually follows serious injury. Consequently, the teacher should always try to prevent shock and recognize its early signs when giving first aid to pupils who are injured. Shock may appear soon after an injury, or it may appear hours later.

Proper first-aid care may greatly reduce the severity of shock. There are a number of signs of shock:

- The face, lips, and nailbeds are paler, blue, or grayish.
- The skin is cool, yet it is covered with moisture, making it feel clammy.
- The shocky person may be nauseated or thirsty or may vomit.
- The person may be partially conscious and complain of feeling cold.
- The person has rapid breathing and fast pulse.

First aid for shock consists of keeping the person lying face up and with legs raised 8 inches higher than the head. *In head or chest injuries, or if breathing becomes more difficult with the head low, the child's head and shoulders should be raised a few inches higher than the feet.* This can be done by placing a pillow or coat under the victim's head and shoulders. If the child develops difficulty in breathing with the head and shoulders elevated, lower them. The pupil should be kept comfortably warm with blankets or coats *but not overheated.* Pain contributes to shock. Unnecessary movement of an injured person makes unnecessary pain. The child should be reassured and should not be bothered with unnecessary questions. The person administering first aid should never give a person in shock any kind of liquids or stimulants.

Fainting

Just before fainting, a child is likely to feel weak and dizzy. Vision becomes blurred, the face becomes pale, and the victim may be covered with a cold sweat. When a child faints, he/she should be assisted to lie down on one side to keep the airway clear. The color of the face indicates, to some extent, the amount of blood being supplied to the brain. If the face is pale, raise the feet 8 to 12 inches until the color of the face improves. On the other hand, if the face is extremely red, it may be desirable to keep the head slightly raised. After the person regains consciousness, he/she should lie quietly for a few minutes. The child should then sit up for a few minutes before standing or walking. A cool, wet cloth may be applied to the face or chest.

Poisoning

Once poison is swallowed and reaches the stomach, it is quickly absorbed. In most cases of poisoning it is important that the poison be diluted and as much of it as possible emptied from the stomach by vomiting. Food "poisoning" is actually a bacterial infection caused by spoiled or partially spoiled foods or by mishandling foods during storage or preparation. Certain types of mushrooms, wild berries, roots, and some types of leaves are actually poisonous. The poisonous type of mushrooms are often called toadstools. Small children are often poisoned by aspirin and petroleum products, such as kerosene and gasoline.

The symptoms of poisoning may vary greatly, depending on the substance swallowed and the time elapsed after ingestion. Some of the general symptoms are nausea, stomach cramps, pain, and sometimes vomiting. Sometimes poisons are absorbed before symptoms become evident. The corrosive poisons, such as acids and alkalis, burn the lips and mouth and cause marked shock. Poisoning caused by foods may cause vomiting, diarrhea, and collapse due to dehydration.

Every school office should post the available Poison Control Center telephone number. The first step is to call the hospital emergency room or the nearest poison control center and follow their directions. You should not induce vomiting unless specifically directed how to do so.

With the number of over-the-counter and prescription drugs available to children in the home, opportunities for poisoning or dangerous overdose are greater today than in past years. Sometimes children will ingest medicines or drugs at home, yet effects may not be noticed until arrival at school.

Diabetic Emergencies*

Diabetes is a condition caused by the inadequate production of a hormone called insulin. One in 600 school-aged children in this nation has diabetes. Consequently, diabetic emergencies are possible in any school. Most students take insulin at home twice a day but need to perform blood glucose (sugar) testing during school hours. The child's doctor or school nurse needs to provide a written care plan to the teacher.

There are two types of diabetic emergencies: diabetic coma (hyperglycemia) and insulin shock (hypoglycemia). Diabetic coma is a rather rare condition of excessive blood sugar resulting from too little insulin because of missed insulin injections, overeating, or the stress of an infection. It is slow in onset and is characterized by frequent thirst or requests to go to the bathroom to urinate, a flushed face, labored breathing, nausea, breath smelling of acetone, and possibly vomiting. If these symptoms appear, the teacher should ask two questions: "What have you eaten?" and "When did you last take your insulin?" The teacher should keep the child in a resting state and follow the care plan, helping the child test his or her blood sugar. It is unusual to have insulin at school. The school nurse, principal, and parents should be notified immediately.

In insulin shock the first sign is general irritability. The student may be weak, despondent, cry readily, or be exuberant or belligerent. In addition, the student may be hungry, perspire excessively, tremble or be unable to concentrate, have a fast pulse, and complain of dizziness. Blood sugar level needs to be tested. The symptoms vary in duration and often disappear in 10 to 15 minutes

---

*Graff J, Ault M, Guess D, Taylor M, Thompson B: *Health care for students with disabilities*, Baltimore, 1990, Paul H Brookes.

by following the student's care plan. Usually the plan involves giving 1 to 2 teaspoons or packets of sugar or 1 to 2 teaspoons of honey, fruit juice, prepackaged glucose in a tube, or cake frosting. After 10 to 15 minutes, a snack with starch and protein is given. If the symptoms do not subside after 15 to 30 minutes, the pupil's parents should be notified.

Seizure Disorders

Most elementary school classroom teachers at one time or another confront epileptic seizures in children. The incidence of generalized seizures, unrelated to fever, is 5 to 7/1000 school-aged children. Epilepsy is a nervous system condition in which seizures occur. A seizure occurs when an abnormal burst of electrical activity in the brain creates a change in alertness or behavior. Generalized epilepsy is usually one of two types: petit mal or grand mal. Petit mal is often not noticed by the teacher. It is marked by such simple signs as a fluttering of the eyelids, lip-smacking, or a glassy stare for 5 to 10 seconds. Often the teacher, student, and student's peers do not know that the student has suffered a seizure.

Grand mal, on the other hand, requires emergency care by the teacher. With grand mal seizures, the individual will most likely fall. The individual's muscles tighten, then relax and tighten repeatedly in jerking movements (convulsions). This phase may last from several seconds to several (usually 5) minutes. After the seizure, the child may become disoriented or fall asleep. Bladder control also may be lost during the seizure.

In giving a child first aid for a seizure, the teacher should not restrain movement. Keep calm and let the convulsion run its course, which it will do in 2 to 5 minutes. The child should be kept in the open where he/she will not be injured by striking any hard or sharp objects. *Do not force anything between the child's teeth.* The child's collar should be loosened to prevent breathing from being obstructed. Turn the victim to one side so that saliva does not fall back into the throat. Place something soft, such as a rolled-up coat, beneath the person's head. After the seizure, the child should be taken to the school's emergency room to sleep. However, the parents should be notified because they may wish to call for the student at once. Ordinarily, if it is known that the child has seizures, a written care plan should state actions to be taken.

Eye Injuries

Because the eyes are delicate organs, they should be treated with the greatest of care. Children should not be allowed to use most sharp-pointed instruments because of the danger of injuring the eye or falling on the instrument. The following points should be remembered in caring for eye injuries:

- If any type of chemical gets into the eyes, it should be washed out immediately with plenty of water for 15 minutes.
- The first-aider should *never* attempt to remove an embedded object from the eye. The eye should be covered with an eye pad.
- If a foreign object gets into the eye, the eye should not be rubbed. Rubbing the eye with a foreign object in it, especially if it is a sharp particle, such as a cinder, may cause a corneal scratch.
- If a child gets a small, foreign object on the eyelid or sclera (white part of eyeball), the teacher may attempt to remove it with a wet sterile gauze. If the object cannot be removed readily, a physician is needed.
- The use of any kind of sharp object should be avoided when removing foreign particles from the eye.

Burns

There are three general types of burns—*chemical, thermal,* and *solar.* Burns and scalds are from heat of such a degree as to cause injury to the skin and tissue of the body. Burns from hot liquids or steam are classified as scalds. Burns are sometimes classified as follows: First-degree (superficial) burns are those in which the skin is reddened; second-degree (partial-thickness) burns are those in which the skin is blistered; third-degree (full-thickness) burns are those in which there is destruction of deeper tissue and are serious, as growth cells that form new skin are destroyed.

First aid for a burn depends somewhat on the extent of the burn. If it is extensive or if tissue has been destroyed, a physician is needed as soon as possible. The main duty of the person administering first aid in this case is to try to prevent and care for shock until a physician is in charge of the individual. Charred fabric should not be removed. Nothing should be put on the burned area. However, relief of pain and control of tissue damage often can be achieved in first- and second-degree burns by immersion in cold water. Do not apply greasy ointments or antiseptic spray to blistered skin. Chemical cold sprays should not be used because of the danger of frostbite. Ice should not be applied because this can aggravate shock.

Fractures

Although there are many classifications of fractures, for the purpose of first aid they can be classed as: (1) simple or closed fractures, in which a bone is broken but the skin is not broken, and (2) compound or open fractures, in which a bone is broken and a wound extends from the break through the tissue and skin.

The symptoms of fracture include site-specific swelling, pain, and bruising or discoloration within 30 minutes. Typically, a fractured limb shows deformity or difference from the one on the opposite side, abnormal motion or position, or loss of voluntary movement. Not all symptoms will necessarily be present in every fracture.

If fracture is suspected, a physician is needed. Because shock may follow a broken bone, first aid for shock should be given. If medical aid is readily available, the child should not be moved and the fracture should not be splinted. Care should be taken, however, not to move the injured part. If it is absolutely necessary to move the patient, a splint should be applied if the arms or legs are involved (Figs. 7-10 and 7-11).

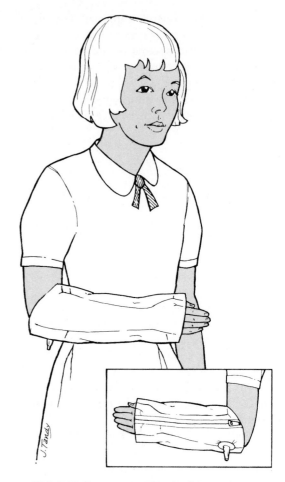

FIG. 7-10 Pneumatic splint for fractured arm.

If the neck or back is involved, extreme care should be used in handling the person. A person with a neck or back injury should be moved only if more danger is imminent. However, if it is necessary to move the injured person with a neck or back injury before medical aid is available, the body, especially the head or neck, should never be allowed to sag. The child should be prevented from moving in any way if at all possible. Rigid material should be used to move the person. Carefully securing the individual to a wide flat board or door will keep the body straight and prevent it from sagging. The person must be securely

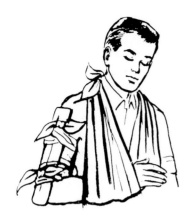

FIG. 7-11 Splint and sling for fracture of upper arm.

strapped to the back board. Plenty of help should be available for carrying the injured person.

Head injury may result from any type of hard blow on the head or by the head striking a hard surface. Some of the symptoms of head injury (e.g., concussion, skull fracture) are bleeding from the nose, mouth, or ears; unconsciousness; pupils of the eyes unequal in size; face flushed or pale, depending on the seriousness of the injury; and evidence of a blow on the head, such as a cut or a bump. All of the symptoms may not be present in every case.

First aid for head injury involves keeping the person in a lying position with the head and shoulders *slightly elevated if the face is flushed.* If the face is pale or ashen, the head and shoulders should not be elevated. The child's body temperature should be maintained, but a heated object should not be applied. A physician should be secured as soon as possible. If a person must be moved before medical aid is available, the victim should be kept in a lying position.

Dislocations

A dislocation is a bone out of place at a joint. The ligaments are injured and torn or stretched. The blood vessels and nerves may be injured, and the ends of the bones may be chipped. A physician is needed to reduce a dislocation safely (this should

never be done by a teacher). The parts of the body that may be dislocated are the fingers and toes, shoulders, jaw, elbows, knees, ankles, and hips. The first-aid care for a dislocation consists of placing an ice bag or cold compress over the joint and securing a physician. Care should be taken not to move the joint, as there is danger of chipping the bone. The general rule is to splint it as it lies.

Sprains

In sprains, ligaments and other tissues may be damaged. Wrists and ankles are most often sprained. In giving first aid for a sprain, the teacher should apply cold compresses or an ice bag for 20 to 30 minutes after the injury. The ice should not be applied directly to the skin, but should be wrapped in a towel, to avoid possibility of freezing the skin. The injured part should be kept elevated above the level of the heart, and the child should not be allowed to put any weight on the sprained part. A sprained ankle may be helped by a crisscrossing bandage, elastic bandage, or adhesive around it to keep it immovable. The usual school procedure to contact parents concerning a physician should be followed.

Insect Stings

Most children are not allergic to bee or wasp stings. First aid involves simply applying ice over the sting, then scraping the stinger out with a plastic card or fingernail. Tweezers should be avoided because they can squeeze the stinger. The child should be observed for at least 15 minutes for an allergic reaction involving breathing difficulty or shock. Emergency medical care should be sought if this occurs. Children known to have sting allergies may have oral or injection medication at school if prescribed by his or her physician.

Ticks

The only way a tick should be removed at school is by *gentle* pulling with tweezers. The bite site needs to be cleaned with soap and water. The incident should be noted in the child's health record. A cold compress can help reduce irritation. The child should be watched for signs of possible Lyme disease.

Splinters

If a splinter can be grasped by tweezers, it should be removed and the skin washed with soap and water. Teachers should not use needles or other objects to further break the skin. A splinter can be left in, but the area should be washed carefully and covered with a sterile bandage. Parents need to be notified to tend to the splinter after school.

Frostbite

In some areas of the country, schoolchildren may occasionally suffer from frostbite. It results from loss of circulation because of constriction of arteries at low temperatures. Consequently, the tissues are deprived of oxygen. Injury from frostbite varies with circumstances and the timing and kind of emergency care given.

The fingers, toes, nose, ears, and cheeks are the parts of the body most likely to be frostbitten. The signs of frostbite are a sensation of intense coldness, stinging followed by numbness, (loss of sensation) in the frozen part. The frostbitten part may be flushed at first and then become white or grayish yellow. Because of loss of sensation, people may not realize that their nose, cheeks, or ears are frostbitten until someone calls attention to it.

In giving first aid for frostbite, the teacher should be careful not to damage the tissue. Rubbing or careless handling of a frozen part may bruise the tissue and cause further damage. If a person is outdoors, the frozen part should be covered with the hand or with cloth, preferably woolen. The child should be brought indoors and placed in a warm room, the frostbitten part should be covered with a warm cloth and immersed in warm water (102° to 104° F). However, hot objects of any kind should be kept away from the frostbitten part.

SUMMARY

The concept of school safety has received a great deal of attention over the past few years. Whenever a child is injured at school, the question, "Who is going to pay for this injury?" arises. There is an increasing trend for people to recover costs from injuries, and the attitude has begun to emerge that parents expect teachers to pay for injuries to students.

The teacher has a duty to care for those who are injured and ill but must realize that the possibility of litigation does exist. In general, teachers should carry personal liability insurance even though school boards may increasingly be sued for damages in injury cases.

The teacher's role in a classroom emergency is at least threefold: First, the teacher must quickly recognize an emergency and provide care when the need arises; second, a teacher must be prepared to render appropriate care by obtaining adequate first-aid training and certification; finally, the teacher must always act in a prudent manner in an emergency.

Although it is best if all teachers are trained and certified in first aid and that these personnel be on duty whenever children are present at school, techniques for handling select emergency situations have been presented in this chapter. Teachers should also be skilled in dealing with students after an illness or emergency. They should help students understand the situation and help the affected student return to the classroom without feeling undue fear or embarrassment. It is hoped that these suggestions will motivate the individual to seek additional first-aid training and that any certification acquired will be kept up to date.

QUESTIONS FOR DISCUSSION

1. Whose responsibility is the promotion of safety in the elementary school?
2. What are the basic components of a school's emergency care procedures?
3. Why should the school emergency plan be a written document?

4. How would you characterize the role of the teacher in emergency care?

5. What is meant by the phrase, "a reasonable and prudent individual?"

6. What is probably the best way to avoid becoming involved in liability litigation?

7. Under what circumstances is the teacher liable in the event of pupil injury?

8. When should students have an individual written care plan for emergency action?

9. Briefly discuss the basic principles that should be followed in administering first aid to the injured?

10. What duties would a teacher be expected to perform in terms of a school safety program?

11. Do you feel that the school board should be exempt from legal liability in cases of pupil injury? Why or why not?

12. Some individuals maintain that school boards should be required to purchase personal liability insurance for all employees. What is your viewpoint on this issue?

13. Why is it desirable that a person certified in first aid be present at all times that students are in the school facility?

14. Why should all pupil injuries be reported on injury or accident report forms?

15. What is meant by "the ABCs of life support?"

16. Why are school personnel admonished not to give a pupil any type of medication unless that medication has been specifically furnished by the student's parent/guardian?

17. Why should a teacher evaluate the scene of an injury?

18. What are serious types of emergencies a teacher may encounter in the classroom?

19. Why is it important that teachers be trained in emergency care procedures?

20. In an emergency, what types of information should a teacher be prepared to provide when calling emergency medical services?

21. As a teacher, what type of emergency plan would you design for your classroom?

22. How will you, as a teacher, remain up to date in emergency care and first aid?

23. What Universal Precautions must be followed by school personnel when dealing with students who are bleeding from an injury?

SELECTED REFERENCES

Airhihenbuwa CO: *First aid and emergency care: procedure and practice,* ed 2, Dubuque, IA, 1989, Kendall/Hunt.

American Heart Association: *Basic life support* (video), Dallas, 1993, The Association.

American Red Cross: *First aid fast,* St Louis, 1994, Mosby–Year Book.

American Red Cross: *Community first aid and safety,* St Louis, 1993, Mosby–Year Book.

American School Health Association, Association for the Advancement of Health Education, and Society for Public Health Education, Inc: *The national adolescent student health survey: a report on the health of America's youth,* Oakland, CA, 1989, Third Party Publishing.

Bender S, Sorochan W: *Teaching elementary health science,* ed 3, Boston, 1989, Jones and Barlett.

Children's Defense Fund: *The state of America's children yearbook 1994,* Washington, DC, 1994, The Fund.

Committee on Trauma Research, Commission on Life Sciences, National Research Council, and the Institute of Medicine: *Injury in America: a continuing public health problem,* Washington, DC, 1985, National Academy Press.

Creswell WH, Newman IM: *School health practice,* ed 10, St Louis, 1993, Mosby–Year Book.

Florio AE, Alles W: *Safety education,* ed 4, New York, 1979, McGraw-Hill.

Graff JC, Ault MM, Guess D, Taylor M, Thompson B: *Health care for students with disabilities,* Baltimore, 1990, Paul H Brookes.

Hafen BQ: *First aid for health emergencies,* ed 3, St Paul, 1985, West.

Healthy people 2000: *National health promotion and disease prevention objectives,* Washington, DC, 1990, US Department of Health and Human Services.

Heimlich HJJ, Uhley MH: The Heimlich maneuver, *Clinical Symposium,* CIBA 31(3):1979.

National Commission on the Role of the School and the Community in Improving Adolescent Health: *Code blue: uniting for healthier youth,* Alexandria, VA, 1990, National Association of State Boards of Education, and American Medical Association.

National Safety Council: *Accident facts,* Itasca, IL, 1994, The Council.

National Safety Council: *First aid and CPR,* Boston, 1991, Jones and Bartlett.

National Safety Council: *School Safety World Newsletter,* Chicago, published quarterly, The Council.

Parcel GS, Rinear CE: *Basic emergency care of the sick and injured,* ed 3, St Louis, 1990, Mosby–Year Book.

Rinke CM, editor: Standards and guidelines for cardiopulmonary resuscitation (CPR) and emergency cardiac care (ECC), *JAMA* 255(21):2905-2894, 1986.

Sorenson E: Plan to prevent accidents: follow this advice and make our schools safer for teachers and kids, *Am School Board J* 72:6, 1985.

Thygerson AL: *First aid and emergency care workbook,* Boston, 1987, Jones and Bartlett.

IV

HEALTH EDUCATION

8

KEY CONCEPTS

Comprehensive school health education programs contribute to the well-being of students.

Health Education Today

Schools offer the most systematic and efficient means available to improve the health of youth and enable young people to avoid health risks.

HEALTHY PEOPLE 2000

Health and education are joined in fundamental ways with each other and the destinies of the nation's children.

RICHARD W. RILEY
SECRETARY OF EDUCATION
DONNA E. SHALALA
SECRETARY OF HEALTH AND HUMAN SERVICES

PROBLEMS TO SOLVE

As a teacher, how might you determine the student and community needs and interests in health-related areas in order to plan and implement a comprehensive school health education program in the elementary school where you teach? As a teacher, how might you convince your school administration that the health education program in terms of the curriculum, the pattern of instruction, and who teaches health should be improved?

HEALTH education in America's schools has been slowly approaching a threshold of awareness, growth, and emphasis that should have a profound future influence on the children and youth of the United States. Acceptance of the need for preventive health care with a focus on adopting life-style behaviors that promote good health is now widely advocated by all leaders in the health and medical community. The concept has received general approval by parents and the general public.

Elementary school health education is supported by governmental, professional, and health and educational organizations, voluntary health agencies, commercial companies, and parents.

In March, 1994, 24 national organizations were funded by the Centers for Disease Control and Prevention to establish national programs designed to assist schools, institutions of higher education, and youth-serving agencies to implement educational programs designed to prevent youth from engaging in behaviors that would place them at risk for several important health problems. In May, 1994, the American Cancer Society released the results of a Gallup poll on the opinions of students, parents, and school administrators toward comprehensive school health education. All groups felt that comprehensive school health education was of equal or greater importance than all other topics taught in school. Further, the American Cancer Society has made comprehensive school health education a major priority of its cancer prevention activities through the year 2000 (Table 8-1). The American Medical Association and the National Association of State Boards of Education have also suggested that comprehensive school health education is a key element in improving the health of the nation's youth.

Approximately 75% of the 50 states have mandated school health education, but its definition and implementation vary widely among school districts. States have required specific curriculum areas, such as alcohol, tobacco and other drugs, safety, and sexually transmitted diseases. Still others have additional permissive legislative provisions. The introduction of health education into schools has been advocated by the American Academy of Pediatrics, the American Association of School Administrators, the American Dental Association, the American Medical Association, the American Public Health Association, the American School Health Association, the Association for the Advancement of Health Education, the Council of Chief State School Officers, the National Association of State Boards of Education, the American Cancer Society, the American Heart Association, and the American Lung Association. The National Dairy Council, the United Way, the Kellogg Foundation, the Henry J. Kaiser Family

TABLE 8-1 Health Topics Considered as a Composite Measure of Comprehensive School Health Education

General topics	Specific issues
Cancer-related	Smoking and tobacco use
	Cancer prevention
	Diet/nutrition/weight control
Implications for cancer	Preventing injuries and accidents
	AIDS and other sexually transmitted diseases
	Alcohol use
	Self-esteem or feeling good about yourself
	Environment and how it affects your health
	Family roles and relationships
	Exercise and physical fitness
	Making decisions about health information and health products
Noncancer-related	Drug use (other than alcohol)
	Suicide and depression
	Preventing violence
	Preventing diseases (other than cancer)
	Dealing with stress
	Taking care of your teeth

From the Gallup Organization: *Values and opinions of comprehensive school health education in US public schools: adolescents, parents, and school district administrators,* Atlanta, 1994, American Cancer Society, p 5.

Foundation, the Robert Wood Johnson Foundation, Metropolitan Life, and Blue Cross and Blue Shield, among others, have also financially supported the development of health education programs in various U.S. communities.

A significant position paper adopted by the Governing Council of the American Public Health Association in 1974 stated that:

The school is a community in which most individuals spend at least twelve years of their lives . . . the health of our school-age youth will determine to a great extent the quality of life each will have during the growing and developing years and on throughout the life cycle.*

In 1981 the Education Commission of the States† proposed that state education agencies should do the following:

- Encourage local school boards and administrators to include health education in the curriculum in elementary and secondary schools
- Promote health education as a responsibility shared by the family, school, and community
- Promote the development of comprehensive school health education programs

Despite the legislative provisions and the efforts of the various organizations and agencies previously identified, health education programs are neither common nor universally found in schools in the United States. The paucity of curricula is caused primarily by the lack of understanding of the need for and the significance of such programs of learning. It is estimated that few comprehensive health instruction programs are in operation in the 15,000 school districts and 90,000 elementary and secondary schools in the United States. However, the number of programs has been increasing in recent years. Most health education programs received emphasis and were probably introduced within the past 30 or 40 years. Although school health programs have been around, in some form, since the turn of the century, nearly 100 years later the development of the concept is continuing to evolve.* Where programs have started, many are fragmented or piecemeal in scope. Some may be broad based (include a variety of topics) but few are what might be considered comprehensive. Some lose their priority status and become obsolete a few years after their initiation. Little has been done to assess the effectiveness of such programs on children's behavior. The situation is best described by the U.S. Department of Health and Human Services in its publication *Better Health for Our Children:*

Many school health education programs at present are neither sufficiently comprehensive nor sufficiently attuned to the influence of peer culture and other important determinants of youthful behavior to be truly effective in promoting good health habits.†

According to Dr. Shirley Jackson, Director of the Office of School Health, U.S. Department of Education, "Comprehensive school health education (CSHE) is a primary prevention strategy for teaching our nation's children and their parents the skills needed for a healthy lifestyle."‡

Teachers, nurses, administrators, and others who desire to or have a duty to develop curricula for their classrooms and schools or those who wish to assume leadership to promote the introduction of health education programs in their districts will find practical material in this text. Programs may be prepared from the information found in the chapters that follow or from the illustrations and sources identified in this chapter.

---

*Governing Council of the American Public Health Association: *Education for health in the school community setting; a position paper,* New Orleans, October 23, 1974. (See Appendix C.)
†Education Commission of the States: *Recommendations for school health education: a handbook for state policymakers,* Denver, 1981, The Commission.

*Stone E: ACCESS: keystones for school health promotion, *J School Health* 60(7):298-300, 1990.
†US Department of Health and Human Services, Public Health Service: *Better health for our children: a national strategy, major findings and recommendations,* vol 1, Washington, DC, 1981, Superintendent of Documents.
‡Jackson S: Introduction. In Jackson SA, editor: *Comprehensive school health education programs: innovative practices and issues in setting standards,* Pub. No. FIRST 93-7006, Washington, DC, 1993, US Department of Education, p 1.

WHY IS HEALTH EDUCATION NEEDED?

Education regarding health should be an essential com-
    ponent of the school curriculum at all grade levels.*

Julius B. Richmond, M.D., former Surgeon
General of the United States, advocated that efforts of the Public Health Service (PHS) of the U.S.
Department of Health and Human Services could
best serve Americans through a preventive approach to health. As a result, the PHS has supported health programs in schools for a number of
years by providing funds for curriculum development and demonstration projects and through
evaluative studies. The importance of school
health was further exemplified by the formation
of the Interagency Committee on School Health,
co-chaired by the Assistant Secretary for Elementary and Secondary Education and the Assistant
Secretary for Health, within the U.S. government,
in April, 1994 (see Appendix L).

There is increasing awareness among the public in general of the need for increased health information and actions that will help persons, families, and communities. State laws mandate instruction in various health categories in curricula.
Parents and many community organizations support the inclusion of health education in school
programs. Controversy has been expressed by
some regarding sexuality education and aspects
of mental health. The numerous student health
problems and conditions identified in Chapter 1,
many of which can be reduced by preventive action, clearly demonstrate the need for health education.

High Cost of Illness and Medical Care

In 1960 only approximately 5% of the gross
national product (GNP) went for health care
costs. Today that figure is estimated to be over
14%,* and it is projected to increase to over 19% by
the year 2000.† Smoking-related illnesses cost
some $65 billion annually. AIDS, an almost en-
tirely preventable disease, costs approximately
$75,000 per person, or $4.3 billion per year; cost estimates run as high as $13 billion for 1992. Treat-
ment for alcohol and drug abuse is at least $16 bil-
lion annually, but the total economic impact of alcohol and drug abuse is more than $110 billion an-
nually.‡ Injury costs well over $100 billion
annually, cancer over $70 billion, and cardiovascu-
lar disease over $135 billion annually (Table 8-2).

The per capita outlay of funds for health care in
1990 was in excess of $2500. The cost of room and
board for a day in a hospital in 1988 exceeded $550
and the average cost per hospital stay was more
than $4200.§ The so-called working poor and the
elderly are the people chiefly affected when a continuing or catastrophic illness causes a severe financial burden.

However, middle-income families also pay a
heavy price for health services because long and
expensive illnesses may reduce them to poverty. It
should be obvious that information provided at an
early age that aids in preventive action could help
reduce the costs of illness and medical care.

Gullible Public

It is estimated that 75 many billions of dollars annually is spent on worthless health products and
services, many of which may even be harmful.
The use of celebrities to promote health care products and lifestyle choices through aggressive marketing has much influence on people. Millions of

---

*US Department of Health and Human Services, Public Health
Service: *Better health for our children: a national strategy, major findings and recommendations,* vol 1, Washington, DC, 1981, Superintendent of Documents.

*Burner ST, Waldo DR, McKusick DR: National health expendi-
ture projections through 2030, *Health Care Finan Rev* 14:1-29,
1992.
†Sullivan LW: Health promotion and disease prevention, *Med
Educ* 26:175-277, 1992.
‡Sullivan LW: *Forward, Healthy people 2000: national health promo-
tion and disease prevention objectives,* Washington, DC, 1990,
US Department of Health and Human Services, Public Health
Service.
§Cornacchia H, Barrett S: *Consumer health: a guide to intelligent
decisions,* ed 5, St Louis, 1993, Times Mirror/Mosby College
Publishing, p 5.

TABLE 8-2 Costs of Treatment for Selected Preventable Conditions

Condition	Overall magnitude (amount/yr)	Avoidable intervention*	Cost per patient†
Heart disease	7 million with coronary artery disease 500,000 deaths 284,000 bypass procedures	Coronary bypass surgery	$30,000
Cancer	1 million new cases 510,000 deaths	Lung cancer treatment Cervical cancer treatment	$29,000 $28,000
Stroke	600,000 strokes 150,000 deaths	Hemiplegia treatment and rehabilitation	$22,000
Injuries	2.3 million hospitalizations 142,500 deaths 177,000 persons with spinal cord injuries in the United States	Quadriplegia treatment and rehabilitation Hip fracture treatment and rehabilitation Severe head injury treatment and rehabilitation	$570,000 (lifetime) $40,000 $310,000
HIV infection	1-1.5 million infected 118,000 AIDS cases (as of January, 1990)	AIDS treatment	$75,000 (lifetime)
Alcoholism	18.5 million abuse alcohol 105,000 alcohol-related deaths	Liver transplant	$250,000
Drug abuse	Regular users: cocaine, 1-3 million, IV drugs, 900,000, heroin, 500,000 Drug-exposed babies: 375,000	Treatment of cocaine-exposed baby	$66,000 (5 years)
Low birth weight baby	260,000 low birth weight babies born 23,000 deaths	Neonatal intensive care for low birth weight babies	$10,000
Inadequate immunization	Lacking basic immunization series: Aged 2 and younger, 20%-30% Aged 6 and older, 3%	Congenital rubella syndrome treatment	$354,000 (lifetime)

*Examples (other interventions may apply).
†Representative first-year costs, except as noted. Not indicated are nonmedical costs, such as lost productivity to society. From Office of Disease Prevention and Health Promotion: *Healthy people 2000: national health promotion and disease prevention objectives*, Washington, DC, 1990, US Department of Health and Human Services, Public Health Service.

dollars each year are wasted on valueless cancer and arthritis remedies. Approximately $150 million is spent on useless and fake remedies ordered through the mails. Over $30 billion is spent on questionable foods, fraudulent weight-reduction schemes, and fad diets, and another $3 billion goes for vitamins and minerals. Over $11 billion per year is spent for over-the-counter drugs and drug products, many of which were unnecessary. Quacks and quackery are rampant throughout the United States. Children and young people need to learn to make intelligent decisions regarding the purchase and use of health products and health services and know how to identify charlatans* (Table 8-3).

Health Misconceptions

Children as well as adults lack accurate scientific health information. Although almost two decades

_____
*Cornacchia H, Barrett S: *Consumer health: a guide to intelligent decisions*, ed 5, St Louis, 1993, Times Mirror/Mosby College Publishing.

TABLE 8-3 Estimated Expenditures for Selected Health Products

Cost	Products
$ 24 billion	Skin and beauty products and aids
2 billion	Cold, cough, allergy, bronchodilators, antiasthmatics
30 billion	Prescription drugs
11.2 billion	Over-the-counter drugs
1.8 billion	Home exercise machines
3.6 billion	Athletic footwear
250 million	Weights and barbells
200 million	Cross-country ski simulators
1 billion	Multi-purpose gyms
200 million	Rowing machines
750 million	Stationary bicycles
282 million	Treadmills
3 billion	Vitamin and mineral supplements
30 billion	Weight control products and services
3 billion	Self-care products, devices, and services

Modified from Cornacchia H, Barrett S: *Consumer health: a guide to intelligent decisions*, ed 5, St Louis, 1993, Times Mirror/Mosby College Publishing, pp 182, 255, 286, 309, 323, 420, 436, 451.

old, one of the largest and most respected efforts to study health practices* and opinions still merits attention. The study, conducted by the U.S. Food and Drug Administration, identified many commonly held misconceptions, among which were the following:

- Extra vitamins give more pep and energy
- The major reason for bad health is that people do not eat the right foods
- Substantial weight loss can occur through perspiring
- A daily bowel movement is necessary for good health
- Most things that advertisements say about health and medicines are true

---

*Food and Drug Administration: *A study of practices and opinions*, Springfield, VA, 1972, National Technical Information Services, US Department of Commerce.

- Most things people buy in drugstores to treat themselves are practically worthless

The 1985 National Health Interview Survey* conducted by the Center for Health Statistics of the U.S. Department of Health and Human Services reported gaps in Americans' practice and knowledge of health habits concerning such things as stress, exercise, tooth decay and tooth loss in children, and alcohol and its relation to throat cancer.

These inaccuracies expressed by adults are unquestionably related to the lack of information they received as children.

Health Information Confusing

Health information that people read or receive from friends, neighbors, and family members may be inaccurate or never clearly defined for a variety of reasons. Testimony from individuals may be based on opinions rather than scientific data. Often factual information becomes distorted in transmission. The causes, prevention, and treatment of many illnesses including arthritis, cancer, and heart disease have not been completely identified nor accurately reported in the media. The media often dramatize the significance of preliminary data from limited scientific studies and mislead the public to believe the information is conclusive. The tremendous expansion of newspapers, magazines, books, and radio and TV advertising and "infomercials" produces an overwhelming amount of health information that is difficult for people to understand and interpret. This information often contains unproved claims. The dissemination of false and inaccurate information by authors and writers is protected by the constitutional provision of "freedom of speech." One study, conducted by the American Council on Science and Health† on the accuracy of nutrition information provided, rated

---

*Gaps found in Americans' knowledge of health habits as reported in the *Nation's Health*, 1,17 July, 1986, American Public Health Association.
†*American Council on Science* and *Health News and Views* 7(5):1, 8-10, November/December, 1986.

25 popular magazines and revealed that 5 were reliable, 14 were generally reliable, 3 were inconsistent in reliability, and 3 were unreliable.

In an analysis of 322 health, nutrition, and psychological articles that appeared over a 3-month period of time in 5 tabloid newspapers, Dr. Stephen Barrett concluded that only 135 (42%) of them contained accurate and reliable information.* Dr. Barrett mentioned that *Time, Newsweek,* and *U.S. News and World Report* generally contained accurate information. He also specified numerous unreliable sources of information (Table 8-4). These factors make it virtually impossible for consumers to determine the reliability and validity of what they read and hear. The question may be asked, "How does one determine fact from fiction?" Young people must learn to locate and use reliable sources of information to be able to identify truths from falsehoods. Teachers must be familiar with ways to distinguish fact from fiction in relation to health information, products, and services.

Media Influence on Behavior

What people read or hear through the media influences their decisions to purchase and use health products and services. Advertising, however, is often unclear, misleading, and deceptive—often deliberately so. The intent is to capitalize on the ignorance of the consumer by describing a product in terms of a mystical ingredient physicians are said to recommend rather than in terms of specific contents and value. Advertising claims have multiple meanings, one or more of which may be false or unsubstantiated from a technical standpoint.

Children need help in learning how to analyze advertising to be able to determine the accuracy of information provided by the media. Even proven medical treatments involve a certain amount of risk. By reading scientific sources of health infor-

*Barrett S: Truth or trash? Health-related information in the tabloids, *Priorities*, Summer, 1989, pp 27-30.

TABLE 8-4 Unreliable Sources of Health Information—Selected Magazines and Newsletters

Alternatives
Better Nutrition for Today's Living
Body, Mind, and Spirit
Cancer Chronicles
The Choice
Delicious!
The Doctors People
East-West Natural Health
Health and Healing
Health Facts
Health World
Let's Live
Longevity
Men's Health Newsletter
Muscle and Fitness
Natural Living Newsletter
New Age Journal
Nutrition News (published by Siri Khalsa)
People's Medical Society Newsletter
Second Opinion
Senior Health
Total Health
Vegetarian Times
Your Health

From Cornacchia H, Barrett S: *Consumer health: a guide to intelligent decisions*, ed 5, St Louis, 1993, Times Mirror/Mosby College Publishing, pp 44-48.

mation and not relying on the "popular press," teachers and students alike can become better informed consumers.

Lifestyle and Disease

American lifestyles contribute to the high incidence of certain diseases such as cancer, heart disease, diabetes, and dental decay. Data reveal that people who exercise regularly, eat nutritious foods, obtain proper sleep and rest, control their weight and the use of alcoholic beverages and drugs, eliminate cigarette smoking, and reduce stress increase their potential to live longer. People who expose themselves to the identified risk factors increase their chances for ill health. One study that assessed the relative contributions of a variety of factors to the 10 leading causes of death suggested that about one half of the deaths were caused by unhealthy behavior and lifestyles.* Schools can help children to eliminate or reduce the risk factors involved through a health education program. If existing behavior is to be altered, students must understand the positive results that can be obtained by making changes. Both short- and long-term benefits need to be demonstrated.

Peer and Adult Pressures

Young people are under pressure from their peers to conform to group behavior patterns in such activities as smoking, alcohol and drug use, and sexual activity. In addition, young people wish to become adults and emulate adult behaviors. Students need to be prepared to know how to deal properly with these pressures as well as those they will encounter as adults. A comprehensive school health instruction program will help pupils acquire the skills needed to cope with the health problems and pressures confronted by both teenagers and adults.

Self-Care

The focus on preventive aspects of health places emphasis on wellness rather than illness. Because good health has a high correlation with lifestyles and behaviors, the concept of self-care needs development and implementation in the health instruction program. Children must increasingly learn to assume responsibility for their own bodies. Young people can learn how to prevent and care for minor health problems and where to go for assistance when more serious complications arise. Because so many children are home alone (see Chapter 4) and may have to take care of

health problems themselves, they must be taught to make intelligent decisions about ways to reduce or eliminate risk factors that lead to poor health or injury.

WHAT IS THE CURRENT STATUS OF HEALTH EDUCATION?

Despite the awareness of the need for health education, the implementation of programs into local schools and school districts continues to leave much to be desired. Furthermore, only 36 states have mandated health education in the schools. Comprehensive curricula are advocated, but their numbers are not rapidly increasing. Most programs continue to be piecemeal and fragmentary. They consist of combining the content of health education with other subject matter, most often with physical education. Only 19 states require that health education be taught sometime during grades 1 through 6, and an additional three states combine the health education requirement with physical education. Twenty-two states require that health education be taught in grades 7 or 8, and an additional four states indicate that the requirement could be met through a combined health and physical education course.* However, the outlook for improvement in the future is optimistic. Events at national, state, and local levels support the positive outlook for school health education. A review of the first edition of *School Health in America*† showed that in 1976, only 17 states had mandated comprehensive health education, compared with the 36 states that were reported in the fifth edition. The indications are that educators in the remaining states are working to make comprehensive health education a reality in the near future. Some

---

Healthy people: the Surgeon General's report on health and disease prevention, Washington, DC, 1979, US Department of Health and Human Services.

---

*Lovato C, Allensworth D, Chan F: *School health in America: an assessment of state policies to protect and improve the health of students,* ed 5, Kent, OH, 1989, American School Health Association, pp 13-14.
†Castile A, Jerick S: *School health in America: a survey of state school health programs,* Kent, OH, 1976, American School Health Association, p 3.

of the impetus for the increased interest in health education and its effects on health behaviors resulted from the identification of education as the most effective way to deal with the AIDS dilemma. In a democratic society, health education is particularly important to ensure that individuals have the information and skills they need to protect and enhance their own health, the health of families for which they are responsible, and the health of the communities in which they live.*

National

A chronology of recent significant legislation, activities, and offices established in support of health education includes:

1973 President Richard Nixon's Committee on Health Education reported that school health education in elementary schools was poor or was not provided.

1974 The Bureau of Health Education was established at the Centers for Disease Control, U.S. Public Health Service.

1975 The National Center for Health Education, a nongovernmental agency, was established to promote health education.

1975 A variety of federal agencies, including the Public Health Service of the U.S. Department of Health, Education, and Welfare, established as priorities for national health planning and resource development the prevention of disease and the development of effective methods for health education of the public. Public Law 94-142,

Education for All Handicapped Children Act, was passed.

1975-1976 The U.S. Congress gave consideration to the passage of the Comprehensive School Health Education Act. The bill did not pass but it gave health education greater visibility, which was reflected in the amendments to the Elementary and Secondary Education Act in 1978.

1976 The Office of Health Information and Health Promotion was created in the U.S. Department of Health, Education, and Welfare (now the Department of Health and Human Services). The first edition of *School Health in America* was published by the American School Health Association.

1978 Amendments to the Elementary and Secondary Education Act of 1965, Title III, authorized funds for states and local districts to develop and implement comprehensive school health education programs. Local school districts now have legal authority to expend funds awarded to states by the federal government under the so-called block grants provision for health education programs.

1979 The Office of Comprehensive School Health was established in the U.S. Department of Education to coordinate the variety of efforts in school health services, instruction, and environmental programs. (The office is not currently operative.) The second edition of *School Health in America* was published by the American School Health Association.

1975-1980 The National Parent-Teacher Association Comprehensive School/ Community Health Education Pro-

---

Healthy people 2000: national health promotion and disease prevention objectives, Pub No (PHS) 91-50212, Washington, DC, 1991, US Department of Health and Human Services, p 249.

ject was contracted for by the Bureau of Health Education to increase community awareness and understanding of health education needs and to develop support for more effective health education.

1980-1981　The U.S. Surgeon General's Office* expressed support for school health education programs. The third edition of *School Health in America* was published by the American School Health Association.

1981　The Centers for Disease Control and the Office of Health Promotion and Disease Prevention contracted to have the National School Health Education Evaluation Study conducted.

1982　The Centers for Disease Control reorganized and included a School Health Section, illustrating a continued federal commitment.

1982　National School Health Education Coalition (NASHEC) was formed as an effort of voluntary health agencies and others to cooperate on a national level for the improvement of school health.

1983　The federal government held an interagency meeting and identified 140 different federal agencies responsible for some aspect of the health of school-age children.

1984　The American School Health Association (ASHA) completed and made available a national marketing kit for school health programs.

1984　The Office of Disease Prevention and Health Promotion (ODPHP) entered into a cooperative agreement with the American Association of School Administrators to disseminate the Oregon Model Health Conference known as the Seaside Health Conference.

1985　ODPHP entered into a cooperative agreement with ASHA to develop model strategies to relate the 1990 health objectives for the nation to the school population.

1985　ODPHP entered into a cooperative agreement with ASHA, Association for the Advancement of Health Education (AAHE), and the Society for Public Health Education (SOPHE) for an on-going national survey of knowledge, attitudes, and practices in school health. Metropolitan Life Foundation announced initiation of the $5 million "Healthy Me" initiative.

1985　National School Health Education Evaluation Study completed and published.

1986　ODPHP approved a study to follow up the 1985 National Youth Fitness Study by evaluating the health status of 6- to 9-year-olds. The fourth edition of *School Health in America* was published by the American School Health Association.

1986　National Center for Health Education cooperated with ASHA and AAHE to publish an evaluation manual for school health programs.

1987　The National Adolescent Student Health Survey was initiated. The Centers for Disease Control and Prevention initiated cooperative agreements with 15 organizations for AIDS education.

---

*US Department of Health and Human Services, Public Health Service: *Better health for our children: a national strategy, major findings and recommendations*, vol 1, Washington, DC, 1981, Superintendent of Documents.

1988 The Division of Adolescent and School Health was established within the National Center for Chronic Disease Prevention and Health Promotion in the Centers for Disease Control and Prevention. The National Commission for Health Education Credentialing was established as a nonprofit agency to develop and administer a national competency-based examination for health educators, develop standards for professional preparation, and promote continuing education for professional growth.

1989 The fifth edition of *School Health in America* was published by the American School Health Association.

1990 *Healthy People 2000: National Health Promotion and Disease Prevention Objectives* were released by Louis Sullivan, M.D., Secretary of the U.S. Department of Health and Human Services. The first national examination for the credentialing of Certified Health Education Specialists was conducted in 15 locations in the United States. *Code Blue: Uniting for Healthier Youth* was published urging implementation of comprehensive school health education programs, K-12. Public Law 101-476, Individuals with Disabilities Education Act, was passed.

1991 Report of the 1990 Joint Committee on Health Education Terminology was released.

1992 American Cancer Society supported a national meeting to develop an action plan to institutionalize comprehensive school health in the nation's schools.

1993 MACRO Systems of Silver Springs, Maryland (supported by the Division of Adolescent and School Health, National Center for Chronic Disease Prevention and Health Promotion, Centers for Disease Control and Prevention) initiated a national study of school health programs.

1994 National School Boards Association released the results of its Comprehensive School Health Project Survey. American Cancer Society released results of a National Gallup Poll of student, school administrators, and parental perceptions of comprehensive school health education in U.S. schools. Interagency Committee on School Health was formed by the U.S. Departments of Education and Health and Human Services. The National Coordinating Committee on School Health was formed.

1995 The American Cancer Society released the results of a national study in which national educational standards for comprehensive school health education in grades 4, 8, and 11 are specified.

State

In 43 states, support for health instruction is included either as a legislated mandate or in the education code. In 40 states, the boards of education have enacted policy statements, regulations, guidelines, and accreditation standards related to health education.* Unfortunately, these programs are not adequately funded or defined in terms of scope, sequence of topic, grade, and time allotment.

A summary of state requirements for health education is found in Chapter 1. Nearly every state

---

*Lovato C, Allensworth D, Chan F: *An assessment of state policies to protect and improve the health of students,* ed 5, Kent, OH, 1989, American School Health Association.

requires certain health topics to be taught. This has led to fragmented rather than comprehensive programs. Alcohol and drug education is required in 29 states and instruction about tobacco and smoking, a major cause of premature mortality in the United States, is required in only 20 states. Nutrition education is a mandated topic of instruction in only 19 states. Unfortunately, the quality of instruction in each of these areas, as well as other areas included in the health education curriculum, is not known.

Local

One of the health goals for the nation for the year 2000 is to increase to at least 75% the proportion of the nation's elementary and secondary schools that provide planned and sequential kindergarten through twelfth-grade quality school health instruction. In the 1995 midcourse review of *Healthy People 2000,* the word "quality" was changed to "comprehensive" to highlight the importance of including the broad range of topic areas included in school health education. As children must attend school in most states until they reach a minimum age of 16, the school offers a natural setting in which quality health education can occur. Through the educational process, young people can attain knowledge and develop skills that will have far-reaching consequences in terms of the decisions that they make related to their health. Naturally the specific program content is and should be locally determined, based on need, even though broad topical areas may be mandated at a state level.

As mentioned, the health education programs found in local school districts vary in nature from individual topical programs to broad-based, comprehensive ones. Their impact on children has not been adequately evaluated on the local level. However, there have been four major national health education evaluations that have been conducted over the years: the School Health Education Study (SHES) in 1961, followed by the National School Health Education Evaluation Study (SHEES) completed in 1984, the National Adoles-

cent Student Health Survey (NASHS) completed in 1989, and the Louis Harris evaluation conducted for Metropolitan Life Foundation in 1988 and published in 1989; these clearly demonstrate the need for and the impact of comprehensive health education. The biannual Youth Risk Behavior Study that is conducted by the Division of Adolescent and School Health of the National Center for Chronic Disease Prevention and Health Promotion, Centers for Disease Control and Prevention, provides more empirical evidence of the potential effect of comprehensive school health education programs.

In order to implement school health education programs, schools have to be creative in their financial support. Although many programs are funded directly from the budget of the school district, many others have been funded primarily through federal and state initiatives, through voluntary health agencies and private foundations, or, a few, through industrial corporations. One of the newer models that seems to be appearing on the national scene is the "Adopt-a-School" program. This program involves the adoption of a school by a local organization, which then provides special funding for health education programs.

Of 251 school districts that reported having a school health program surveyed by the National School Boards Association (NSBA)* organized in 1994, only 52% of them had adopted a school health mission or policy statement. Although many states indicate that they have mandated school health education, the lack of funding for support of state- and local-level personnel to assist in the development of the programs has left health education fragmented in most local school districts across the nation. This fragmentation is further proliferated by categorical funding by the government for such efforts as Drug Free Schools and HIV/AIDS preven-

---

*National School Boards Association: *School board member knowledge of and attitudes regarding school health program,* Alexandria, VA, 1994, The Association.

tion programs. Based on the NSBA survey, 92% of the school districts surveyed stated that substance abuse was included; 85% included personal health, nutrition, and disease prevention. The topics least likely to be included were consumer health, community health, and environmental health. Additional material about evaluation of school health program may be found in Chapter 13.

Preschool Children

A major responsibility of society is to educate the young before they enter school in order to equip them to become functioning members of society. This is exemplified in the first National Education Goal: All children in America will start school ready to learn.* According to the National Education Association, the children of baby boomers are reporting to preschools in droves. From 1981 to 1986, the enrollment in nursery school and kindergarten jumped 25%.† The question of what to provide in more formalized educational settings becomes even more formidable when one considers that over 30 states now have 4-year-olds in their public school programs.‡

The increasing number of families with both parents in the work force has also necessitated the development of child-care centers. The introduction of early education and child-care has resulted in new opportunities for health-related education for over 4 million pupils. Those who are entrusted with the education of very young children must not tolerate watered-down elementary programs, compartmentalized, highly structured lessons, authoritarian methods, standardized tests, competition, drills, and other "dehumanistic" procedures.* It is also clear that the three Rs are not enough. New basics include the ability to analyze, solve complex problems, think critically, and adapt to change.† It has been suggested that health education should become the fourth "R." As noted by U.S. Secretaries Riley and Shalala, health and education are inexorably joined. One must have health in order to learn as well as possible, and one must be educated to be able to make positive lifestyle decisions (see Appendix L). Programs that meet only the custodial needs of children do not take into consideration the preschool child's potential to learn skills and adopt behaviors once reserved for early elementary school-age children.‡

It is obvious that maintenance of good health is essential if children are to grow normally and engage in meaningful activity. Although many years old, the words of Lemuel Shattuck in his Report on the Sanitary Commission of Massachusetts§ are as applicable today as when they were originally written:

Every child should be taught early in life that to pursue one's own life and one's health and the lives and health of others is one of the most important and constantly abiding duties. Everything connected with even the greatest duties of morals and religion are performed more acceptably in a healthy than in a sickly condition.

Evidence supports the fact that unhealthy students do not get the most from their educational experience. We must look at both long- and short-range goals so that we can facilitate the early establishment of skills, practices, and attitudes that will be applicable to a lifetime of decision making.

---

*America 2000: an educational strategy, Washington, DC, 1991, US Department of Education.
†Hanson M: Early childhood: the national scene, Reston, VA, 1989, American Alliance for Health, Physical Education, Recreation, and Dance.
‡American Alliance for Health, Physical Education, Recreation, and Dance: Children's programs' annual report, Reston, VA, 1990, The Alliance, p 2.

---

*American Alliance for Health, Physical Education, Recreation, and Dance: Children's programs' annual report, Reston, VA, 1990, The Alliance, p 2.
†Pipho C: Stateline, Phi Delta Kappan 84:229, 1982.
‡Hendricks C, Echols D, Nelson G: The impact of a preschool health curriculum on children's health knowledge, J School Health 59(9):389-392, 1989.
§Shattuck L: Report of the Sanitary Commission of the State of Massachusetts, Cambridge, MA, 1850, Harvard University Press (facsimile).

Children begin making decisions relative to many aspects of their health at increasingly early ages. If a child makes unhealthy decisions and his or her health suffers as a consequence, that child may begin to develop a poor self-concept that could affect the behavior of the child and ultimately the ability of the child to learn. Clearly it is easier to develop positive health habits during initial behavior development than it is to try and alter existing behavior.

We would do well to remember that infants do not smoke, do not take drugs, and do not deliberately risk their health for pleasure or convenience. These decisions occur much later in life. Our task is to prevent these behaviors from developing.* The early years of education are crucial, for it is in the early years that children gain the foundation for later successes. Education for decision making that will lead to maintaining a healthy lifestyle should begin at the earliest age possible. This education, in order to be most effective, must be planned, sequential, and appropriate to the developmental level of the child. The federal government has advocated instruction and has developed health instruction materials for use in such programs as Head Start. Stress has been placed on the development of habit patterns relating to such areas as nutrition, safety, disease control, and dental health. In this text, the content material for teachers in Chapter 11 and the teaching/learning activities in Chapter 12 are useful in the development of health instruction programs for preschool children.

Special Services for Handicapped Children

The passage of Public Law 94-142, the Education for All Handicapped Children Act of 1975, placed greater emphasis on providing equal educational opportunities for handicapped young people. This Act was amended in 1983 and 1986. In 1986,

Public Law 99-457 broadened the range of students who were covered, and, in 1990, the passage of Public Law 101-476, Individuals with Disabilities Act (IDEA), replaced the term "handicap" with "disability." This Act also served to draw schools and parents closer together to develop Individualized Family Service Plans (IFSP) for children needing special services. The act enables children with disabilities to be integrated (mainstreamed) into regular academic classes, including providing health instruction for these students. Suggestions for content may be found in Chapters 11 and 12.

WHAT ARE THE ADMINISTRATIVE PROBLEMS?

The major administrative problem is the low priority given to health education as a subject field by superintendents and school boards despite the increased recognition of need and the progress made in program development. Although a recent Gallup* poll showed that 85% of the administrators surveyed felt that comprehensive school health education was just as or more important that other topics taught in school, the problem is compounded by these concerns now facing all U.S. public schools: (1) the questioning by the community of the quality of education, (2) the desire of parents for a return to an emphasis on basic subjects (reading, writing, arithmetic) in the curriculum, (3) the curtailment of federal and state financial support, (4) legislative mandates that constrain developmental efforts.†

These difficulties are formidable but are not insurmountable. Health instruction can be introduced into school curricula despite existing problems. School boards make the decisions regarding the adoption of health instruction as well as any

---

*Hochbaum G: Behavior change as the goal of health education, *The Eta Sigma Gamman,* Fall/Winter, pp 127-130, 1981.

*Seffrin J: *America's interest in comprehensive school health education.* Paper presented to the Second Annual School Health Conference, Atlanta, June 8, 1994.
†National School Boards Association: *School board member knowledge of and attitudes regarding school health programs,* Alexandria, VA, 1994, The Association, p 14.

other curriculum. As community representatives, school board members are expected to serve the people they represent. Coordinated pressures by parents and health professionals can affect such decisions.

The presence of a health instruction program in a school is no assurance that it will have a positive effect on children. A quality program depends on the thorough consideration of a variety of administrative problems that follow.

How Should Health Instruction Be Included in the Curriculum?

The question of whether to have a pattern of instruction that includes *direct* teaching or *integrative* teaching or both must be answered.

Direct teaching. The direct teaching approach is one in which health is identified as a separate subject in the curriculum with a specified amount of teaching time allocated in the school day similar to that given to other subjects. It is planned and sequentially arranged to consider the needs, interests, and developmental levels of students. Direct teaching provides status to health instruction as a necessary curriculum area. Direct teaching in health education allows for the attainment of attitudes and practices of healthful living by students that will enable them to develop lifestyles conducive to good health.

The direct method of teaching must receive priority as the best approach to use in health instruction (Fig. 8-1). However, the use of direct teaching does not guarantee that a health education program is comprehensive.

Integrative teaching. Integrative teaching involves having health taught throughout the many subject fields in the curriculum. For example, social studies may include information about health organizations and personnel—health departments, physicians, and nurses. When covering addition, subtraction, multiplication, and division in arithmetic, the teacher can relate these procedures to the numbers of oranges and apples in boxes or to determining the cost of 1 day's food supply; the structure and function of muscles and body or-

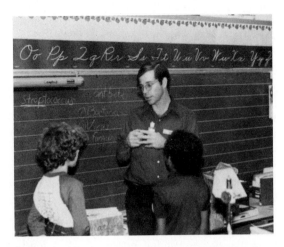

FIG. 8-1 Direct teaching is important in health education. (Courtesy Austin Independent School District, Austin, Texas.)

gans may be included in science; language arts may include reading and writing about "Who am I?" or a show-and-tell visit to the dentist; and the physical education program may cover safety on apparatus or on the playground. Actually, health-related matters can be integrated with any school subject.

The integrative approach presents two important problems for health instruction: (1) the major emphasis in teaching may be on a special subject area rather than on health, and (2) the learning objectives stressed may be on the acquisition of information, factual data, or the skills of writing, reading, or computation rather than on healthful living. By way of illustration, a lesson in reading from a nutrition text may focus on teaching students how to read rather than on eating a nutritious diet. If the objective of the health program is to get pupils to eat nutritious foods, reading may be used to help students analyze the nutritional content of breakfasts, lunches, and dinners.

The integrative method can provide positive health learning, especially when used for reinforcement and repetition. It should not be the basic, nor the only, approach to the teaching of health. Integrative health teaching requires careful planning so that health concepts are included throughout and across courses, thereby eliminating unnecessary duplication of content from year to year although some reinforcement of content is advisable.

Integrative health teaching is the only health program found in many schools that claim to have a health education program. Sometimes the program is so well integrated it cannot be located. The quality of such programs in terms of their impact on student health lifestyles can often be questioned. They are rarely, if ever, evaluated in terms of their impact on children's behavior.

Informal teaching. Informal health teaching has always existed in schools when, for example, students go to visit the nurse or ask a teacher about a specific health problem. This generally occurs incidentally, on an unplanned basis. Although the word *informal* connotes actions that take place spontaneously, there is need for a limited amount of planning. In recent years, except perhaps in drug education, little informal health instruction has occurred. Drug counselors or people knowledgeable about drugs have been available to meet with students individually or in small groups on a voluntary basis for information or guidance. In a few schools, voluntary student group meetings, in which opportunities are provided for pupils to ask questions or to engage in discussions on specific health problems, have been held after school hours. Informal gatherings of this nature need to be included in health instruction programs, although planning will need to be limited in an informal learning setting. These gatherings should be correlated with the direct teaching program. Presently there are no guidelines for conducting this kind of instruction.

What About Grade Placement?

The determination of grade placement for any or all of the health instruction areas in the curriculum is a complex task. It has not been clearly defined by professional health educators or by curriculum specialists. The reason is probably because of the variety of pupil and community health problems that must be locally identified and introduced. In addition, grade placement is an imperfect but expeditious manner of organizing schools. There is no single grade arrangement that will function best for all school districts. The pattern to be used must be selected on an individual basis. The suggestions that follow are based on our many years of curriculum experience.

Grade placement in health education is determined through the use of several curriculum principles and a number of additional factors. Three principles in need of attention are that (1) student needs and interests are fundamental, (2) instructional areas should be sequentially organized through the grades, and (3) periodic repetition of subject areas is necessary for the reinforcement of learning. This means consideration must be given to both horizontal (within a given grade) and vertical (across grades) sequencing.

Students may not always be able to identify health needs and interests for use in curriculum development. Therefore, in addition to pupil involvement through surveys and other means, information must be derived from state laws (some mandate specific content areas by grades or grade level groups); review of the growth and developmental characteristics of children; examination of local community health problems; identification of ethnic, religious, and racial factors; observation of pupils by parents; and data from physicians, dentists, and other health professionals.

The sequence of subject areas in health instruction through the grades must follow a pattern that is related to children's growth, development (e.g., dental health at the first grade level because of the appearance of the 6-year molars; menstruation for girls at the fourth-, fifth-, or sixth-grade level), and to their felt and unfelt needs and interests. The curriculum information presented to pupils must flow from simple facts to more complex concepts as students move upward in grade level.

The content and objectives provided in the sequence of learning must give consideration to reinforcement of learning without undue repetition throughout the grades. It may be advisable to space or cycle some health areas. For example, nutrition can be introduced in kindergarten or earlier and repeated in grades 1, 3, 5, and 7. Although perhaps desirable, not every health area needs to be taught at every grade. There may not be enough time in the total school curriculum for such consideration.

Adequate amounts of time are needed in the formal instruction program for direct teaching to have a positive effect on student lifestyles. Such provision will enable the spacing procedure to be introduced into the health curriculum and help reduce the problem of excessive repetition of information, yet allow for the necessary reinforcement of learning to take place.

The chart found in Table 11-1 (pp. 276-278) provides an illustration of grade placement for health instruction. The content areas were determined through a survey of pupil needs and interests, with consideration given to growth and development characteristics, and through the use of a variety of other information and procedures. The areas have been cycled and are not taught at every grade; however, the individual teacher in any given grade can repeat health areas in immediate higher grades if it seems necessary, depending on student needs. This curriculum provides for direct teaching within the formal instructional program.

How Much Time Should Be Allotted?

The amount of time needed to teach health instruction adequately at any given grade level or throughout the grades has not been sufficiently researched. Therefore most of the information available today is based solely on professional opinions.

The School Health Education Evaluation Study (SHEES)* provided excellent insights about many important questions concerning implementation of effective health education programs, including how much time should be allotted to the teaching

of health for effective results. This study involved more than 30,000 children (grades 4 to 7) in 1071 classrooms from 20 states.

Figure 8-2 contains a summary of the SHEES data that shows the relationship between classroom hours of health education and the extent of the resultant effects on student health knowledge, practices, and attitudes. The information in this figure highlights several items of interest in relation to the question of "How much time should be spent in health instruction?":

- More classroom hours are required to produce significant attitude change than are needed to produce either knowledge or practice change.
- "Large" effects (greater than 0.8 standard deviation) are achievable for general health knowledge gain, but only after more than 50 classroom hours. Conversely "large" gains in specific subsets of health knowledge are achievable in far fewer hours.
- "Medium" effects are achievable for general health practices when more than 40 hours of classroom instruction is provided.
- "Small" effects are achievable for general health attitudes, but these emerge only after 30 hours of classroom instruction is provided.
- Effects for all three domains reach generally stable levels at about 50 classroom hours.*

Thus the data from this study suggest that there is a definite association between student effects and classroom hours across all three domains. Furthermore, the evidence seems to indicate that a minimum of 50 hours of instruction time is required to reach the maximum total effect. This is not unreasonable as there are usually 36 weeks in a school year.

Traditionally most health education experts have recommended instructional time configurations ranging from 40 hours per year in the primary school grades to 75 to 80 hours in the middle school grades. Although local schools and school districts must individually determine the amount of time to allot for health instruction, data from the SHEES and expert opinion do provide excel-

*Connell DB, Turner RR, Mason EF: *School health education evaluation, final report,* vols I-VI, Washington, DC, 1985, Centers for Disease Control and Office of Disease Prevention and Health Promotion, Public Health Service, US Department of Health and Human Services.

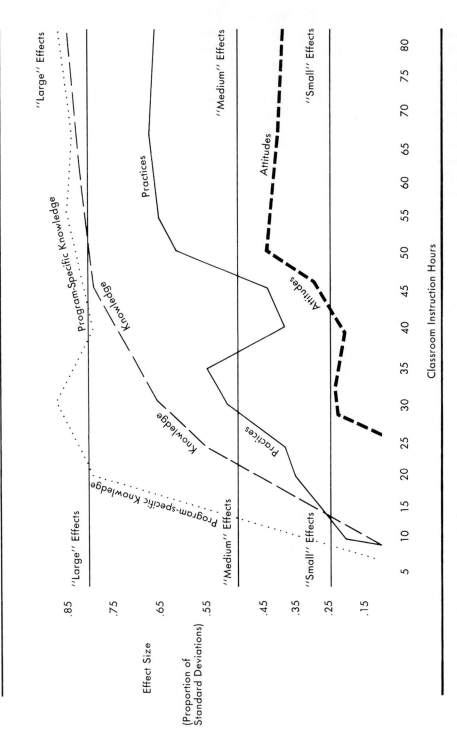

FIG. 8-2 Relationship of effect size and instruction hours for health knowledge, attitudes, and practice. (From Connell DB, Turner RR, Mason EF: Summary of findings of the school health education evaluation: health promotion effectiveness, implementation, and cost, *J School Health* 55(8):316-324, 1985.)

lent guidance. Although school administrators feel that comprehensive school health is important, less than a fourth of them feel more time should be devoted to school health than is devoted to other topics in the curriculum.*

If one examines the data collected by the American School Health Association relative to time allotted for health instruction (Table 8-5) for those states where health education is required at some point during grades 1 to 6, the average number of hours required per year was 53.15, clearly above the 50 hours suggested by the SHEES. However, in grades 7 and 8 the average number of hours required decreases to 49.3 hours per year.

Who Is Responsible for the Program?

The development, maintenance, and continuance of a health instruction program will take place most effectively if one person in the school or school district has supervisory or administrative responsibility. This individual should be professionally qualified in the field of health education. A person designated as the health coordinator, supervisor, or consultant could be a health educator, a physician, a registered nurse, or a qualified teacher. The Carnegie Council on Adolescent Development specifically recommended that a health coordinator should be present in every middle school. Someone is needed who has access to the school superintendent and the school board. This person must be given the responsibility and authority to (1) develop the curriculum, (2) seek funds for support of the program, (3) conduct in-service teacher preparation programs, (4) communicate with parents and community organizations and agencies, (5) order and help select teaching aids and equipment, and (6) supervise and administer the program. Clearly the best situation would be to have a person who was profes-

TABLE 8-5 Average Number of Health Education Hours Required per Year in States with a Specific Time Requirement, Grades 1 to 6 and 7 to 8

States	Grade range	
	1-6	7-8
Alaska	0	0
Arkansas	60.00	60.00
Arizona	30.00	19.00
District of Columbia	86.00	54.00
Delaware	60.00	30.00
Florida	0	0
Georgia	30.00	30.00
Hawaii	*	45.00
Idaho	0	35.00
Illinois	*	45.00
Indiana	54.00+	60.00+
Kentucky	60.00	30.00
Louisiana	90.00	180.00+
Maine	0	0
Minnesota	36.00	20.00
Montana	*	72.00+
North Carolina	*	*
North Dakota	0	0
New Hampshire	0	0
New Jersey	90.00+	90.00+
Nevada	*	*
New York	0	30.00
Ohio	0	48.00
Oregon	0	0
Pennsylvania	*	15.00
South Carolina	45.00	37.50
Tennessee	*	90.00
Texas	*	0.00
Utah	*	45.00
Virginia	0	72.00
Wisconsin	*	15.00
West Virginia	34.00	54.00
Total	691.000	1182.000
Mean†	53.154	49.271
S.D.	24.351	35.871

0 = No hours
+ = Hours combined with PE
* = Health Education required but unable to determine hours
† = Mean is based on the states that reported a requirement
From Lovato C et al: *School health in America, ed 5,* Kent, OH, 1989, American School Health Association, p 14.

---

*The Gallup Organization: *Values and opinions of comprehensive school health education in US public schools: adolescents, parents, and school district administrators,* Atlanta, 1994, The American Cancer Society, p 89.

sionally prepared as a health educator and who is a certified health education specialist (CHES) as the health education coordinator. Unfortunately, except perhaps in some large districts, there are not many such people employed in local school districts.

Many school nurses have become qualified in the field of health education, have become certified health education specialists, and have assumed health education responsibilities in schools. These are some of the ways nurses may provide assistance:

- Assist in curriculum development
- Serve as school health committee members
- Consult with teachers regarding instructional possibilities of health services programs
- Assist in lesson planning
- Occasionally teach selected classes
- Help with the selection and location of teaching aids
- Locate resources for community materials and speakers
- Aid in evaluation of the programs

Despite the lack of administrative or nurse assistance in schools that have no program, competent individual teachers who wish to introduce health instruction into their classrooms will find sufficient information in this text to develop a program. These teachers should also understand that the variety of state and local government offices, health departments, and voluntary and professional health agencies and organizations in the local community have many services to provide on request. Teachers and nurses who wish to implement health education programs should also request that specific in-service education programs be offered on a regular basis within the school.

Who Should Teach Health Education?

The cornerstone of a successful, comprehensive health education program is an adequately prepared and interested teacher. Based on information from a recent Gallup poll* of 809 school administrators, 56% felt that teachers are not being adequately prepared to present health information and skills to children. At the elementary level the primary responsibility for the teaching of health should rest with the classroom teacher. This person is familiar with teaching methods and is in the best position to maintain, coordinate, and integrate the program into the curriculum. Where nurse services are available, teachers should use them as a resource in many ways, including bringing them into the classroom to discuss specific health topics. School administrators should provide in-service education opportunities for all school personnel in health-related matters, including health content and methods. On the other hand, teachers should also take the initiative to specifically request in-service programs that deal with health-related topics.

Although some nurses are qualified to teach health education, for them to serve on a full-time basis and in all classes would be logistically impossible. Many districts may provide only limited nurse services. Besides, if nurses are expected to be involved in the health services program and possibly the environmental health aspect of the program, the extent of their responsibilities would not permit them to participate extensively in health education.

Special in-service training programs should be provided for teachers who are expected to teach health but are not qualified. Those teachers who wish to become prepared in health education or desire to upgrade their competencies can do so by taking college and university courses and workshops, reading current health literature, attending conferences and seminars, requesting in-service programs, and seeking help from the many available community health resources.

It should be noted that as of 1988, only 21 states offered certification for elementary health educa-

---

*The Gallup Organization: *Values and opinions of comprehensive school health education in US public schools: adolescents, parents, and school district administrators,* Atlanta, 1994, The American Cancer Society, p 40.

tion teachers. Ten of these states offered separate certification, eight offered dual certification in health and physical education as well as separate health certification, and one offered only dual health and physical education certification. However, only one state required certification in health education in order to teach the subject in elementary schools.*

Should Parent Education Be Included?

The need for both formal and informal education of parents is justified on the basis that many health behaviors occur outside the classroom, in the home and the community. Without parental support and cooperation, the effectiveness of school health instruction will be greatly reduced. Parents should have the opportunity to review and comment on the objectives of the program. They need to understand the nature of the school program.

Parent education, although difficult to make operational, can be achieved through planning and concerted effort. Formal education can take place through lectures, films, group discussions, newsletters, and other procedures. Information regarding the inclusion of controversial areas must be communicated to parents.

Informal education may occur through parent-teacher, nurse-parent, or nurse-parent-teacher conferences; special bulletins; telephone calls; notes sent home; newspaper articles; radio and TV presentations; and in many other ways. Counseling and guidance can be effective in handling individual student problems.

The extent of parent health education is believed to be sporadic in U.S. schools, and its effectiveness is not known. There are ways, however, to help ensure a successful parent education program (Table 8-6).

---

*Lovato C, Allensworth D, Chan F: *School health in America: an assessment of state policies to protect and improve the health of students,* ed 5, Kent, OH, 1989, American School Health Association, p 11.

TABLE 8-6 Making Parental Education Programs Successful

In order to help ensure the success of parental education programs, the following guidelines should be considered:

- Parents should feel that what they have to say will be heard by school personnel; involve them in decision making.
- Begin with parents who are already involved and have them help you reach other parents.
- Be sure that the activity for which you are requesting parental involvement has meaning—don't waste parents' time.
- Create activities that make parents want to become involved.
- Don't be afraid to reach out to parents who are at home; get away from the concept that everything must be done at school. Consider planning neighborhood programs.
- Maintain open channels of communication between the school and parents.
- Offer courses for parents that parallel what is being taught to students. This will foster parent-student-school communication.
- Consider the development of a newsletter for parents that contains information about how they can become involved in school-related activities and programs.
- Develop cooperative learning strategies that will necessitate students and parents working together.
- Conduct in-service training programs for teachers to help them learn how to involve family members in classroom activities.

Modified from Birch D: Involving families in school health education: an essential partnership. In Cortese P, Middleton K, editors: *The comprehensive school health challenge,* vol 2, Santa Cruz, CA, 1994, ETR Associates, pp 687-707; Davies D: Schools reaching out, *Phi Delta Kappan* 72 (5):376-382, 1991; Redding S: Creating a school community through parent involvement, *Educa Digest* 57:6-9, 1991.

What Controversial Areas Should Be Included in the Curriculum?

As mentioned in Chapter 2, many health education topics may be considered controversial. Sex education and education about sexually transmitted diseases (including AIDS), drug education (including alcohol and tobacco), death education, education about suicide, and values clarification are curriculum areas parents generally have the greatest concern about including in the health instruction program. The primary arguments raised in the controversy are:

- Students will be encouraged to experiment with sex and drugs.
- The home and/or church should be responsible for this education.
- Schools are not capable of dealing with moral and ethical issues, that is, with values education.
- Schools may teach values that are in conflict with those of the home or church.
- Parents generally prefer only the teaching of abstinence in the use of drugs and sexual involvement rather than intelligent decision making.
- Teachers are not competent to teach these subjects.

Many student problems are connected with these controversial areas. Unfortunately, numerous parents are unable, unwilling, or lack the information to provide the counseling and guidance their children need. Schools have a responsibility to attempt to help students and parents cope with these problems through programs of instruction and in other ways. Should schools decide to introduce any or all of the controversial areas into the curriculum, these factors must be considered:

- Written policies about curriculum and material selection, parental and community involvement, and acceptance and review of complaints/concerns should be available and distributed.
- Parents, with community support from health departments, physicians, voluntary health agencies, religious institutions, and others, should provide input to identify those curriculum areas to be included. Involvement of these individuals and organizations in the preparation of the curriculum will provide understanding and enhance the chances of approval by the school board.

- Curricula must be approved by the school board and must adhere to legal mandates. School board members are representatives of the people and must supply the funds to implement and support the program.
- Teachers must be qualified to teach the subject areas. In-service programs may be necessary to develop curricula and teacher competencies. Teachers must be interested in, feel comfortable with, and be capable of teaching the subject to which they are assigned.
- Teachers should be well-adjusted, emotionally stable, mature persons with a wholesome and positive outlook on life. Parents should be provided the opportunity to meet the teachers who will conduct the instructional programs. Parents need to feel comfortable and assured that these teachers will give proper professional treatment to the instructional program.
- Parents should be provided the opportunity to view teaching materials. This is mandatory for sex education in some states.
- The curriculum objectives, content, and materials should be periodically reviewed by parents and appropriate community groups. School districts cannot expect that a program approved in any given year will have support in later years. The needs and problems of students and the nature of families and community representatives are constantly changing.

Controversial areas have been approved for inclusion in the curriculum and have generally been successful in school districts where these factors have received adequate consideration. For those interested in implementing a program in the area of sexuality education, the American School Health Association has developed a set of useful guidelines.*

---

*American School Health Association: *Sexuality education within comprehensive school health education*, Kent, OH, 1991, The Association.

What Should Be the Role of the Community?

The school as a part of the community must involve parents and health and safety organization representatives in the development, maintenance, implementation, and assessment of health instruction programs. The extent and nature of their specific participation must be determined by each school or school district. The critical factor is the development of school/community partnerships. By doing this, material taught in school can be reinforced in home and community settings.

Parents can provide valuable assistance in a variety of ways that include (1) identification of student health problems, (2) help in conducting pupil need and interest surveys, (3) service on health instruction committees, (4) organization of community support for instructional programs, (5) persuasion of school boards to develop and conduct health education, (6) assistance with evaluation procedures, and (7) serving on school health advisory committees or on community health councils. Health departments, voluntary health agencies, medical and dental organizations, and individual physicians and dentists can participate in parent activities and in addition can help to (1) determine the nature and accuracy of the curriculum content, (2) determine the feasibility of the program objectives, (3) provide, recommend, and assess teaching aids, and (4) serve on the school health advisory committee or on the community health council.

Is Evaluation Necessary?

Periodically the health instruction program should be quantitatively and qualitatively evaluated to determine the extent to which objectives have been achieved. Quantitatively it is important to know whether the curriculum is adequate. Some of the questions that should be answered include:

- Are the subject areas provided sufficient to meet student needs?
- Are the curriculum guides useful?
- Are the teaching aids effective?

It is more important, however, to discover the quality of the program in terms of its impact on student behavior. It is necessary to know lifestyle changes in terms of student practices, attitudes, and knowledge.

The evaluation process in health education has not been greatly used or adequately developed. In fact, an ineffective evaluation process undoubtedly has been a factor in the failure of many health education programs. Qualitative, organized assessment of the health program to determine the achievement of student behaviors has rarely occurred in schools. Chapter 14 contains information that will help with the evaluation process.

SUMMARY

The awareness of the need for health instruction programs, although fairly well established, continues to require development. Many parent and community health organizations and agencies support the inclusion of health education in school curricula. Despite the establishment of several national and governmental health education agencies and organizations, as well as the existence of numerous state requirements, few comprehensive health instruction programs may be found in schools. Fragmented curricula consisting of one or more content areas are evident in many school districts. Health instruction programs may be justified because of the spiraling costs of medical care, health misconceptions, a gullible public, confusion about health information, the media influence on behavior, the relation of lifestyle to disease, and the need for self-care. The increased use of child-care centers and the increasing number of children who enroll in preschools provide unique opportunities to develop educational programs that will help give these students a good foundation for making health-related decisions. The implementation of effective programs in schools can be achieved through the resolution of a variety of administrative problems, by considering the controversial nature of some topics included in health education, and by having written policies and open communication so that parents and the community can become involved.

QUESTIONS FOR DISCUSSION

1. What evidence exists that indicates there is increased support for health instruction programs in U.S. schools?
2. What factors identify the need for the health education of both preschool and elementary school children?
3. What is the current status of health education in the United States at the national, state, and local levels?
4. What are the administrative problems in need of school attention to ensure effective health instruction programs?
5. Identify and describe two basic patterns of health instruction that may be used in schools. What are the advantages and disadvantages of their use? Illustrate their application to health instruction.
6. What principles are used in the determination of the grade placement of health education in schools? Illustrate their application to the health instruction program.
7. How much time should be provided in the elementary school curriculum for health education? What factors are used in determining the amount of time for health education?
8. Who should teach in the elementary school health instruction program? Why? How might teachers become better prepared to teach health education?
9. Why should parents be included in the elementary school health education program? How can this be achieved?
10. What are some ways the community can become involved in the school health program?
11. Why are some topics considered to be controversial in health education? What factors need school consideration for decisions to include these topics in the instruction program? What might teachers do to avoid "getting into trouble?"

REFERENCES

America 2000: an educational strategy, Washington, DC, 1991, US Department of Education.

American Alliance for Health, Physical Education, Recreation, and Dance: *Children's programs' annual report,* Reston, VA, 1990, The Alliance.

American Association of School Administrators: *Why school health,* Arlington, VA, 1987, The Association.

American Council on Science and *Health News and Views,* 7(5):1, 8-10, November/December, 1986.

American Public Health Association: Gaps found in Americans' knowledge of health habits, *Nation's Health* 1, July 17, 1986.

American Public Health Association, School Health Section: *Education for health in the school-community setting,* Washington, DC, 1975, The Association.

American School Health Association: *Sexuality education within comprehensive school health education,* Kent, OH, 1991, The Association.

Birch D: Involving families in school health education: an essential partnership. In Cortese P, Middleton K, editors: *The comprehensive school health challenge,* vol 2, Santa Cruz, CA, 1994, ETR Associates, pp 687-707.

Brun J, Murray J, Parcel G: Preschool health education program (PHEP): analysis of education and behavioral outcomes, *Health Educa Quart* 10(3/4):149-171, 1984.

Burks A, Fox E: Why is inservice training essential? In Cortese P, Middleton K, editors: *The comprehensive school health challenge,* vol 2, Santa Cruz, CA, 1994, ETR Associates, pp 783-799.

Burner ST, Waldo DR, McKusick DR: National health expenditures projections through 2030, *Health Care Finance Rev* 14:1-29, 1992.

Cleary M, Gobble D: The changing nature of public schools: implications for teacher preparation, *Journal School Health* 60(2):53-55, 1990.

Coalition of National Health Education Organizations: *Incentives for strengthening elementary school health education.* A position paper by the delegates to the Coalition of National Health Education Organizations, Chapel Hill, NC, 1990, School of Public Health, University of North Carolina at Chapel Hill.

Connell DB, Turner RR, Mason EF: *School health education evaluation, final report,* vols I-VI, Washington, DC, 1985, Centers for Disease Control and Office of Disease Prevention and Health Promotion, Public Health Service, US Department of Health and Human Services.

Connell DB, Turner RR, Mason EF: Summary of findings of the school health education evaluation: health promotion effectiveness, implementation and cost, *J School Health* 55(8):316-324, 1985.

Cornacchia HJ, Barrett S: *Consumer health: a guide to intelligent decisions,* ed 5, St Louis, 1993, Times Mirror/Mosby College Publishing.

Davies D: Schools reaching out, *Phi Delta Kappan* 72(5):376-382, 1991.

Redding S: Creating a school community through parent involvement, *Educa Digest* 57:6-9, 1991.

Drolet JC: Professional preparation. In Cortese P, Middleton K, editors: *The comprehensive school health challenge,* vol 2, Santa Cruz, CA, 1994, ETR Associates, pp 801-834.

Education Commission of the States: *Recommendations for school health education: a handbook for state policymakers,* Denver, 1981, The Commission.

Food and Drug Administration: *A study of practices and opinions,* Springfield, VA, 1972, National Technical Information Service, US Department of Commerce.

The Gallup Organization: *Values and opinions of comprehensive school health education in US public schools: adolescents, parents, and school district administrators,* Atlanta, 1994, American Cancer Society.

Hanson M: *Early childhood: the national scene,* Reston, VA, 1989, American Alliance for Health, Physical Education, Recreation, and Dance.

Hausman AJ, Ruzek SB: Implementation of comprehensive school health education in elementary schools: focus on teacher concerns, *J School Health* 65(3):81-86, 1995.

Healthy People 2000: national health promotion and disease prevention objectives, Pub No (PHS) 91-50212, Washington, DC, 1991, US Department of Health and Human Services.

Healthy people: the Surgeon General's report on health and disease prevention, Washington, DC, 1979, US Department of Health and Human Services.

Hendricks C, Echols D, Nelson G: The impact of a preschool health curriculum on children's health knowledge, *J School Health* 59(9):389-392, 1989.

Hochbaum G: Behavior change as the goal of health education, *The Eta Sigma Gamman,* Fall/Winter, 1981, pp 127-130 .

Jackson S: Introduction. In Jackson SA, editor: *Comprehensive school health programs: innovative practices and issues in setting standards,* Pub No FIRST 93-7006, Washington, DC, 1993, US Department of Education.

Lovato C, Allensworth D, Chan F: *School health in America: an assessment of state policies to protect and improve the health of students,* ed 5, Kent, OH, 1989, American School Health Association.

McGinnis JM: Health problems of children and youth: a challenge for schools, *Health Educa Quart* 8(1):11-14, 1981.

Nagy C, Nagy MC: Administrative perceptions of health education in the special education curriculum, *Teacher Educa Special Educa* 10:121, 1987.

National Commission on the Role of the School and the Community in Improving Adolescent Health: *Code blue: uniting for healthier youth,* Alexandria, VA, 1990, National Association of State Boards of Education, and American Medical Association.

National School Boards Association: *School board member knowledge of and attitudes regarding school health programs,* Alexandria, VA, 1994, The Association.

Noak M: *State policy support for school health education: a review and analysis,* report No 182-1, Washington, DC, 1982, Education Commission of the States.

Pipho C: Stateline, *Phi Delta Kappan,* 84:229, 1982.

Resnicow K, Cherry J, Cross D: Ten unanswered questions regarding comprehensive school health promotion, *J School Health* 63(4):171-175, 1993.

Seffrin J: *America's interest in comprehensive school health education.* Paper presented to the Second Annual School Health Conference, Atlanta, June 8, 1994.

Shattuck L: *Report of the Sanitary Commission of the State of Massachusetts,* Cambridge, MA, 1850, Harvard University Press (facsimile).

Siri DK: Community/school partnerships: a vision for the future. In Cortese P, Middleton K, editors: *The comprehensive school health challenge,* vol 2, Santa Cruz, CA, 1994, ETR Associates, pp 881-887.

Stone E: ACCESS: keystones for school health promotion, *J School Health* 60(7):298-300, 1990.

Sullivan LW: *Forward, Healthy people 2000: national health promotion and disease prevention objectives,* Washington, DC, 1990, US Department of Health and Human Services, Public Health Service.

Sullivan LW: Health promotion and disease prevention, *Med Educa* 26:175-177, 1992.

US Department of Health, Education, and Welfare; Health Services and Mental Health Administration: *The Report of the President's Committee on Health Education,* Washington, DC, 1973, Superintendent of Documents.

US Department of Health and Human Services, Public Health Service: *Better health for our children: a na-*

tional strategy, major findings and recommendations, vol 1, Washington, DC, 1981, Superintendent of Documents.

US Department of Education: *What works; schools without drugs,* Washington, DC, 1980, The Department.

Varnes JW: Preservice education: providing health knowledge for all teachers. In Cortese P, Middleton K, editors: *The comprehensive school health challenge,* vol 2, Santa Cruz, CA, 1994, ETR Associates, pp 763-781.

9

The Learning Process and Health Education

KEY CONCEPT

Use of fundamental learning principles will have a favorable impact on student health behavior.

Learning seldom comes from passively sitting still in the water with sails flapping.
R.S. BARTH*

Health education programs must be theoretically consistent. . . . they should be designed so that their goals, objectives, interventions [methods and techniques], and evaluative measures are consistent with the basic theories of learning.
M.A. VOJTECKY†

PROBLEM TO SOLVE

As a fifth-grade teacher you desire to change the way you have been teaching health because the present approach has not had a positive effect on student behavior. You have concluded that the use of the basic principles of learning are essential. What methods might you select that would illustrate the application of each of the principles to the following areas: nutrition, dental health, safety, and drug abuse?

*Barth RS: A personal vision of a good school, *Phi Delta Kappan* 71:512-516, 1990.
†Vojtecky MA: An adaptation of Bigge's classification of learning to health education and an analysis of theory underlying recent health education programs, *Health Ed Quart* 103:247-261, 1984.

HEALTH education learning must focus its efforts on helping young people develop practices, habits, and skills that prevent illness and promote and maintain good health. A great deal of health learning that has occurred in schools has emphasized anatomical and physiological knowledge. Learning solely about the effects of the intake of legal and illegal substances or the use of fats, cholesterol, and fiber will not achieve the desired behavioral changes. Some of this information is necessary for understanding. Learning, however, must stress ways to cope with social and environmental conditions and provide understanding of the psychological factors that influence behavior. Awareness of the influences that come from peers, the home, the media, and other sources is extremely important. Children and youth need to develop a positive self-image and be confident in their ability to handle the pressures that will influence their decisions whether to smoke, drink, or engage in sexual activity.

Human health behavior is a complex process resistant to change, especially when habit patterns have been established. Susser* stated that the task of developing or changing behavior is both difficult and slow. It is exceedingly more difficult for adults. The achievement of the present changes in habit patterns related to smoking, diet, and exercise has taken more than two decades to occur in the United States.

Health behavior is influenced by a variety of factors previously identified in the concept of health (see also Chapter 1). These factors include physiological, psychological, social/cultural, and spiritual components (holistic health focus).† Home atmosphere; racial, ethnic, or cultural background; peer influences; self-image; adequacy of housing and food intake; affection received; achievements; self-respect; and bias and prejudice all have a specific impact on children and youth. Pupil needs, motivations, beliefs, values, experiences, and environmental influences all affect their health habit patterns. These influences affect the ability of people to make responsible health decisions and to cope with or adjust to problems they face in the society in which they live. These factors are in need of recognition and use if educational programs are to achieve high levels of wellness in individuals.

Modification of health behavior in terms of health knowledge, attitudes, and practices is necessary to enable individuals to live in a healthful manner. However, when to attempt to modify the health behavior of people and, more importantly how to modify behavior has not been adequately resolved. Health behavior involves an internal process that is influenced by personal needs and environmental exposures. It is not something done to pupils but rather includes educational procedures or methods used to help individuals adapt, adjust, solve problems, or cope with situations in regard to their health. Health education should attempt to aid students to make intelligent and responsible decisions about exercise, disease prevention and control, drugs, sexual activity, safety, and so on.

The question of the extent to which educators should try to modify health behavior is moot. Should the use of alcohol or tobacco, including smokeless tobacco, be condemned or condoned? Should all individuals exercise at regular intervals and in the same manner? Should the use and distribution of contraceptives be promoted? Should pupils reduce their consumption of foods containing high levels of salt, sugar and cholesterol? Should the flossing and brushing of teeth be universally advocated? In the early elementary grades, health behaviors to be achieved do not demand extensive explanation. Children need to receive positive directions that are easy to understand. However, in the middle and upper grades, young people should start to learn how to make their own decisions. They need to learn how to solve problems, especially those involving peer pressures.

---

*Susser M, editor: Editorial: the tribulations and trials—interventions in communities, *Am J Pub Health* 85:156-158, 1995.
†Holistic health is a concept used in health education that refers to the consideration given to all the factors that affect the health of the individual and not merely those that are physiological.

Hochbaum* identified a fundamental principle of learning some years ago that continues to be applicable; in controversial aspects of health behavior, no attempt should be made to make modifications in line with rigid criteria (not to drink, not to smoke). He believed that students should be informed adequately and accurately and helped to develop skills and motivation that would enable them to arrive at rational and intelligent decisions.

The purpose of this chapter is to help the reader gain insight into the process for influencing health behavior. Information will be provided that will enable the teacher to (1) become better informed about the learning process and its application to health education and (2) that will introduce and apply the essential principles of learning needed in the selection of methods and materials (see also Chapters 12 and 13) for effective health instruction programs.

WHAT IS LEARNING?

Learning is a complex process that depends on factors taking place both inside (psychological/spiritual) and outside (social) the individual. It refers to the physical, intellectual, and emotional changes that occur in human organisms as a result of their interaction with the environment. It is the growth and development process that goes on within individuals as a result of their participation in a variety of experiences, feelings, attitudes, and interests. The health-educated pupil, having been exposed to a variety of health opportunities and activities, is better able to promote and maintain good health.

The process of learning happens within the individual but is influenced by the experiences to which pupils are exposed through the teaching methods, techniques, and material aids (see also Chapters 12 and 13) selected by the teacher. Knowledge of the nature, conditions, and the principles of learning is basic to an understanding

*Hochbaum GM: Behavior modification, *School Health Rev* 2:September, 1971.

and implementation of the teaching process in the health instruction program.

HOW DO CHILDREN LEARN?

The specific scientific nature of learning cannot be clearly identified. However, the process does involve a series of rewards and punishments. Positive reinforcements may include money, candy, privileges, grades, peer approval, praise, attention, and self-interest. Negative reinforcement that results in the elimination or modification of behavior may be the result of loud sounds, disapproval, punishment, poor grades, peer and other pressures, and use of unpleasant substances. It is believed that learning takes place most efficiently and effectively when someone *wants* (favorable attitude) to learn something (positive learning). This person is then said to be motivated to action—to be goal directed. A diagram best illustrates the learning process as it probably occurs (Fig. 9-1).

The process of learning may be illustrated by the example of the teacher who desires to have a student learn procedures that will help prevent and control communicable disease. The teacher attempts to stimulate interest in student learning by identifying a school problem in which a large number of children have been absent and there is an existing need to protect those now in school from illness. The goal or goals are established whereby students will know and realize the importance of, and will behave in a manner to control and prevent, disease. The teacher selects a variety of activities to aid in the achievement of this objective. These experiences may include having students (1) read and report on how bacteria are transmitted and the hazards to their health, (2) participate in cooperative learning to solve the problem of prevention and control of disease, (3) wash hands before lunch, (4) prepare a bulletin board display or artwork for classroom and school about hazards and preventive procedures, and (5) conduct experiments in growing bacteria in class.

However, such activities may create emotional tension or conflict in the students. The amount of tension or conflict will depend on a number of fac-

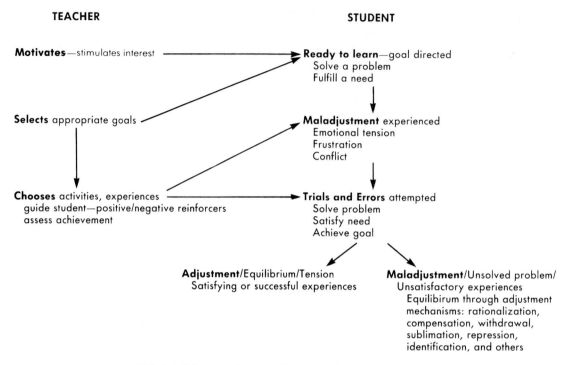

FIG. 9-1 Schematic diagram illustrating the learning process.

tors such as the intensity of the motivation, the difficulty encountered in reaching a solution (failure of ill children to remain at home, insufficient nurse services to check ill students, or inadequate supplies and equipment in school or at home), the amount of work required, and the desire for a good grade. In the process the teacher guides the pupils individually or collectively to try to reduce the errors, to resolve the problem, and to provide individual help where necessary. If the motivation is effective and the activities and guidance are appropriate, the goal will be reached, pupils will feel satisfied, and the needed equilibrium will be attained. Should the goal not be reached, pupils may react through a variety of adjustment mechanisms by making excuses such as: "There was too much work to do," "The teacher didn't help enough," "I didn't understand what to do," "We didn't have the proper supplies and facilities."

Learning occurs when a learner encounters new experiences in the environment. There are students who can learn without teachers; however, teacher guidance serves to motivate this learning and reduce the errors a pupil may make in the learning process by controlling, manipulating, and selecting the appropriate kinds of activities.

LEARNING AND THE CONCEPT APPROACH TO HEALTH EDUCATION

One effective approach to teaching health is through the emphasis on concepts. It is important to help students develop big ideas or reach conclusions about health that will enable them to take positive action and make wise decisions regarding their own, their families', and their community's health. Teachers must be aware of these generalizations and help students to achieve them. Such concepts—smoking may be harmful to the human body, drugs are mood modifiers, certain foods are needed for proper growth and development, there are ways to protect ourselves from disease—help teachers determine more relevant and effective health education goals (see also Appendix B, Partial Health Units). These "big ideas" are more likely to be remembered and hopefully will provide greater potential for pupil action.

LEARNING AND THE GOALS OF HEALTH EDUCATION

Clear identification and awareness of the objectives of health education are important to the learning and teaching process. Goals give direction to the learning that enables pupils to acquire the concepts and behaviors needed for healthful living. It is necessary, therefore, that teachers clearly understand the purposes of health education for the most effective teaching. Precisely defined health objectives have particular meaning since learning should be centered on behavior outcomes as well as on factual achievements. Learning should lead students to the acquisition of health education concepts.

The present aim of health education is to develop practices, skills, and attitudes of safe and healthful living through the understanding of scientific health information. Individuals should be able to make intelligent decisions about the physical, mental, spiritual, and social aspects of health. Health be-

haviors are therefore related to and depend on the cognitive learning acquired by pupils.

The precise relationship of knowledge and attitudes to practices is not known. Phi Delta Kappa's Center on Evaluation, Development, and Research stated that there had been no significant research to indicate the consistent nature of these relationships.* Present evidence, however, indicates there is an interdependency. However, the possession of understanding by itself does not necessarily result in good health habits. A 6-year follow-up educational study of the use of alcohol, tobacco, and marijuana revealed that students had acquired knowledge but there was no detectable impact on behavior.†

Knowing how to brush your teeth does not mean that this practice will be followed. Knowing that some snack-time foods are more nutritious than others is no assurance that they will be eaten. Knowing that immunizations protect against diseases does not always result in these preventive measures being obtained. Knowing the physiological effects of drugs does not necessarily reduce their usage. *Although knowing may not always lead to doing, there will be no doing without knowing.*

Lawrence and McLeroy‡ advocated the importance of attitudes in health teaching as a means of bridging the gap between "knowing" and "doing." They claimed that self-efficacy (one's belief in the ability to do a specific behavior) is the principal connection because it usually precedes behavior. Brubaker and Loftin,§ in a study on the use of smokeless tobacco by middle-school male students, stated that behavioral attention is based on individual attitudes toward performing the behavior and the individual's perception of whether others would or would not approve.

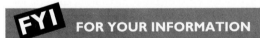

FOR YOUR INFORMATION

The National Institute for Development and Administration at the University of Texas reported that individuals remember only:

  10% of what they read
  20% of what they hear
  30% of what they see
  50% of what they see and hear
  70% of what they say
  90% of what they say and do

From Lapp DC: (Nearly) total recall, *Stanford* 20:48-51, 1992.

---

*Practical application of research, *Newsletter, Phi Delta Kappa's Center on Evaluation, Development, and Research* 5:4, 1983.
†Preventing substance abuse: rethinking strategies, *Am J Public Health,* 83:793-795, 1993.
‡Lawrence L, McLeroy KR: Self-efficacy and health education, *J School Health* 56:317-322, 1986.
§Brubaker RF, Loftin TL: Smokeless tobacco use by middle school males: a preliminary test of the reasoned action theory, *J School Health* 57:64-67, 1987.

A hierarchy of attitudes, ranging from those of lesser to greater intensity, is presented in Table 9-1. Strong attitudes that have been internalized, such as beliefs and values, and that are of great significance probably will have the greatest impact on health actions. Appreciation and feelings about health matters expressed in opinions of a lesser intensity may or may not lead to favorable health behaviors. However, such interests or opinions may be used as motivational devices. A person who is interested in preventing dental decay because it may affect one's appearance is more likely to brush his or her teeth or to visit a dentist. Someone who believes in and values these practices will more likely behave appropriately. Strong attitudes such as beliefs and values that have been internalized undoubtedly will have the greatest impact on actions. Teachers must be aware of the importance and use of attitudes in learning about health.

Research evidence has shown that health habit patterns may be developed without attitudinal involvement and with little or no knowledge. This evidence is particularly applicable to young children, especially those in the lower grades. Adult statements that certain foods are important for growth, that safe practices on the playground prevent injuries, and that use of cigarettes is hazardous to health may result in the desired behavior if sufficient repetition and reinforcement are provided and if there is parental support for these concepts.

In the home, children's nutritional, dental, sleep, and other behaviors are usually established by parents. In school, habit patterns may occur through rules and regulations issued by the teacher or principal as they relate to safety (bicycle, playground), nutrition (school lunch, snack machine contents), and control of disease (washing hands before lunch and after toilet use, sneezing, or coughing).

Consideration must be given to the fact that behavioral and attitudinal changes in health do not necessarily take place immediately after teaching. It may take considerable time and repetition before they become established. Cultural, social, and other values and beliefs that pupils bring from home and the community make the changing of health habits extremely difficult or impossible to achieve during school time. However, some behavior changes may be observable in the classroom and are subject to measurement; those oc-

TABLE 9-1 Hierarchy of Attitudes

	Attitude	Definitions	Behavioral manifestations
Overt action	Interest	Emotional responses to stimuli; feelings	Attention, awareness, appreciation by listening, talking, reading, writing, and other ways
	Opinion	—	Verbal or written expression
Internalization	Belief	Emotional acceptance of a concept, proposition, or doctrine; a preference; a decision about something; a conviction to or about something	Willingness to be identified with a proposition, or concept; self-expression with verbal, written, or performance action
	Value	A high, deep, and long-lasting degree of emotional acceptance and commitment to a concept, proposition, or doctrine; to cherish or prize; a faith; a potential goal	Pursues, seeks, and wants; takes action in satisfying ways through participation—convincing others, spending time, effort, and funds

Modified from Rosser JM: Values and health, *J School Health* 41:386-390, 1971; and Cornacchia HJ, Smith DE, Bentel DJ: *Drugs in the classroom: a conceptual model for school programs,* ed 2, St Louis, 1978, Mosby.

curring in the home and elsewhere outside of school may not be seen (unobservable) and may be extremely difficult to assess. Kirby* states that changing behavior outside the classroom is difficult to achieve. It should be recognized that the impact of health learning often takes time to affect children.

Habits established in the early years need reinforcement and repetition in a sequential program throughout the school years. Additional support and repetition in the home are necessary. Peer pressure and influence as well as other social factors, including the mass media, can interfere with the establishment of good health behaviors. Despite these difficulties, the acquisition of appropriate health behaviors depends on accurate information and understanding.

Good health behavior is significant only in terms of its effect on the lives of pupils. Good health, therefore, should be a means to an end and not an end in itself. Being healthy should enable children to obtain a better education, be happier, have fun, be able to play for longer periods of time without undue fatigue, be more productive in the world, and be better citizens in the community. But when good health is an end in itself, it may lead to neurotic health behavior or other problems.

Teachers should be aware that all students may not be able to acquire the same health levels because of hereditary and environmental factors. Children who are blind or deaf may never have these senses restored. Children who suffer with allergies may need special medical attention. Boys and girls with uncorrectable heart defects may never have the stamina to play strenuous games. Students without adequate food may be hungry and malnourished. Despite these handicaps, students need to maintain the best health status possible within their own limitations. Numerous examples of handicapped people leading well-adjusted, happy, and productive lives are found in society. The goals in health education, therefore, may need to be modified to fit the individual differences of children.

Inspection of the specific outcomes of health education that teachers should seek to achieve may be categorized into the following:

- Practices, habits, skills—action domain
- Attitudes, feelings, ideals, interests, appreciations, beliefs, values—affective domain
- Knowledge, understanding, information—cognitive domain

Practices and habits are synonymous health education terms that refer to behaviors performed with regularity. Some practices, however, also require special expertise in muscle-motor action (skills). Therefore, although some skills are necessary for some practices, the ability to perform a skill does not mean it will be established as a habit or a practice. Brushing the teeth, exercising properly, or caring for wounds resulting from injuries are skills that must be learned but may not become practices.

The *decision-making process* (see "Ability to Solve Problems," p. 243) must receive attention by teachers in the health instruction program. Pupils are growing and developing organisms who are exposed constantly to environmental influences

FOR YOUR INFORMATION

Substance Abuse Prevention

Prevention may be encouraged through social reinforcement, focusing on social pressures to develop skills to:
- Recognize the pressures to use drugs
- Develop skills to resist those pressures
- Identify social and physical risks

Some of the methods to achieve prevention include discussions, behavior modeling, role-playing, and extended practice.

From Bruvold WH: A meta-analysis, *Am J Public Health,* June, 1993.

*Kirby D: Reduce risk-taking behaviors, *J School Health* 62:280-287, 1992.

affecting health and about which decisions must be made. Adolescents are faced with problems that involve decision making, such as sexual activity, teen pregnancy, peer pressures, and stress. Young people must have the opportunity to make their own decisions and not be expected to follow the dictates of the teacher. However, such decisions must be based on accurate scientific information and complete awareness of the consequences. To make wise decisions, it is important that students be exposed to the possible alternatives for action without teacher bias or prejudice. Such teacher consideration is vital to health teaching because it aids in the establishment of credibility, it allows for the free choice of action, and it prepares students to think and act for themselves. It is teaching for the future. By way of illustration, young people find cigarettes available in their communities and are constantly being persuaded by their peers and the media to use them. If these individuals are to be able to determine intelligently whether to smoke or not to smoke, they must learn the positive as well as the negative effects of smoking on the human organism. They must learn how to react to peer pressures. Merely condemning cigarettes may create distrust among students who talk to peers and adults and obtain conflicting evidence regarding the beneficial or detrimental aspects. This is not to imply that the use of tobacco is not hazardous but rather to emphasize that wise decisions will more likely come about when the total spectrum of tobacco's effects is provided by the teacher; when trust in the truthfulness of teacher information is achieved.

HOW CAN TEACHERS RELATE KNOWLEDGE TO BEHAVIOR IN THE INSTRUCTION PROGRAM?

The importance of health practices and habits points to the need for the use of teaching procedures that will help bridge the gap between knowledge and behavior in order to preserve and maintain health. Unfortunately, the precise methods are not known today. However, significant evidence indicates that attitudes play an important role in student health behavior. It is believed that the acquisition of feelings, interests, and appreciation will motivate students to turn their basic understanding into desirable practices.

An attitude refers to a mind set for action; it is an internal readiness to perform or behave. Therefore what pupils believe, feel, or value affects what they do. Young people who do not perceive the risks of using smokeless tobacco may believe it is safer than smoking cigarettes. Adolescents who engage in sexual activity may not think they are susceptible to STDs (sexually transmitted diseases), pregnancy, or AIDS. Pupils who do not believe that excessive sugar consumption might lead to dental decay may not eat nutritious snacktime foods. Boys and girls who do not realize the dangers of jay-walking may cross streets at the improper places. Young people may need to be helped to develop an interest in the concept of improving self-esteem. Effective learning in health education, therefore, must give consideration to including teaching methods that will attempt to develop appropriate student health attitudes as well as proper understanding.

A health education program that tries to stress the development of health attitudes is difficult to achieve, particularly because children come to school with ideas, interests, values, and feelings developed and influenced by their home and community experiences. For example, in arithmetic or spelling, the child may come to school lacking any information. Yet in matters relating to health and safety, the child may not only lack scientifically sound information but also, and more importantly, may have strong beliefs affirmed by family and community that may be false and perhaps even dangerous. Getting pupils to take responsibility for their own lives, whereby they seek to protect and maintain good health, is difficult and takes much teaching skill and thoughtful planning. It involves initiative, ingenuity, creativity, and fortitude on the part of teachers who aspire to reach this goal. It also involves parental participation and support.

Learning about health and safety does not always start with the provision of information or knowledge. There will be occasions when students will be expected to behave in certain ways and develop habit patterns of conformity that precede understanding from which positive or negative attitudes will emerge. These occasions may be especially necessary in the early grades before students have learned to make their own decisions. There will be situations in which adults take authoritative or arbitrary action that is considered to be in the best interests of students (for example, a fire breaks out in the school, the candy and soft drink machines are removed from the halls, a school lunch program with a balanced, nutritional meal is provided for all children, or an accident occurs to the school bus that is taking pupils home).

Many theories have been advanced by psychologists about learning. Numerous health educators and other health specialists have conducted research on segments of the learning process. They have generalized about its application to health behavior. Despite these efforts, a consistent, effective approach to learning applied to health instruction has not emerged. The need for such an approach is increased by current problems such as substance abuse, AIDS, violence, and sexual activity.

The principles of learning contained in this chapter are an attempt to provide a consistent approach for use in health education. They provide the fundamentals needed for effective health education. They represent the result of a thorough and careful review of pertinent literature and the extensive school health experiences of the authors. They have been found to be successful in the development and implementation of health education curricula. They were used in the development of the partial units found in Appendix B. Teachers who use these principles in the selection of their teaching methods will improve learning and thereby help students to acquire favorable health practices and attitudes.

WHY ARE PRINCIPLES OF LEARNING IMPORTANT IN HEALTH?

Knowledge of the principles of learning is important to teachers in health instruction programs because:

- Learning is a complex process
- Behavior-centered emphasis in learning compounds the complexity of the learning process; attitudes are difficult to modify and assess and many practices occur outside the school and are, therefore, not observable in the classroom
- Understanding about motivation and behavior is necessary for effective teaching
- Teaching methods and learning are interrelated

WHAT ARE THE PRINCIPLES OF LEARNING?
Motivation Is Essential to Learning

Health behavior is determined by individuals' motives and beliefs or values about various courses of action open to them. Because all behavior is motivated, the extent to which the health behavior of individuals can be understood, predicted, or controlled depends upon the ability of teachers to identify these motives and beliefs and to use them in their health teaching (Fig. 9-2).

Positively, motives refer to those drives, needs, urges, or inner compulsions that stimulate individuals to want certain things. They are classified as the following:

- Physiological needs, such as food, water, sleep, rest, air, sunshine, and exercise
- Psychological needs, such as security, love, achievement, independence, responsibility, and authority

Motives may also be considered in a negative sense, presenting cultural, social, or economic barriers to health that individuals must overcome.

Values are the strong beliefs or attitudinal concerns that have influence on positive or negative motives. The use of alcohol and tobacco and other

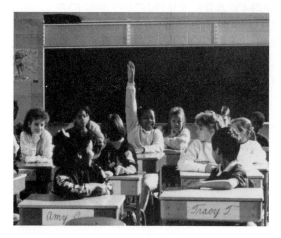

FIG. 9-2 Motivation is important. (Courtesy Michigan Department of Education.)

drugs, the control of disease, periodic visits to physicians, daily exercise, playing safely, and care of eyes and ears depend on individual belief in the importance of these actions. People have to feel that their practices will enable them to play longer, have more fun, and be more productive citizens.

Values are acquired from a variety of sources including the family, social groups, TV and other mass media, adults admired by children, and peer cultures in school. When they are consistent with the goals of health education, they will reinforce learning, but when they are in conflict, learning may be limited or restricted. They are not completely resistant to change, despite the cultural and social factors that may have influenced their formation. The earlier in the lives of children that attempts are made to instill proper health behaviors, the greater are the possibilities that these practices will be highly valued by pupils. The school, therefore, has both a responsibility and an opportunity to modify beliefs and attitudes as well as develop new ones that will promote and maintain good health.

Principles of motivation. The fundamental principles of motivation that influence health decision behaviors are:

- Degree of the threat of the problem to the individual

- Resolution of the conflict of motives
- Related and unrelated health behaviors that may occur
- Fear that may cause rational or irrational behavior
- Risk-taking that is normal and necessary but demands selectivity

Preventive health action is determined by the degree to which a person sees a health problem as threatening in terms of the following:

- Its probability of susceptibility or occurrence. Will smoking cause lung cancer?
- Its seriousness, severity, or urgency of the consequences. Are dental caries sufficiently important to warrant attention? Will an infection be painful?
- Its benefits or courses of action to reduce or remove the threat to the individual's health. What health practices should individuals follow and will these practices be beneficial? Is peer approval helpful? Are nurse or counseling services available?

Individual motives and beliefs about various courses of action are often in conflict with each other, and behavior emerges as the conflicts are resolved. The kinds of conflicts referred to include:

- When two motives compete with each other for dominance, the one of greater importance or the more highly valued one will become dominant. A family may spend what little money it has for food, shelter, and necessities rather than on medical or dental visitations. Candy may taste better than an apple. Sexual activity may be pleasurable. A child who must wear glasses because of poor eyesight may not wear them because the peer group at school ridicules this practice. A pupil will smoke cigarettes to gain social acceptance.
- If a pupil is motivated to act in a healthful manner (sees a course of action open), but the action is unpleasant, painful, time-consuming, or inconvenient, the pupil may not complete the action.
- A pupil may not accept a teacher's beliefs or opinions that there are ways to prevent or help a specific health condition and, there-

fore, does not see an effective way (course of action) to resolve the problem. For example, a girl with an infection on her leg may have been advised to visit a physician but fails to do so because she may not believe the condition is serious or because she does not see how this action can help her. She may try self-medication, but as the infection grows worse she may find that her concerns and fears increase because she is not sure what action she should take.

Health-related motives may sometimes lead to behavior unrelated to health, and conversely some behavior that has the appearance of being health related may in fact be determined by motives unrelated to health. A hungry child may not reveal hunger to a teacher and may be untruthful when asked whether he or she has eaten any food. An illustration of the converse part of this principle is one in which a child may drink milk in class because other students are drinking it. An abused child may be embarrassed or afraid to reveal the abuse.

It should be evident that teachers play an important role in health instruction programs by motivating children to seek appropriate health goals as well as by helping boys and girls to acquire beliefs and values related to these motives. Teachers must provide pupils with experiences and activities that will improve their values of good health so that they will be better prepared to resolve conflicts in motives when they occur.

Fear can lead to rational as well as irrational behavior. It serves to protect, and it can be destructive to individuals. The fear of cancer may help students to refrain from smoking. The fear of becoming overweight may lead pupils to reduce food intake. However, a teenager with a genital sore or infection may be afraid to learn that a sexually transmitted disease has been contracted and may not have the condition checked by a physician.

Risk-taking is normal and necessary and demands selectivity on the part of individuals after determination of benefit and harm. Everything people do involves risks of varying degrees. The decision to take them depends on whether the rewards outweigh the penalties. Crossing the street or eating food in a restaurant or lunchroom involves risk. However, they are minimal in comparison to the advantages. Surgery is hazardous, but if the chances of survival are increased, the benefits predominate in the decision. The risk of sexual activity leading to disease or AIDS may not seem important. The dangers of using cocaine or driving an automobile when under the influence of alcohol may be greater than the pleasures derived. Young people need to be taught to compare the advantages and disadvantages of risk-taking behavior in order to make responsible decisions.

Subprinciples of motivation. The subprinciples of motivation must receive consideration and will assist teachers in the learning process.

Cultural and social factors may be barriers to learning. The traditions and practices in the home, at play, in social groups, with adults, in the peer culture at school, in the community, and in the total environment in which children live affect and influence the values, prejudices, and perceptions that pupils bring to class. Families that rank highest economically generally spend more of their income on health services and products. Some families may not have funds to purchase glasses, toothbrushes, or adequate food or to provide health examinations for children. Some parents may not be concerned with immunizations or dental care. The nutritional and dress habits of certain ethnic and racial groups may differ somewhat from those advocated in school. Working parents may not be able to adequately supervise the eating habits and activities of their children. Certain religious groups may not believe in health examinations and appraisals, treatment, services, or fluoridation of the water supply. If both parents smoke cigarettes, the smoking rate among their children is higher than among those whose parents do not smoke. Social pressures of peers, parents, and the media have an influence on children's use of alcoholic beverages.

Teachers should be cognizant of the impact of cultural and social factors and realize that they may have an effect on the health education program. They may support the health instruction program, or they may adversely affect it.

Size of objects and use of color and movement in instructional materials may aid in attracting attention and developing interest in learning. The principle concerning size, color, and movement emphasizes the importance of using a variety of teaching aids in the health instruction program. These materials aid in gaining attention, increasing interest, and helping make teaching more effective, therefore making learning more concrete and specific.

The use of a variety of films, filmstrips, tape recorders, cassettes, CDs, TV/Cable TV and radio programs, computer programs, videos, exhibits, flannelboards, magnetic boards, objects, specimens, graphs, and charts will stimulate interest in the learning experiences provided by the teacher.

Models of the human torso, heart, eyes, ears, and teeth serve as valuable teaching tools. Exhibits of the contents of first-aid kits or the hazardous objects found in the home help to create interest in the area of safety. Use of food models and flannelboards will increase attention when nutrition is being taught.

Chapter 13 provides detailed information about teaching aids usable in the health instruction program.

Extrinsic motivation is less effective than intrinsic motivation. Should children engage in good health habits because of some material reward they will receive or because of the inherent values of the practices performed? Should teachers award gold stars to children who come to school with tissues, when they have brushed their teeth, and for other such reasons? Is it advisable to present a special scroll to classrooms that report 100% attendance of their pupils? Should pupils receive candy or toys as rewards for visits to dentists or physicians? The external stimuli described may encourage the health action desired, but the results usually are temporary. Also, learning may be interfered with because the reward becomes the motivation. The procedures described are questionable because:

- Some parents do not give their children tissues to bring to school.
- Some parents do not buy toothbrushes for their children nor do they take their children to physicians.
- Pupils not able to have tissues or brush their teeth may be embarrassed when special focus on these practices occurs in class. The mental health implications may be of greater importance than the rewards themselves.
- When children come to school who are ill, they may infect others.

Many educators believe that the best motivation is self-motivation. Teachers should motivate children to good health practices through the use of meaningful experiences and other approaches that develop intrinsic values for good health rather than through the use of artificial stimuli. This kind of health teaching will more likely produce the lasting behaviors desired. Further illustrations of this point will be found in other principles of learning.

Moderate tension facilitates learning, but severe tension may inhibit learning. Individuals generally perform better under some tension. However, the degree of pressure that pupils can handle is an individual matter. Teachers often question the degree to which they should pressure children into desirable health behaviors and practices. The illustrations that follow provide examples that give some guidance.

The cause of a child's dislike for or never having tried celery and carrot sticks may be related to some unpleasant home experience involving pressure or punishment. This same pupil, however, is more likely to try these foods in the classroom during a tasting party where the pressures of group approval are not quite as severe and there is an accompanying pleasant experience.

The teacher who is consistently sarcastic, rude, and unfair, who expects absolute quiet at all times, or who seldom has a sense of humor or permits pupil planning, participation, or decisions in the classroom undoubtedly provides a mental health environment that is less conducive to learning. However, the teacher who is generally courteous and fair and who frequently uses democratic procedures in class presents a more permissive atmosphere that will provide a better balance of tension that will facilitate learning.

The fear approach in health education, in which the teacher exhorts and admonishes children by saying, "If you don't do this, here's what will happen," may create tensions that will inhibit the acquisition of the desired health behaviors. The teacher who strongly urges tetanus shots following a deep puncture wound caused by a nail or knife, because failure to do so will cause a serious infection that may require surgery, may create considerable fear resulting in students' refusal to receive such injections. Although children may be afraid of having a needle injected into the skin, they are more likely to obtain injections if they understand their nature, value, and the minimal pain involved when administered.

Learning is generally greater when praise is used more often than blame or reproof, when success occurs more often than failure. Success and praise reinforce learning, but constant frustration and failure adversely affect learning. The importance of the application of this statement to the mental health of children is extremely significant for classroom teachers. It emphasizes the need for teachers to recognize improvement based on individual standards rather than on general levels of achievement. Pupils with poor vision, defective hearing, or other physical ailments may need special praise or opportunities for success experiences in the classroom or on the playground. The balance between success and failure differs with individuals.

Achievement standards should be individual. From a mental health viewpoint, the expectation level of children toward the health goals established should be consistent with their powers of accomplishment. A few specific illustrations of the application of this principle to a behavior-centered health education program include the following:

- Children's needs for amount of sleep may vary
- The brushing of teeth after meals may not be possible in homes that do not provide toothbrushes or dentifrices

- Some children may be allergic or diabetic and should not be expected to drink milk or eat all the foods prepared by the cafeteria at lunch

Knowledge of results is a strong incentive to learning. The principle of knowledge as a strong incentive to learning refers to evaluation of the instructional program in terms of the achievement of the health education goals discussed earlier. Teachers as well as pupils want to know whether they are progressing toward the attainment of these purposes. They will want to know whether the practices, attitudes, and knowledge of healthful living have been acquired. This assessment of learning serves as a stimulus as well as an aid in redirecting the learning when necessary. Through the use of paper and pencil tests, demonstrations, observations, surveys, and other such techniques, some of the following questions may be answered:

- Are children receiving the appropriate immunizations?
- Do children know what to do when injured or ill at school?
- Can children identify hazardous play areas?
- Do children know how to administer simple first aid?
- Are children getting adequate sleep, rest, and exercise?

A more complete discussion of evaluation can be found in Chapter 14.

Summary of Motivation

Awareness and use of the principles and subprinciples of motivation identified in this chapter will help children to behave in a healthful manner. Teachers should use the principles of learning to help children (1) understand the probability of, seriousness of, and benefits or courses of action open to deal with a health problem; (2) resolve conflicts of health action; (3) realize that health-related motives may lead to unrelated health behavior and behavior that appears to be health-related may be unrelated to health; (4) appreciate that fear may lead to both rational and irrational

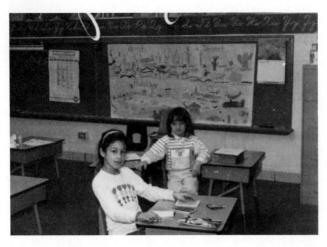

FIG. 9-3 Readiness can affect learning. (Courtesy Galeton Area School District, Galeton, Pennsylvania.)

behavior; and (5) understand the benefits and dangers of risk behavior.

The following subprinciples of learning should be guidelines for selecting health teaching methods to be used in health instruction: (1) cultural and social factors may be barriers to learning, (2) attractive and appealing teaching aids help with attention and interest, (3) intrinsic motivation is more lasting than extrinsic motivation, (4) moderate tension and the use of praise more often than blame is advisable, and (5) achievement standards should be based on individual needs (based on periodic assessment) to stimulate learning.

The principles for learning that come next are all related to the concept of motivation previously discussed. They should be considered as additional ways to stimulate learning. They are essential guidelines for effective health education.

Maturation and Readiness of the Child Affect Learning

Heredity, or the genetic makeup of the pupil, sets the limits of learning for that individual by determining the individual's native intelligence and other capacities as well as his or her physical and mental disabilities. However, maturation, or the physiological growth and development of the pupil, is also a determining factor whether the pupil is mentally, physically, socially, or emotionally ready to learn. It provides useful information when determining grade placement of content in curriculum development and helps to determine a state of readiness important in health education as well as in all learning (Fig. 9-3). The following illustrations offer applications of this principle to learning.

In dental health, 6- and 7-year-old children may have difficulty learning proper toothbrushing techniques. The coordination involved requires use of the small muscles of the fingers and hands, and pupils may not be ready to learn this difficult procedure as completely or as accurately as desired. Although the brush is a fairly large implement, expertness of performance will take time and may be delayed until the child physically matures. Nevertheless, the brushing habit needs to be started early, and teachers should introduce this motor skill in school.

In the area of safety, children may not be ready to learn to manipulate sharp-pointed implements, use apparatus safely, operate bicycles safely, or perform other motor skills. Teachers need to be aware of these pupil limitations in their educational programs.

Taking heights and weights in school is a time when pupils are ready to learn about their individual physical and emotional growth patterns. Pupils will be able to better understand their hereditary limitations in weight, height, size, and shape at this time.

The menstrual process generally begins in girls in the fifth and sixth grades, and an educational program is appropriate when this growth change appears.

Adolescence is a time when students are interested in the growth changes taking place in their bodies. Youths are under peer pressure to engage in the use of alcohol, tobacco, and other drugs, and in sexual activity.

In the early grades, especially, pupils are not completely ready to learn to be social individuals. However, it becomes necessary for children to learn to get along with others, respect authority, and cooperate in school if they are to grow into emotionally healthy individuals (see also Appendix K).

Experiences and the Environment Affect Learning

Despite the variety of health behaviors that children bring to school, provisions must be made for learning experiences and environmental conditions that are conducive to good health. Teachers and other personnel have responsibilities to control the daily activities and conditions under which pupils learn. Some of the health experiences and conditions that should be included are the following:

- The curriculum should provide opportunities for children to learn how to live healthfully and safely.
- Nutritious snacktime foods should be sold at lunchtime or used at parties and social gatherings, rather than the frequent use of candy and cakes. Excessive soft drinks may not be conducive to good nutrition and dental health.
- Provision of a nutritionally sound hot lunch at noon may help develop good habits.

- Playgrounds, classrooms, halls, and other places should be free of hazardous conditions and should be safe areas for learning.
- Classrooms, halls, and playgrounds should be maintained in a neat, clean, and sanitary fashion.
- Lavatories should provide soap and water for use when necessary.
- Teachers and staff should be free of communicable diseases and should be in good physical and mental health.
- Adequate lighting, heating, and ventilation should be provided.
- A friendly, supportive, and democratic atmosphere in the classroom and the school will result in greater learning than an autocratic atmosphere where discipline is severe or nonexistent.
- Assistance and support of adolescents regarding such matters as nutrition, nonuse of alcohol, tobacco, and other drugs, and safety should be provided.
- The learning environment and the academic achievement of students should be improved as a logical violence prevention strategy.
- The hours schools are open should be expanded to offer students a safer haven and an alternative to violent streets.

Guidance Is Necessary for the Most Effective Learning

Health instruction must be a part of the school curriculum if the greatest health learning is to occur. A comprehensive health education program is necessary if children are to learn to play fairly and get along with others, understand fears, know how to prevent and control diseases, know what to do when injured, realize the importance of adequate sleep and rest, and follow numerous other health practices and attitudes. Inclusion of this program means that schools must make teachers available to teach the subject area and must also provide materials that will enable them to carry out this teaching responsibility. These items should include teachers' guides or units that have been developed around pupils' health problems and needs as well as a variety of teaching aids and materials.

Teachers help children in the health instruction program by motivating them to learn, selecting the goals to be achieved, determining the content to teach, and choosing and arranging the experience or activities to be used. Teachers help them learn to wash their hands properly, brush their teeth properly, assume responsibilities, have successful experiences, and ride bicycles safely by using a variety of experiences and techniques including dramatizations, demonstrations, experiments, and discussions. The teacher facilitates learning by providing motivation, distributing the learning at appropriate intervals, and organizing the learning process. Use of the learning principles found in this chapter will aid in this organization process.

Parental guidance is necessary in the development of all student health behavior but especially in behavior regarding smoking, drinking, and use of other drugs. Parents can help pupils in their decisions regarding the use of such substances. Newman and Ward* stated that parental attitudes in which parents clearly express their opposition to risky behaviors such as cigarette smoking should be encouraged.

Learning Is a Self-Active Process

The behavior-centered emphasis of health education makes the active participation of the learner particularly important and appropriate. Merely telling pupils "you should eat the proper foods," "you should take the safest route home," or "you should play fairly" will not achieve the desired health behaviors. Bridging the gap between knowledge and practices is more likely to come through pupil participation and attitude involvement. Children must feel, see, discuss, act out, ma-

nipulate, and even taste things if the attitudes that affect good health practices are to be developed. The teacher has the important role of determining the nature of the experiences to be used in the learning process. *Whenever possible, children should have two, three, or more of their senses involved in learning.* It is believed that the greater the pupil participation, the greater will be the possibility of developing the appropriate behaviors (Fig. 9-4).

To illustrate the application of this principle, the following specific activities are recommended:

- Have children learn about good snacktime foods by conducting a tasting party in which they eat appropriate nutritious foods.
- Have children learn the proper way to brush their teeth by actually performing the exact

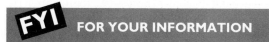
FYI   FOR YOUR INFORMATION

Cooperative Learning Ideas

Numbered Heads Together	Questions are posed by teacher. Students consult on answer in small groups, and one student in the group responds when called by teacher.
Think-Pair-Share	Students think to themselves on a question or issue raised by teacher. Student discusses thoughts with a partner. The pair then shares thoughts with class.
Roundtable	Each student, in turn, writes one answer on a piece of paper passed around the group regarding a question or issue. Teacher or pupils read group responses followed by discussion.

*Newman IM, Ward JM: The influence of parental attitude and behavior on early adolescent cigarette smoking, *J School Health* 59:150-152, 1989.

From Cinelli B et al: Applying cooperative learning, *J School Health*, 64:99-102, 1994.

Fluoridation: friends and foes

Can the Mind Help Cure Disease?

Crack Smoking Seen as a Peril to Lungs

Health Claims:
Separating Fact From Fiction

The Dark Side of Worshiping the Sun

Pot smokers may be high cancer risks

THESE SHOES ARE MADE FOR WALKING

Cigarette makers are assailed for targeting the young

EATING GOES BACK TO BASICS

FIG. 9-4 Learning is a self-active process—students prepare a bulletin board of current newspaper/magazine articles with topical headings: "What's in Health News." Students can be prepared to briefly summarize the article they post in class.

procedure in class. Merely demonstrating this technique will not be satisfactory.

- Have children make a survey of the unsafe conditions in the school and help develop solutions for their elimination.
- Take the class on a field trip and actually follow the safest way to the home of one class member.
- Teach fair play, honesty, getting along with others, or waiting turns by including these values in a softball game, a tag game, or as part of apparatus play.
- Have pupils collect and analyze a variety of advertisements relating to health products.
- Use peer leaders to help with drug abuse prevention.
- Use cooperative learning procedures in the instructional program.

Most Effective Learning Occurs When There Are Good Personal Relationships between the Pupil and the Teacher

The dominant factor in any learning situation is the combination of personal and social relationships that exist between the pupils and the teacher in the classroom. Learning should take place in a democratic setting with the opportunity for free expression and participation by all children. Consideration must be given to the fair, just, and humane treatment of all pupils, regardless of race or ethnic background. The school and classroom should provide a warm, comfortable, and friendly environment. The teacher should be understanding and permissive but must also provide guidance and security. The emotional climate that pervades a school is extremely important to the effectiveness of the learning process.

Teachers should realize that their personal values, beliefs, prejudices, enthusiasms, and perceptions of health are brought to the classroom. They may affect the human relationship if they conflict with their pupils, peer groups, or families. They may influence the health behavior of children in a way that is contrary to best practice. Illustrations of these differences include:

- Cleanliness and appropriate clothing
- Amount of sugar consumed and significance to dental health
- Appropriate foods for parties and snack times
- Food faddism—use of vitamins and other food supplements
- Food aversions—spinach, milk, liver
- Fluoridation of the water supply
- Use of alcohol and tobacco
- Exercise and play
- Choice of medical practitioner or health adviser

Teachers who make conscious efforts to avoid permitting their prejudices to influence pupils' health and who are willing to objectively permit children to look at scientific evidence do not necessarily have to compromise their own beliefs and values. This approach should enable teachers to maintain the good relations previously established.

Much Learning Is Soon Forgotten and Only a Fraction of What Was Once Learned Is Ultimately Remembered

Studies reveal the greatest forgetting by pupils occurs when emphasis in learning is placed on the recall of factual material; evidence shows that meaningful information related to attitudes and practices is more easily learned and is remembered more completely and for longer periods of time. Understanding and knowledge should be provided in a context other than that of unrelated, isolated, factual information. Mere memorization or regurgitation of the names of the teeth, the process of the digestion of foods, or the body systems will not be remembered unless the facts are more closely associated with the attitudes and habits of healthful living. Lessons should lead to the acquisition of big ideas or generalizations, to concepts of health (see Chapter 11 and Appendix B). They should also address student problems and needs.

This principle emphasizes the need to stress the psychological approach over the logical or structure-and-function approach to teaching. It indicates the importance of the greater use of problem solving in helping students make intelligent decisions in the health instruction program. It demonstrates the importance of learning centered around health needs and problems of pupils. Here are several illustrations to demonstrate this principle:

- Pupils' appreciation of the possible hazards of using tobacco and other drugs must be more meaningfully related to the ingredients in tobacco and various drugs. Pupils must feel that these substances may affect their performances in athletics, in recreation, and in school as well as their growth and health. Teachers should explore with students the "why" of tobacco and other drug use, including peer pressure and the need for acceptance. Pupils should learn the strategies needed to "say no" to the use of substances.
- Students will be able to understand and resist advertising pressure for health products they use after learning how to analyze ads.
- Pupils' appreciation for eating proper foods and a balanced diet will be increased when information is related to their own "snack-time" and "mealtime" food and to the school lunch program.

Well-Organized, Meaningful Material Is More Easily Learned and Remembered Longer Than Meaningless or Nonsense Material

The content of the health education program should be based on the needs and interests of pupils if it is to be meaningful. Various studies indicate the following areas are representative of these needs and interests: cleanliness and grooming; community health; consumer health; dental health; control and prevention of disease; care of the eyes, ears, and feet; exercise and fitness; family health; growth and development; mental health; nutrition; rest, sleep, and fatigue; safety; and alcohol, tobacco, and drugs. Learning that is organized around these areas will result in the most effective health behaviors.

Schools should have teacher guides for health education that contain units of instruction focused around the health areas identified in the previous paragraph. These manuals should define the learning that should take place at the various grade levels. They should provide a grade level sequence of learning that avoids excessive overlapping and duplication of content.

Teachers should capitalize on incidents that occur at school or in the home and use these "teachable moments" (see Chapter 12) in their instruction programs, thus making health education practical as well as functional. Such incidents as the following are usable:

- The class is going to use the playground apparatus
- The nurse is coming to do the vision screening
- Fire Prevention Week is emphasized in the community
- A child reports a visit to the dentist
- Children wash their hands before lunch and after going to the lavatory

Ability to Solve Problems, to Reason, to Make Intelligent Decisions, and to Do Reflective Thinking Involves Training and Must Be Learned

The ability to solve problems and to make intelligent decisions must be learned. Elias and Kress[*] claim children need to learn "life's skills" (reasoned disagreement, negotiation, compromise) to be able to solve problems, to be able to think clearly.

Children should be taught how to think rather than what to think. Wasserman[†] states that factual information has little influence on critical think-

---

[*]Elias MJ, Kress JS: Social decision-making and life skills development, *J School Health* 64:62-66, 1994.
[†]Wasserman S: Teaching for thinking: Louis E. Raths revisited, *Phi Delta Kappan* 68:460-465, 1987.

ing. Learning should include such goals as comparing, interpreting, observing, summarizing, classifying, suggesting, hypothesizing, inquiring, creating, criticizing and evaluating, and investigating. Learning should include activities such as role-playing, cooperative learning, brainstorming, class discussions, and small group participation.

Duryea* identified these steps in decision making (problem solving): (1) appraise the challenge (review of problem), (2) survey alternatives, (3) weigh alternatives (advantages/disadvantages), and (4) determine commitment (select alternative). The decision then needs to be implemented and evaluated.

The many quacks, charlatans, and pseudomedical people who live in our communities, together with the millions of dollars spent yearly on unnecessary drugs, vitamins, patent medicines, and many other health products and services, make it necessary that children begin to be able to do reflective thinking in health as they do in other phases of learning. Children and adults need to know whether the health information they are hearing is valid and to know what are reliable sources of health facts.

Illustrations of problems that teachers may use for children to solve may include the following:

- What should you do when you are injured?
- What should you do when you are ill?
- Who can help you when you are ill or injured?
- How can you make friends?
- What kinds of clothing should you wear to protect your body?
- How does the health department protect the health of the people?
- Should we believe what we read and hear about health products?
- What hazards in the home may cause accidents?
- Where can you get help if you have a sexually transmitted disease?

---

*Duryea EJ: Decision making and health education, *J School Health* 53:29-30, 1983.

- How can we analyze the newspaper and TV advertisements for health products we use?
- How can you learn to say "no" to peer pressure regarding alcohol, tobacco, and other drugs?
- How can you resolve a conflict without using violence?

Learning Process Must Specifically Include Teaching for Transfer of Training or Learning if This Transfer Is to Occur

Health knowledge that carries over into or transfers to pupil activities outside of school and into the home is the most significant kind of learning. This unobserved health behavior is difficult to assess and to achieve. Transfer does not happen by chance but rather by design. Teachers must include teaching for carryover in their planning if school health activities are to occur in the home and community.

The most effective transfer of learning happens when the learning in school is as near real-life situations as possible. Learning, therefore, must be lifelike to obtain the greatest transfer.

When teaching pupils about safety at street corners, it may be necessary either to go to the corner itself and perform the safe behavior or to simulate a street corner on the school grounds using traffic lights, small cars, and other props with the children participating in a role-playing activity.

To obtain the greatest safety in the home, it may be necessary for children to survey the hazards therein with their parents and mutually suggest ways to reduce or remove these hazards.

To expect children to eat balanced meals at home, it may be advisable to provide such meals in school at noontime.

To expect children to reduce their consumption of sugars and sweets, it will be necessary to curtail, or remove, their availability at lunchtime, at snacktime, during parties, and during other social occasions in school. However, some health educators believe that foods containing sugars should be available but controlled as an educational means of teaching children their proper use.

Parental involvement in the identification of two ways to leave the house when a fire occurs should be part of home fire safety. To expect students to resist peer pressures regarding the use of drugs, strategies that identify and resist social pressures must be provided and must have parent and community support.

Use of Repetition and Reinforcement Is Necessary in Learning

Health learnings must be repeated and reinforced if they are to have the greatest effect on the health behavior of individuals and if they are to be useful in the daily lives of children. A brief exposure in a classroom, or elsewhere, to a discussion, demonstration, or report on the safest way home from school, the safe way to act on the bus, the use of hand signals when riding a bicycle, the importance of eating the proper foods, the hazards of smoking, what to do when someone is injured, or the proper way to brush teeth does not ensure that these actions will be followed consistently for any length of time. Activities used to achieve health and safety objectives must be used on several occasions either during the unit, during the semester, or during the entire school year. They must be repeated for reinforcement at appropriate grade-level intervals through all the years pupils are in school. Where skills such as proper toothbrushing and first-aid and safety procedures are involved, repetitive practice becomes necessary for reinforcement. These skills must be transferred to the home and community for effective health education. Bruvold* reported that a meta-analysis study of 94 adolescent smoking prevention programs indicated the greatest behavioral effect occurred through interventions involving social reinforcement orientation, recognition of social pressures, developing skills to resist tobacco use, and social and physical consequences of smoking.

In psychological terms, this type of learning is often referred to as spaced learning—a repetition of what has been taught after intervals of time have elapsed. These time intervals may occur during or at the end of a lesson, in the middle or end of a unit, during the semester, or there might be longer spacing. To illustrate, when teaching the proper technique for brushing the teeth during a unit on dental health, a demonstration of the correct procedure might have to be made again during the lesson and be followed by the pupils actually performing the correct technique. The entire sequence, or some modification, may have to be repeated one time or more during the unit and possibly reviewed during the semester. Had this learning occurred in the first or second grade, it may be advisable and necessary to repeat or reinforce it in the third or fourth grades and possibly again in the fifth, sixth, or seventh grades. In a comprehensive health education curriculum this procedure is referred to as cycling—sequential placement of specific health areas at a variety of grades throughout the school years. The failure of schools to achieve their objectives in numerous preventive programs undoubtedly is correlated with the nature and frequency of the repetition of learning.

The nature, extent, and degree of repetition will vary and depends on any or all of the following:

- The desired health behaviors to be achieved
- The individual differences in pupils' ability to learn
- The nature and frequency of the reinforcement procedures
- The grade level and sequential curriculum patterns
- Parent and community support and assistance
- The health values pupils bring to schools

SUMMARY

Learning is a complex process that must be internalized by pupils and is influenced by external experiences. How children learn is not clear, but it is clear that pupils learn when teachers motivate

---

*Bruvold WH: A meta-analysis of adolescent smoking prevention programs, *Am J Public Health* 83:872-880, 1993.

TABLE 9-2 Principles of Learning and Their Reference to Text Information

Principles	Text references by chapter
Motivation	
Principles	
Preventive action threatening	1 - Prevention
	8 - Gullible public, health misconceptions, health information conflict, media influence, peer pressure
Conflict in beliefs	1 - What is health? Factors influencing pupil health
	2 - Controversial areas
	8 - Controversial areas, lifestyle
	11 - Values
Health-related motives, unrelated behavior, etc.	1 - Social and lifestyle-related problems
Fear: rational/irrational behavior	8 - Prevent action, peer pressure
Risk taking	1 - Social and lifestyle-related problems
	8 - Controversial areas, peer/adult pressure
Subprinciples	
Cultural/social factors	1 - What is health? Factors influencing pupil health, social and lifestyle-related problems
	2 - Controversial areas
	8 - Lifestyle and disease, peer/adult pressure, media influence, selfcare. Why health education?
	11 - Values
	12 - Incidents as methods
Size of objects, etc.	13 - Instructional aids (see Appendixes D, E, F, and H)
Extrinsic/intrinsic	8 - Why health education?
	12 - Methods and techniques
Moderate tension	11 - Taxonomy of objectives, units (objectives)
	12 - Methods and techniques
Praise/blame	12 - Methods and techniques
	14 - Evaluation (see also Good personal relations)
Individual achievement	2 - Individual differences
	6 - Guidance, adjustment of program
	12 - Methods and techniques
	13 - Instructional aids
Knowledge of results	14 - Evaluation
Maturation/readiness	1 - Health problems of children
	5 - Appraisals—growth and development characteristics
	11 - Interest/needs of students, values
	12 - Incidents as methods
Experiences/environment	3 - Environment—physical aspects
	4 - Emotional climate
	5 - Emergency care
	8 - Role of community
	11 - Values; Why health education?
Guidance	2 - Individual differences
	6 - Guidance/counseling
	8 - Patterns of instruction, grade placement, time, concepts

TABLE 9-2 Principles of Learning and Their Reference to Text Information—cont'd

Principles	Text references by chapter
	10 - Health education approaches
	11 - Taxonomy of objectives, unit teaching, lesson planning, scope and sequence
Self-active process	12 - Methods and techniques
	13 - Instructional aids (see also Appendixes D, E, F, and H)
Good personal relations	2 - Health of personnel
	3 - Environment—physical aspects
	4 - Emotional climate (see also Guidance)
Much learning soon forgotten	11 - Taxonomy of objectives
	12 - Methods and techniques
	13 - Instructional aids
Well organized/meaningful	1 - What is school health? What is health?
	10 - Health education approaches
	11 - Scope and sequence, unit teaching, lesson plans
	12 - Incidents as methods (see also all other principles)
Problem solving (decision making)	11 - Needs/interests of pupils
	12 - Methods and techniques
	13 - Instructional aids
	9 - Units, lesson plans (see also all other principles)
Transfer of training	11 - Needs/interests of pupils (see also all other principles)
Repetition/reinforcement	11 - Scope and sequence, units, lesson planning
	12 - Methods and techniques
	14 - Evaluation (see also Guidance, and Well organized/meaningfulness)

students, select the appropriate goals related to pupils' needs and problems, and choose activities and experiences that will enable pupils to live in a healthful manner. This learning must involve more than the provision of health knowledge. Bridging the gap between health practices and health knowledge probably occurs through the development of favorable attitudes. However, some practices may be learned without attitudinal involvement. The variety of principles of learning described in the text will be helpful to teachers when planning and teaching health education. They are of special use in the selection of teaching methods and activities. Application of the learning principles to the information found in this text is presented in Table 9-2. The principles of learning also have specific use in the development of the health education curriculum.

QUESTIONS FOR DISCUSSION

1. What are the factors that influence the establishment of human health behaviors?
2. What is learning and how is it believed that children learn?
3. How does the concept approach relate to health?
4. What are the basic goals of health education? What are their relationships to learning? Illustrate.
5. What are the differences and relationships between the objectives, practices, and skills? Illustrate their application to health education.
6. What is the hierarchy of attitudes and its relationship to learning about health?
7. What is meant by the term *teaching for decision making*? Illustrate its application to health education.

8. How can teachers relate knowledge to behavior in health education?
9. What is meant by "bridging the gap" between health knowledge and health behavior?
10. Why are the principles of learning important in health teaching?
11. What are the principles of learning that will help the teacher in the health instruction program? Provide illustrations of the application of each principle to several content areas in health education.
12. What are the principles of motivation that have an effect on learning in health education?
13. Why are good teacher/student relationships important and necessary for effective health teaching?
14. What are several illustrations of ways the teacher can make health learning a self-active process?
15. What is the significance of fear and risk taking in behavior modification in health education?
16. What is the meaning of "spaced learning?" Illustrate its application to health education.

SELECTED REFERENCES

Bosworth K, Sailes J: Content and teaching strategies in 10 selected drug abuse prevention curricula, *J School Health* 63:247-253, 1993.

Botvin GJ: Substance abuse prevention research: recent developments and future directions, *J School Health* 56:369-374, 1986.

Brubaker RG, Loften TL: Smokeless tobacco use by middle school males: a preliminary test of the reasoned action theory, *J School Health* 57:64-67, 1987.

Bruvold WH: A meta-analysis of adolescent smoking prevention programs, *Am J Public Health* 83:872-880, 1993.

Cinelli B et al: Applying cooperative learning in health education practice, *J School Health* 64:99-102, 1994.

Clarke KS: Values and risk-taking behavior; the concept of calculated risk, *Health Ed* 6: November/December, 1975.

Crocket SJ et al: Parent nutrition education: a conceptual model, *J School Health* 58:53-57, 1988.

Duryea EJ: Decision making and health education, *J School Health* 53:29-30, 1983.

Elias MJ, Kress JS: Social decision-making and life skills development: a critical approach to health promotion in the middle school, *J School Health* 64:62-66, 1994.

Ellickson PL et al: Preventing adolescent drug use: long-term results of a junior high program, *Am J Public Health* 83:856-861, 1993.

Engs RC, Fors SW: Drug abuse hysteria: the challenge of keeping perspective, *J School Health* 58:26-28, 1988.

Galli N et al: Health education and sensitivity to cultural, religious and ethnic beliefs, *J School Health* 57:177-180, 1987.

Gilchrist LD et al: The relationship of cognitive and behavioral skills to adolescent tobacco smoking, *J School Health* 55:132-134, 1985.

Hochbaum G: *Research in behavioral sciences.* Presented at the Regional Institute on the Science of Health Education at the University of California at Los Angeles, June 12-14, 1961.

Hochbaum G: Learning and behavior: alcohol education for what? *Alcohol Education Conference Proceedings,* March 1966, US Department of Health, Education, and Welfare.

Hochbaum G: *Effecting health behavior.* Presented at the annual meeting of the New York State Public Health Association, Buffalo, May 23, 1967.

Hochbaum G: How we can teach adolescents about smoking, drinking, and drug abuse? *J Health, Physical Ed, Recrea* 39:October, 1968.

Hochbaum G: Changing health behavior in youth, *School Health, Rev* September, 1969.

Hochbaum G: *Health behavior,* Belmont, Calif, 1970, Wadsworth.

Hochbaum G: Human behavior and nutrition education, *Nutrition News* 40:February, 1977.

Hochbaum G: Should health behavior change be the objective of health education? *J School Health* 51:379-380, 1981.

Hovell MF et al: Modification of student snacking: comparison of behavioral teaching methods, *Health Ed* 19:26-33, 1988.

Kirby D: School-based programs to reduce risk-taking behavior, *J School Health* 62:280-287, 1992.

Klepp K et al: The efficacy of peer leaders in drug abuse prevention, *J School Health* 56:407-411, 1986.

Lapp CC: (Nearly) total recall, *Stanford* 20:48-51, 1992.

Lawrence L, McLeroy KR: Self-efficacy and health education, *J School Health* 56:317-322, 1986.

Lewis CE, Lewis MA: Peer pressure and risk-taking behaviors in children, *Am J Public Health* 74:580-584, 1984.

Motivations, practical applications of research, *Newsletter, Phi Delta Kappa's Center on Evaluation, Development, and Research,* 5:1-3 September, 1982.

Newman IM, Ward JM: The influence of parental attitude and behavior on early adolescent cigarette smoking, *J School Health* 59:150-152, 1989.

Petosa R: Enhancing the health competency of school-age children through behavioral self-management skills, *J School Health* 56:211-214, 1986.

Preventing substance abuse: rethinking strategies, *Am J Public Health* 83:793-795, 1993.

Protheow-Stith D: Setting sights on violence, *America's Agenda* 4:42-49, 1994.

Susser M, editor: Editorial: the tribulations of trials—intervention in communities, *Am J Public Health* 85:156-158, 1995.

Van Reek J et al: The influence of peers and parents on the smoking behavior of schoolchildren, *J School Health* 57:30, 1987.

Wasserman, S: Teaching for thinking: Louis E. Raths revisited, *Phi Delta Kappan* 68:460-465, 1987.

10

Health Education Approaches

KEY CONCEPT

Despite the varying approaches used in the development of school health education programs, effective comprehensive health education curricula need to be constructed that use a sound and consistent educational philosophy.

Health education works; it works better when there's more of it; and it works best when it is implemented with broad-scale administrative and pedagogic support for teacher training, integrated materials, and continuity across grades.

SCHOOL HEALTH EDUCATION ADVISORY PANEL
NATIONAL SCHOOL HEALTH EDUCATION EVALUATION STUDY

PROBLEM TO SOLVE

You have been placed on a school district subcommittee to study and make recommendations about the inclusion of a comprehensive elementary school health education program in the district where you work. Identify several illustrative, reportedly useful, and effective programs that will help in the preparation of your recommendations.

SELECTED CURRICULA IN ELEMENTARY SCHOOL HEALTH EDUCATION

Many elementary school health education programs in the United States have been developed by health education and curriculum specialists, voluntary health agencies, state departments of education, and commercial companies without the use of a consistent procedure or educationally sound philosophy. Few individuals, including health educators, understand completely the process of curriculum development; know how to prepare functional programs using pupils, teachers, and community resources; have been engaged in successful experiences in terms of completion and implementation; or have been able to assess the effectiveness of their programs. Often programs and curricula have been prepared based on what others have done without adequate consideration of the quality or the nature of their impact on children. A basic set of principles and procedures that are universally acceptable or that can be generally implemented by professionals has not emerged. The development of health education curricula cannot take place without such guidelines. The first major organized effort in this regard that used talented health education experts occurred in the 1960s in the School Health Education Study (SHES) project directed by Dr. Elena Sliepcevich. Since that time numerous curricula have been prepared at national, state, and local levels. These curricula have been found useful, have gained popularity, and show promise of fulfilling the basic principles for development found in Chapter 11.

The purpose of this chapter is to provide illustrations of selected programs that could be reviewed by districts planning to develop health education programs. The resources provided should encourage the examination of additional curricula before the adoption of a particular one.

Numerous approaches to curriculum development have been used, and many programs are available. Each program must be reviewed in terms of its particular strengths and weaknesses. Schools wishing to introduce a health education curriculum should peruse other successful programs to be certain they are sufficiently flexible to meet local student and community needs and interests as well as the legal mandates of the state. Adaptation of a program that has proved to be successful is one way school districts can begin to develop health education curricula. One way to begin is to become familiar with the National Diffusion Network, a federal dissemination system specifically designed to assist schools in locating exemplary programs in all areas of curriculum, including health instruction.

NATIONAL DIFFUSION NETWORK

The National Diffusion Network (NDN) is a federally funded system that makes exemplary and proved educational programs available for adoption by schools, colleges, and other institutions. Formed in 1973 under the Elementary and Secondary Education Act (ESEA) of 1965, the NDN has become the nation's primary means of sharing proved educational programs.

Whereas many locally developed programs are extremely successful in helping children learn, few of these projects have been used away from the sites where they were first developed. Because of this, a need exists for a nationwide means of disseminating information about the programs. The NDN was formed in response to the desire of Congress to formulate such a dissemination system.

The basic purpose of the NDN is to offer local schools the chance to adopt high-quality, cost-effective education projects that have been developed by classroom teachers.

The goals of the NDN are as follows:

- To stimulate positive educational change in local schools
- To help parents, teachers, and administrators find programs for children that match local needs
- To move programs quickly and cost effectively to classrooms nationwide

- To help public and private schools secure information about new programs and support for their implementation in the district
- To ensure that nationwide communication about these programs continues among local school districts, intermediate service agencies, and state departments of education

By achieving these goals, the NDN supports the flow of new ideas and increases the impact of educational investments that have already been made.*

The NDN can provide limited funds to help create an awareness of exemplary school programs, aid schools with adoption decisions, provide in-service training and follow-up assistance, and in selected instances, purchase teaching aids for classroom use. At present, over 400 exemplary programs are available through the NDN.

What Is an Exemplary Program?

To be considered "exemplary" by the NDN, a program must have proved itself educationally effective for children and be cost-effective with reasonable per pupil cost. If a program developer feels that the program meets these criteria, the developer can submit the program to the NDN for consideration.

The Program Effectiveness Panel

Before being accepted for inclusion as an NDN-approved program, the program is reviewed by the Department of Education's Program Effectiveness Panel (PEP) or Joint Dissemination Review Panel (JDRP). These panels were created specifically to review evidence (generally research) presented by program developers to show that what they developed is effective in attaining the goals set forth for that particular program and that this

---

*The information contained in this section comes in part from: *EPTW Educational Programs That Work,* the catalogue of the National Diffusion Network (NDN), ed 19, Longmont, CO, 1993, Sopris West.

same effectiveness will occur for others in similar educational settings.

Consisting of approximately 50 education and evaluation experts from the U.S. Department of Education and other areas of educational research practice, the JDRP and the PEP convene periodically to review programs that have been nominated as exemplary.

If a project is approved, it becomes eligible for funds either from the NDN or through other federal funding programs. If the program is not approved, the reasons for rejection are explained. In the case of rejection, the project can be revised or new evidence of effectiveness can be prepared and the project resubmitted for consideration at a later date.

An approved program receives several direct benefits including (1) recognition of the program by both professionals and the public through awareness workshops, (2) increased chances for obtaining competitive federal funds, and (3) entry into a federal diffusion system.

NDN State Facilitators

Each state has at least one individual specifically designated as State Facilitator for the NDN. This person is in a key position to aid local school district planners who want to examine a variety of approaches to a given curricular area before the development of a local curriculum. The state facilitator will be able to convene an awareness workshop of proved programs for districts that ask to see exemplary projects available through the NDN. These "showcases" generally prove quite useful because they provide information about a wide range of programs in any given curricular area.

The state facilitator may also help a local school district match its needs with appropriate NDN projects, help develop and plan local workshops, and help search for alternate sources of funding. The state facilitator also has limited funds to support school personnel who wish to visit sites of demonstration projects.

SELECTED ELEMENTARY SCHOOL HEALTH INSTRUCTION PROGRAMS

Presented here are some examples of elementary health education programs available in the United States. This listing is in no way meant to be exhaustive. It should also be pointed out that inclusion of a given program does not suggest endorsement of the program nor does omission of a program suggest rejection. These programs are presented as examples of nationally validated programs (included in the NDN), state-based programs, locally based programs, programs available through various health-related agencies, and commercially prepared programs. Educators interested in evaluating specific elementary health education curricula are urged to seek advice from their respective state department of education, which may be able to provide additional examples of appropriate curricula.

Programs Included in the NDN

In May 1979 the *School Health Curriculum Project* became the first health instruction program to be nationally validated for inclusion in the NDN. One year later, the *Primary Grades Health Curriculum Project*, a companion to the *School Health Curriculum Project*, was also approved for inclusion in the NDN. These two programs subsequently merged to form *Growing Healthy.* This program is the only comprehensive health instruction program currently approved for inclusion in the NDN. Several programs have been approved that emphasize individual subject areas and include content dealing with nutrition, cardiovascular health, fitness, smoking, and alcohol and drug abuse.

Growing Healthy. Originally called the *Berkeley Project* and the *Seattle Project* and subsequently the *School Health Curriculum Project* and the *Primary Grades Health Curriculum Project*, these two companion projects have merged to form *Growing Healthy*, a K through 7 program that is student focused and broad based in scope (Fig. 10-1).

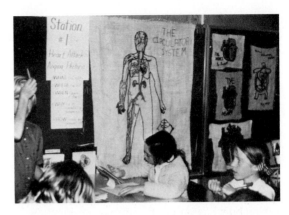

FIG. 10-1 The *Growing Healthy* program in action.

The goals of *Growing Healthy* are to:
- Increase students' knowledge and decision-making abilities about a wide range of behaviors and in a number of health education areas
- Help students learn how their bodies function and how their personal choices affect their health
- Integrate classroom learning with other life situations
- Offer students and teachers an experience-based understanding of the physical, mental, and emotional dimensions of their own health

Designed primarily as a direct method of teaching health, the units of instruction also lend themselves to integration with other elementary school curricular topics. *Growing Healthy* is a broad-based program that includes an intensive 30- to 60-hour teacher-training component; a wide variety of teaching methods; strategies for involving both parents and the community; and a variety of useful teaching aids. It has been called a student-centered, hands-on, multimedia approach to health instruction.

The program content at the various grade levels has been developed around central themes with these titles:
- Kindergarten: Happiness Is Being Healthy
- Grade 1: Super Me

- Grade 2: Sights and Sounds
- Grade 3: The Body: Its Framework and Movement
- Grade 4: About Our Digestion and Our Nutrition
- Grade 5: About Our Lungs and Respiration
- Grade 6: About Our Hearts and Circulation
- Grade 7: Living Well with Our Nervous System

The pattern for health teaching at each grade level follows this organizational sequence: introduction (motivational activities), awareness (body interactions), appreciation (proper function of body parts contribute to well-being), structure and function (in a healthy state), diseases and disorders, prevention, and culmination (overview of learned concepts presented by students at a special parents' night).

Growing Healthy has developed an ongoing program of research to determine its effectiveness. The K through 3 segment of the program has been evaluated in selected demonstration centers across the United States. Reports of this evaluation are available from the American Lung Association.

Have a Healthy Heart (HHH). *Have a Healthy Heart* has been included in the NDN since December 1980. The program was recertified in January 1985. This limited-focus program, designed for grades 4 through 6, deals with cardiovascular health. It was developed in cooperation with sports medicine physicians, cardiologists, biomedical researchers, dietitians, and the American Heart Association's Heart, Health, and the Young Committee. Presented as a supplement to existing programs, this project incorporates an aerobic fitness component designed to be taught 1 to 2 hours per week during a 2- to 3-month period. The basic goal of the program is to help students learn and practice health habits that will help decrease their risk of incurring heart disease.

A one-day workshop for teachers was developed to acquaint them with the philosophy and materials used in the curriculum. The American Heart Association and the American National Red Cross often participate in the workshops and help provide follow-up services for workshop participants.

The classroom implementation phase begins with the administration of a walk-run test and the studying of a fitness booklet developed specifically for the program. Students participate in aerobic exercise 3 times each week for 15 to 20 minutes. At the end of each month, the walk-run test is readministered so students can see the progress they have made relative to cardiovascular fitness. On completion of the fitness booklet, students begin working on a lifestyle booklet that is designed to acquaint them with the cardiovascular risk factors of smoking, overweight, stress, heredity, exercise, cholesterol, hypertension, and the methods they can use to reduce those risk factors in their personal lives.

The results of various evaluations of *Have a Healthy Heart* suggest that student knowledge about cardiovascular risk factors and performance on general fitness tests increase significantly as a result of exposure to the program.

Social Decision Making and Problem Solving. Approved in July 1989 by the PEP, *Social Decision Making and Problem Solving* is a program developed specifically for teachers, administrators, guidance counselors, child study team staff, and parents of elementary students in grades K-6. The purpose of the program is to train educators and parents to help children develop self-control and group participation skills. The focus is to assist children to "think clearly" when they are under pressure. Central to the project is the development of self-control and group participation and social awareness skills, particularly when confronted with potential violence or substance abuse situations. An 8-step decision-making strategy is used to help students apply newly developed skills in real life interpersonal and academic situations.

Specialized training is provided at a cost and is generally limited to no more than 30 people. These teachers generally participate in a 2-day workshop designed to acquaint them with the project goals, objectives, and processes. Districts or buildings are asked to form a Social Decision-Making Committee that assumes a leadership role and oversees the development of the program. The Social Decision-Making Committee generally consists of key teachers, administrators, and specialists, including guidance counselors, drug and alcohol prevention specialists, and those in special education. These individuals undergo one additional day of training so that they can learn how to involve parents in the program, as well as to train them how to serve as resources for teachers who will be implementing the program in classrooms.

Me-Me Drug and Alcohol Prevention Education Program. A limited focus program for grades 1-6 dealing with substance abuse, the *Me-Me Drug and Alcohol Prevention Education Program* was initially approved in May, 1975. Since then, the program has undergone revisions that have made it even more effective.

Over 100 specific activities are included in the program. These activities are designed to complement activities already present in schools that have a comprehensive drug/alcohol education program in place, a requirement for becoming involved in the *Me-Me* program. A 6-hour training component for teachers is provided at a small cost to the district. Central to the program is the parental component, which includes parental feedback and involvement in their child's decision not to use drugs. The central purpose of the program is to help improve students' self-esteem and help them say NO to drugs.

State-Based Programs

A total of 43 states* require some sort of health instruction to be included in the curricula of their schools and an additional 7 states require some combination of health and physical education. Selection of subject matter to be included, however, is an individual school district decision. As such, there is a great deal of latitude in how health education is viewed by school districts. Commonly the teaching of drug, alcohol, and tobacco use and misuse is mandated although for varied amounts

of time (see Chapters 8 and 11). Going beyond merely stating that health education should be taught, most states have developed general guidelines for local school districts to use when developing health education programs. Some states have passed legislation allowing the State Superintendent of Public Instruction to set minimum guidelines for the development of health instruction programs. Some states, such as California, have developed rather detailed frameworks for health instruction. Still other states, such as Michigan, Minnesota, and North Carolina, have drawn from many programs and have developed validation processes for recognizing exemplary programs within the state.

Health Framework for California Public Schools, Kindergarten Through Grade Twelve. Approved in 1994, the *Health Framework** calls on educators, parents, and community members to unite to support the health of young people. The *Framework* was developed as a blueprint for action and undergirds the philosophy that "as a society we are all responsible for supporting the health of young people." The *Framework* is based on the premise "that health literacy is as important in today's complex, challenging world as linguistic, mathematical, and scientific literacy. The goal of the *Framework* is to describe health education and schoolwide health promotion strategies that will help children and youths become health-literate individuals with a lifelong commitment to healthy living." Four unifying themes pervade the *Framework:*

- Acceptance of personal responsibility for lifelong health
- Respect for and promotion of the health of others
- An understanding of the process of growth and development
- Informed use of health-related information, products, and services.

---

*American School Health Association: *School health in America,* ed 5, Kent, OH, 1989, The Association.

*Modified from California State Board of Education; *Health framework for California public schools: kindergarten through grade twelve,* Sacramento, CA, 1994, California Department of Education.

These four themes appear as foci within the *Framework* and are reinforced through various grade-level activities. Throughout the *Framework,* nine basic content areas are emphasized:

- Personal health
- Consumer and community health
- Injury prevention and safety
- Alcohol, tobacco, and other drugs
- Nutrition
- Environmental health
- Family living
- Individual growth and development
- Communicable and chronic diseases

Within each of the content areas, mental and emotional health concepts appear, thus reinforcing the idea that mental and emotional health are an integral part of all aspects of health.

Each of the nine basic content areas is explained and expectations, by grade level and content area, are specified. Within each grade level and content area, examples of skills and behaviors are provided. Specific materials to be used within the *Framework* are not specified, but guidelines that can be used in the selection of materials are included.

Michigan Model. Also called the *Wellness Curriculum, the Michigan Model for Comprehensive School Health Education* represents the efforts of many individuals over more than 10 years. The curriculum is a structured wellness program that brings together state government, schools, community groups, and parents to provide children with the information and skills that they need to make positive and healthy lifestyle decisions (Fig. 10-2).

In the early 1970s the Michigan State Board of Education and State Department of Education developed specific performance objectives to help ensure that students would at least meet minimum competencies within essential educational disciplines. These objectives have been evaluated and revised three times since their initial development in 1976. The most recent revision was in 1991.

In 1980 a position statement regarding comprehensive school health was adopted. Within this document was a definition of school health education that was subsequently adopted by the State Board of Education to avoid fragmentation and misinterpretation by the myriad of agencies within the state that were developing materials to be used within the educational program.

In 1981 the *Comprehensive School Health Plan* was published. This document placed an emphasis on cooperative planning and implementation to attain its goals. At present, the *Michigan Model for Comprehensive School Health Education* is a cooperative effort of seven state agencies.

The curriculum consists of approximately 60 lessons per grade level, K through 6, and approximately 50 lessons per grade level 7 through 8 in 10 broad health education topics. The basic philosophy of the program is to provide a solid foundation for subsequent decision making. Included are safety, nutrition, family health, consumer health, community health, growth and development, substance use and abuse, personal health practices, emotional and mental health, and disease prevention and control.

The model incorporates teacher training as a mandatory component for all teachers who use the curriculum. The teacher training component requires a minimum of 30 hours. Included in this training time is time for making classroom materials. The training is designed to provide teachers who will be implementing the *Michigan Model*

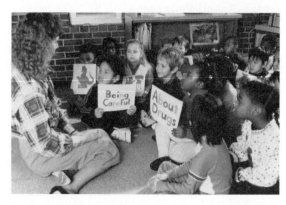

FIG. 10-2 *The Michigan Model.* (Courtesy Michigan Department of Education.)

with the philosophy of the program as well as with information needed to teach the material accurately using appropriate teaching strategies.

Two forms of evaluation are used: a determination of implementation progress and informal surveys within districts that have implemented the model about the attitudes of parents, administrators, and others regarding the value of the program. Currently Michigan State University is conducting a 10-year evaluation of the program to assess the overall impact of the program on selected student populations.

Minnesota School Health Education 110 Program. In Minnesota, health education is required in all grades, K-6, and one or more health education courses (60 clock hours) are required at the middle/junior high level. In an attempt to assist those responsible for planning school health education, The Minnesota Department of Education developed one model that was made available to all schools in the state. Although not specifically mandated, this particular model has been made available on computer disk so that it can be easily accessed by program developers. Based on the *Minnesota Department of Education Health Education Model Learner Outcomes,* the project was initially developed in 1991 and was reviewed by over 700 health teachers, school administrators, and school nurses. The project name, *110 Program,** was based on the development of 110 individual grade and content cells; 10 grade levels (K-6, middle/junior high, and senior high) and eleven content area strands contained within the project. The eleven major content area strands are:

- Prevent tobacco use
- Prevent and control injuries
- Prevent and reduce alcohol and other drug problems
- Improve dietary practices
- Improve health-related physical fitness
- Prevent, reduce risks, and control disease and disorders

- Prevent and reduce sexual health problems
- Improve personal health practices
- Improve social, emotional, and mental health
- Improve family living
- Improve community and environmental health

Within each program goal, by grade level, end products are presented as student competencies. The competencies have been developed both vertically and horizontally. This allows program developers to examine the curriculum by content area across grade levels or by grade level across content areas.

Multiple teaching strategies are referenced for each competency. The final selection of specific goals, instructional methodologies, and resource materials are left to the discretion of each individual school district, thus making the program responsive to local needs.

North Carolina Standard Course of Study for Healthful Living Education. Adopted by the State Board of Education in June, 1993, *Healthful Living Education** incorporates health education and physical education in an integrated manner. The course emphasizes high-risk behaviors and the skills of behavior management, communications, self-esteem building, and resource use. The purpose of the course of study is to provide appropriate instruction so that students can acquire behaviors that contribute to a healthy lifestyle. It is hoped that through implementation of the course, all students will gain information and skills about issues important to their age level and apply these skills to a variety of their own health-related behaviors including:

- Involvement in violent acts
- Consuming excessive fat, calories, and sodium; insufficient fiber, and variety of foods
- Using tobacco
- Engaging in sexual intercourse, which could lead to pregnancy and disease
- Insufficient exercise

---

*Modified from Minnesota Department of Education: *Minnesota School Health Education 110 Program,* Minneapolis, MN, 1992, Minnesota Department of Education.

*Modified from North Carolina Department of Public Instruction: *Standard course of study for healthful living,* Raleigh, NC, 1994, North Carolina Department of Public Instruction.

- Attempting suicide
- Driving while under the influence of alcohol and other drugs, traveling as a passenger with a driver who is under the influence, driving too fast, and not using passenger restraints or bicycle helmets
- Injecting drugs
- Engaging in water-related recreation without appropriate flotation devices or supervision, or without skill in swimming and staying afloat, or while using alcohol or other drugs

Skill development occurs both through the study of the skills and through application of the skills to personal health issues and behaviors. The specific *Healthful Living Education* skills areas include:

I. Self-esteem building
   A. Self-perception
   B. Self-acceptance
   C. Self-efficacy
II. Behavior self-management
   A. Self-awareness/self-monitoring
   B. Ethics development
   C. Decision making/problem solving
   D. Planning behavioral strategies
III. Communicating
   A. Empathy
   B. Assertion
   C. Conflict resolution
   D. Responding to persuasion
IV. Using appropriate resources
   A. Assessing the need for help
   B. Locating sources of help
   C. Exercising rights
   D. Overcoming obstacles

For each grade level, K-12, specific educational descriptors are provided that indicate the goals and objectives found within the program at each grade level. The descriptors deal with each of the 10 basic areas included in the total *Healthful Living Education* program. The 10 basic areas included within the program are:

- The nature of health, health risks, and health education
- Stress management
- Substance abuse
- Nutrition and weight management
- Self-protection
- Relationships
- Personal fitness
- Recreational dance
- Games and sports
- Developmental gymnastics

Through implementation of the various activities suggested, the program should result in:

- Fewer risk-taking behaviors that contribute to disease, injury, and death
- Desirable social behaviors and increased levels of self-image
- Establishment of the positive behaviors that promote higher levels of health
- Higher morale and productivity and less absenteeism by students
- Development of appropriate levels of personal fitness and an understanding of the importance of physical activity for maintaining a viable and productive life
- Fewer instances of dropping out of school due to health-related behaviors (e.g., pregnancy, alcohol and drug use)
- Lower health-care expenses
- An increased awareness and respect for cultural diversity
- Better health-educated citizenry, equipped to handle personal, social, environmental, safety, and medical care decisions
- The development of appropriate skills and behaviors that will enable students to be proficient in at least three lifetime activities.

Major emphases for each progression level (K-3, 4-5, 6-7, and 9-12) are listed. In addition, specific goals and objectives, by content area and progression level, are presented. Guidelines specific to HIV/AIDS education are contained within the standard course of study.

Locally Based Programs

A number of local school districts have developed health education programs. Some of these programs are considered to be comprehensive, and others have a more limited focus.

Sunflower Project. The *Sunflower Project* was developed over 10 years ago in the Shawnee Mission, Kansas School District. As did the *Michigan Model*, the *Sunflower Project* evolved from the cooperation of many health agencies as well as the University of Kansas Medical School and the Department of Health, Physical Education, and Recreation of the University of Kansas.

Four major units of instruction are included: fitness, nutrition, cardiovascular health, and respiratory health. The basic goals of the program are to teach children the fundamentals of good health, create a positive attitude within students in terms of nutrition and their lifestyle, and provide each student with positive experiences that will demonstrate the feeling associated with good personal health and fitness.

Specifically developed for grades K through 6, the project contains basic content within each of the four areas, test materials, and suggested teaching materials. The program was designed as a supplement to the health education curriculum already available in Shawnee Mission.

Battle Creek (Michigan) Healthy Lifestyles Program. Funded by the W.K. Kellogg Foundation, the *Healthy Lifestyles Program* represents the efforts of four school districts that simultaneously submitted proposals to the W.K. Kellogg Foundation. Four risk factors were eventually selected for inclusion in the program: nutrition, substance abuse, stress management, and physical fitness. Later, family planning and sexually transmitted diseases were added to the program.

Currently in operation in four school districts in the Battle Creek area is a Healthy Lifestyles Task Force that assists in the coordination of the program. Activities included in the project include health fairs, runs, special contests, adult wellness programs, and classroom presentations.

The mission of the project was to promote change in attitudes and behavior consistent with a healthy lifestyle and to improve the quality of life by focusing on the total well-being of the individual. Central to the project is the opportunity for individuals to gain knowledge that will assist them in making positive lifestyle choices, particularly in

the areas of nutrition, substance abuse, stress management, and physical fitness, and to adopt healthy behaviors in those areas.

It's Up To You. *It's Up to You* is a state-validated broad-based 1-6 grade health education program that was developed in Brattleboro, Vermont. Initially developed under a Title IV C grant, the program has attained a regionalized status. The program focuses on the concept that individual responsibility and awareness of one's values is paramount to the development of a health-promoting lifestyle. The program is "hands on" oriented with both content and concepts developed from grade to grade in a sequential fashion. The program incorporates a "cookbook" core approach that teachers have found excites students. Included in each grade level teacher's guide are activities and materials that can extend the basic core activities so that health can be integrated into other areas of the curriculum. The program has stated goals in physical, social, and mental health areas.

CHAMPS HIV/AIDS Prevention Program. The *CHAMPS* (Champs Have And Model Positive Peer Skills) program was designed for students K-12 to help develop student leadership skills, prevent negative behaviors, and provide students with information about HIV/AIDS in a nonthreatening manner. A secondary purpose is to help students understand that they can remain safe from HIV/AIDS and still respect and retain compassion for those who have contracted the virus.

The program represents a cooperative venture between governmental agencies, voluntary health agencies, and private business and industry. Included in this coalition are the Arizona Departments of Drug Policy, Education, and Economic Security; the Arizona Supreme Court; American Express Company; United Dairy Council; U.S. West Communications; and the Centers for Disease Control and Prevention.

Peer leadership is emphasized and puppets are used as a key training process. Students who become a part of the peer leadership program are trained as puppeteers to present grade-level specific programs to younger children. Prerecorded cassette tape scripts are used, and specific classroom activities, developmentally appropriate for various grades, follow the puppet presentations. Incentives are provided to the students who become involved in the program, as well as for students who observe the puppet shows.

Feeling Good. *Feeling Good* is a combination physical fitness and cardiovascular health education program designed for students in grades K-7. Funded in part by the W.K. Kellogg Foundation, the program was implemented in Jackson County, Michigan. The program is designed to be taught twice a week for 30 minutes per meeting over a 13-week time period. The physical fitness component of the program includes four 30-minute aerobic workouts each week for the entire 13 weeks of the program. Evaluation of the program has shown that students' health knowledge, attitudes, and selected behaviors all improved. Of particular note was the decrease in cholesterol levels, diastolic blood pressures, and the improvement in cardiovascular endurance among students who participated in the program.

3Rs and HBP. Developed through local funding from the Georgia Affiliate of the American Heart Association, 3 *Rs and HBP* is a 2-week, limited-focus program specifically designed for grades 5 and 6. The program is aimed at helping students understand high blood pressure. A parental outreach component is incorporated whereby students have the opportunity to borrow medical equipment from their school and become "health messengers" to their parents and other family members to discuss the relationships between high blood pressure and lifestyle while actually measuring the blood pressure of the family members. A 6-hour teacher in-service program is designed to show the teachers how to implement the curriculum most effectively and teach the process of measuring blood pressure. Knowledge inventories, skills tests, and community involvement, including hospital tours for classes involved in the curriculum, are incorporated into the program.

Hazelwood School District Comprehensive School Health Education Program. The *Hazelwood School District Comprehensive School Health Education Program* was developed using local school district funding in Florissant, Missouri. This K-6 broad-based health education program includes eight major content areas (substance abuse, safety and first aid, mental and emotional health, personal health, drunk driving, nutrition, environmental health, and community health). As with other health education programs, individual responsibility is stressed at each grade level. Unique to this program is a segment designed to foster an appreciation in the students of the progress that has been made in health research and the health professions.

A detailed scope and sequence outline identifying the major areas of content for each grade level is central to the program. Specific grade-level objectives, learning experiences, and evaluative activities have been developed for each unit within each grade level. The program uses community resources as well as 16-mm films, slides, filmstrips, overhead transparencies, posters, and games. The *Hazelwood Program* was also one of the recipients of Metropolitan Life Foundation's Healthy Me awards in 1988.

Here's Looking At You, 2000. *Here's Looking At You, 2000* is a nationally recognized K-12 alcohol and drug education program. It is based on recent research studies that identify characteristics of potential drug users. These "risk factors" include early drug use, association with friends who use drugs, lack of positive social skills, chemical dependency in the family, and failure in school, among others. Each lesson focuses on one or more of these risk factors.

Here's Looking At You, 2000 was created with input from subject area experts. It has been extensively pilot tested by master teachers and is being used throughout this nation and in many other countries. Teachers are guided through at least 15 lessons at each grade level. The program includes strong "no use" messages, opportunity for parental involvement, focus on "gateway" drugs (tobacco, alcohol, and marijuana), social skill training, and opportunities for cross-age teaching.

A kit containing all the materials necessary to teach each lesson is available for each grade level. The program can be taught as a 3-week unit in a regular health instruction program or can be integrated throughout the school year. A training workshop for classroom teachers, school counselors, nurses, and school administrators is designed to acquaint these persons with the methods, materials, activities, and content of the program.

Here's Looking at AIDS and You. *Here's Looking at AIDS and You* was developed to help students recognize and avoid situations that put them at risk for getting AIDS and other sexually transmitted diseases. The curriculum begins early (grades 4-6), and it involves the student's family as well as school and community resources.

Instructional aids for the total program are contained in three separate grade-grouped kits (4-6, 6-9, and 9-12). In the upper elementary program, students learn about basic anatomy, the immune system, and the ways AIDS can and cannot be transmitted. They also learn a social skill—how to stay in control when their friends try to get them in trouble.

Middle school or junior high students (grades 6-9) learn about basic anatomy, the immune system, the ways AIDS and other sexually transmissible diseases can and cannot be transmitted, abstinence, and people whose lives have changed as a result of AIDS. They also learn social skills—how to make good decisions, how to stay in control when their friends try to do something that is not right, and how to stay in control when they themselves are tempted to do something that is not right.

A training program is available for teachers and for those who seek to train teachers in the curriculum.

HIV/AIDS Prevention Programs*

The HIV/AIDS epidemic has spurred the development of numerous limited focus programs that deal with this particular disease. Presented in this

*The materials mentioned in this section are available from The Association for the Advancement of Health Education (AAHE), AAHPERD Publications, PO Box 704, Waldorf, MD 20604, (800) 321-0789.

section are several programs that will assist local school districts in developing a health instruction program to address this pressing health issue. Several of these programs are available from the Association for Health Education located in Reston, Virginia.

HIV Prevention and AIDS education. This particular program was specifically developed for use by teachers in grades 5-7. A multicultural approach is emphasized and students are educated before initiation of behaviors that would place them at risk for HIV/AIDS. Included in the program is a detailed instructor's guide that contains teaching strategies, grade level activities and lesson plans, and strategies for getting parents involved with the program.

AIDS: What Young Adults Should Know. Supported in part by the Centers for Disease Control and Prevention, this program was designed specifically for students in grades 7-12. Printed in both English and Spanish, the instructor's manual contains teaching strategies, student activities, worksheets, handouts, and examination questions. Student materials are made available as a workbook that students can keep for future reference.

HIV Prevention and AIDS Education: Resources for Special Educators. The first of its kind, this particular resource was developed in cooperation with The Council for Exceptional Children (CEC). The basic information about HIV/AIDS has been adapted for presentation to special population groups. Included is a checklist so those who are teaching special education can recommend materials that might be added to the resources already present. This resource is particularly useful for those who are faced with the problem of ensuring that all students within a school system are exposed to information about HIV/AIDS.

Programs Available through Various Health-Related Agencies and Associations

The American Heart Association, the American Cancer Society, the National Dairy Council, the

National Fire Protection Association, the American Health Foundation, and the United Way are some of the many health agencies that have developed programs that can be integrated into an existing health instruction program.

Putting Your Heart into the Curriculum. *Putting Your Heart into the Curriculum,* developed by the American Heart Association, is specifically designed as a series of teaching modules and strategies to be used in grades K-12 by teachers as an addition to their regular health instruction program. It is designed to affect those attitudes and value judgments of young people that may have an effect on their behaviors.

The following areas are included:

• Choosing not to smoke
• Making informed and healthy food choices
• The importance of having a blood pressure within normal limits
• Recognizing the various risk factors of cardiovascular disease and how to lessen their impact on the individual
• Developing and keeping a regular program of weight control and physical exercise

In-service training for teachers is available from the Association or through selected universities that participate in the program. Teaching aids and materials are available free of charge from local chapters of the American Heart Association.

An Early Start to Good Health. *An Early Start to Good Health* instruction program for grades K-3, developed by the American Cancer Society, consists of four separate units and includes teacher guides, filmstrips, posters, phonograph records, and activity sheets. It is designed to develop health awareness and to supplement existing programs.

The four units of instruction include the following:

• Unit 1: My Body—introduction to basic body organs
• Unit 2: My Self—the difference between the inner and outer self
• Unit 3: My Health—activities needed to maintain health

• Unit 4: My Choice—personal choices and the effects of those choices

Health Network. *Health Network* was also developed by the American Cancer Society and is designed as a companion to the *Early Start to Good Health* program. *Health Network* consists of three units of instruction designed specifically for use in grades 4, 5, and 6. Each unit contains a filmstrip and either a phonograph record or tape cassette that provides the story for the unit. Also included are a teacher's guide with an introductory lesson and several group activities, reproduction masters to make handouts for the students, and either a game or poster that exemplifies the basic content of the unit.

The three units of instruction each have objectives for students that aid the teacher in planning to use the program. The three units of instruction are as follows:

• Unit 4: Special People—cigarettes don't improve one's self-image, and one need not be a "star" to be a valuable person
• Unit 5: Health News—a simulated television news broadcast that reports on how the respiratory system uses oxygen in the process of breathing
• Unit 6: Starga's World—a girl from outer space visits Earth and learns how to make decisions about herself and her health

Food: Your Choice. The National Dairy Council designed *Food: Your Choice,* a nutrition education program, for students in grades K-6. The program is sequential and activity oriented. Its purpose is to (1) foster an understanding of key concepts of nutrition, (2) convey the importance of nutrition in preventing health problems, and (3) encourage maintaining a healthy body.

The program consists of three levels:

• Level 1: Specifically designed for use in grades K-2, nutrition concepts are learned through hands-on experiments and meal preparation.
• Level 2: Designed for use in grades 3 and 4, this level is designed to further expand the concepts learned in Level 1. Students have the opportunity to examine more closely the

role of food in society. They classify foods and learn the consequences of poor food selection and eating habits.

- Level 3: Designed for grades 5 and 6, this level focuses on a study of nutrients in food as well as analysis of those factors that influence eating patterns, food selection, and food advertising. Special materials have been developed to integrate nutrition teaching into social studies, science, and home economics.

Most state dairy council office staff members will conduct teacher-training workshops designed to acquaint school personnel with the program.

Learn Not to Burn. The *Learn Not to Burn* program was developed between 1975 and 1978 by the National Fire Protection Association (NFPA) to provide a comprehensive fire prevention program for grades K-8. A survey revealed that little coordination between fire departments and school districts in terms of fire prevention curricula existed in the United States. The program is unique in that it involves parents as well as fire department personnel.

The basic goals of the program are as follows:

- Protection of persons from fires
- Prevention of fires
- Motivation of persons to practice fire prevention and safety

The program consists of three major segments that are reflected in the program goals. It includes 25 key fire prevention and protection behaviors in the three major segments of protection, prevention, and persuasion. Each of the 25 behaviors has at its core an action domain determined to be the most direct means of saving life and property together with knowledge and attitudes necessary to achieve the action.

The NFPA* reported it had documented evidence that 298 lives had been saved in 118 fires as a result of the introduction of the *Learn Not to Burn* curriculum in over 50,000 classrooms reaching several million students (estimated). Supplementary curriculum materials for grades pre-

school and K-3 are available that include special class activities—songs, hand puppets, and an evaluation instrument.

Know Your Body. *Know Your Body* is a broad-based, nationally available and PEP-approved (in 1989) curriculum developed by the American Health Foundation through funding provided by the National Cancer Institute, the National Heart, Lung and Blood Institute, and the W.K. Kellogg Foundation. Developed for grades K-6, this program is designed to:

- Increase student health knowledge about selected health factors
- Develop values and attitudes that promote a healthy lifestyle
- Promote behavior that will enhance personal health
- Increase student ability to alter personal health practices

The overriding objective of *Know Your Body* is to provide health education that helps students realize that health is a personal, relevant, and enduring concept. Based in social learning theory, such things as role modeling, goal orientation, and positive health behavior reinforcement are central to the program. Designed as a 1-year program taught once or twice a week for 40 to 50 minutes each class, students participate in a personalized health screening program to learn about basic concepts of wellness and health behaviors. Through this process they are encouraged to alter their behavior through personal decision making so that their total well-being is enhanced. The concepts of self-responsibility and self-care are stressed as they relate to a core of decision making, goal setting, and communication skills in the areas of nutrition, physical fitness, self-esteem, family living, AIDS, dental health, first aid, accident prevention, risk factor reduction, environmental health, consumer awareness, and avoidance of use of tobacco, alcohol, and drugs. Instruction in how to prevent some of the major health problems of today (accidents, cancer, and heart disease) is also stressed.

A sequentially arranged spiraled scope and sequence has been developed to better articulate grades K-3 and 4-6. As students progress through

---

*Barbara Dunn, Manager, Public Education, National Fire Protection Association: Personal communication, February 2, 1995.

the curriculum, new concepts are introduced and prior learnings are reinforced. Printed teachers' guides and student worksheets for each grade level are available for teachers who participate in the training workshops conducted by *Know Your Body* staff. Promoting school-wide activities that create a health-conscious school culture is a central component of the *Know Your Body* curriculum.

Health Education Curriculum Guide. Developed in 1974 by a committee of teachers, health educators, health agency personnel, and parents, the *Health Education Curriculum Guide* is a special project of the United Way of Central Stark County, Ohio. The main content areas of this K-6 broad-based curriculum include family living; growth and development; alcohol, drugs, and tobacco; safety; environmental, community, and mental health; and nutrition. A teacher's guide containing content, learning activities, and suggested evaluation activities and resources for each of the six content areas is available for each grade level. Nearly 400 learning activities across the seven grade levels are presented in the program.

Science for Life and Living: Integrating Science, Technology, and Health. This is a year-long program for each of seven grades, K-6. It includes at least 8 weeks of health instruction at each grade level. It was developed with grants from the National Science Foundation, the Gates Foundation, Coors Foundation, and IBM as an innovative, alternative approach to both science education and health education. At each grade level the focus of the health component is on healthy behavior, such as practicing safety, eating nutritiously, or engaging in regular, appropriate exercise. Research linking behaviors with wellness guided the choice of behaviors. The concepts, information, and skills presented at each level relate directly to the targeted behavior, as do the attitudes that are addressed. Although the authors targeted certain behaviors, the approach is discovery-based. Students participate in hands-on experiences that help them discover for themselves why certain behaviors are valuable. Then the program teaches specific skills that students need to engage in the behavior.

In addition to the integration with science and technology, the behavioral focus, and the depth versus breadth approach, this program has other innovative features. It builds cooperative learning into the program; the teacher does not need to decide how to structure group work. Students do much of the work in teams, so they learn to depend on themselves more and on the teacher less. This frees teachers to spend time with students who need help with the content or with group process. It also enhances students' self-esteem. Another feature of the program is that it uses an instructional model based on a constructivist theory of how children learn. In addition, in the health units the authors used the health belief model, social learning theory, and the PRECEDE* (Predisposing, Reinforcing and Enabling Causes in Educational Diagnosis and Evaluation) model as the bases for curricular decisions.

The 7-year program is a comprehensive health education curriculum. The program, however, is not comprehensive at any one grade level. It consists of a teacher's guide for each grade level K-6, student texts for each grade level 1-6, kit materials for each grade level K-6, and an implementation manual. Training is available through the publisher, usually in collaboration with teacher-training institutions of higher learning.

Commercially prepared programs. Many school health instruction programs rely on commercial companies for the teaching aids and other materials they use in their programs. Therefore some of these business firms have prepared curricula that incorporate the variety of teaching aids they manufacture for sale. Five such programs are *Beltman*, developed by Film Loops, Inc.; *Health Skills for Life*, developed in Oregon; the *Health Activities Project*, distributed by the Hubbard Scientific Company; the *BEST Campaign*, developed by the Agency for Instructional Technology; and the *Contemporary Health Series*, published by ETR Associates.

---

*Green L, Kreuter M, Deeds S, Partridge K: *Health education planning: a diagnostic approach*, Palo Alto, CA, 1980, Mayfield.

Beltman. *Beltman* is a multimedia program specifically designed for students in grades K-2. Designed for 9 to 10 lessons, the purpose of the program is to teach young children pedestrian safety and to increase their seatbelt use. The program objectives include:

- Teaching children how to use seatbelts and motivating them to use the belts
- Teaching children proper pedestrian behavior, including the safe way to cross streets
- Developing within children an appreciation for safety as a lifestyle

A teacher's guide, five cassette tapes, three filmstrips, and other teaching aids are included in the kit. Such things as iron-on decals are included as motivational devices. Independent evaluation of the *Beltman* program indicated that when it was combined with parental involvement, the program could develop safety consciousness and more consistent use of seatbelts in children.

Health Skills for Life. Although developmental funding for *Health Skills for Life,* a skill-based, comprehensive K-12 health education program came from the Oregon State Department of Education and from a Title IV C grant, it is now available through a private, commercial company that carries the same name as the project. The project itself consists of 122 separate teaching packages that address 10 major content areas (alcohol, tobacco, and other drugs; disease prevention; environmental health; dental health; fitness; consumer and health services; mental health; safety and first aid; growth and development; and nutrition). Within the 10 areas, concepts about family, life, and human sexuality are introduced in appropriate places. Each grade level contains 8 to 12 units, a teacher's guide, a performance indicator poster, and a parent poster. Each of the grade level units is packaged separately so a school system can select those units that are responsive to the specific needs of the district.

The purpose of the program is to provide students with opportunities to practice health behaviors in the areas of physical, mental, social, and emotional health. Each of the 122 skills were written as competencies that were to be demonstrated by the student exposed to the units of instruction. This facilitates the evaluation of the unit of instruction. Combined with the skills are performance indicators, health content, and a set sequence of activities that help direct the student toward the skill. Suggestions for integrating the specific skills and content with other curriculum areas such as mathematics, reading, and writing are included.

A detailed scope and sequence chart is available, as are administrators' guides and optional resource materials that could be included in the program. A 3½-hour teacher training program and a 2-hour administrator training program are offered by the project developers.

Health Skills for Life has been validated by the Oregon State Department of Education and was selected in 1985 as 1 of the 20 programs honored by Metropolitan Life Foundation as an exemplary health education program in the United States.

Health Activities Project. The *Health Activities Project* gets students involved with personal health and safety using hands-on, discovery-type activities. It is assumed that students can realize how to improve their health and safety by learning how their bodies function.

The program uses a variety of teaching aids for the 58 different activities. The teacher's guide contains a description of each activity, the health background for it, the space requirements necessary to conduct the activity, and the materials that are needed. The activities are specifically designed to supplement and enrich existing school health, physical education, and science curricula.

The BEST Campaign. This limited focus program is a cooperative program that involves the school, parents, and the community, so that a consistent message that life is better without using drugs, alcohol, or tobacco is conveyed. Developed by the Agency for Instructional Technology, the *BEST (Bringing Everybody's Strength Together) for a Drug-Free Tomorrow Campaign* contains three basic components. The first component "Just for Me" was designed to be used in grades 2-4. This component consists of six 15-minute videotapes, a facilitator's manual that contains extension activities, a peer helper handbook, and a home component that uses three videotapes, a parental guide, and a parental workshop leader's manual. For grades 5 and 6, the program is entitled "Your Choice . . . Our Chance." In this segment, ten 15-minute videotapes are included. There is also a teacher's guide, an information videotape, and a facilitator's guide. As with the "Just for Me" segment, there is a community component that consists of three 30-minute videotapes and a community organization handbook. The final component of the program, "Project Alert," contains 13 weekly lessons, 10 for grade 7, and three booster lessons for grade 8. As with the other components, the program is designed around the use of videotapes, posters, and homework assignments. Across the three components are the tenets of basic skill development in resisting peer pressure, developing good communication skills, engaging in critical thinking, and practicing good decision making that will help youths live an alcohol, drug, and tobacco-free life. The videotape components contain simulated "real-life" scenarios in multicultural settings that facilitate student discussion and allow students to immediately apply what they have learned. Recently the Association for the Advancement of Health Education (AAHE) has been offering specialized training that is conducted over a 2-4 hour period so that there is a project director in each state for those states that take advantage of the training. These project directors help organize, publicize, and conduct additional teacher training for districts that wish to implement The BEST Campaign in their schools and communities.

Contemporary Health Series. Available from ETR Associates in Santa Cruz, California, the *Contemporary Health Series* was developed and designed by health educators as a K-12 comprehensive program. The three basic components of the series, "Actions for Health," "Into Adolescence," and "Entering Adulthood," were designed for K-6, middle school, and high school, respectively. There are 10 basic content areas included in the program (nutrition, growth and development, mental and emotional health, family life and health, disease prevention and control, personal health and hygiene, consumer health, injury prevention and safety, and community and environmental health). Lesson plans, specific objectives, teaching strategies, references to materials, implementation strategies, evaluation processes and optional follow-up or extension activities are contained in the instructor's guides for the series. Each lesson plan also contains major objectives and a timetable for implementation so that the greatest impact of the program on students can be attained.

SUMMARY

The programs described in this chapter represent but a few of the different types of health instruction programs available in the United States. The critical elements in each program that must be identified are flexibility in terms of meeting student and community needs and how local teachers can use the program in terms of direct and integrated health instruction. For those faced with having to develop a health instruction program, these illustrations provide suggestions for use in newly developed curricula.

We recognize that anyone who is not familiar with health education curriculum development and desires to develop a program should obtain expert assistance before undertaking such a project. This aid might be obtained from the state department of education, professional health educators in colleges or universities, or neighboring school districts. Programs should be developed that are responsive to student and community needs and that are based on sound principles of curriculum development such as those presented in Chapter 11. Finally, regardless of whatever program is used, it will only be effective if it is supported administratively and implemented by faculty who value the importance of health education throughout the curriculum.

QUESTIONS FOR DISCUSSION

1. Why do you think that no clear-cut procedures for developing and implementing health instruction curricula in U.S. schools have been developed?

2. What do you perceive is the value of the National Diffusion Network?

3. Why might state National Diffusion Network facilitators be considered the most important links in the network?

4. What are the different ways a program might be considered for inclusion in the National Diffusion Network, and what is the basic process for including a program in the network?

5. How would *you* define an "exemplary" health instruction program? How does your definition differ from that used by the Joint Dissemination Review Panel?

6. What benefits might accrue to a program that is included in the National Diffusion Network?

7. You have been asked to make a recommendation to a school district about how to initiate a comprehensive school health instruction program. Identify the components of several illustrative programs found in this chapter that you will include in your recommendations.

8. What factors appear to have been key elements in the success of specific programs illustrated in this chapter?

9. What factors do you feel have kept many state legislatures from enacting comprehensive school health instruction legislation?

10. What factors exist in common among the various locally based health instruction programs presented in the text?

11. What factors exist in common among the various programs available through health-related agencies that are discussed in the text?

12. In your opinion, why have commercial companies produced health education materials?

SELECTED REFERENCES

American Association of School Administrators: *Healthy kids for the year 2000: an action plan for schools,* Arlington, VA, 1991, The Association.

Association for the Advancement of Health Education: *Summary of the national forum on HIV/AIDS prevention education for children and youth with special education needs,* Reston, VA, 1989, The Association.

Association for the Advancement of Health Education: *Cultural awareness and sensitivity: guidelines for health educators,* Reston, VA, 1994, The Association.

Association for the Advancement of Health Education: *Healthy networks: models for success,* Reston, VA, 1992, The Association.

Association for the Advancement of Health Education: *Strengthening health education for the 1990s,* Reston, VA, 1991, The Association.

American Cancer Society: *National action plan for comprehensive school health education,* Atlanta, 1992, The Society.

Association for Supervision and Curriculum Development: *ASCD yearbook,* Alexandria, VA, 1994, The Association.

Brown LK, Fritz GK: AIDS education in the schools: a literature review as a guide for curriculum planning, *Clin Pediatr* 27:311-316, 1988.

California State Board of Education: *Health framework for California public schools: kindergarten through grade twelve,* Sacramento, CA, 1994, California State Board of Education.

Centers for Disease Control and Prevention: *Cooperative agreement for national programs to strengthen comprehensive school health programs and prevent health problems among youth: project summaries for national organizations,* Atlanta, 1994, Centers for Disease Control and Prevention.

Cohen JH, Weiss HB, Mulvey EP, Deerwater SR: A primer on school violence prevention, *J School Health* 64(8):309-313, 1994.

Council of Chief State School Officers: *Beyond the health room,* Washington, DC, 1991, The Council.

Downey AM, Frank GC, Webber LS, Harsha DW, Virgikio SJ, Franklin FA et al: Implementation of "Heart Smart": a cardiovascular school health promotion program, *J School Health* 57(3):98-104, 1987.

DuShaw ML: A comparative study of three model comprehensive elementary school health education programs, *J School Health* 54:397-400, 1984.

Frank C: Helping health education to grow: the New York City experience, *Health Ed* 19(5):57-60, 1988.

Frank C, Goldman L: Growing healthy in New York City, *Phi Delta Kappan* Feb:454-455, 1988.

Fredisdorf M: Alcohol and drug abuse prevention in Wisconsin public schools, *J School Health* 59(1):21-24, 1989.

Green L, Krueter M, Deeds S, Partridge K: *Health education planning: a diagnostic approach,* Palo Alto, CA, 1980, Mayfield.

Guttmacher A: *Today's adolescents: tomorrow's parents: a portrait of the Americas,* New York, 1991, The Alan Guttmacher Institute.

Hammes M: Guidelines to assist classroom teachers in designing and implementing student involvement techniques, *Health Ed* 17:48-50, 1986.

Lloyd-Kolkin D, Hunter L: *The comprehensive school health sourcebook,* Menlo Park, CA, 1990, Health and Education Communication Consultants.

Lovato C, Allensworth D, Chan F: *School health in America: an assessment of state policies to protect and improve the health of students,* ed 5, Kent, OH, 1989, American School Health Association.

Metropolitan Life Foundation: *Healthy me: a compendium of award winning programs, 1985-1989,* New York, 1990, The Foundation.

Metropolitan Life Foundation: *Health: you've got to be taught: an evaluation of comprehensive health education in American public schools,* New York, 1988, The Foundation.

Minnesota Department of Education: *Minnesota School Health Education 110 Program,* Minneapolis, MN, 1992, Minnesota Department of Education.

National Diffusion Network (NDN): *EPTW educational programs that work,* ed 19, Longmont, CO, 1993, Sopris West.

National Professional School Health Education Organization: Comprehensive school health education, *J School Health* 54(8):312-315, 1984.

North Carolina Department of Public Instruction: *Standard course of study for healthful living,* Raleigh, NC, 1994, North Carolina Department of Public Instruction.

Parcel GS, Erickson MP, Lovato CY, Gottleib NH, Brink SG, Green LW: The diffusion of school-based tobacco-use prevention programs: project description and baseline data, *Health Ed Res* 4(1):111-124, 1989.

Perry C, Klepp K, Sillers C: Community-wide strategies for cardiovascular health: the Minnesota heart health program youth program, *Health Ed Res Theory Prac* 4(1):87-101, 1989.

Price J: Learn not to burn: a K-8 curriculum, *J School Health* 51:543-547, 1981.

Resnicow K, Orlandi M, Vaccaro D, Wynder E: Implementation of a pilot school-site cholesterol reduction intervention, *J School Health* 59(2):74-78, 1989.

Scheer JK: *HIV prevention education for teachers of elementary and middle school grades,* Santa Cruz, CA, 1992, ETR Associates.

Seffrin JR: *America's interest in comprehensive school health education.* Paper presented to the Second Annual School Health Leadership Conference, Atlanta, 1994.

Taggart V, Bush P, Zuckerman A, Theiss P: A process evaluation of the District of Columbia "Know Your Body" project, *J School Health* 60(2):60-66, 1990.

Task Force on Education of Young Adolescents: *Turning points: preparing American youth for the 21st century,* Washington, DC, 1989, Carnegie Council on Adolescent Development.

The Adolescent Suicide Awareness Program, *School Interv Reports* 1(1):5, 1987.

The Gallup Organization: *Values and opinions of comprehensive school health education in US public schools: adolescents, parents, and school district administrators,* Atlanta, 1994, American Cancer Society.

The National Commission on the Role of the School and the Community in Improving Adolescent Health: *Code blue: uniting for healthier youth,* Alexandria, VA, 1990, National Association of State Boards of Education.

United States Public Health Service: *Healthy people 2000: national health promotion and disease prevention objectives,* Washington, DC, 1990, US Government Printing Office.

Williams P, Kubik J: The Battle Creek (Michigan) schools' healthy lifestyles program, *J School Health* 60(4):142-146, 1990.

11

Organizing for Health Teaching

KEY CONCEPT

Developing, organizing, teaching, and evaluating comprehensive health education programs using basic principles of curriculum development and instruction are shared responsibilities of teachers, administrators, and community members.

Instruction for healthful living is essential for every student.

AMERICAN MEDICAL ASSOCIATION
MEDICINE/EDUCATION COMMITTEE
ON SCHOOL AND COLLEGE HEALTH

Automobile accidents, suicide, homicide and other injuries—all problems linked to health behaviors that are strongly influenced by school health education—are the leading killers of today's youth.

CENTERS FOR DISEASE CONTROL AND PREVENTION

PROBLEM TO SOLVE

You have accepted a position to teach a fourth grade class in a growing suburban area. One of your new responsibilities is to teach appropriate health education lessons. To your dismay, you discover the district has neither curriculum guides nor textbooks for health education. Describe how you would go about developing and organizing a yearly plan for your fourth grade health teaching. Include your rationale for each major organizing step. As part of your plan, create an original unit on a health topic of your choice. Include a minimum of three, logically sequenced, student-centered lesson plans.

THERE is general agreement among authorities on the importance of planning and organizing for health education. Both are critical to achieve objectives in the cognitive (knowledge), affective (attitudes), and action (behavior) areas of child development in schools. Clear definitions should be provided in curricula in terms of what pupil goals teachers should be seeking, what content should be included, what methods and materials are to be used, and whether the established purposes have been achieved. Ideally, experiences for pupils should be both scientifically oriented and student centered. This chapter provides information and direction toward this end.

Health education must be organized in both formal and informal ways if the differing needs and interests of students are to receive proper consideration. Pupils with drug problems (including alcohol and tobacco), sexual (including gender identity) concerns, and emotional and psychological difficulties often cannot be helped, except on a one-to-one or small group basis. To date, insufficient attention has been given to the informal approach in schools. Chapter 6 contains a variety of ways to guide and counsel young people. This chapter and succeeding chapters focus on organizing for formal health teaching.

Curriculum development and implementation is basic to organizing for formal health teaching. A variety of tasks need attention, including determination of what shall be taught and the preparation or selection of units for teacher reference and use. In addition, teachers need help in developing their own plans for teaching and guidance through illustrative units.

Before presenting material in this text in regard to curriculum development and teacher planning, the teachers and administrators must understand some of the basic principles involved in curriculum development and lesson planning, be familiar with the conceptual approach to learning, be aware of the usefulness of values clarification as a strategy in health education, and have some knowledge about personal and shared responsibility for the preparation of the curriculum.

WHAT ARE THE BASIC PRINCIPLES FOR CURRICULUM DEVELOPMENT IN HEALTH EDUCATION?

For any educational function to proceed on a sound basis, it must be predicated on certain valid principles or assumptions. If we begin with a firm foundation of fact and philosophy, we cannot stray far from the path of excellence.

Fundamentally, a sound curriculum must be based on the needs, problems, and opportunities of society and the individual. Beyond this broad approach are certain principles and assumptions that may be used as guidelines for curriculum planning and development in health education:

- Providing a sequential, comprehensive program that includes an ascending spiral effect to facilitate increasing depth of information and development of higher level skills and thought processes from kindergarten through grade 12 (Fig. 11-1).
- Providing repetition of content areas without excessive duplication by cycling content areas across grade levels or in other appropriate ways.
- Including learning focused on thinking and meaning while retaining a central place for factual knowledge.
- Considering adaptability and flexibility, thus allowing for changes and modifications to be made, new content and information to be included, and new materials to be used (e.g., technologies) as they develop and evolve in society.
- Using a conceptual approach in developing the curriculum, with emphasis on health concepts and objectives.
- Emphasizing the preventive aspects of health within the instructional program, with a particular focus on self-care responsibilities
- Keeping a balanced emphasis on physiological, sociological, psychological, and spiritual aspects of health
- Emphasizing the needs and interests of students and society as the basis for the curriculum, thus ensuring it will be appropriate for

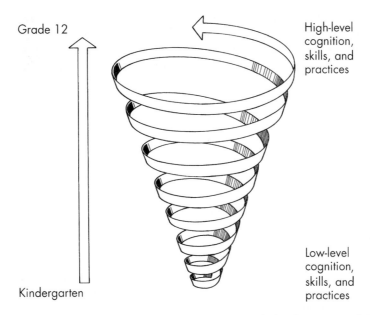

FIG. 11-1 Student health education learnings increase by grade level. Learning of the needed knowledge, skills, and practices for good health should start with low levels of achievement and then incrementally build and broaden as pupils move up the grade level ladder.

the local community or communities and the social climates in which pupils reside; special consideration must be given to the health needs of minorities, the underserved, and those with economic, ethnic, and cultural differences.

- Providing written objectives in behavioral terms, including objectives in the cognitive, affective, and action domains.*
- Developing objectives that are observable in the classroom, as well as action domain ob-

jectives that are nonobservable and that might take a longer time to attain.

- Providing goals with differential emphases at various grade levels (e.g., primary grades—focus on physiological aspects of health with limited psychological and social aspects—; intermediate grades—focus on physiological aspects of health with greater inclusion of psychological and social aspects, and limited spiritual emphasis—; and upper grades—focus primarily on psychological and social aspects, with decreasing emphasis on the physiological aspects, but with concern for the spiritual component).
- Including a diversity of alternatives to action and mastery of social skills, thus facilitating student ability to make intelligent decisions regarding behavior.
- Allowing students to make personal decisions, which do not impinge on the decisions of others, regarding behavior when appropriate.

---

*The student drug problem resulted in new educational terminology (such as affective and confluent education) and emphasis being introduced in schools. The need for students to develop positive self-concepts, express feelings and aspirations, reach social maturity, and participate in values clarification has led authorities to support affective education. It is believed such emphasis will enable persons to more effectively cope with life's problems. Confluent education refers to the integration of affective and cognitive elements in learning. These are worthwhile directions for inclusion in health education. The objectives found in the units in Appendix B include these new ideas.

- Including current, accurate, and nonbiased content that has been derived from scientific sources, including both the positive and negative aspects whenever possible.
- Using the principles of learning (see Chapter 9) to select methods and techniques of teaching that stress student involvement, decision making, critical thinking, discussions, problem solving, self-direction, clarification of values, and responsibilities
- Using a variety of resource materials that are interesting, current, accurate, carefully screened, culturally diverse, and appropriate for the students.
- Involving students, parents, and community representatives in developing and evaluating the curriculum.
- Providing periodic assessment (evaluation [see Chapter 14] of various aspects of the curriculum, including organization, content, methods, and materials).

These principles and assumptions may seem to be self-evident, yet often elementary school programs of health education omit one or more of these guidelines. These principles are applied in the sections that follow.

THE CONCEPTUAL APPROACH

For years researchers in psychology and education have attempted to increase their knowledge of how children learn so they can help pupils learn more effectively. The concept approach is one of the more promising methods to evolve from their efforts.

Concept Formation

Learning involves thinking. The thinking process may include one or more of these six types of thinking: *perceptive, associative, inductive-deductive, creative, critical,* and *problem-solving.* The formation of concepts involves the use of the perceptive process.

Percepts are simplified conclusions that students obtain from seeing, hearing, touching, tast-

ing, and smelling. They are the raw materials of thinking that result from environmental stimuli. In the classroom these stimuli are generally provided and controlled by the teacher and may include the teacher's oral presentations; other pupils' comments; content of health textbooks, films, videos, software, and bulletin board information; and many others. Perception is essential to concept formation.

Children's ability to understand broad concepts or generalizations and abstractions depends on their ability to have direct sensory experiences. These experiences help them construct and reconstruct percepts. Research shows that sensory-motor experiences (for example, manipulation and construction) are most effective in developing percepts. Then, through use and application of these raw materials of health instruction, children can understand and deal with more abstract concepts. For example, "use of substances that modify mood and behavior arises from a variety of motivations," is a concept. It is a rather obtuse statement that necessitates specific sensory experiences for understanding and comprehension. Pupils may need to have discussions, hear comments by teachers, and review literature about why people use drugs to understand the meaning of the concepts.

Thus children are exposed to, screen, and select stimuli. The stimuli produce percepts that lead to the formation of concepts, which are conclusions or generalizations about what they have experienced.

Concepts Applied to Health Education

The concept approach to health education was introduced in the mid-1960s and emerged from the School Health Education Study (SHES) conducted under the leadership of Dr. Elena Sliepcevich. It continues to be a valid and useful procedure for use in curriculum development. An innovative project, the study was prepared using futuristic educational philosophy. It was also the first attempt to scientifically develop a health education curriculum that followed the basic principles used for all other educational curricula. Many health curriculum efforts since publication of the SHES have direct roots in this landmark work. It is fundamental to the eclectic plan identified in this text, which gives consideration to a variety of other significant prevalent ideas, including the concept of holistic health (physiological, psychological, social, and spiritual), student needs and interests, prevention, and ecology.

Health concepts are conclusions or generalizations that result from learning experiences to which students have been exposed. Concepts cannot be taught directly. They emerge from exposure to the variety of activities introduced by teachers from which students derive perceptions. They serve as an organizing framework that can be used to determine content and to develop the objectives of the curriculum. Thus after students have completed their learnings, they should be able to conclude that "use of substances that modify mood and behavior arises from a variety of motivations."

Examples of realistic and effective applications of the conceptual approach are exemplified in the partial health education curriculum units presented in Appendix B.

VALUES IN THE CURRICULUM

Family lifestyle changes, the influence of the mass communications media, technological innovations, world events, materialism, conflict of conformity and self-reliance, ethics, and affluence are among the factors that create difficulties in the establishment of values by young people. As a result, youth are searching for meaning in life. They are asking themselves questions such as, "Who am I? Why am I here? What really matters?" They desire to cope with daily problems, develop life-coping skills, understand themselves, and be able to make wise decisions. Because of the failure to answer these questions, a variety of behavioral problems have been appearing in school-aged children. Such problems include apathy, inconsistent behaviors, dropping out, violence, and depression. Schools have a major role in helping chil-

dren and youth at early ages begin to clarify their values.

Leaders in the field of psychology have indicated that individuals need to have a sense of purpose in their lives. People actively search for meaningfulness and identity in life, although some may never be able to clearly define or achieve such a goal. The achievement or failure to achieve a sense of purpose may affect an individual's mental health either positively or negatively.

There is no single, clear definition of values. They have been said to be deep, long-lasting commitments to a concept or doctrine that is highly prized and about which action will be taken in satisfying ways. They are characteristics or attitudes about human experiences that are strongly desirable to an individual or group of individuals. Values give direction to life and are influential in determining behavior. They aid in the making of decisions and judgments. They have been identified in the concept of health described in Chapter 1 as part of the *spiritual* aspect of health (see Fig. 1-2). They have been included in the units in Appendix B in the affective domain objectives.

Values may be learned through a variety of meaningful experiences and through interaction with the environment. Thus the sources of values include adults, peer cultures, the family, religious leaders, the communications media, friends, social groups, and the school.

Raths and colleagues* have said the focus—probably starting in the intermediate grades—should be on *value* clarification and not on the teaching of values per se. They believe values will emerge through this process. Didactic value clarification involves a series of strategies or methods for helping students learn to identify values. They state that a value must meet these seven criteria:

I. Choosing
   A. Choosing freely—individual should not be coerced and should have freedom of selection

---

*Raths LE, Harmin M, Simon S: *Values and teaching,* ed 2, Columbus, OH, 1987, Charles E Merrill.

B. Choosing from alternatives—a variety of alternatives must be provided

C. Choosing thoughtfully—consideration should be given to the consequences of each alternative

D. Affirming—when something is cherished, it is publicly and verbally supported: doing something

II. Prizing

A. Prizing and cherishing—choice has a positive tone and is held in high esteem

III. Action

A. Acting on choices—life is affected through reading, spending money, and budgeting time

B. Repeating—persistency and endurance become a pattern of life

Value clarification has a place in health education as part of both content and methodology. It has particular application to the areas of mental health, drugs, human sexuality, alcohol, smoking, consumerism, health care, and environment; but it is also useful in other health areas. The outlines of content found in the illustrative units in Appendix B contain suggestions. Some of the strategies useful for value clarification are presented in Chapter 12.

The inclusion of value clarification in any teaching may be considered controversial by some parents. Things to be considered when deciding on whether to include them in the curriculum are found in Chapter 8.

Beane* claimed that the value clarification process may only superficially treat values. It cannot be assumed that students will evaluate or decide on their own values. The conceptualization and organization of values may require cognitive elements for analysis, synthesis, and evaluation. The method does generate interest and stimulate student discussion, but Beane raises serious questions about the contribution of the method of values education.

The wise teacher will remember that students arrive at school with many values already formed. The key is not to force or push the teacher's values on students, but rather to help students clarify and organize their existing values so that good decision-making skills, based on positive values, will emerge and enhance students' health.

WHO IS RESPONSIBLE FOR DEVELOPING THE CURRICULUM IN HEALTH?

Curriculum development and improvement have become major functions of modern education. Not too long ago the curriculum was shaped largely by experts in the various disciplines. In recent years, however, these experts have been joined by teachers, pupils, parents, and others in planning curricula. This does not imply that the opinions of experts are minimized or disregarded. It means that a curriculum can be developed to fit a certain school and community best if opportunity is provided for teachers, pupils, and lay groups to adapt the curriculum to local interests and needs.

For example, an elementary school in Florida might want to provide time in the curriculum to hookworm infestation and "creeping eruption" (a skin infestation caused by dog and cat hookworms), instead of spending time on frostbite and winter sport safety. An impoverished area school in the inner city might decide to stress the problems of teen pregnancy and sexually transmitted disease at an earlier grade level than a suburban school. A rural school might emphasize the importance of water purity, sanitation, and farm safety, whereas an urban school might take more time for air pollution. A school whose pupils come from families where ethnic and racial backgrounds shape their daily meals would surely want to stress the place of various ethnic foods as they apply to choosing a balanced diet.

Thus we find real need for adapting the curriculum to best meet local problems in many areas of health. Fundamentally, however, the subject matter is the same for all schools and all children. It is the fringe areas and the manner of illustrating

---

*Beane JA: The continuing controversy over affective education, *Educ Leadership* 43(4):26-31, 1985/1986.

basic concepts that offer the best opportunity for adaptation.

Curriculum development is a shared responsibility. Even though the approach may differ from one community to another, the curriculum in health and safety should reflect the interests, concerns, and efforts of teachers, pupils, parents, physicians, dentists, public health specialists, law enforcement officials, civil defense authorities, school board members, fire department officials, representatives of voluntary health agencies, school nurses, principals, curriculum specialists, and school health coordinators. These people, working together at the local level, can fashion the most fundamental and functional curriculum for their local school situation while retaining the common learnings in health and safety. Often the local group will need to make only a few minor changes in a course of study that has been prepared by the state department of education, regional education service unit, or another school district.

Cooperative planning and action can be helpful. The school health council at the district level, under the direction and guidance of the health coordinator or consultant, can give considerable support to the curriculum development program. The health council usually represents the thinking of concerned persons and organizations. Moreover, it provides a mechanism for resolving variances in philosophy and for implementing group decisions.

Few school districts throughout the country have the personnel resources to develop a sound, up-to-date health education curriculum on their own. If a professionally qualified health coordinator is not available, schools should seek guidance from state or local colleges and universities or private consultants.

Critical analysis of the curriculum in health education must be a continual process if the instructional program is to be functional in the lives of children. Rapid advances in the health sciences no longer permit schools to "stand pat" for very long on content. Sequence also is affected by increasingly frequent medical and health science developments and problems. These are reported in newspapers, magazines, telecasts, and other media. Often such health science reporting provides the teacher with a "teachable moment"—a time when pupils are more likely to be motivated—for a topic that had not been planned. Examples are many: AIDS, hazardous waste, new hepatitis A and B vaccines, sexually transmitted diseases, population growth, elimination of smallpox, toxic shock syndrome, the energy crisis, radiation hazards, violence, new drugs being used and abused, quackery and fraud in the health marketplace, the emergence of new diseases such as those caused by the Ebola virus, and a host of others.

The wise and imaginative teacher will be flexible enough to depart from the lesson plan and take full advantage of the heightened interest of pupils when these media stories "break." Remember, curriculum guides will provide the "what," but it is teachers who provide the "how." Chapter 12 is a useful resource for teachers looking for innovative ways to teach health education.

HOW IS THE CURRICULUM DETERMINED?

Many factors must be considered in determining a district's health education curriculum. The most significant factors are those directly related to the students. Therefore to determine what should be taught in health education, it is necessary to identify the health interests and needs of pupils. Once they have been identified, a scope and sequence chart is prepared. This chart is used to determine which units need to be constructed at each grade level.

Sample scope and sequence charts based on National Health Education Standards and from local school districts are found in Tables 11-1 and 11-2. Scope and sequence charts provide a logical basis for further program refinements for the general student population, but consideration must also be given to the special problems and unique needs of minority, non-English speaking, economically deprived, the physically and mentally challenged, and other special groups.

Interests and Needs

The following is a variety of information sources useful in determining the scope and sequence of the curriculum.

Student interests. Pupils learn better when they have interest in the subject matter. In essence, interest is an attitude favorable to learning. Beyond this, interest hinges on the values, desires, wants, and purposes of the pupil. As children perceive the relationship of a topic to their personal

TABLE 11-1 National Health Education Standards

Standard	Performance indicators	
	K-4	**5-8**
Students will comprehend concepts related to health promotion and disease prevention	• Describe relationships between personal health behaviors and individual well-being • Identify indicators of mental, emotional, social, and physical health during childhood • Describe the basic structure and functions of the human body systems • Describe how the family influences personal health • Describe how physical, social, and emotional environments influence personal health • Identify common health problems of children • Identify health problems that should be detected and treated early • Explain how childhood injuries and illnesses can be prevented or treated	• Explain the relationship between positive health behaviors and the prevention of injury, illness, disease, and premature death • Describe the interrelationship of mental, emotional, social, and physical health during adolescence • Explain how health is influenced by the interaction of body systems • Describe how family and peers influence the health of adolescents • Analyze how environment and personal health are interrelated • Describe ways to reduce risks related to adolescent health problems • Explain how appropriate health care can prevent premature death and disability • Describe how lifestyle, pathogens, family history, and other risk factors are related to the cause or prevention of disease and other health problems
Students will demonstrate the ability to access valid health information and health-promoting products and services	• Identify characteristics of valid health information and health-promoting products and services • Demonstrate the ability to locate resources from home, school, and community that provide valid health information • Explain how media influences the selection of health information, products, and services • Demonstrate the ability to locate school and community health helpers	• Analyze the validity of health information, products, and services • Demonstrate the ability to utilize resources from home, school, and community that provide valid health information • Analyze how media influence the selection of health information and products • Demonstrate the ability to locate health products and services • Compare the costs and validity of health products • Describe situations requiring professional health services

TABLE 11-1 National Health Education Standards—cont'd

Standard	Performance indicators	
	K-4	**5-8**
Students will demonstrate the ability to practice health-enhancing behaviors and reduce health risks	• Identify responsible health behaviors • Identify personal health needs • Compare behaviors that are safe to those that are risky or harmful • Demonstrate strategies to improve or maintain personal health • Develop injury prevention and management strategies for personal health • Demonstrate ways to avoid and reduce threatening situations • Apply skills to manage stress	• Explain the importance of assuming responsibility for personal health behaviors • Analyze a personal health assessment to determine health strengths and risks • Distinguish between safe and risky or harmful behaviors in relationships • Demonstrate strategies to improve or maintain personal and family health • Demonstrate ways to avoid and reduce threatening situations • Demonstrate strategies to manage stress
Students will analyze the influence of culture, media, technology, and other factors on health	• Describe how culture influences personal health behaviors • Explain how media influence thoughts, feelings, and health behaviors • Describe ways technology can influence personal health • Explain how information from school and family influences health	• Describe the influence of cultural beliefs on health behaviors and the use of health services • Analyze how messages from media and other sources influence health behaviors • Analyze the influence of technology on personal and family health • Analyze how information from peers influences health
Students will demonstrate the ability to use interpersonal communication skills to enhance health	• Distinguish between verbal and nonverbal communication • Describe characteristics needed to be a responsible friend and family member • Demonstrate healthy ways to express needs, wants, and feelings • Demonstrate ways to communicate care, consideration, and respect of self and others • Demonstrate attentive listening skills to build and maintain healthy relationships • Differentiate between negative and positive behaviors used in conflict situations • Demonstrate nonviolent strategies to resolve conflicts	• Demonstrate effective verbal and nonverbal communication skills to enhance health • Describe how the behavior of family and peers affects interpersonal communication • Demonstrate healthy ways to express needs, wants, and feelings • Demonstrate ways to communicate care, consideration, and respect of self and others • Demonstrate communication skills to build and maintain healthy relationships • Demonstrate refusal and negotiation skills to enhance health • Analyze the possible causes of conflict among youth in schools and communities • Demonstrate strategies to manage conflict in healthy ways

Continued.

TABLE 11-1 National Health Education Standards—cont'd

Standard	Performance indicators	
	K-4	**5-8**
Students will demonstrate the ability to use goal-setting and decision-making skills to enhance health	• Demonstrate the ability to apply a decision-making process to health issues and problems • Explain when to ask for assistance in making health-related decisions and setting health goals • Predict outcomes of positive health decisions • Set a personal health goal and track progress toward its achievement	• Demonstrate the ability to apply a decision-making process to health issues and problems individually and collaboratively • Analyze how health-related decisions are influenced by individuals, family, and community • Predict how decisions regarding health behaviors have consequences for self and others • Apply strategies and skills needed to attain personal health goals • Describe how personal health goals are influenced by changing information, abilities, priorities, and responsibilities
Students will demonstrate the ability to advocate for personal, family, and community health	• Describe a variety of methods to convey accurate health information and ideas • Express information and opinions about health issues • Identify community agencies that advocate for healthy individuals, families, and communities • Demonstrate the ability to influence and support others in making positive health choices	• Analyze various communication methods to accurately express health information and ideas • Express information and opinions about health issues • Identify barriers to effective communication of information, ideas, feelings, and opinions about health issues • Demonstrate the ability to influence and support others in making positive health choices • Demonstrate the ability to work cooperatively when advocating for healthy individuals, families, and schools

This table represents the work of the Joint Committee on National Health Education Standards, 1995. Copies of *National Health Education Standards: Achieving Literacy* can be obtained through the American School Health Association, Association for the Advancement of Health Education, or the American Cancer Society.

advantage and well-being, they become interested. *Active interests* are those that relate here and now to the child's daily life and world. *Latent interests* are those that the child may have had at an earlier age, but that were stifled because parents and other adults would not or could not encourage and develop them.

Finally, because interests depend heavily on past experiences, there are many areas in which pupils have practically no interest. It is one of the central purposes of education to amplify and diversify the interests of children. Thus pupil interests, although vital to motivation, cannot be considered in themselves as complete indicators of the relative importance of topics in health and safety.

TABLE 11-2 Second Grade Scope, Sequence, and Teacher Plans for Health Education—Ellensburg, Washington, Public Schools

Month	Area	Concepts	Learning activities	Teaching aids	Integration
September	Mental health	New experiences may give satisfaction Home, school, church, and community can be warm, safe places	Have children act as "big brother" or "big sister" to new students Encourage drawings about things they love, how it feels when hurt or scared, how to be helpful Encourage art work to relieve tensions Discuss leaders and followers, forgiveness, and other topics Dramatize putting self in others' shoes Films	Films: We play and share together Courtesy at school Health text: second and third grade	Language arts: write short experiences Music: listen to quiet music if tense Physical education: suggest activities to relax Social studies: discover community helpers
October	Dental health	Daily care promotes dental health Dentists help maintain healthy teeth Community resources provide for dental care	Demonstrate (using model) brushing teeth Make toothpowder in class Show films and filmstrips and discuss them Survey for number of dental visits Have vocabulary bingo game Write creative story about detergent foods	Films: The beaver tale Learning to brush Salt and baking soda Toothbrush dental kit Pictures: detergent foods and other foods	Mathematics: count teeth; subtract missing teeth Social studies: characterize dentist as community helper Art: make detergent-food mobile

Continued.

TABLE 11-2 Second Grade Scope, Sequence, and Teacher Plans for Health Education—Ellensburg, Washington, Public Schools—cont'd

Month	Area	Concepts	Learning activities	Teaching aids	Integration
November	Family health	Families help each other in the community	Make pictures of the family Tell experiences List ways neighbors can be helpful Arrange bulletin board about good neighborhood	Health text Record: Community helpers, Bowman Family fun with familiar music	Language arts: employ creative dramatics Music: play records and songs Art: draw pictures
January	Consumer and community health	Doctors and dentists who help us are our friends Hazards of the environment can cause discomfort and problems Many people keep water and air safe Individuals can improve their surroundings	Keep home duty chart Use atomizers to show how odors disperse Show films and filmstrips Make notebook on community helpers' relation to environment Dramatize how children help at home Locate on map local family and health agencies Decorate flannelboard with creative story with characters Leave food out, covered and uncovered, to relate to improper storage	Film: Magic touch Filmstrip: Dentist School nurse Record: Community helpers Personal pictures Map of community	Social studies: relate to community helpers unit Language arts: encourage reports or notebooks Art: make mural of community helpers
February	Nutrition	There are many kinds of foods Some foods may be better than others for you	Try new foods at tasting party Experiment with white rat Make vegetable soup	Film: Eat for health Filmstrip: The food we eat Transparencies: See unit Food models of card-	Art: draw basic 4 food groups; prepare mural Mathematics: sell items in grocery store and add costs

Month	Topic	Understandings	Activities	Materials	Correlation
			Make grocery store; use food models and shop for nutritious foods Make clay or paper maché fruit Select basic 4 foods, using magazine pictures	board cutouts Health text	Science: Experiment with white rat Social studies: take trip to store
March	Anatomy-physiology	Good posture helps prevent fatigue, enables the body to work better, and makes you more attractive	Use horizontal ladder for proper alignment Use plumbline to check posture Decorate bulletin board with stick figures or pipe cleaners Show film and discuss	Film: Beginning good posture Filmstrip: Let's stand tall	Physical education: relate to apparatus activities Art: make silhouettes and individual pictures Language arts: show and tell
April	Disease control	Good health habits help to keep us well When ill, certain practices help us get well We depend on others for good health	Use poster to illustrate ways to protect others Stage choral reading and speaking Use chart to show ways germs are transmitted Write reports Grow germs on cloth in warm and cool places Dramatize going to doctor for help Experiment with potato and agar in Petri dish	Films: Common cold; Soapy the germ fighter Milne: We are six (Wheezie and Sneezie)	Language arts: relate to experiences when sick, effects of care, creative stories Science: experiment with potatoes and agar
May	Family health	An egg grows into a baby	Discuss charts of mammal reproduction Prepare chart on life cycle of animal reproduction Hatch egg in incubator Chart and discuss fish egg development Make mural of animals caring for own babies Show films and filmstrips	Eye Gate charts of mammal reproduction series and fish egg development Films: Baby animals; Animals growing up Filmstrip: The zoo trip	Science: hatch egg; relate to insect unit Art: prepare mural

Prepared by a group of special education teachers in Ellensburg, Washington.

Teachers should identify pupil interests and emphasize those already developed. This is simply good motivation. Latent health interests (for example, "What makes me grow?" "Where do I go when I sleep?" "Where do babies come from?") will have to be further developed and new interests created for effective health teaching.

A 1984 report* by the Washington State Department of Education provides remarkable insight into the health interests, concerns, and problems of elementary school pupils. This study, entitled *Students Speak*, involved more than 5000 students from kindergarten through the twelfth grade. It showed, among other things, that basic health interests were common to all pupils whether they lived in a city, rural, suburban, or high socioeconomic environment. The questions and comments of elementary school-aged children were grouped according to grade level.

Responses were obtained by structured and unstructured methods. Written questionnaires were the source of the structured data. The sources of unstructured data were:

- Classroom observation by teachers and Washington State Medical Association Auxiliary volunteers
- Audiotapes and open classroom discussions stimulated by questions
- Voluntary responses by individual students
- Voluntary oral comments made after students finished the written questionaires

Sample summaries of structured and unstructured responses follow that illustrate, on a grade-level basis, some of the findings of this study.

KINDERGARTEN PARTIAL SUMMARY OF INTERESTS

HUMAN BODY/GROWTH AND DEVELOPMENT—A HIGH INTEREST

Unstructured:

In kindergarten, a big interest was the human body. Questions related to parts of the body, systems of the body, physical handicaps, the kindergartners' own growth, and prenatal growth and development.

Structured:

The number one interest, as shown on the written questionnaire, was about the body and its parts. Tied for second in interest was how the kindergartners' ears and eyes are made and work and how they grow as human beings.

SAFE LIVING/FIRST AID—A HIGH INTEREST

Unstructured:

The most frequently recited responses centered around accident prevention, what to do in case of a fire, and first aid; there was also interest in poisoning.

Structured:

Of the six written questionnaire items on safe living/first aid, all are in the top 15 interests: What to do if there were a fire (tied for first in interest); what to do when one is hurt at school or home (tied for second); how to prevent younger brothers and sisters or neighbor children from eating and drinking things that could poison them (tied for second); what to do if one is lost, how to prevent accidents at school, and how to prevent getting hurt going to and from school (all tied for fourth).

PHYSICAL WELL-BEING—A HIGH INTEREST

Unstructured:

When asked about topics relating to their physical well-being, kindergartners seemed to be interested in everything—especially dental care, sleep, and exercise.

Structured:

First in interest to kindergartners on the written questionnaire was how to stay healthy. Tied for second was how to take care of one's teeth and what food one should eat to play, learn, and grow.

FIRST GRADE PARTIAL SUMMARY OF INTERESTS

HUMAN BODY/GROWTH AND DEVELOPMENT—A HIGH INTEREST

Unstructured:

This health area was of highest interest to first graders. They wanted to know all about such things as how the

---

*Trucano L: *Students speak*, Seattle, 1984, Comprehensive Health Education Foundation. (Most recent published study)

body looks, works, breaks down, heals, and grows inside and out.

Structured:

The written question receiving the highest percentage of interest by first graders was the one dealing with the body and its parts. In second place was how ears and eyes are made and work.

SAFE LIVING/FIRST AID—A HIGH INTEREST
Unstructured:

First aid and accident prevention was an area of high interest to first graders. They imagine all kinds of circumstances in which they might find themselves and wonder what they should do. They were even concerned about preventing accidents from rockets.

Structured:

Four of the six written questions on safe living/first aid were in the top 15 interests of first graders. These four were: preventing younger brothers and sisters from ingesting poisonous substances (tied for first place); what to do in case of a fire (second most interesting item); what to do if lost (in third place); and how to prevent harm to themselves as they go to and from school (tied for fourth place).

MENTAL HEALTH—A HIGH INTEREST
Unstructured:

First graders were interested in understanding why people behave as they do, causes of feelings, and dealing with feelings. Friendship and decision making also held concern for them.

Structured:

The six written questions on mental health show 82% to 86% interest by students.

SECOND GRADE PARTIAL SUMMARY OF INTERESTS

HUMAN BODY/GROWTH AND DEVELOPMENT—A HIGH INTEREST
Unstructured:

The health area, human body, held an interest at all elementary grade levels, but second graders' responses seemed to indicate that this was *their* main interest. Second graders wanted to know all about body parts,

how they work, how they grow, and how babies grow inside mothers. They wanted details, including limits of vision, why wrinkles occur, how one learns to talk, how organs relate to each other, and how a cell starts. Types of handicaps and the reasons for them also brought forth a lot of questions. They were interested in their own beginnings and endings. Typical questions were, "How does God invent people?" "How long can you stay alive?" and "Why do people die early?"

Structured:

Three of the four written questions for this health area were in the top 15 interests. The questions were how the ears and eyes work (95%); about the body and its parts (93%); and how one grows (92%).

MENTAL HEALTH—A HIGH INTEREST
Unstructured:

Four topics brought forth the most questions: friendship, death, feelings, and behavior. On the topic of behavior, second graders wanted to know why they act as they do and how to control behavior that is negative.

Structured:

The mental health question in the top 15 interests concerned why people act the way they do. Not in the top 15 questions second graders wanted answered, but with an 85% interest, concerned how what one does or says affects other people, and what makes one feel good and bad; 89% of the second graders were interested in ways to get along with others; 87% in how handicapped people feel; and 86% in getting over sad, angry, or fearful feelings.

PHYSICAL WELL-BEING—A HIGH INTEREST
Unstructured:

Second graders were most interested in how to stay healthy, exercise, and keep teeth healthy.

Structured:

The number one interest of second graders was in learning how to stay healthy, with 97% of the students indicating they were interested. Other items in the top 15 were: what foods one should eat so one can play, learn, and grow (93%); how food affects teeth (92%); and why one needs to rest and exercise (90%).

THIRD GRADE PARTIAL SUMMARY OF INTERESTS

HUMAN BODY/GROWTH AND DEVELOPMENT—A HIGH INTEREST

Unstructured:

Third graders wanted to know much about the body and its parts, especially the brain and heart, and about their own growth and development. They were interested in fetal development. They wanted to know what happens to make things go wrong and cause handicaps such as deafness, dumbness, and paralysis. There was some interest in aging, senility, and how and why people die.

Structured:

Written questionnaire items appearing in the top 15 interests were learning about your body and its parts (95%); how the ears and eyes are made and work (90%); and how one grows (88%).

SAFE LIVING/FIRST AID—A HIGH INTEREST

Unstructured:

Although there were a lot of questions and comments by students on accident prevention—from snake bites, to lead poisoning—no one topic dominated this health area.

Structured:

Five of the six written questions in this health area were in the top 15 interests. What to do if lost had 95% interest; preventing younger brothers and sisters from ingesting poisonous substances had 95% interest; knowing what to do if hurt at home or school had 94% interest; what to do in case of a fire had 93% interest; and preventing accidents at school had 87% interest.

DISEASE CONTROL/PREVENTING HEALTH PROBLEMS—A HIGH INTEREST

Unstructured:

Disease was another area where there was a considerable number of questions but no pattern except for a commonly expressed interest in how people become sick or why some people get one disease and not another. There were many questions about specific diseases—especially about arthritis, cancer, and heart attacks. Several questions also were asked about immunization.

Structured:

Three written questions concerning this health area appear on the list of the top 15 interests. One question concerned home medicines—how they may help or hurt a person (90%); a second indicated an interest in certain illnesses, like colds (87%), and the third concerned immunizations (87%).

FOURTH GRADE PARTIAL SUMMARY OF INTERESTS

MENTAL HEALTH—A HIGH INTEREST

Unstructured:

Fourth graders showed much concern about their own feelings and the feelings of others (Fig. 11-2). They wanted to help others feel good about themselves. They wanted to like themselves, make friends, and avoid excessive worry and fear. Several commented on the deaths of friends, family members, and pets. They were concerned about how to make the right decisions.

Structured:

In the written questions, how a good friend should act was one of two mental health items in the top 15. The reasons why people might misuse drugs was the other item.

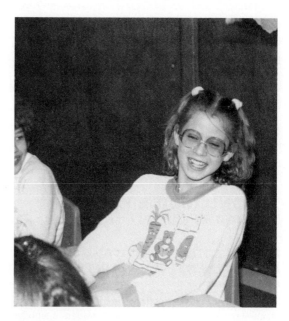

FIG. 11-2 Feelings are important. (Courtesy Galeton Area School District, Galeton, Pennsylvania.)

FAMILY RELATIONSHIPS—A HIGH INTEREST
Unstructured:

Fourth graders had a lot of interest in family. There was deep concern for the happiness of their families—how they could help make the family happy and keep the family together. Many questions were asked about divorce and the effect of divorce on them. They were interested in how babies come about, develop, and are born.

Structured:

Two written questions on family relationships were considered of top interest to fourth graders. They were concerned about how to help their families be happy; and closely tied to this was the concern of how problems may affect their families.

DRUGS—A HIGH INTEREST
Unstructured:

Fourth graders were interested in the effects of drugs on the human body and mind and on relationships; they wondered why people use them; they were concerned about the dangers and whether experimentation is dangerous and leads to habituation or addiction.

Structured:

All four written questions on drugs appeared in the top 15 interests of fourth graders: they wanted to know about drugs and what they do to the body; why people misuse drugs; how drugs affect the way people act; and how the wrong use of drugs may affect the family and community.

FIFTH GRADE PARTIAL SUMMARY OF INTERESTS

MENTAL HEALTH—A HIGH INTEREST
Unstructured:

Students asked about reasons for and how to deal with feelings. They were concerned about friendships, self-concept and decision making. Of lesser interest were how people are alike and different and how to deal with death and grief.

Structured:

Written questionnaire items on mental health from the top 15 interests were: reasons people misuse alcohol and medicine, how drugs affect how people act, how a good friend should act, and how the wrong use of drugs may affect the family and community.

HUMAN BODY/GROWTH AND DEVELOPMENT—A HIGH INTEREST
Unstructured:

Fifth graders wanted to know how the body works and why it works—from why there is swelling after an injury to how the body heals. Prenatal growth patterns and their own growth patterns brought forth many questions.

Causes of handicapping conditions and problems relating to the handicapped were mentioned often. Many questions on heredity also were asked.

Structured:

The top 15 interests that fifth graders expressed on the questionnaire included the causes of handicaps, changes occurring at puberty, the development of the unborn, and the mechanics of the human body.

FAMILY RELATIONSHIPS—A HIGH INTEREST
Unstructured:

One of the most frequently recited responses concerned family happiness. Students wanted to know how to keep a family happy, how to prevent divorce, and how to get over the hurt of divorce. There was some interest in how babies come to be. There was a beginning recognition of boy-girl relationships. There was also concern about child abuse.

Structured:

How to help the family be happy and how problems affect the family were in the top 15 interests from the written questionnaire.

DRUGS—A HIGH INTEREST
Unstructured:

Fifth graders' individual responses were numerous about legal and illegal drugs. Mostly they were interested in the effects of drugs on the mind and body, and in why people take drugs. They were interested in the reasons drugs exist, which drugs were illegal and which ones were harmful, and in how to help people stop taking drugs.

Structured:

All written questions on drugs related to other health areas and appeared here as well as in the other areas. Questions relating to drugs from the top 15 interests were about drugs and what they do to the body; why people misuse alcohol and medicine; how drugs affect how people act; and how the wrong use of drugs may affect the family and the community.

SIXTH GRADE PARTIAL SUMMARY OF INTERESTS

MENTAL HEALTH—A HIGH INTEREST

Unstructured:

The major interests of sixth graders in the area of mental health concerned personal relationships (liking and being liked) (Fig. 11-3), fears and worries (about family, dark, crime), suicide (causes, prevention, helping friends), and feelings (helping others, controlling emotions, effects on health, releasing emotions without hurting others, and understanding behavior of others).

Structured:

The item, "Ways to say no if your friends are pressuring you to use drugs," was the second highest item of interest on the written questionnaire.

FAMILY RELATIONSHIPS—A HIGH INTEREST

Unstructured:

Teenage pregnancy concerned sixth graders; they wanted to know why it happens and the effect on all concerned. A high interest topic was family; family harmony, parenting (caring for children), and child abuse. There was some interest in boy-girl relationships.

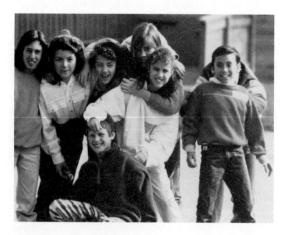

FIG. 11-3 Friendships contribute to mental health. (Courtesy Michigan Department of Education.)

Structured:

Appearing in the top 15 interests from the written questionnaire were the effects of pregnancy on the unwed teenaged girl, the responsibility of the boy, and others.

DRUGS—A HIGH INTEREST

Unstructured:

The interest in drugs, including alcohol and tobacco, was high. The topics of concern centered on the effects of drugs and why they are being used. Sixth graders expressed concern about why drugs are sold and how to avoid them, or how to help others avoid them.

Structured:

The top two interests of sixth graders on the written questionnaire concerned how drugs, including aspirin, alcohol, and speed, affect people's minds and bodies, and ways to say no if friends are pressuring one to use drugs.

PHYSICAL WELL-BEING—A HIGH INTEREST

Unstructured:

The major topics that emerged were exercise (its effect, types, how much), grooming (skin care, evaluating products, relationships to health and stress), and being healthy in general (how one becomes healthy and how one knows if one is healthy).

Structured:

How to be physically fit was the third most popular item on the written questionnaire.

HUMAN BODY/GROWTH AND DEVELOPMENT—A HIGH INTEREST

Unstructured:

Sixth graders wanted to know about prenatal growth and development (how food, drugs, and disease affect healthy development), and about how they themselves mature (the differences, reasons for changes, and the effect these changes will have on their future). They asked about the structure and function of the body (how it grows, looks, works, and changes—especially the reproductive system). There was high interest in the handicapped person (what help is available, including changing environmental barriers; how handicaps affect people's lives and their families, and how they all cope emotionally and physically). There was expressed interest in genetics (inherited diseases, feelings about incurable hereditary diseases, birth defects, and what one can inherit).

Structured:

In the top 15 interests of sixth graders from the written questionnaire was the item, "What causes changes in the body when a girl becomes a woman and a boy becomes a man?"

SEVENTH GRADE PARTIAL SUMMARY OF INTERESTS

MENTAL HEALTH—A HIGH INTEREST
Unstructured:

Seventh graders seemed to have a preoccupation with suicide. They wanted to know why people do it, how to prevent it, and how to talk people out of it. They stated high interest in stress—its causes, effects, and prevention—and in coping mechanisms. Many comments appeared on worries and fears: how to get rid of them, facing them, and whether or not to share them. How to be a good friend was high on the students' interest list. They wanted to know how to select a good friend. Other topics that received comments were: self-concept, feelings, coping with problems, peer pressure, and relating to others.

Structured:

Two items appeared in the top 15 interests from the written questionnaire: the causes and preventions of suicide, and ways to say no if one's friends are pressuring the use of drugs.

FAMILY RELATIONSHIPS—A HIGH INTEREST
Unstructured:

The major topic of concern for seventh graders was the unmarried pregnant teenager. They were concerned about why such pregnancies occur, how to help a friend who is pregnant, the effect on all involved, and having healthy babies. Family relationships were of high interest. They wanted to understand problems families have, how they could help and not hurt family members, and how they themselves affect their families. Areas of medium interest were child abuse, babies, and child care.

Structured:

Two written questionnaire items relating to family were on the list of the top 15 interests of seventh graders. One

item was the effects of pregnancy on unmarried teenagers and all concerned. The other item was what love is and how one might know if he/she is really in love.

DRUGS—A HIGH INTEREST
Unstructured:

Seventh graders were interested in the effects of drugs, including alcohol and tobacco. They were interested in why people use drugs and abuse drugs. They wanted to know about types of drugs and about the legal control of drugs.

Structured:

Three questionnaire items were in the top 15 interests of seventh graders. The number one interest was how drugs, including aspirin, caffeine, alcohol, and speed affect people's minds and bodies. The other two items concerned ways to say no if friends are pressuring one to use drugs; and how drugs, including alcohol, tobacco, tranquilizers, and marijuana, might cause injury to self or others.

EIGHTH GRADE PARTIAL SUMMARY OF INTERESTS

DRUGS—A HIGH INTEREST
Unstructured:

Eighth graders wanted to know everything about legal and illegal drugs, especially how they affect the mind and body. The impression given by the students' comments was that they wanted information, not advice. They were not too eager to try drugs, but they wanted to know what drugs really do, why people take them, how to help people in trouble with drugs.

Structured:

Three written questionnaire items were on the list of top interests of eighth graders. They were how drugs, including aspirin, caffeine, alcohol, and speed affect people's minds and bodies; ways to say no when friends are pressuring one to use drugs; and how drugs might cause one to injure oneself or others.

NUTRITION—A HIGH INTEREST
Unstructured:

Eighth graders wanted to know the effect foods have on the body, which foods are best, the amount needed, how food and disease are related, and the effect of nutrition on a developing baby. There was special interest in weight control, such as why people have trouble controlling weight, how to diet for physical fitness, how to lose weight in a healthy way, why some labels do not list calories, the effect of dieting, what are healthy snacks, how to diet when eating out, and the effects of candy on appetite. Another topic of some interest was world hunger.

Structured:

Questionnaire items of most importance to eighth graders included: how to determine if one is eating so one will grow and stay healthy; how exercise, work, and stress affect food eaten; world hunger and its effects; the importance of breakfast; and fast foods, food processing, and food additives.

FAMILY RELATIONSHIPS—A HIGH INTEREST

Unstructured:

Eighth graders were extremely interested in family, the effect on one's lifespan, how families influence children, how to promote closeness, exploration of "rules for fighting" to prevent hurting family members, how to be honest among family members, how to raise children properly, effective discipline, divorce and its effects on family members, child abuse (why it occurs, options, where to go for help), and adoption.

Another big topic of interest was human sexuality. The topic of most concern dealt with problems surrounding pregnancies of unmarried teenagers. Students wanted to know how it affects the child, the parents of the teenagers, and the teenagers themselves—including the boy. There was some interest in birth control; that is legality, types, vasectomy. They recognized the need to know the consequences of early sexual behavior; they wanted some understanding of how changes in feeling occur and how to handle them. They also wanted to discuss the responsible boy-girl relationships, and especially how to say "no" to sexual activity.

Structured:

Two written questionnaire items appeared on the list of the top 15 interests: the effects of pregnancy of unmarried teenagers on all concerned, and what love is.

MENTAL HEALTH—A HIGH INTEREST

Unstructured:

Students were interested in suicide, stress, relating to others, coping skills, and understanding feelings. They wanted to know causes and preventions of suicide, indications that someone might try suicide, and how to cope after a friend has committed suicide. In regard to stress, they wanted to know both the physical and mental effects, how to overcome it, and how peer pressure creates it. Relating to others seemed to revolve around brother-sister relationships, coping with bullies, what love is, making and keeping friends, and expressing oneself comfortably. Coping skills related to peer pressure, shyness, understanding oneself (what is normal, how to be happy), and how to reduce fears and worries were important. Understanding feelings include how to express them responsibly, how to control one's temper, depression, and causes of fears and worries.

Structured:

Eighth graders placed the causes and prevention of suicide in their top 15 items of interest. Also of concern were ways to say "no" if one's friends are pressuring one to use drugs.

Student needs. Student needs generally fall into two groups: those that are *felt* by children and those that are prevalent health and safety problems but are *unfelt* by children. *Felt needs* are the wants and desires of students that can be expressed in *interest surveys* such as the one completed in Washington state. *Unfelt needs* are health problems and concerns from other sources and those expressed by people other than pupils. Such information comes from mortality and morbidity statistics; accident statistics; growth and development characteristics of children; state laws regarding health instruction areas; local, state, and national health departments; voluntary, commercial, and professional health agencies and organizations; pupils' health and absenteeism records; and other sources. Some of the people who can provide information about health problems of children include parents, teachers, nurses, physicians, dentists, and officials in health departments and health agencies.

Although large school districts and those in charge of statewide curriculum projects may be able to conduct extensive surveys of student interests and needs, smaller districts may have to rely on other sources of data. Some of these data sources include governmental agencies (particularly the Division of Adolescent and School Health of the Centers for Disease Control and Prevention), state departments of health and of education, various voluntary and private health agencies, and even private foundations. Regardless of where students live, some basic needs are common to all. Such things as the need to feel safe, good nutrition, intellectual stimulation, good dental care, and being nurtured all should be foundation elements when planning curricula.

In an effort to identify some basic standards that would represent minimal attainments for health education by school children and adolescents, the American Cancer Society sponsored a national effort to identify what is being proposed as National Health Education Standards: Achieving Health Literacy.* The work of a special joint committee of representatives from the Association for the Advancement of Health Education, the American School Health Association, and the School Health Education and Services Section of the American Public Health Association resulted in the creation of seven basic standards that can be used to provide a strong basis for the development of a comprehensive school health education program. Each standard includes suggested performance indicators that may be used to assess whether the standard is attained by students (Table 11-1). At present, a specific effort is underway to develop a series of evaluation instruments that can be used in conjunction with the National Standards.

Several unmet health needs surfaced in the National Adolescent Student Health Survey. The health behaviors and beliefs of over 11,000 students in grades 8 and 10 were reported in this study. Areas covered in the study included injury prevention; suicide; AIDS; sexually transmitted diseases; violence; the use of tobacco, drugs, and alcohol; nutrition; and consumer skills. The following examples illustrate how unmet needs can be identified from this type of survey.

*Joint Committee on National Health Education Standards: *National health education standards*, Atlanta, 1995, American Cancer Society.

AIDS. Students had much correct information about AIDS that might be attributed to intensive campaigns at the national, state, or local levels to combat the spread of the disease. However, the findings reveal some common misconceptions about AIDS transmission and dangerous attitudes related to AIDS. Instruction must focus on surfacing and correcting misconceptions that increase the risk of contracting AIDS (see Appendix A).

Suicide. The percentage of students who reported that they have "seriously thought" about committing suicide and have "actually tried" to commit suicide underscores the importance of suicide prevention efforts. More than half the students have known someone who tried to commit suicide. Suicide prevention therefore must focus not only on those who might contemplate suicide, but also on students who might have to deal with suicide by others. More than half of all students could not locate a community resource for suicide prevention. This suggests a need to make students aware of existing resources and also to motivate them to use community services.

Nutrition. The survey revealed that the eating habits of students are often incongruent with their nutrition knowledge. Although 73% of students knew that eating fatty foods may cause heart problems, they reported diets high in fat content. In addition, many respondents did not know that the maximum safe weight loss per week is 1 to 2 pounds. This information suggests that decision-making skills and access to healthy food and accurate information should be addressed in nutrition education.

The illustrative units found in Appendix B include a broad approach to pupils' interests and needs.

SCOPE AND SEQUENCE

To determine the scope and sequence of health teaching in the elementary school program, it is necessary to consider the needs and interests of children of all age levels from kindergarten throughout the elementary school. Many state departments of education produce sample scope and sequence charts to provide guidance to local school districts. These state documents are usually based on research, literature reviews, and advice from teachers, parents, and other experts. They provide an excellent point of reference for people charged with the responsibility of developing health education programs in local districts. Table 11-3 contains an illustrative scope and sequence chart published by the Wisconsin Department of Public Education.*

Organized health instruction should be provided at all grade levels throughout the elementary school. There are a number of important reasons why it should be offered at all levels. First, the body of knowledge concerning health and healthful living in the modern world is so extensive that it is necessary to offer it over a period of years to adequately impart the knowledge needed. Second, there is a need for a certain amount of health knowledge at all grade levels, including kindergarten. The degree of maturity of children in the elementary grades is such that they should not receive the extensive knowledge needed for adult life. Yet it is very important that instruction be given and that the various phases of health and healthful living be introduced to the children as rapidly as their maturity and level of intelligence will permit.

Logic indicates that it is much easier to establish proper habits of health and healthful living early in the child's life. Also, the child needs to practice good health and safety habits just as much at an early age as later. Therefore it seems sound to teach as much about health as early as possible, considering the stages of maturity of the children. An example of this is in the area of nutrition, which is a part of the health education program at practically all grade levels. The subject of nutrition should be introduced and developed as far as the ability of the children at any particular

age level permits, for nutrition is a functional part of the life of the primary-age child just as it is of an older child. Even though primary-age children are not mature enough to be given all the safety information they need for life, it is very important that they know as much about safety as possible to safeguard their lives while growing up. As an example, the failure to teach elementary schoolchildren certain facts about pedestrian, bicycle, and traffic safety could result in a child's death or permanent disability.

What then can we consider to be properly included in the course of study for health and safety in our elementary schools? As we know, the needs of communities, states, and regions may differ somewhat in that some problems are specific for certain localities.

In general, research, experience, and surveys have shown that the elementary health curriculum should include units on nutrition; consumer health; growth; exercise; sleep; rest and relaxation; dental health; eyes and ears; family life and health; mental health; safety; first aid; alcohol, tobacco, and other drugs; body mechanics; structure, function, and care of the body; control of diseases; medical and dental care; community health problems; and chronic diseases. All of these areas are also easily integrated throughout the National Health Education Standards (see Table 11-1). Many of these areas are covered in the illustrative material found in Appendix B.

Special Education

Although often mainstreamed into regular classrooms, students in special education need to be provided with learning experiences in health education. They have problems and interests similar to those of the so-called normal students. For those with mental disabilities, much of what is used in the regular program in sexuality education can be adapted to a simpler presentation. Also the use of more visual aids and repetition is necessary. For those who have cerebral palsy, special toothbrushes and prophylactic implements can be prepared for oral health. Teachers and therapists can develop their own items, make adapta-

---

*Wisconsin Department of Public Instruction: *A guide to curriculum planning in health education,* Madison, WI, 1985, The Department.

TABLE 11-3 Wisconsin State Level Scope and Sequence and Recommended Time Allotment for Specific Grade Levels

	Recommended number of periods per year* 1 year = 34 weeks				Recommended number of periods per semester	
	K	1-2	3-4	5-6	7-8-9	10-11-12
	45 min per wk. 1 period = 15 min	75 min per wk. 1 period = 25 min	100 min per wk. 1 period = 25 min	125 min per wk. 1 period = 50 min	1 course, meeting 90 periods in a semester. 1 period = 50 min	1 course, meeting 90 periods in a semester. 1 period = 50 min

	Grade levels								
School health education Major content areas for classroom instruction	**15-min periods**	**25-min periods**				**50-min periods**			
	K	1	2	3	4	5	6	7-8-9	10-11-12
I. Accident prevention and safety	15	12	12	15	15	6	5	5	14
II. Community health	0	0	0	6	6	5	5	5	5
III. Consumer health	0	0	0	6	6	5	5	10	8
IV. Environmental health	0	0	0	6	6	5	5	10	10
V. Family life education	6	9	9	12	12	10	10	15	12
VI. Mental and emotional health	18	18	18	18	18	13	15	12	8
VII. Nutrition	18	18	18	18	18	10	10	5	5
VIII. Personal health	18	18	18	18	18	13	12	10	9
IX. Prevention and control of disease	6	6	6	6	6	3	3	3	4
X. Substance use and abuse	6	9	9	15	15	15	15	10	10
Total periods	87	90	90	120	120	85	85	85	85

*The recommended periods for a year or semester *do not* necessarily mean that all instruction should be completed in that specific content area in consecutive lessons.
Reprinted with permission from the Wisconsin Department of Public Instruction.

tions, and work with school nurses to explore community resources for assistance.

Many mainstreamed students are limited in social skills and have low self-esteem. Increasingly teachers report that when mainstreamed students are placed in small, heterogeneous cooperative learning groups and are assigned specific roles, their achievement and self-esteem increases. Additional information about cooperative learning is found in Chapter 12. A suggested health educa-

tion program usable in a classroom where children have physical and mental disabilities is in Table 11-4.

Health Education Curriculum for Preschool Programs

American educators, encouraged by parents, political leaders, and public officials, have been moving quickly to accept new levels of responsibility

TABLE 11-4 Health Education for Special Children

Areas	Levels*				
	I	**II**	**III**	**IV**	**V**
Safety	*Emergencies* Awareness and simple first aid Communication Report	*Traveling* Pedestrian Passenger Bicycle	*School* Classroom Building Playground	*Home* General Fire and electricity Appliances and equipment	*Recreation* Environment Use of equipment and games Bicycle and camping
Mental health	*Self-acceptance* Physical abilities and limitations Mental abilities and limitations Cultural and social differences	*Acceptance of others* Physical abilities Mental abilities and limitations Cultural and social differences	*Values* Personal Home and school Community and national	*Adjustment to stress* School Home Community	
Family living	*Roles in family* Recognizing roles Learning roles Accepting changing roles	*Home management and maintenance* Supervised responsibilities Simple independent responsibilities Self-directed responsibilities	*Family and child care* Supervised responsibility Simple independent responsibilities Self-directed responsibilities	*Sex education* Sex organs Reproduction	
Nutrition	*Foods* Sources Types Components	*Diet* Selection of basic food Planning of daily menus Effects of components	*Preparation and preservation of foods* Cleaning and storing Preparation of food for meals Preservation of foods	*Health problems* Weight Vitality Allergies	
Body care and personal hygiene	*Cleanliness* Routine Grooming Body changes	*Respect and protection of body parts* Dental care	*Rest and exercise* Awareness of need Understanding of need Ways and means	*Proper clothing and shelter* Awareness of need Understanding of need Ways and means	

TABLE 11-4 Health Education for Special Children—cont'd

Areas	Levels*				
	I	**II**	**III**	**IV**	**V**
Disease and illness	*Communicable disease* Symptoms Causes Treatment	*Sanitation* Personal Home and school Community	*Personal care* Awareness Communication Treatment	*Health services* Knowledge of community Knowledge and location of services When and how to use	

*Refers to stages of learning progression. Children move from level to level upward when ready regardless of grade.
Prepared by a group of special education teachers in Ellensburg, Washington.

for the education of young children. No longer the exclusive province of the very rich or the very poor, preschool education now holds the potential for greater academic achievement, less at-risk behavior in the teen years, and enhanced educational opportunity for children from all economic sectors. Although experts differ about the specifics of formal education programs for preschoolers, there appears to be general acceptance that (1) children should be offered learning opportunities consistent with their levels of development; (2) the curriculum must provide for all areas of the child's physical, emotional, social, and cognitive development; (3) the educational experiences should match the child's abilities and interests; (4) language development opportunities—including both speaking and listening comprehension—must be emphasized; (5) activities should progress from simple to complex, from concrete to abstract; and (6) there should be a balance between spontaneous child-initiated experiences and teacher-initiated experiences.

Preschool programs should include planned curricula in health education. The types of information in this chapter, including the unit materials that are categorically listed in Appendix B and the activities in Chapter 12 at the primary grade levels, are useful. Teachers will need to select the applicable sections and organize them into suitable units and lessons. Some years ago the U.S. Office of Child Development Project Head Start prepared a curriculum guide useful to teachers. The following represents a suggested content outline adapted from that reference.

All About Me

My body (inside, outside, functions of body systems)
Who am I? (sex, race, ethnic group)
Real me (How do I feel inside? happy, sad, angry, afraid, lonely, and so forth)

Accident Prevention and First Aid

Home
Fire
Playground
To and from school
Dangerous strangers

Disease Control

Germs
Infections
Colds
Coughs
Immunizations and other control

Dental Health

Decay
Brushing and flossing
Sugar foods

Nutrition

Selection of nutritious items

Rest, Sleep and Exercise

Need for and adequate amounts

Who Helps to Take Care of Health

Family (parents, physician, teacher, school nurse, others)

THE UNIT IN HEALTH TEACHING

The unit approach is one of the best methods available for organizing more meaningful learning experiences. Beyond this, the unit helps ensure a sound, logical presentation of subject matter. It represents an effective blending of psychological and logical organization of topics and concepts.

In preparing the objectives for the units found in this chapter, the taxonomy (classification) of educational goals developed by Bloom and associates* and widely utilized in curriculum development in the United States was used. Although developed decades ago, it continues to provide an effective basis for preparing behavioral objectives.

TAXONOMY OF OBJECTIVES

COGNITIVE DOMAIN (KNOWLEDGE/UNDERSTANDINGS)

Know—define, name, relate, list, recall, explain, state, recite, tell

Comprehend—predict, draw conclusions, diagram, illustrate, discuss, classify, recognize, identify, report, review, describe

Apply—solve, translate, demonstrate, dramatize, illustrate

Analyze—identify, distinguish, establish criteria, conclude, interpret, translate, classify, criticize, debate, question, examine

Synthesize—plan, integrate, summarize, develop, compare, design, create, prepare, construct, formulate, compose

Evaluate—compare, contrast, differentiate, judge, rate, appraise, select, assess, measure, estimate

---

*Modified from Bloom B, editor: *Taxonomy of educational objectives. Handbook I: cognitive domain,* New York, 1956, David McKay; Krathwohl DR, Bloom BS, Masia BB: *Taxonomy of educational objectives. Handbook II: affective domain,* New York, 1964, David McKay.

AFFECTIVE DOMAIN (ATTITUDES: FEELINGS, APPRECIATIONS, VALUES)

Attend (be receptive)—talk about, be supportive, listen, display interest, be attentive

Respond (be impressed)—ask questions, react, give opinions, bring things to class

Value (rate highly)—accept, support

ACTION DOMAIN (PRACTICES)

Act, eat, wash, brush, buy, avoid, refrain from, demonstrate, choose, place, obey

Illustrative Partial Units for Primary, Intermediate, and Upper Grades

The illustrative partial units in Appendix B cover many of the important health content areas teachers may use in planning for health instruction. Note that they follow the basic principles previously identified and give consideration to the new definition of health, the concept approach, and values.

Appendix B is designed to help those teaching elementary school health. It saves many hours of work by providing an outline of general content in each area plus hundreds of sample concepts and objectives. In essence it provides the raw material for each teacher to begin planning for his/her basic health lessons. This material has the additional advantage of covering the entire K through 8 grade sequence. Thus a teacher who faces a grade level assignment change can turn to the material in Appendix B to help reduce the burden of creating health units appropriate for his/her new assignment.

HOW DOES THE TEACHER PLAN?

Teachers can plan for health instruction programs in schools in several ways. They involve procedures that organize learning experiences into a number of useful patterns. The materials presented in this chapter together with those provided in Chapters 9 and 12 through 14 and Appendixes B, D, E, and F will be helpful. The guidelines should be followed in the sequence listed for the *direct* teaching of health in classrooms where there are no health curricula:

1. Identify the needs and interests of students and use this information to establish a scope of topics
2. Determine a logical sequence for each topic
3. Identify student learning objectives
4. Identify school and community resources for health instruction curriculum guides, teaching aids, and health education specialists
5. Prepare a series of units from the scope and content previously identified
6. Prepare lesson plans or modules from the units

In those school districts where curriculum guides are available, teachers may wish to start with procedure 3 or 4. Regardless, it is important that teachers and school district administrators alike take heed of what the National Commission on the Role of the School and the Community in Improving Adolescent Health stated in *Code Blue,* "Provide a new kind of health education at the earliest appropriate age, an education that ensures students have the knowledge and skills to lead healthy lives and avoid health-risking behaviors."*

Classroom Scope and Sequence

Using the material or one of the procedures described in this chapter will enable a teacher to identify students' needs and interests. A meeting with the school nurse may help to obtain this information quickly. These data can then be grouped into topical areas as illustrated in Table 11-1 and Table 11-2 (under *Area*). The sequence in terms of a monthly schedule as seen in Table 11-2 is merely illustrative and may need modification during the school year. The teacher may desire to organize unit teaching in accordance with many of the Health Observances in the box on pp. 296-297.

---

*National Commission on the Role of the School and the Community in Improving Adolescent Health: *Code Blue: uniting for healthier youth,* Alexandria, VA, 1990, National Association of State Boards of Education.

The mental health unit permeates the entire school curriculum, and portions may be covered whenever it is deemed appropriate. Teachers should feel free to modify this arrangement if a teachable moment arises that will permit introduction of an area when it will have greater student interest and motivation.

Unit Construction

By definition, unit construction refers to a procedure that organizes learning experiences related to a particular topic or unifying purpose—for example, nutrition or dental health. The content of a unit generally includes these elements: topic, grade level, number of lessons or time, concepts, goals or objectives, content, teaching/learning activities, teaching aids, evaluation, and integration possibilities. The partial illustrative units in Appendix B contain content, concepts, and objectives. The teaching techniques, the teaching aids, and the evaluation suggestions can be selected by the individual teacher from the material found in Chapters 12 through 14.

Table 11-2 is a partial illustrative unit or a series of units that may also be used by the individual teacher as a yearly scope-and-sequence arrangement prepared by an individual teacher. This unit outline can help teachers plan a health instruction program for a semester or for an entire year. It will be necessary to develop lesson plans or modules from this material that will also include the objectives to be achieved and other relevant information.

It might be advisable to provide information about ways to integrate this unit into language arts, social studies, science, and other curriculum areas. Table 11-2 provides an illustration of how this material might be included.

In planning the development of the unit, the teacher should check local school and community resources for material that will help in unit construction or lesson planning. Some of the items that need to be identified include resource personnel, curriculum guides, films, videos, software, models, charts, books, pamphlets, and other

Calendar of Health Observances

Following is a list of month-, week-, and day-long health observances.

JANUARY

Birth Defects Prevention Month
National Eye Health Care Month
National Volunteer Blood Donor Month
National Autism Awareness Week
National Glaucoma Awareness Week
Sight Saving Sabbath
School Nurse Day

FEBRUARY

American Heart Month
AMD Awareness Month
National Children's Dental Health Month
National Cardiac Rehabilitation Week
National Child Passenger Safety Awareness Week
National Girls and Women in Sports Day

MARCH

Cataract Awareness Month
Hemophilia Month
Mental Retardation Month
National Kidney Month
National Chronic Fatigue Syndrome Awareness Month
National Eye Donor Month
National Nutrition Month
Red Cross Month
National PTA Drug and Alcohol Awareness Week
Save Your Vision Week
National School Breakfast Week
Children and Hospitals Week
National Poison Prevention Week
National Pulmonary Rehabilitation Week
American Diabetes Alert

APRIL

National Alcohol Awareness Month
National Cancer Control Month
National Child Abuse Prevention Month
Occupational Therapy Month
Sports Eye Safety Month
National Building Safety Week
National Medical Lab Week
Minority Cancer Awareness Week
National Organ and Tissue Donor Awareness Week
National Preschool Immunization Week
Alcohol-Free Weekend
World Health Day

MAY

Asthma and Allergy Awareness Month
Better Hearing and Speech Month
Better Sleep Month
Clean Air Month
Correct Posture Month
Huntington's Disease Awareness Month
Mental Health Month
National Arthritis Month
National Bike Month
National Digestive Disease Awareness Month
National High Blood Pressure Month
National Melanoma/Skin Cancer Detection and Prevention Month
National Neurofibromatosis Month
National Physical Fitness and Sports Month
National Sight-Saving Month
National Trauma Awareness Month
Older Americans Month
Stroke Awareness Month
Tuberous Sclerosis Awareness Month
Buckle America Week
National Alcohol- and Other Drug-Related Birth Defects Awareness Week
National Hospital Week
National Nursing Home Week
National Osteoporosis Prevention Week
National Physical Education and Sports Week
National Running and Fitness Week
National Safe Boating Week
National Senior Smile Week
Safe Kids Week
The Great American Workout
National Employee Health and Fitness Day
World No Tobacco Day
World Red Cross Day

Calendar of Health Observances—cont'd

JUNE

Dairy Month
Firework Safety Month
National Scleroderma Awareness Month
Helen Keller Deaf-Blind Awareness Week
National Safety Week

JULY

Hemochromatosis Screening Awareness Month
National Therapeutic Recreation Week

AUGUST

Foot Health Month
National Water Quality Month

SEPTEMBER

Bed Check Month
Children's Eye Health and Safety Month
Christmas Seals Campaign
Leukemia Society Month
National Cholesterol Education Month
National Pediculosis Prevention Month
National Sickle Cell Month
Teen Sleeplessness Month
Treatment Works Month
National Rehabilitation Week

OCTOBER

Celiac Sprue Awareness Month
Child Health Month
Family Health Month
National Breast Cancer Awareness Month
National Dental Hygiene Month
National Family Sexuality Education Month
National Disability Employment Awareness Month
National Liver Awareness Month
National Lupus Awareness Month

National Physical Therapy Month
National Spina Bifida Month
National Spinal Health Month
Sudden Infant Death Syndrome Awareness Month
Talk About Prescriptions Month
Auto Battery Safety Month
Mental Illness Awareness Week
National Nurse-Midwifery Week
Child Health Day
American Heart Walk
National Fire Prevention Week
National School Lunch Week
National Infection Control Week
National School Bus Safety Week
National Collegiate Alcohol Awareness Week
World Food Day
National Mammography Day
American Heart Association's Heartfest
National Adult Immunization Week
National Red Ribbon Week

NOVEMBER

Child Safety and Protection Month
Diabetic Eye Disease Awareness Month
National Alzheimer's Awareness Month
National Diabetes Month
National Epilepsy Month
National Hospice Month
Great American Smokeout
National Home Care Week

DECEMBER

National Drunk and Drugged Driving Prevention Month
Safe Toys and Gifts Month
National Aplastic Anemia Awareness Week
World AIDS Day

Courtesy American School Health Association, PO Box 708, Kent, OH 44240.

teaching aids. School nurses can often be of considerable help in this regard.

Lesson Plans/Modules

Lesson plans or modules are step-by-step procedures to be followed by the teacher in one session or for a given period of time. They, therefore, may not be completed in one day. Lesson plans/modules are segments of instruction that are related to a particular subject matter area. They are prepared from the units that have been developed, and their content may include concepts, objectives, content, and other information (see p. 298). They should

LESSON PLANS

Illustration of a Lesson Plan

Unit: Prevention and control of disease
Level: Grade 6
Specific topical key: Causes of premature death
Approximate time: 50 minutes
Objective: The students will name the four most common causes of early death of Americans today:
Activities: Following a lecture on the most common causes of early death of Americans—heart disease, cancer, stroke and accidents—the students will create an original theme advertising campaign
   The students will work in cooperative teams to plan their campaign. They must include promoting healthy behaviors that can help reduce the risk for the four major causes of early death.
Resources needed: Magazines, video clips of television advertisements.
Evaluation focus:
   ☒ Knowledge   ☒ Attitude   ☒ Problem solving   ☒ Teamwork
Teacher's notes (things to change):

also provide for a presentation or learning sequence that enables teachers to know exactly what to do at any time, how to introduce content, how to use various teaching aids, and how to involve students. An important component of the lesson plan is the teacher's notes. Here is where the teacher can make suggestions about what worked well or not so well, and what might be done differently the next time this particular lesson is taught. A module may differ somewhat from a lesson plan in that it contains all of the teaching aids such as charts, illustrations, tests and other materials ready for use by any teacher. A teacher may have to prepare a lesson plan without all of the items found in a module and therefore must develop them before using the lesson plan. In some instances a single unit around an instructional area may not be prepared, but rather several modules centering on a given subject area are developed. This arrangement could be considered to be equivalent to a unit in organization.

Illustrations of lesson plans containing varying degrees of detail, beginning with a minimum of information and progressing toward a greater amount of detail are provided on pp. 300-303.

SUMMARY

Effective health teaching in the classroom revolves around a well-organized curriculum conceived from a scope and sequence based on known growth and developmental patterns and student needs and interests. The curriculum itself must be founded on sound principles applicable to all subject area disciplines. It must also include those factors that are unique to the teaching of health such as physiological, sociological, psychological, and spiritual aspects of health.

The conceptual approach, first applied to health teaching by a team of health educators under the leadership of Dr. Elena Sliepcevich, has produced a number of landmark papers and documents that still serve as the basis for much of today's curriculum work in health. The conceptual approach is fundamental to the eclectic plan identified in this text. It legitimizes the inclusion of value clarification, holistic health, and decision making into the curriculum.

A relatively new approach to health curriculum development combines content area authorities with teachers, nurses, and parents in collaborative efforts to develop subject matter. This allows for the development of curriculum tailored to specific local needs. However, the fundamental subject matter in health is primarily the same for most schools.

The needs and interests of students are basic sources of information for determining the health curriculum, including the scope and sequence. Local surveys can be undertaken or reference can be made to existing data such as those contained in Students Speak. Another benefit of using these data is that misinformation and misconceptions are often revealed. Attention should be given to all grade levels and to the needs of all students, including children enrolled in preschools.

The unit is a method of organizing lessons within a specific health program. Hundreds of sample concepts and objectives are included in Appendix B for the teacher. Content is outlined in general, but each teacher must seek out additional content for his/her own lessons. This is as it should be, as content in health topics changes rapidly and teachers need to consistently upgrade their knowledge.

Illustrations of lesson plans containing varying degrees of detail are provided to assist the teacher in deciding which might work best. The samples share one common philosophy—they are all student centered. Information contained in this and succeeding chapters has been developed to provide guidance and aid for the teacher so that every lesson is important, relevant, and student centered.

LESSON PLANS

Illustration of a Lesson Plan

Unit: Mental and emotional health
Level: Grade 1
Specific topical key: Self-concept
Approximate time: 50 minutes
Objective: The students will list positive qualities in themselves and others.
Activities: Read the story *The Little Rabbit Who Wanted Red Wings* by Carolyn Sherwin Bailey to your class or, if you prefer, show them the filmstrip that is available.
   Afterward, discuss the book and ask children to fill out the answer sheets.
Script: Do you remember the story of *The Little Rabbit Who Wanted Red Wings?* He always wanted to be anything but what he was. He found out that the best thing to be was himself—a rabbit! There was only one rabbit like him and he decided to be the best he could be. Your job is to be the best that you can be. Just think, there is only one person like you in the whole world. Isn't that great? Now, the little rabbit would like to know more about that special you. Please fill out your answer sheet for him.

Answer sheet:

1. My first name is _____

2. My last name is _____

3. I am _____ years old

4. I am in _____ grade
5. (Really think about this before you write your answer down.) I am special because

_____

_____

6. Draw a picture of "that special me."

Teacher note: This can lead to a discussion about positive qualities others display.
Resources needed: The book and/or filmstrip entitled *The Little Rabbit Who Wanted Red Wings.*

Evaluation focus:
   ☐ Knowledge   ☒ Attitude   ☐ Problem solving
Teacher's notes (things to change):

LESSON PLANS—cont'd

Illustration of a Lesson Plan

Unit: To smoke or not to smoke
Level: Grade 7 or 8
Time needed: About 45 minutes
Previous lesson: Strategies used in advertising
Concept: Advertising may influence the use of tobacco

Goal: The student:

1. Realizes the importance of slogans and advertisements in influencing the use of cigarettes

Objectives: The student:

1. Identifies the appeals and slogans used to influence the use of cigarettes
Content: Advertising appeals: attractive people; glamour and elegance; sex or love; macho image; better taste; beautiful scenery; better filter; low tar and nicotine; sign of adulthood
   Slogans: "You've come a long way, baby"
        "The coolest taste around"
        "Where a man belongs"
   Some reasons for use: sell more cigarettes by trying to appeal to people's psychological needs through social influences—adulthood, peer acceptance, love, beauty, less hazardous to health, strong/powerful/controlled person
   What are advertisers trying to sell? Hope; to be like others

Learning Activities/Procedures:

1. On chalkboard teacher introduces some slogans and appeals obtained from cigarette advertisements brought to class by students.
2. Organize class into small discussion groups with one student as chairperson in charge of each and provide each group with three advertisements. Ask each group to take 20 minutes to analyze the advertisements in terms of: (1) identification of the advertising appeals and slogans and (2) the reasons why these slogans and appeals are used.
3. Reassemble the class, have chairpersons report their information, and tally the findings on the blackboard.
4. Teacher summarizes the essential points and students put information in notebooks.
Evaluation: Teacher observations of student interest in lesson together with the extent of pupil participation
Materials and resources needed: Numerous magazine and newspaper cigarette advertisements; chalkboard
Assignment: Students bring empty cigarette containers to class and are prepared to orally comment on the meaning of the "warning against smoking" found on the package. Also identify the amount of tar and nicotine in the brand of cigarettes. Read appropriate chapter in the assigned text.
Next lesson: Alternatives to use of cigarettes: develop own personality; better self-care; self-image; success in school, job, and recreational skills.
Vocabulary: glamour, elegance, beautiful, nicotine, advertisements, adulthood, attractive

---

Modified from Middleton K: Back to some basics in health lesson planning, *Health Ed* 12:4-8, 1981.

LESSON PLANS—cont'd

A Drug That's Not a Medicine—Grade 3

READY

The student will demonstrate the ability to

1. Describe the physical and behavioral effects of nicotine.

2. List reasons why people use and don't use drugs.

SET

Resources

From the kit

Message poster, "Be smart—don't start"
Definition card, "Nicotine"
Nicotine puzzle and outline

From the guide

Fact sheet, "Nicotine"
Read the **fact sheet**

New Vocabulary

stimulant a drug that speeds up the functioning of the body
tobacco a plant made into products that are often smoked or chewed
nicotine a stimulant drug found in tobacco

GO

Review

1. Remind the class that yesterday they learned about some of the medicines that are used a lot in your community.

Introduction

2. Explain that today you have a special puzzle that will help them learn some important facts about a drug found in tobacco that isn't used as medicine.

3. Ask students if they have ever put something in their mouth that tasted terrible. Ask:
   • What was it?
   • Would you put it in your mouth again?
   Explain that tobacco is like the substances they named because it tastes terrible, but people keep using it because it's hard to stop using it once you start.

Objective

4. Explain that today students will learn about a drug found in tobacco; the drug is called *nicotine.* Explain that they are also going to learn why people use nicotine.

Activity

5. Explain that tobacco has been around for a long, long time. Ask students what products have tobacco in them (*cigarettes, pipes, cigars, chew, snuff, etc.*).

6. Explain to students that nicotine is a *stimulant* drug, which means that taking it speeds up the body.

7. Distribute pieces of the **puzzle** to students in the class so that each student has at least one piece.

8. Place the large **puzzle outline** sheet on the floor (or large table) so that students can gather around the sheet and have easy access to it. Have students come around the puzzle and look over the outline to try and locate where their piece should be placed.

9. Have students start at the head and place their pieces on the outline until the head and messages around the head are complete. Have the students whose pieces made up this area of the puzzle read the statements they created out loud and in unison to the rest of the class. Continue this process for the other parts of the anatomy.

LESSON PLANS—cont'd

Closure

10. Ask students to share a new fact they learned about tobacco (nicotine). Encourage them to make positive, healthy choices like not smoking. Show the **message poster,** "Be smart—don't start." Display the **definition** card.

Extension

11. Have students talk with any adult in his/her home who has used nicotine, asking when and how the adult got started. Have students write down the reasons. If there is no one at home who has used nicotine, the student can ask an adult to share any stories about people he/she knows who have used it. Make a list of the reasons and talk about them with the students. Discuss ways of avoiding starting to use nicotine.

From Roberts HC et al: *Here's looking at you, 2000,* Seattle, 1986, The Comprehensive Health Education Foundation.

QUESTIONS FOR DISCUSSION

1. Who should be responsible for curriculum development in the school?
2. What are the basic principles on which the health curriculum should be based?
3. Why is both formal and informal health education necessary in schools?
4. What is the meaning and significance of the inclusion of values in the curriculum?
5. What is the meaning of the concept approach to curriculum development, and how can it be applied to health education?
6. How is the curriculum in health education determined?
7. To what extent could you use the health interests of children as shown by the Washington study (Students Speak)?
8. What are some of the sources of helpful information in determining health content for elementary pupils?
9. How might the development of National Health Education Standards help those who are responsible for developing the health and safety curriculum?
10. Why is it important to have procedures to follow when developing a health and safety curriculum for schools? What procedures might be followed?
11. What is the fundamental purpose of the unit in health teaching?
12. What is the meaning of the phrase *scope and sequence?*
13. What are the common, essential elements of a good *teaching* unit?
14. What should be the nature of the health education curriculum for students in special education and preschool programs?
15. What must the teacher do to plan for health instruction?
16. How can the broad concept of health (holistic) identified in Chapter 1 be utilized in the development of the health education curriculum?
17. What does the phrase *taxonomy of objectives* mean as identified by Bloom and others, and how can it be used in health education?

SELECTED REFERENCES

American School Health Association, Association for the Advancement of Health Education, and The Society for Public Health Education: *National adolescent student health survey,* Reston, VA, 1989, The Association.

Ames EE: Instructional planning for health education. In Cortese P, Middleton K, editors: *The comprehensive school health challenge,* vol 1, Santa Cruz, CA, 1994, ETR Associates.

Agustine DK, Gruber KD, Hanson LR: Cooperation works! *Educational Leadership* 47(4):4-7, 1989/January, 1990.

Beane, JA: The continuing controversy over affective education, *Educ Leadership* 43(4):4-7, 1985/1986.

Bloom B, editor: *Taxonomy of educational objectives. Handbook I: Cognitive domain,* New York, 1956, David McKay.

Bradley C, editor: *A guide to curriculum planning in health education,* Madison, WI, 1985, Wisconsin Department of Public Instruction.

Cornacchia HJ, Barrett S: *Consumer health: a guide to intelligent decisions,* ed 6, St Louis, 1993, Mosby–Year Book.

Cornacchia HJ, Barrett S: *Shopping for health: an essential guide for products and services,* St Louis, 1982, Mosby–Year Book.

DeFriese GH, Crossland CL, Wilcox BMP, Sowers JG: Comprehensive school health programs: prospects for change in American schools, *J School Health* 60(4):182-187, 1990.

Harmin M: Value clarity, high morality: let's go for both, *Educ Leadership* 45(8):24-31, 1988.

Hawkins DJ, Catalano RF: Broadening the vision of education: schools as health promoting environments, *J School Health* 60(4):178-181, 1990.

Jackson SA, editor: Comprehensive school health education program: innovative practices and issues in setting standards, Washington, DC, 1993, Office of Educational Research and Improvement, Fund for the Improvement and Reform of Schools and Teaching, US Department of Education.

Health and Safety Division: *Health: you've got to be taught,* New York, 1988, Metropolitan Life Insurance.

Krathwohl DR, Bloom BS, Masia BB: *Taxonomy of educational objectives, Handbook II: Affective domain,* New York, 1964, David McKay.

Joint Committee on National Health Education Standards: *National health education standards,* Atlanta, 1995, American Cancer Society.

Kane WM: Planning for a comprehensive school health program. In Cortese P, Middleton K, editors: *The com-*

prehensive school health challenge, vol 1, Santa Cruz, CA, 1994, ETR Associates.

Lieberman A: Collaborative work, *Educ Leadership* 43(5):4-8, 1986.

Maranzo RJ et al: *Dimensions of thinking: a framework for curriculum and instruction*, Alexandria, VA, 1988, Association for Supervision and Curriculum Development.

Middleton K: Back to some basics in health lesson planning, *Health Educ* 12:4-8, 1981.

Nader P: The concept of "comprehensiveness" in the design and implementation of school health programs, *J School Health* 60(4):133-138, 1990.

National School Boards Association: *School health: helping children learn, Leadership reports*, Alexandria, VA, 1991-92, The Association.

Novello A, DeGraw C, Kleinman D: Healthy children ready to learn: an essential collaboration between health and education, *Public Health Rep* 107(1):3-10, 1992.

Perry CL: A conceptual approach to school-based health promotion, Cooperative Edition, *Health Educ* 15(4) and *J School Health* 54(6):33-38, 1984.

Pine P: *Promoting health education in schools—problems and solutions, Critical Issues Report*, Arlington, VA, 1985, American Association of School Administrators.

Raths LE, Harmin M, Simon S: *Values and teaching*, ed 2, Columbus, OH, 1987, Charles E Merrill.

Resnick LB, Klopfer LE, editors: *Toward the thinking curriculum: current cognitive research*, Alexandria, VA, 1989, Association for Supervision and Curriculum Development.

Roberts HC et al: *Here's looking at you, 2000*, Seattle, 1986, The Comprehensive Health Education Foundation.

School Health Education Study, Inc: *Health education: a conceptual approach*, St Paul, 1967, 3M Educational Press.

Stone E: ACCESS: keystones for school health promotion, *J School Health* 60(7):298-300, 1990.

The National Commission on the Role of the School and the Community in Improving Adolescent Health: *Code blue: uniting for healthier youth*, Alexandria, VA, 1990, National Association of State Boards of Education.

Trucano L: *Students speak*, Seattle, 1984, The Comprehensive Health Education Foundation.

Wang MC, Rubenstein JL, Reynolds MC: Clearing the road to success for students with special needs, *Educ Leadership* 43(1):62-65, 1985.

Warger C, editor: *A resource guide to public school early childhood programs*, Alexandria, VA, 1988, Association for Supervision and Curriculum Development.

V

METHODS AND MATERIALS IN HEALTH EDUCATION

12

Methods and Techniques in Health Teaching

KEY CONCEPT

Achievement of positive student health attitudes and practices is increased through the use of pupil-centered methods and techniques in health instruction.

Health cannot be given to people, it demands their participation.

RENE SAUD

PROBLEMS TO SOLVE

You will soon begin your student teaching at the grade level you desire. You have already been told that the first lessons you are expected to teach will be in health. After writing a personal analysis of your strengths and weaknesses as a teacher, identify four teaching methods you are likely to use during your student teaching experience. Explain why you chose these four methods and how they relate to your strengths and weaknesses. Also, identify any additional information you will want before actually using the methods you have selected. What information will you collect as you broaden the various teaching methods you use in the classroom?

HAVING discussed the learner in health education in Chapter 9 and having covered ways to organize for health teaching in Chapter 11, it is now necessary to look at the role of the teacher in changing behavior with specific reference to the learning process.

The teacher is the most important factor in the health education program. The responsibility for organizing, guiding, and directing the learning toward health objectives rests with the teacher. This is accomplished through a familiarity with a wide assortment of teaching activities and experiences. Selection of a variety of methods and techniques that will most efficiently and effectively aid learning and lead to health-educated pupils is necessary. The variety of procedures used by teachers to achieve the practices, attitudes, and knowledge goals of healthful living are called methods or methods of teaching.

WHAT IS METHOD?

Method is a broad term in teaching referring to the organized and systematic ways used by teachers to achieve purposes or objectives. Method is often said to be the "how to" of teaching. It represents what the teacher does. *Technique* is a concrete word describing more specific ways to attain goals. Techniques may be called activities, experiences, or teaching/learning activities. These represent what the student does to attain behavioral objectives. Together, methods and techniques are procedures designed to help interpret and translate scientific information to pupils.

The mere selection of appropriate activities or experiences by the teacher does not ensure effective learning. These related factors must also receive consideration:

- The maintenance of good pupil relationships provides an atmosphere conducive to learning. Understanding children's physical, emotional, social, and intellectual characteristics; treating pupils fairly and firmly; and using democratic procedures contribute to an appropriate social climate in the classroom.

- Teachers must recognize and provide for differences in abilities, aptitudes, and achievements in pupils. For example, some students may need more help in learning how to floss and brush their teeth, whereas others may require special guidance to complete survey and research projects.

- Methods may be teacher or pupil centered. Teacher-centered methods are those dominated by the teacher and are usually more formal in approach. They may include recitations, question-and-answer sessions, and lectures. Pupil-centered methods refer to the nondirective processes that allow for greater student participation. They may include demonstrations, excursions, constructive activities, discussion, and small group involvement. Greater emphasis must be given to those activities involving pupils if health attitudes and behavior changes are to occur.

WHAT ARE THE TYPES OF METHODS?

Methods are difficult to categorize because the variations and combinations used by teachers are so numerous. In addition, their close relationship to instructional materials adds to the complexity of grouping. Although methods may be categorized differently, the types listed here are classifications that have been found effective and useful in health instruction programs in elementary schools.

- Problem solving
- Construction activities
- Creative activities
- Demonstrations and experiments
- Discussions
- Dramatizations
- Field trips
- Individual and group reports
- Illustrated presentations
- Resource people—guest speakers
- Show and tell time
- Surveys

Problem Solving

The development of the ability to think rationally by students involves application of knowledge to the problems with which they are confronted in the social atmosphere in which they live. Therefore, problem solving is a very important and practical method in health education that will help students make decisions and enhance their achievement of positive pupil health behaviors. It is a general process whereby children learn to solve personal and community health problems through the use of the scientific approach. Pupils learn how to investigate, reason, and think reflectively so that they can differentiate facts from fiction and truths from superstition.

Problem solving is a teaching technique whereby children are presented with specific health questions or situations and they attempt to provide solutions through class discussions. For example, a teacher may present the following situations for pupil reactions:

- What would you do if you were injured at school?
- What would you do if you were injured a long way from home?
- What would you do if a friend tried to persuade you to smoke a cigarette? (Fig. 12-1).

A modification of this procedure would be to present a problem in written form, such as the following:

You were playing in the school yard at lunchtime and cut your leg on a sharp object. The wound was bleeding quite a bit, and you were in pain. Place a check in the box beside the statement below that would best describe what you would do. Be prepared to tell why you would take this action.

1. Obtain a clean cloth and wrap it around the cut ☐
2. Wash the cut with water ☐
3. Press my hand on the cut to try to stop the bleeding ☐
4. Report to the nurse or to my teacher ☐
5. Wait until I arrived at home before doing anything ☐
6. Not do anything ☐
7. Go home ☐

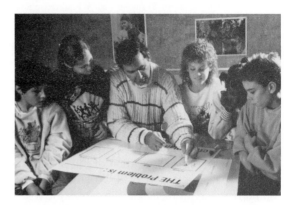

FIG. 12-1 Problem solving and decision making. (Courtesy Michigan Department of Education.)

The teacher may permit pupils to check more than one box and also list sequence of action. Critical review of quotations found in the literature and analysis of newspaper articles, lyrics from popular songs, scenes from movies, and value strategies are additional problem-solving possibilities.

Several illustrations of health problems that may be solved are: How can we protect ourselves from disease? Who are some of the people who help us stay healthy? What foods do we need for growth? How can we prevent accidents? How can we deal with the pressure to use drugs and alcohol? (See Fig. 12-1.) What can be done to stop people from using tobacco products?

The sequential steps that teachers can use to guide pupils in solving health problems are as follows:

- Recognition of the problem
- Definition of the problem
- Consideration of alternative ways to proceed
- Selection of methods of procedure
- Collection of pertinent data
- Selection, interpretation, and organization of data
- Preparation of conclusions or alternatives
- Application of conclusions or alternatives to the solution, problem, or plan of action
- Evaluation of solution or solutions

Practice is necessary for the acquisition of problem-solving skills. Repetitive involvement develops student confidence when confronted with having to make health decisions. Problem solving techniques include brainstorming, clarification of values, and cooperative learning activities,

Brainstorming—a type of problem solving. Brainstorming is a group attempt to solve a well-defined problem by offering any solution that comes to mind, no matter how extreme. The purpose is to generate ideas quickly and in large quantity by the free association of ideas. Following a stated time period of discussion, students should rank the problem solutions from the worst to the least acceptable.

These procedures should be followed:

- Encourage a free flow of ideas no matter how far out; permit free thinking
- Do not permit critical judgments, negative comments, or evaluations
- Restate the problem and start sorting out and refining ideas
- Evaluate the ideas objectively and narrow them to one or more solutions
- Summarize and assign responsibilities

These problems are suitable for brainstorming. How can we encourage people to refrain from smoking cigarettes? How can we improve safety at school? How can we convince people to refrain from the use of drugs? How can we persuade people to eat a balanced diet of foods?

This procedure has value because it allows for freedom of expression, an exchange of ideas, and creative thinking. It has limitations in that the teacher may find it difficult to maintain class control, and it may not be productive if the class is quite large. It also demands clarification of ideas, well-planned organization, and follow-up for effective results.

Values clarification—a type of problem solving. All students bring to school a variety of differing values from their environmental experiences and the cultures in which they are born. Students can easily be confused about their own values and may have prejudices regarding those of their classmates. Teachers are in a position to help provide understanding about pupils, values and respect for the values of others.

Values clarification involves a series of strategies or methods for helping students learn about values. It does not attempt to teach values per se.

Values clarification strategies are designed to help students review and understand their own as well as society's values. It will help pupils identify the concept of self and search for meaning in life.

It should be understood that although it is often useful to accept students' value statements nonjudgmentally, values clarification theory does not require the teacher to accept *all* student statements in that manner. Nor does it suggest that teachers cease acting as moral leaders. When using this method, teachers should help students learn to think through personal values and understand what it takes to live a committed, value-directed life. Students can be helped to personalize and internalize health education.

In addition, teachers must realize that what they do is as important—maybe even more important—than what they say. For example, the teacher who says "All those turning in their work late will lose ten points" supports values of individual responsibility and punishment. If the teacher says "Let's discuss better ways of getting everyone to turn in work on time," emphasis is given to the values of cooperative responsibility and problem prevention.

When using the value clarification method, teachers should anticipate that students will want to know what values their teacher holds. The teacher should be prepared to respond honestly to the students. The teacher's daily actions should reflect consistency with stated values.

Cooperative team learning. There is a well-established principle of social psychology that people working together toward a common goal can accomplish more than individuals working alone. Practical cooperative learning strategies for classroom use have been developed, researched, and found to be instructionally effective.

Cooperative learning in its basic sense refers to a set of instructorial methods in which students work in small, mixed-ability learning groups. These groups usually have four members—one high achiever, two average achievers, and one low achiever. The students in each group are responsible not only for learning the material being taught, but also for helping their group mates learn it. The group's task is almost always to prepare group members to succeed on individual assessments. This focuses the group activity on explaining ideas, practicing skills, and assessing all members to ensure that they will all be successful. Each student has a role such as recorder, reader of the problem, checker to see that everyone participates, and reporter. It is a good idea for the teacher to keep track of the role of each student so that each student is provided the opportunity to serve in each of the roles over time.

Five basic elements are included in the cooperative learning method.

Positive interdependence. Students must believe they are responsible for both personal learning and the learning of the other members of their group. This is achieved through mutual goals; division of labor; dividing materials, resources, or information among group members; assigning students different roles; and by giving group awards. For a learning situation to be cooperative, students must perceive that they are positively interdependent with other members of their learning group. This makes the concept of **TEAM** (Together Everyone Achieves More) become a reality.

Face-to-face promotive interaction. Students must have the opportunity to explain what they are learning to each other and to help each other understand and complete assignments. The patterns of interaction and verbal interchange among students promoted by positive interdependence affect educational outcomes.

Individual accountability. Each student must demonstrate mastery of the assigned work. The purpose of a learning situation is to maximize the achievement of each individual student and demonstrate the importance of that achievement to the team's achievement.

Social skills. Each student must communicate effectively, provide leadership for the group's work, build and maintain trust among group members, and resolve conflicts constructively within the group. These skills must be taught and students must be motivated to use them for cooperative learning to be successful. Each student must finish his or her assignment before the team or group progresses to the next task. This re-emphasizes the concept of cooperating and working together to attain mutually acceptable and agreeable goals.

Group processing. Groups must stop periodically and assess how well they are working and how their effectiveness may be improved. The teacher may also intervene when necessary to assist the group with the assessment.

To increase the effectiveness of this methodology, the teacher must do some careful planning. Paramount are the identification of objectives and decisions about placing students in groups. The teacher must:

I. Clearly specify the objectives for the lesson
   A. Academic objectives or student outcome objectives
   B. Collaborative skills objective—note the collaborative skills that will be emphasized in the lesson
II. Make decisions about placing students in groups before the lesson is begun
   A. Size of group—usually four to six students per group
   B. Materials available or specific nature of tasks may dictate size of group
   C. The shorter the period of time available, the smaller the learning group should be

Once the learning groups are working, the teacher must monitor their activity. Just because students are in groups does not ensure that they will stay on track. Much of the teacher's time must be spent in observing group members to see what problems they are having in completing the assignment and in working cooperatively.

Things to look for include the following: contributing ideas, asking questions, expressing feelings, active listening, expressions of support and acceptance toward ideas, encouraging others to participate, summarizing, checking for understanding, and giving direction to the group's work.

While monitoring groups, the teacher should look for opportunities to clarify instructions, review procedures and strategies, and answer questions. However, teachers should not intervene in the group any more than is absolutely necessary.

Case studies—a type of problem solving. Case studies also can be used to help students develop problem solving skills. Case studies can be hypothetical or real. Situations that have appeared in the newspaper, in professional literature, or on television can provide case studies that can be used in class. Students should be instructed to examine the case carefully, decide what additional information they would like to have, review the solution that was presented within the study, determine what might have been done differently, and determine what might have occurred, if alternative strategies had been used.

Construction Activities

Construction activities involve pupil and teacher planning as well as pupil participation in the preparation of a variety of items (using paper, wood, cardboard, glue, crayons, and other materials). Construction activities can involve the development of bulletin boards, exhibits, flannel boards, mobiles, models, murals, and posters, to specify but a few. Illustrations of specific items that may be made include a fire alarm box; a traffic light standard with stop and go signals; papier-mâché models of fruits and vegetables; clay models of teeth, the heart, and other organs of the body; and construction of paper models. These items have use in dramatic play, exhibits, bulletin board displays, and other techniques of teaching.

Creative Activities

The free expression of children's thoughts, ideas, and feelings through such media as stories, poems and verses, dramatic plays, murals, music, cartoons (see Fig. 12-5), and other creative activities may be useful and productive in the health instruction program. (See Teaching Techniques, for illustrations.) Creative activities build on the varied and unique abilities of students. By providing

students the latitude to be creative in learning about being healthy, the teacher fosters an atmosphere of freedom where each child can use his or her abilities and experience the self-satisfaction of success.

Construction and creative activities offer the additional advantage of providing meaningful learning opportunities for those students who tend to learn more efficiently by manipulation of objects and creative thought processes. This important fact has gained considerable attention through recent research on how people learn, and it holds great promise in the teaching of thinking skills. Good teachers have long known that creative and constructive activities work and have applied this knowledge to health activities, as well as other subjects.

Demonstrations and Experiments

Demonstrations and experiments are methods that help make abstract verbal descriptions and symbols more concrete and meaningful in health education. They may include involvement of the visual, tactile, and auditory senses (Fig. 12-2). They are helpful ways to improve the teaching process and may be performed by teachers or pupils.

Five important reasons for the use of demonstrations and experiments in teaching are the following:

- They stimulate interest and thereby motivate learning
- They help clarify learnings
- They help improve and accelerate the learning process
- They may be used to initiate a unit
- They provide a visual image helpful in the retention of learnings

Experiments are procedures that use the scientific method to test suggested truths or to illustrate known truths. They are ways to solve problems and also may be classified as demonstrations. They differ from demonstrations because the techniques used are more exacting and precise, and

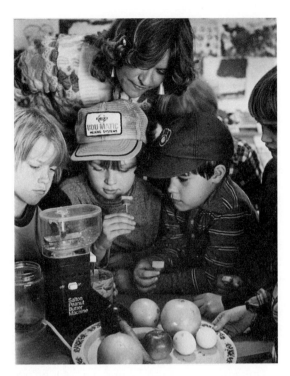

FIG. 12-2 Tasting party—making peanut butter. (Courtesy Wisconsin Department of Public Instruction, Madison, Wisconsin.)

controls are used to ensure valid results. The specific sequential steps may include the following:
- Define the problem to be solved or the hypothesis to be tested
- Select the methods of procedure to be used
- Identify and assemble the necessary materials
- Conduct the experiment
- Collect and record data
- Select, organize, and interpret the data
- Prepare conclusions

Experiments stimulate interest and attention in learning. They provide realism to abstract concepts and make learning more meaningful.

Following are illustrations of experiments that have been helpful in the health instruction program:
- The effect of good and poor diets on growth development may be shown by the white rat

feeding experiment, details of which are available from the National Dairy Council.* This demonstration may be completed with kindergarten or first-grade children to encourage good nutrition and discourage the excessive consumption of sweets.
- The importance of washing hands with soap may be demonstrated through the use of a series of sterile agar plates (Petri dishes from science department). Children touch one dish with fingers before washing with soap and water and a second dish after washing. The dishes are then incubated or kept in a warm place for 24 hours or longer, and the extent of germ growth can be compared in the two dishes.

Demonstrations and experiments may be performed individually or in groups. Demonstrations have an expected outcome, whereas with experiments the outcome may vary. Demonstrations and experiments may be performed in learning centers and students can "rotate" through the various learning centers. For the technique to be successful, all necessary equipment and supplies should be readily available, and the teacher should have "practiced" the demonstration or experiment to ensure that it actually will work, if performed correctly. The teacher must watch carefully to ensure that each student in the group has the opportunity to participate in and contribute to the demonstration or experiment. If students are to present the demonstration to the rest of the class, the teacher must provide time for students to practice the demonstration beforehand.

Some demonstrations usable in health education are (1) the importance of oxygen in fires; (2) the proper way to brush teeth; (3) the safest way to ride a bicycle on sidewalks, streets, and highways; (4) specific first-aid procedures by students to class; and (5) the proper use of fire extinguishers.

---

*National Dairy Council, 6300 North River Road, Rosemont, IL 60018-4233.

Discussions

The discussion as a method of teaching is probably the most familiar and commonly used procedure in health instruction. Discussions generally begin with a lecture by the teacher, students, or a resource person. Regardless, all activities and methods used in health instruction should include some type of discussion. These methods generally permit children to ask questions, make recitations, perform surveys, and participate in numerous other ways in the learning process. They provide opportunities for the exchange of information between pupils and teachers. Group discussion is especially valuable because it is conducive to helping children gain understanding and respect for each other's feelings and viewpoints. To achieve this, the teacher must foster an open and trusting classroom environment where students will feel comfortable in expressing their own thoughts and feelings.

Discussions need teacher guidance. The following points should aid in directing the conversation along constructive channels:

- Encourage and stimulate pupil questions, because they provide information about needs, interests, and concerns. Pupils should be helped to think through their own experiences and relate them to the discussion.
- Try to get all children in the class to participate or be involved.
- Do not hurry the discussion, but do not let it drag
- Listen carefully to all contributions and relate them to the topic. Compliment and encourage children who make remarks. It may be necessary to have students amplify their statements.
- When groups are reluctant to engage in discussions, mention of a personal experience or anecdote or asking a pertinent question may help get children to participate.

Discussions may take place in a variety of ways, and the suggestions that follow merely illustrate some of the numerous variations and formats that may be used in the health instruction program.

Questions and answers. Questions may not only introduce a health area, they may also be part of the teaching process used during the presentation of a unit or lesson, and they may serve as a review or summary of a class discussion.

The best results are obtained when careful thought, planning, and organization are given to building sets of questions. As a general rule, question-and-answer sessions should be planned in advance as carefully as other teaching procedures.

Question box. Occasionally, children are reluctant to ask questions in class because they fear embarrassment or for other reasons. This situation can be solved by having a receptacle of some kind available where pupils may anonymously place questions of interest or concern. This procedure may be especially appropriate when the topic of sexuality education or social hygiene is being considered in class.

Quizzes. Quizzes can be oral, written, or performance based. They have value when used for drill, review, or grading purposes. They motivate learning and are important in the instruction program. They have evaluation limitations as they tend to measure only the cognitive learning (understandings) acquired by pupils.

Self-tests. Self-tests are a series of teacher-prepared, easily answered questions that help stimulate discussion about a particular health topic. The number and difficulty of questions can vary depending on the purpose of the test and the grade level in which it is used. Self-tests help students focus on themselves. They are for personal use or information only and are a good way for students to reflect on what they know, feel, and do.

These tests are not given for grading purposes. They have value because they can be duplicated and distributed at the start of the class and immediately get all pupils participating and thinking about the lesson. They also may be used to initiate a unit, as well as to help determine additional class activities.

The following is an illustration of a partial self-test without grade level identification:

What Do You Know About Tobacco?

Please circle the correct answer to the statements that are listed below. If you do not know the answer, circle the letter "D."

1. The drug in tobacco is caffeine.   T   F   D
2. Smoking has been linked to lung   T   F   D
   cancer.
3. The use of tobacco increases the heart   T   F   D
   rate.
4. Smokeless tobacco has no bad health   T   F   D
   effects.
5. Smoking cigarettes irritates linings in   T   F   D
   the body.
6. Smoking has no link to heart disease.   T   F   D
7. Nicotine is a drug that slows the body   T   F   D
   down.
8. Blood pressure goes down when a   T   F   D
   person smokes.

Word searches, crossword puzzles, picture puzzles. Nearly every topic in health education lends itself to the development of word searches and crossword puzzles. These activities can be made rather easily by the teacher by using computer packages that are currently on the market. Use of these types of activities helps students learn vocabulary while having fun at the same time. Care must be taken to define terms carefully so that the student is not confused by conflicting definitions. In constructing word searches, the difficulty can be varied by grade level (Fig. 12-3). Having the words all move from left to right rather than in a random fashion may be best for students in the intermediate grades, and random placement of words will work well for those in the upper

NUTRITION

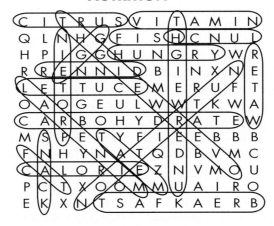

WORD LIST: NUTRITION

BREAKFAST	FAT	MINERAL	VITAMIN
CALORIE	FISH	NUTRITION	WATER
CARBOHYDRATE	HUNGRY	OVERWEIGHT	
CITRUS	LETTUCE	PROTEIN	
DINNER	LUNCH	SNACK	
EGG	MEAT	UNDERWEIGHT	

FIG. 12-3 Word search.

grades. These types of activities can be used as culmination activities to review words that have been used within a unit of instruction. Health words also can be part of the language arts program.

Use of picture puzzles is good to help younger children understand spatial relationships, as well as conveying health messages. These puzzles may be large "floor" puzzles, or smaller, desktop type puzzles. Several excellent, health-related picture puzzles can be purchased at local teacher or school supply houses.

Experience charts and records. Experience charts and records are lists of phrases or brief stories or synopses dictated by children to the teacher, who records the suggestions, ideas, or thoughts on the chalkboard, on large sheets of paper, or on a computer. This procedure has been used in the primary grades to introduce reading, but it also is a good technique when teaching health education. It is usable at other grade levels as a way to list or record questions that need to be answered about a particular health topic. It also may be considered part of the problem-solving technique in teaching.

Buzz groups. The buzz group method is often used as a cooperative learning strategy. The class is divided into heterogeneous groups of from five to eight pupils to discuss a specific problem or series of problems for a limited time, usually 3 to 5 minutes. Each subgroup selects a chairperson to keep the discussion on the topic and give everyone an opportunity to speak. A recorder is chosen who jots down key points. A reporter works with the recorder and is prepared to present these orally to the entire class on request. The teacher's role during the buzzing is to move from group to group to be certain that the topic is being discussed, see that students know what is expected of them, and clarify questions relating to the problem under discussion. At the conclusion of the exercise, the teacher requests the spokespersons to report their answers, and a pupil summarizes the main points on the blackboard. Further discussion is encouraged by the class members during the summary period.

This technique has a number of important advantages for use in the health instruction program:

- It provides a way to have several committees in class study different aspects of a given topic
- It allows greater pupil participation in the discussion
- It provides an atmosphere conducive to discussion
- It may serve as a diagnostic procedure to find out what pupils know about a particular topic
- It may lead to further pupil activities or experiences
- It helps students see how to break a problem into smaller parts, then see how problem solving each part helps solve the major problem.

Buzz groups may be used (1) to discuss a particular problem or question, (2) to determine what action to take regarding a particular problem or question, and (3) to determine questions to ask a resource person who may be invited to class.

This procedure has limitations, especially if pupils have no background information about the discussion topic; it may result in a rehash of ignorance. Also, a buzz group takes careful planning to produce optimal results, to prevent a few students from dominating the conversation, and to confine the comments to the topic being discussed. Selection of a subject about which students have controversial and varying opinions increases the chances of success when using this method.

Panels and debates. Panels and debates provide students the opportunity to explore different sides of various issues. For both of these strategies, heterogeneous groups of three to five students are placed in a group and given a topic or issue. In the case of a debate, one group is given the responsibility to debate for the issue, and one group is given the responsibility to debate against the issue. For panels, students are given a general topic and discuss various aspects, both positive and negative, about the issue.

In general, 15 minutes is sufficient for a panel presentation or a debate. The topics and the time devoted to the presentation vary with the grade level and developmental level of the students who are participating. The advantage of these methods is that students all have a chance to participate and make their views known. After the panel presentation or debate, there could be a general classroom discussion of the material presented.

In these types of activities, the teacher serves as a facilitator to ensure that all students are participating and that presentations remain focused on the relevant issues. The teacher also should have basic material available for student use to ensure that the information is current and accurate. After the presentation and subsequent discussion, the teacher can summarize the information so that salient points are reinforced with the students.

Dramatizations

Dramatizations provide ways for children to express their feelings and ideas through make-believe, imitation, and imagination. By having students portray different roles, they begin to project personal feelings into those roles. It is believed that children are more likely to remember facts when they are portraying them. These procedures are interesting to children and apparently contribute to the development of health attitudes and values, including the concepts of diversity and multiculturalism, as pupils tend to identify themselves with characters in the situations. Care must be taken not to control the dramatization. Teachers are not psychological counselors, and sometimes students may portray culturally insensitive positions. Those who oppose health education in schools could use this event as a way to argue against including health education in the curriculum.

Dramatic play. Dramatic play is an informal, spontaneous, natural way for children to act out what they have been reading, discussing, or seeing in health.

Children who have visited or read about a fire station may construct an imaginary station in the classroom and play fire fighter. A visit to a grocery store may result in such a store being established in school. The presence of the school physician may encourage children to establish a corner in the room as a physician's office.

Role playing. Role playing is a more formalized procedure than dramatic play, but it still relies on spontaneity. The teacher determines the focus and assigns the roles. It is spontaneous and unrehearsed and focuses on a health problem of interest or concern. Students have the opportunity to explore divergent viewpoints and practice both communication and listening skills. It provides a considerable amount of realism that apparently communicates to individuals.

The steps to follow in conducting role playing generally include the following:

- Selection of a problem of interest and importance to children
- Explanation of the technique in simple terms
- Provision of enough of the story to set the scene
- Selection of children to participate
- Definition of the problem and role of each pupil
- Definition of the audience role
- Provision of cues to begin or opening remarks needed by first actors to get started
- Cessation of role playing at the point where action drops or when discussion should be started (maybe after a 2- or 3-minute presentation)
- Conduction of discussion afterward, asking such questions as: "What was being presented?" "What was good about the way the situation was handled?" "What might have been changed in the situation?"

Illustrations or dramatizations suitable in health education include (1) walking across the street, (2) riding a bicycle on the street, (3) helping a person who is lost, (4) showing how a person feels and behaves when teased or threatened by someone, and (5) describing how to say "no" and resist peer pressure without losing friends. Role playing also provides students with the opportunity to develop and practice assertiveness skills.

Plays. Plays are more formal because they have a prepared script and involve memorization of dialogue. They may or may not be pupil written. They can serve as culminating activities with presentations made to parent groups or school assemblies.

Puppet shows. When children are involved in making the puppets and planning the stories for puppet shows, the effect on health behaviors can be beneficial. These experiences are enjoyed by young children both as spectators and as participants. When students are involved in making the puppets, it also helps them to exercise their creative abilities. Puppets have great attitudinal effects on pupils. Puppets also may be used in dramatic play or with spontaneous dialogue.

Many areas including mental health, nutrition, and safety provide suitable materials for these shows.

Stories and storytelling. Children enjoy stories* and storytelling to the extent that various health topics can serve as themes. They can be used to initiate a unit in health, or they may be part of the ongoing activities. They help stimulate questions and answers.

Some illustrations of how this procedure may be used are: (1) read stories about fear, courage, honesty, truthfulness, and other phases of mental health; (2) read stories about fire and traffic safety; (3) prepare a puppet or a construction paper character having some such name as Bozo the dog, Chippy the chipmunk, or Ronny the raccoon and create a story in which this animal discusses mental health or nutrition; (4) prepare a flip chart with a series of humorous or otherwise interesting drawings that relate to how to take care of the eyes, ears, or feet; (5) show pictures of toothbrushes, wash cloths, combs, and other such items and encourage pupil discussions relative to the importance of these items to health. Having students develop endings to stories, either individually or in small groups, helps them to understand how different actions can produce different results and that not everyone has to do the same thing. Storytelling can be enhanced through the use of visual materials such as flannelboards and flat pictures or overhead transparencies.

---
*See Appendix D for specific story references.

Field Trips

Field trips are designed to enrich classroom teaching procedures by making health more meaningful. Field trips may be limited to the school plant and the school neighborhood, or they may be distant journeys requiring bus transportation. In general, field trips should be used as final, not introductory, activities.

Some places to visit that may be part of the health instruction program are the school lunchroom, the school grounds, a grocery store, the corner crosswalk, the first-aid station, a dairy, a water treatment plant, a fire station, a hospital, a dentist's office, and the health department. If it is not possible for an entire class to go on a field trip, perhaps the teacher could visit the site and videotape or take slides of the visit. These slides can then be used in the classroom by the teacher, or even by a resource person from the facility that was visited.

Individual and Group Reports

Individual and group reports are methods whereby oral or written reports, or both, are made about assigned or special interest health topics by individual pupils or groups of pupils. They involve critical reading and analyses, research, independent study, interviews, investigations, and excursions or field trips. Questions and answers become necessary as they may precede, be part of, or follow the reports. They may include panel and forum presentations and independent study. When using this material the teacher may be relatively sure that the student or students learned from preparing the report.

Illustrated Presentations

Illustrated presentations are activities whereby teachers present phases of health using visual materials such as charts, models (Fig. 12-4), pictures, graphs, and specimens. Children should be encouraged to participate in discussions and ask questions.

An example of this procedure would be the use of food models on a flannelboard to illustrate the basic food groups or appropriate breakfasts, lunches, and dinners.

Chalk could be used effectively to make cartoons, sketches, and schematic drawings of germs, body parts, foods, maps, illustrated slogans (such as "Germs hate soap"), charts, and a variety of other valuable and useful visual presentations.

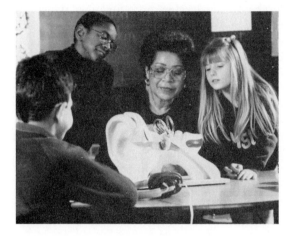

FIG. 12-4 Teacher helps children learn about the ear. (Courtesy Michigan Department of Education.)

Presenting a cartoon and having children prepare captions combines knowledge with creative activities (Fig. 12-5).

Resource People—Guest Speakers

The use of community resource people who are experts in their chosen fields often enriches the health instruction program. Such individuals may include physicians, dentists, health officers, police officers, fire fighters, and nurses.

The following points should be discussed with resource people or guest speakers who are invited to schools:

- The choice of a topic appropriate to that being covered in class
- The grade level of the class
- The material covered in class before and what will happen after the speaker departs
- The nature of the vocabulary to use
- The use of audiovisual aids whenever possible
- The use of demonstrations, experiments, and illustrations whenever possible

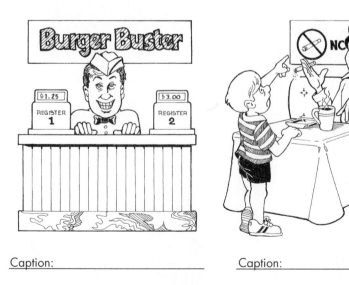

FIG. 12-5 Having students produce captions for cartoons combines knowledge and creative abilities. (Original art concept by Larry M. Olsen, drawn by Donald P. O'Conner.)

- Permission for children to ask questions; pupils should prepare their questions in advance

It is not a good practice to invite a recovering alcoholic or drug user as a single, assembly-type speaker. Students may see the person and think, "Well, he or she got off of drugs or alcohol and doesn't look so bad." This type of guest speaker should be used as one component of a total unit in any given health topic area.

A small group of students or the entire class may be responsible for inviting and hosting the resource person. They also may prepare the questions to ask the guest.

Cross-age teaching. This is a method whereby older students prepare materials for use or are able to discuss one or more health topics with younger children in formal and informal educational settings. By way of illustration, these procedures may include preparing audiovisual materials for presentation, conducting rap sessions, par-

ticipating in and leading a variety of discussions, and writing and producing newspaper articles and special bulletin materials for distribution. Careful selection of the students who will serve as peer teacher, and providing them with good training and supervision will help ensure a successful cross-age teacher program.

Some lessons are readily adaptable to cross-age teaching. The teacher may find it a rewarding change of pace, as well as an opportunity to get a different perspective, by bringing in an older student to help teach some health lessons (Fig. 12-6). Older students who have recovered successfully from operations, who are drug free, or who have other health-related experiences can be very influential when they share their experiences. A senior high or junior high class can stage a health-related play for younger children. Refusal skills, making friends, and staying out of trouble are topics that lend themselves well to cross-age teaching. This idea is worthy of consideration in the upper

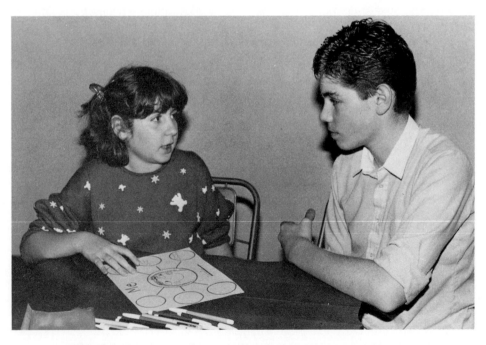

FIG. 12-6 Cross-age teaching. (Courtesy Jay Schupack, Seattle, Washington.)

grades and possibly also in the intermediate grades.

Show and Tell Time

Show and tell is an appropriate time to discuss health matters as well as other topics. This activity is especially useful in the primary grades for children to tell about visits to dentists or physicians, accidents at home, or fires that happened in the community. The teacher must be aware that children may begin to discuss private matters. Thus they should be prepared to refocus the student's presentation or to terminate the presentation tactfully without embarrassing the student. Some children with parents who are physicians, dentists, fire fighters, police officers, or health officers may have special health items such as stethoscopes, models, charts, books, and pamphlets that they will bring to school and share with their classmates.

Surveys

Surveys are procedures in which students use checklists, interviews, questionnaires, and opinionnaires to collect information about the nature and extent of pupil or community health problems or practices. They may be considered part of the problem-solving process. Some consider this method as *guided discovery.*

The survey provides excellent opportunities to integrate health with language and mathematics. The survey forms will need to be prepared by pupils, and oral and written reports and research also may be necessary. In addition, mathematic tabulations and computations must be completed.

Some areas in health that lend themselves to surveys are (1) the types and amounts of snack-time foods consumed by pupils; (2) how students spend leisure time; (3) the kinds of foods eaten for breakfast, lunch, and dinner by children; (4) the extent to which students use tobacco; and (5) the safety hazards in the school or home.

Others

Many variations of the methods of teaching described in this chapter can be used in health education. Teacher ingenuity and creativity are necessary to develop the variety of other possible techniques. Communication media including television, radio, tape recordings, films, filmstrips, videotapes, videodiscs, computers and slides, as well as models, charts, exhibits, displays, bulletin boards (Fig. 12-7), posters, flannelboards, and other audiovisual aids may be combined with the procedures just presented to provide numerous additional activities and experiences. Chapter 13 contains details about the use of these teaching aids in the school health program.

WHAT METHODS SHOULD TEACHERS USE?

There is no one best method or combination of methods to use in the health instruction program. If any procedure is to be singled out as a basis from which to start selecting, perhaps the problem-solving approach must be given first consideration. This method is a meaningful and scientific way to teach health education, it involves other activities, and it is behavior centered, as well as pupil centered.

The process of developing health-educated individuals is complex and difficult. The techniques teachers use should help pupils understand the concepts needed to acquire the practices, attitudes, and knowledge for healthful living. It is important therefore that teachers use and be familiar with the nature, values, and limitations of many methods so that they may choose those that will aid pupils to achieve their objectives. Using a variety of methods will help ensure that the teacher has been responsive to the variations in learning styles of students in the classroom.

Many criteria could be used to select a method to use within health instruction. Answers to the questions listed below will help the teacher make

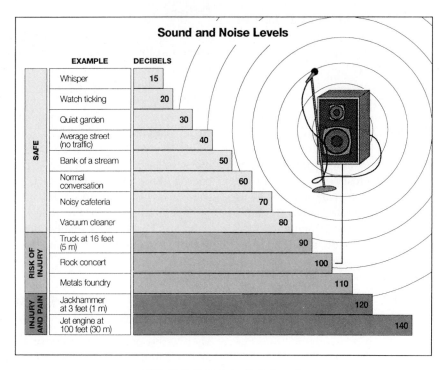

FIG. 12-7 Sample bulletin board.

a wise selection of which method or combination of methods to use.*

- Does the method contribute to the objectives of the lesson and unit?
- Does the method have educational value?
- What are the basic skills or knowledge to be gained from using the method?
- Does the method provide students the opportunity to practice a skill, use basic knowledge, or develop new knowledge?
- Does the method appeal to the needs and interests of the students?
- Is the teacher familiar with the method, including its advantages and disadvantages?

- Does the method involve active or passive learning on the part of the student?
- Is the method appropriate for the abilities, aptitudes, and developmental level of the students?
- Is more than one sense involved when using the method?
- Does the method help students develop or understand the concept of the lesson?
- Is the method economical in terms of time and materials costs?
- Is the method adaptable to the supplies, equipment, and facilities that are readily available?
- Is more than one desirable outcome addressed when using the method?

Kindergarten and Primary Grades

The health education program in kindergarten and the primary grades should center around

---

*Modified from Ames EE: Instructional planning for health education. In Cortese P, Middleton K, editors: *The comprehensive school health challenge*, vol 1, Santa Cruz, CA, 1994, ETR Associates; Cornacchia HJ, Olsen LK, Nickerson CL: *Health in the elementary school*, ed 8, St Louis, 1991, Mosby–Year Book; Pollock MB, Middleton K: *School health instruction*, ed 3, St Louis, 1994, Mosby–Year Book; Sorochan WD, Bender SJ: *Teaching elementary health science*, ed 3, Boston, 1989, Jones and Bartlett.

daily activities in school, the home, and the community such as safety, disease control, nutrition, rest and sleep, the physician, the police officer, the fire fighter, and the nurse.

Health can be integrated easily into other areas of the curriculum, such as language arts, social studies, and science (Fig. 12-8); however, there will always be the need for direct teaching.

The methods selected for these grades should include doing, experiencing, and observing. The techniques that will achieve the best results will probably include reading, stories, games, problem solving, excursions, discussions, show and tell periods, creative activities, construction activities, questions and answers, experience charts and records, and dramatizations.

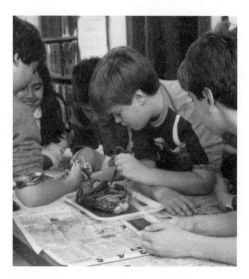

FIG. 12-8 Dissecting—examining an animal heart.

Intermediate Grades

Children in intermediate grades have acquired a new level of curiosity and enthusiasm. They begin asking more questions and want to know the "why's" of health. They are seeking more exact answers to their questions.

The growth changes occurring in pupils provide the need for learning about the structure and functions of the human organism (see Appendix K). Girls particularly need information about menstrual hygiene.

The beginning of group activities and the wider use of community resources and problem-solving procedures become possible and should be considered for use by teachers in their health instruction programs.

Health continues to be integrated to some extent with other subjects, but more direct teaching is necessary. Some administrators frequently need reminders that health content often lends itself to subject areas such as reading, arithmetic, and social studies.

The methods that teachers may use in intermediate grade programs include discussions, problem solving, cooperative learning, educational games, surveys, excursions, illustrated lectures, role playing, experiments, demonstra-

tions, computer-assisted instruction, videodisks, resource people, and individual and group reports.

Upper Grades

Children in the upper grades are adventuresome, want to experiment, and desire more activity than ever before in their lives. Therefore the health experiences must go far beyond the confines of the textbook. Pupils can be involved in cooperative planning and sharing of experiences (see Fig. 12-8).

The early adolescent period indicates the need for additional content areas to be included in the health instruction program. The use of tobacco, alcohol, and drugs begins to have added meaning for these children, although these areas should receive consideration in the lower grades. In addition, exercise takes on importance, with dental and nutritional problems, interpersonal relationships, and sexually transmissible disease having special significance.

Some of the methods that may be included in the health instruction program are surveys, panels, debates, excursions, peer group action, exhibits, tape recordings, independent study, cooperative learning, demonstrations, experiments, buzz groups, and problem solving.

ARE INCIDENTS METHODS?

Incidents by themselves are not methods. However, they are teachable moments that stimulate learning by setting the stage for meaningful health education. They can initiate units or lessons. They may be considered as health problems that lend themselves to solutions through the use of the problem-solving process and other procedures. They lend themselves to both formal and informal educational approaches. Therefore they may be considered a part of method.

Teachers must be constantly alert for the numerous occasions that happen in schools, homes, and communities and that are usable in health instruction programs. Newspapers, magazines, and TV are sources of these incidents, as are student and adult reports. Teachers should consistently capitalize on these motivating events.

The teacher must recognize that there are values as well as limitations when using incidents in health teaching. When they are improperly used, they may result in serious emotional disturbances among children. A teacher who discusses the cleanliness habits or the decayed teeth of a particular pupil in class not only may embarrass the child, but also may make the child unnecessarily conspicuous before the other students. In addition, this action would constitute questionable ethical practice. From a psychological viewpoint therefore this action may be harmful to the child. The teacher must use discretion in choosing incidents, as well as the appropriate occasion for capitalizing on such situations. Incidents in health teaching may be used in several ways:

- To discuss individual health problems with pupils in private or with parents.
- To discuss health and safety problems that have been observed in school or elsewhere without reference to any special pupil or groups of pupils (e.g., violence).
- To discuss special events or occasions involving health and safety that will take place in the school or community (e.g., walkathons for health causes such as March of Dimes).
- To discuss a particular pupil health problem when the child is not in the room. This is probably the rare occasion but may be necessary for the protection of the child. For example, if a child has had an epileptic seizure in class, it will be necessary for the teacher to seek the support of the child's classmates to help the pupil when necessary. A seizure could occur on the playground or on the way home when the teacher or other adult is not nearby. Therefore a brief explanation of the nature of seizures and first-aid procedures is important. This action may help to prevent the pupil from being injured and being rejected by the other classmates. It is important to secure permission from the parents before discussing a child's problems in class.

The following incidents that occur in the school setting illustrate opportunities available for health instruction:

- Students using tobacco products in school
- Many children absent because of influenza
- Pupils come to school with colds
- Children prepare refreshments for a party at school
- A student tells how a friend's hand was burned while playing with matches
- The school conducts a fire drill
- A child reports a visit to the dentist
- Pupils make fun of children wearing eyeglasses or hearing aids
- The food served for lunch at school
- Children have their vision and/or hearing screened at school
- A student asks about dental health or nutrition claims in TV commercials
- A child is bitten by a dog
- A student has a seizure in class
- An accident occurs to a student on the way to, from, or at school
- School fund raising activities involving selling candy

A third-grade teacher who took advantage of a report in the newspaper of a bicycle accident that occurred to a schoolchild and resulted in a broken arm illustrates how to use an incident in the instruction program. The morning after the accident the teacher asked the class how it happened. Discussion brought out such matters as careless riders, unsafe conditions, and unsafe equipment. The conversation led the pupils to list the actions that often lead to accidents: bicycle riding, car driving, walking, behavior in school, and behavior at home. The teacher then asked the question: "If these may lead to accidents, how can we act safely?" The pupils began to mention safety rules but finally decided they needed more information to be able to answer this question satisfactorily. At this point the teacher suggested that continued planning go on the next day.

When the discussion resumed the following day, the children decided to participate in a variety of experiences to learn more about safety. These are some of the activities they selected:

- Read stories in safety books and pamphlets
- Create bulletin board displays of safety posters
- Create a checklist of "Ways to make my home safe"
- Invite a police officer to visit the class to discuss safety
- Conduct a culminating activity that dramatizes a typical day of children who do not practice safety and a typical day of children who do

Special community and school events are also important occasions that can be used as a part of health education in schools. The Calendar of Health Observances presented in Chapter 11 (see box, pp. 296-297) contains many possible events that could be used to motivate students.

Seasonal events also offer opportunities for health education: (1) when children return to school in the fall may be the appropriate time to discuss safety to and from school, bicycle safety, and playground safety; (2) fall and winter may be significant times to discuss respiratory diseases and other communicable diseases; and (3) spring may be the time when camping, picnic, and water safety become important.

IS THE USE OF THE HEALTH TEXTBOOK A METHOD?

The health textbook is an important teaching aid that provides a reference or resource for information necessary to solve health problems. It should be used in conjunction with a variety of pupil-centered activities and experiences and therefore may be considered a part of or related to method. It may be used in the preparation for discussions, panels, individual and group work, and so on. It can help provide continuity and direction to learning experiences.

A textbook, however, should not be used as a passive reading lesson. Children will not acquire necessary health skills and behaviors if their experiences are limited to a 10- or 15-minute daily reading assignment in a health text. This procedure is contrary to the principles of learning discussed in Chapter 9. Teachers must be more imaginative and creative and use a variety of the methods and activities described in this chapter if the goals of health education are to be achieved. Additional information about selecting textbooks is found in Chapter 13 and Appendix H.

WHAT ARE THE RELATIONSHIPS BETWEEN METHODS AND MATERIAL AIDS?

Material or teaching aids, such as models of the teeth, health videos, flannelboards, exhibits, or displays of the contents of first-aid kits, are valuable supplementary items that enrich learning experiences. They are aids to learning that make abstract health concepts specific, concrete, and meaningful in the lives of students; they attract and maintain attention; they help stimulate interest in the teaching process; and they assist in encouraging greater student participation in the learning process. Teachers should be familiar with the variety of such items that are available and use many of them in their teaching. Chapter 13 provides comprehensive coverage of the nature of these aids.

Instructional aids should not be considered teaching methods in themselves. However, they are important supplementary and complementary aspects of the procedures used in learning. They are part of the "how to" methods of teaching.

At times it is difficult to distinguish between methods and teaching aids. An example or two best illustrates this point. A film by itself is a teaching aid. When children are expected to look for specific information as they view the film and, after its showing, discuss what they saw, then it becomes part of the teaching process. Therefore discussion may be the method used in the learning, with the film being a part of this procedure. A flannelboard and food models are teaching aids. When these items are used in a discussion to demonstrate the food items needed for an adequate breakfast, they become part of the method.

Using a variety of teaching aids can greatly contribute to the emphasis on pupil-centered teaching. They will assist in providing more pupil participation in the learning process.

WHAT TEACHING TECHNIQUES ARE USABLE IN HEALTH INSTRUCTION?

The wide variety of specific teaching techniques* that are presented next will aid the teacher in the achievement of the objectives in health education. They include more than 1200 ideas for use in the instructional program. They are organized alphabetically into 15 subject areas, and the appropriate grade level group for each activity is identified.

---

*An excellent culminating activity that involves much student, parent, and community participation is a *health fair*. The references at the end of this chapter related to health fairs are worthy of review.

When the procedures for health teaching are selected, it will be helpful to keep in mind these essentials:

- The purposes of health education go beyond an emphasis on information alone; they also consider the development of health attitudes and practices.
- The principles of learning described in Chapter 9 are important.
- The specific technique or combination of techniques to be used should help achieve a desired goal or goals.
- Activities should be continually evaluated to determine the extent of learning taking place.

Despite the many types of activities presented, the procedures that follow do not provide a comprehensive coverage of all health teaching experiences. Rather they serve a fourfold purpose:

- To provide specific, tested techniques that will give spark and vitality to the health instruction program (the numerous experiences listed have been used by many teachers in their classrooms)
- To provide a broad selection of activities
- To provide suggestions of teaching techniques that will stimulate the creative and imaginative teacher to modify, change, or devise completely new procedures
- To provide methods that may be used to initiate new units or as culminating activities

It should be noted that the following teaching procedures have been organized in a functional and practical manner for easy reference by the teacher. The letters or numbers found on the right side of the page in the activities or experiences that follow refer to the *suggested* grades or grade level in which they may be used: *P*, primary; *I*, intermediate; *U*, upper.

TEACHING TECHNIQUES

Alcohol

			Grades
Bulletin board	1	Illustrated display of accidents and other losses attributed to alcohol.	U
	2	Illustrated display of the alcohol content of the various kinds of beverages.	U
Buzz group	3	Conduct a buzz session on the questions "What should be the punishment for driving while intoxicated?" "Why do people drink alcoholic beverages?"	U
Chart	4	Prepare a chart or poster that shows the effects of alcohol on the body and the level of alcohol in the blood after beverages with alcohol are consumed.	U
Demonstration	5	Place a small (3-inch) goldfish in a solution of ½ ounce of alcohol in ¾ pint of water (the amount in a 12-ounce bottle of beer). In almost 20 minutes the fish will be "under the influence" (floating to the surface). When the effect of the alcohol can be seen, remove the fish, and place it in fresh water to be revived.	I, U
Discussion	6	The physiological, psychological, and sociological effects of alcohol on the human body.	U
	7	The nutritional elements of a glass of milk, an ounce of whiskey, and a bottle of beer.	U
	8	The nature of the alcohol in beer, wine, and whiskey.	U
	9	Collect ads from newspapers and magazines on alcoholic beverages and analyze them in class.	U
	10	Safe and unsafe use of alcohol.	U
	11	Predisposing factors to alcoholism.	U
	12	Effects on families of individuals with alcohol problems.	U
Dramatization	13	High school drama class depicts scenes of pressures put on sixth-, seventh-, and eighth-grade students to drink alcoholic beverages. Follow with discussion of junior high school pupils' suggestions for handling such situations.	U
Exhibit	14	Display whiskey, wine, and beer glasses and discuss the amount of alcohol contained in each beverage and in each glass.	U
	15	Display a variety of magazines, pamphlets, and other materials for students to read, do research, and prepare oral and written reports on alcohol.	U
	16	Pupils display labels taken from medicine bottles and other containers and prepare a list of the amount of alcohol found in these substances.	U
Graph	17	Compare the amount of money spent nationally on alcohol and the amount spent on education, cancer, heart disease, and other health projects.	U
Guest speakers	18	Invite a member of Alcoholics Anonymous to discuss services rendered by this organization to help alcoholics.	U

TEACHING TECHNIQUES: ALCOHOL—cont'd

		Grades
Guest speakers— cont'd	19 Invite a physician to discuss the physiological effects of alcohol on the human body.	U
Individual and group reports	20 Pupil committees write letters to organizations having materials on alcohol and request copies for use in class.	I, U
	21 Pupils prepare oral and written reports on recent magazine articles about alcohol.	I, U
	22 Pupils prepare oral and written reports on the effects of alcohol on a person participating in sports, driving an automobile, flying an airplane, typing, and using industrial skills.	U
	23 Pupils prepare individual and group reports on such topics as the preserving quality of alcohol, alcohol as fuel, alcohol in medicine, and alcohol as a disinfectant.	U
Interview	24 Interview a member of the sheriff's office or police department to find out the effect of alcohol on the crime rate and the "crash" rate in the community.	U
	25 A pupil committee interviews a physician and a health officer on the benefits and adverse features of the use of alcohol.	U
Panel	26 Have a panel discussion on the topic: "Why people drink alcoholic beverages."	U
Problem solving	27 Pupils do research and prepare oral and written reports about a series of problems such as: "Why do people drink? Why do some people pressure others to drink? What effect does alcohol have on the body? What effect does alcohol have on the mind? Is alcohol a food? What are the uses of alcohol?" These may also serve as introductory questions to stimulate student discussion to determine ways to find solutions.	U
Reports	28 Pupils prepare reports on Alateen and Alanon programs; relationships of alcoholism and nutritional problems; state laws; community resources to treat alcoholism; and alcohol and its use in religious ceremonies.	U
Resource persons	29 Have a police officer talk about alcohol intoxication tests.	U
Role playing	30 Saying no when offered an alcoholic beverage.	U
	31 Pressures of peer groups to consume alcoholic beverages.	U
Scrapbook	32 Pupils make scrapbooks to include pictures, magazine and newspaper articles, stories, and other items about the use and effect of alcohol.	U
Self-test	33 Pupils complete a self-test and conduct a discussion afterward.	U
Survey	34 Conduct a survey among pupils to find out their views on alcohol use.	U
Tape recording	35 Have students interview a recovering alcoholic about attitudes toward use of alcoholic beverages.	U

TEACHING TECHNIQUES

Care of the Ears

		Grades
Bulletin board	1 Display drawings or pictures that show how the ears help us to hear.	P, I
	2 Prepare a bulletin board showing the head of a clown and place a large pupil-drawn ear on the clown. Put a caption at the top of the display "We use our ears to:" and then put various other statements around the clown, such as "use the telephone," "hear bells," "hear danger signals," and "enjoy music."	P, I
Cartoons	3 Draw cartoons illustrating rules about the care of and hazards to the ears.	P, I
Demonstration	4 The proper way to wash the ears.	P
	5 The proper way to blow the nose. Have children practice the procedure following the demonstration.	P
	6 Show a drum and relate it to the functions of the eardrum and sound vibrations.	P, I
	7 Demonstrate lip reading to show how handicapped a deaf person might be. Discuss the importance of protecting one's hearing.	P, I
	8 How a drum head may be punctured from a severe blow and relate the possibility of this occurring to the eardrum from a loud noise or blow.	P, I, U
	9 Sound vibrations using a tuning fork. Drop a rock in water to show how vibrations travel in all directions.	I, U
	10 Test hearing using the whisper and watch test.	I, U
Discussion	11 How infections, accidents, and foreign objects may affect hearing.	P, I
	12 How the ear helps us to hear.	P, I
	13 The need for reporting pains or other symptoms of ear problems.	P, I
	14 The dangers of putting objects in the ear.	P, I
	15 How we hear. Use rhythm instruments to produce sounds and relate these to hearing.	P, I
	16 How to protect ears from loud noises, such as yelling in someone's ear or the TV or radio being turned on too loud.	I, U
	17 The structure and function of the ear using charts and models to illustrate.	I, U
	18 The prevention of ear injuries when swimming, blowing the nose, cleaning the ears, playing, and receiving blows to the ears.	I, U
	19 How colds and other diseases may result in deafness.	I, U
	20 How to help the person with poor hearing: hearing aids, talking into the good ear, making distinct words for the lip reader, and removing wax from the ears.	I, U
	21 Motion sickness.	I, U
Dramatization	22 Dramatize hearing testing or a doctor's examination of the ears.	P

TEACHING TECHNIQUES: CARE OF THE EARS—cont'd

		Grades
Dramatiza-tion—cont'd	23 Have children dramatize the following procedures: proper way to blow nose, wash ears, whispered conversation, loud voice, and normal conversation.	P, I
	24 Dramatize a situation in which a person is wearing a hearing aid and is overly conscious of it. Bring out the relationships of hearing problems to emotional stability and the importance of understanding on the part of friends.	U
Exhibit	25 Display an otoscope (instrument to look into ears) and discuss how the doctor uses this instrument.	P, I
	26 Permit children to examine an ear model.	P, I
	27 Display several types of hearing aids.	I, U
Experience chart	28 Prepare an experience chart on the care of the ears.	P
Game	29 Play "listening" game. Have each child blindfolded or with closed eyes and ask individual players to identify different sounds: bell, bottle half full of water being shaken, horn, clock, crumpling of paper, and others.	P
	30 Have pupils learn basics of sign language and create games using only signing.	I, U
Guest speaker	31 Invite an audiometrist or school nurse to demonstrate hearing testing and discuss care of the ears.	P, I, U
	32 Invite a teacher for the hard-of-hearing to discuss hearing.	I, U
Individual and group reports	33 Pupils prepare written reports on care of the ears.	I, U
	34 Pupils prepare oral and written reports about people who have succeeded in life despite hearing difficulties.	U
Posters	35 Prepare a series of posters showing how the ear may be injured.	I, U
	36 Prepare drawing of the ear and label the major parts.	I, U
Pretest	37 Give a pretest to determine the extent of pupil understanding of the structure, function, and care of the ears.	I, U
Story	38 Children and teacher cooperatively write stories about the care of the ears.	P

TEACHING TECHNIQUES

Care of the Eyes

		Grades
Bulletin board	1 Display pictures and drawings about care of the eyes.	P, I
Chart	2 Prepare a chart containing important terms to know about the eye.	I, U
	3 Have pupils complete the names of the parts of the eye on a diagram.	I, U
Demonstration	4 The correct way to carry objects such as sticks, knives, and tools.	P, I
	5 The procedure for removing foreign objects from the eye.	P, I, U
	6 The proper lighting for reading and working.	P, I, U
	7 Have a child read or look at a book or picture in direct sunlight or under a bright light. Discuss such questions as "Why is it difficult to read?" "Do your eyes hurt?" "Must you squint or frown to see?"	P, I, U
	8 Blindfold a child and have him/her try to walk to different places in the room. Discuss blindness.	P, I, U
	9 The importance of sight by having children cover their eyes and explain their reactions to a variety of situations.	P, I, U
	10 Teacher or nurse demonstrates the vision screening procedure.	P, I, U
	11 Demonstrate the blinking response using one student in class. With the corner of a soft paper, touch the lashes near the inner corner of one eye. Have children note the blinking reaction. Discuss the closure of the eyelid when sand lands on the eyeball, which is accompanied by a flow of tears to try to flush away the particle.	P, I, U
	12 Completely darken the room for a few minutes and then lighten it. Discuss what happens to sight when you first enter a darkened movie theater and also when later you first come into the bright sunlight.	P, I, U
	13 Demonstrate or draw a comparison between the function of the eye and a camera.	I, U
	14 Display various types of paper showing those with low and high gloss and discuss their importance in vision.	I, U
	15 Use a light meter to show the amount of light in the classroom.	I, U
	16 Have students hold one of their thumbs at arm's length and look at it. Have them close their right eyes and line up the thumbs with the corner of the room. Without moving the arm, have them close their left eyes and look with the right eyes. Students should see a different view with each eye, demonstrating that binocular vision helps to adjust to space relationships.	I, U
	17 Have students close one eye and hold a pencil from 12 to 14 inches from the other eye. Have students look at the pencil and then at a distant object and report how the pencil appeared in each instance. Pencil looks blurred when the eye is focused on a distant object or the reverse is true. This indicates the need for occasional resting of the eyes because muscles are involved in eye-focusing changes.	I, U

TEACHING TECHNIQUES: CARE OF THE EYES—cont'd

		Grades
Demonstra- tion—cont'd	18 Have students look at a neighbor's eye in a darkened room. Lighten the room quickly and have students note contractions of the pupils of the eye. The eye must adjust to various amounts of light; therefore, a well-lighted room involves fewer eye adjustments and is less fatiguing.	I, U
	19 Where the optic nerve enters the eyeball there is a blind spot that can easily be demonstrated. Have students draw a black dot (¼ inch in diameter) on a white sheet of paper, and about 1½ inches to the right draw a black cross (¼ inch). Have the students close their left eyes and stare steadily at the black dot with their right eyes while the paper rests on the table. Have students pick up the sheet of paper and move it slowly toward the eye while staring at the dot. They will find a point where the image of the cross to the right will disappear. The blind spot for the left eye can be found by closing the right one and staring at the cross. When the sheet is brought close to the eye, the black spot will disappear.	I, U
	20 With curtains or blinds drawn, hold a lighted 40-watt electric lamp exactly 2 feet above an open book. This is approximately the amount of illumination needed for comfortable reading. Show that light rapidly diminishes as the lamp is moved further away. At a distance of about 3 feet, a 100-watt bulb is needed to provide the same illumination that a 40-watt bulb gives at 2 feet.	P, I, U
Discussion	21 The possible danger to the eyes of throwing things including sand, rocks, and dirt.	P, I
	22 The importance of vision to animals, showing pictures to illustrate.	P, I
	23 An accident on the playground that resulted in an injury to a child's eye.	P, I
	24 The importance of wearing safety glasses when necessary.	P, I, U
	25 Show pictures of artists, surgeons, pilots, and others and discuss the importance of vision in their work.	P, I, U
	26 Care of the eyes and TV.	P, I, U
	27 Have children roll a sheet of paper to make a cylinder and look through it with one eye. Discuss tunnel vision.	P, I, U
	28 The importance of symptoms of vision difficulties such as inability to see the blackboard, words look fuzzy, or vision is blurred. Emphasize importance of notifying parent or teacher when these signs appear.	P, I, U
	29 The hazards to vision of looking directly at the sun.	P, I, U
	30 The ways eyes are protected in various sports.	P, I, U
	31 The structure and function of the eye, using charts and models.	I, U
	32 The importance of periodic eye examinations.	I, U
Dramatization	33 Dramatize the school nurse doing the vision screening test on a child.	P, I
	34 Dramatize the correct sitting distance and lighting for various TV viewing.	P, I
	35 Dramatize good reading habits and a visit to an eye doctor.	P, I

TEACHING TECHNIQUES: CARE OF THE EYES—cont'd

			Grades
Exhibit	36	Display a model of the eye and permit children to take it apart and put it together.	P, I
	37	Display samples of Braille material and discuss how a blind person uses it to learn to read.	P, I, U
	38	Display various materials used in the vision screening program and discuss.	P, I, U
	39	Display pamphlets, magazines, and other reading materials on vision and make available for reading and research.	I, U
	40	Display different styles of glasses including sunglasses and goggles used to protect the eye in various activities.	I, U
Experience chart or record	41	Make an experience chart or record about the care of the eyes.	P
Game	42	Play the game "Pin the tail on the donkey" and discuss the importance of vision.	P, I
Guest speaker	43	Invite the school nurse to discuss vision screening.	P, I, U
	44	Invite an eye doctor to discuss care of the eyes.	I, U
Individual and group reports	45	Students prepare oral or written reports about signs and symptoms of vision problems as well as common eye difficulties.	I, U
	46	Students prepare oral or written reports on eye infections: conjunctivitis, styes, and others.	I, U
	47	Students prepare oral or written reports on the various kinds of eye specialists in the community.	I, U
	48	Students write reports on the various ways eyes are protected in sports.	U
Mural	49	Make a mural on care of the eyes or hazards to the eye.	P, I
Panel	50	Have a panel discussion of the various ways eyes are protected in sports. Get opinions on football, basketball, baseball, and others from appropriate sources.	U
Poems, stories, and plays	51	Create poems, stories, and plays about care of the eyes.	P
Posters	52	Make a series of pictures or drawings about proper lighting for reading as well as care of the eyes.	P, I
Role play	53	Role-play parents and children watching a TV program, a visit to an eye physician, having to wear glasses, and others. Discuss the significance to vision.	P, I

TEACHING TECHNIQUES: CARE OF THE EYES—cont'd

		Grades
Self-test	**54** Give self-test on the structure and function of the eye.	I, U

Self-test illustration

eyeball   pupil   retina
iris   lens   optic nerve

Fill in the blanks using the words above.
_____ Small, dark, round hole in center of eye.
_____ Carries pictures from retina to brain.
_____ Moves up, down, and sideways.
_____ Light passes through lens, falls on lining at back of eyeball.
_____ Front part of eyeball, blue, brown or gray (in color) in circle.
_____ Behind the pupil and inside the eye.

Show and tell	**55** Children relate a visit to an eye physician or tell how wearing glasses helps those who need them.	P
Survey	**56** A student committee determines the amount of light in the classroom, halls, and other areas of the school using a light meter.	I, U

TEACHING TECHNIQUES

Care of the Feet

		Grades
Bulletin board	**1** Prepare a bulletin board display using magazine pictures and drawings of appropriate types of shoes for play, school, parties, and other occasions.	P, I, U
Chart	**2** Prepare a chart listing the important rules to consider when purchasing shoes.	P, I, U
	3 Prepare a chart listing the important rules to consider in caring for the feet.	P, I, U
Demonstration	**4** The proper way to walk with the feet parallel. Have children practice this method.	P, I, U
	5 The proper way to wash and dry the feet.	P, I, U
	6 To demonstrate the proper way to walk, have a pupil make footprints on paper and make cutouts of these prints. Draw a straight line on the floor with chalk and have the pupil tape the footprints to the floor so that the inside of each print is parallel to the line and the toes point straight ahead. Now permit the child to walk the chalk line stepping in the footprints.	I, U
	7 Have pupils trace the outline of their shoes on a piece of paper. Have them remove the shoes and trace the outline of the foot on top of the shoe outline. Compare the two drawings and determine whether the shoe is the proper size.	I, U
	8 The importance of the feet to posture. Illustrate how walking with pronated or inverted feet may cause undue back and leg pressures with the possible result that posture will be affected.	I, U
	9 High and low foot arches by having pupils walk on pieces of paper with wet feet.	I, U
Discussion	**10** The importance of changing shoes and socks when wet.	P, I, U
	11 The proper way to cut toenails.	P, I, U
	12 The importance of drying the feet properly.	P, I, U
	13 The proper care of the feet.	P, I, U
	14 The importance of shoes and socks or stockings that fit well and provide the best protection for the feet.	P, I, U
	15 The signs and symptoms of foot problems and who to see when they appear.	P, I, U
	16 How posture is affected by shoes that do not fit properly or are in poor condition.	P, I, U
	17 How to prevent athlete's foot and what to do about it when you have the condition.	I, U
	18 The importance of the bones and arches of the feet to posture and walking using a chart, drawing, or model.	I, U
Dramatization	**19** Dramatize buying a new pair of shoes.	P, I, U

TEACHING TECHNIQUES: CARE OF THE FEET—cont'd

			Grades
Exhibit	20	Display a variety of shoes for different kinds of activities.	P, I
	21	Display various types of materials found in socks, such as wool, nylon, and cotton, and discuss their significance in foot care.	I, U
Experience chart or record	22	Prepare an experience chart or record to show the proper ways to care for the feet.	P
Guest speaker	23	Invite a shoe salesman to discuss the way to select a properly fitting shoe.	I, U
	24	Invite a podiatrist to discuss the care of the feet.	U
Poems and plays	25	Children write poems, jingles, and plays about the proper care of the feet.	P
Posters	26	Make drawings or posters illustrating the importance of properly fitting shoes and socks.	P, I
Scrapbook	27	Prepare a scrapbook of magazine pictures and drawings of different styles of shoes for various activities and also stories about the care of the feet.	P, I
Story	28	Have children create a story about the kinds of shoes to wear for various types of weather.	P

TEACHING TECHNIQUES

Community Health

		Grades
Bulletin board	1 Display illustrated drawings or pictures of the functions of various community health agencies.	I, U
	2 Show the life cycle of the mosquito or the fly.	I, U
Chart	3 Make illustrated charts and posters about community health helpers.	P
	4 List ways children can help promote good health in the community.	P, I
	5 Make a chart listing the professional, official, and voluntary health agencies in the community.	I, U
Checklist	6 Prepare a checklist for use in rating the school health environment and the community health environment.	U
Construction	7 Make a bear's head out of papier-mache and a large ice cream carton; have the mouth open for paper deposits—"Litter Bear."	P, I
Demonstration	8 The correct way to use the drinking fountain.	P, I
	9 How water may be purified by filtration as illustrated in Fig. 12-9.	I, U

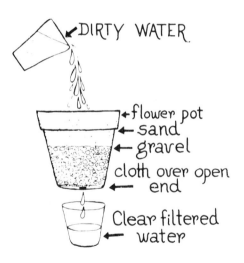

FIG. 12-9

10	Have pupils examine some swamp water under a microscope and a second sample of this same water after it has been treated with chlorine.	U
11	Show how a small amount of oil on water forms a thin layer that causes mosquito larvae to die because they cannot penetrate the film to breathe. Obtain swamp or other stagnant water containing mosquito larvae for this demonstration.	U

TEACHING TECHNIQUES: COMMUNITY HEALTH—cont'd

			Grades
Diorama	12	Prepare a diorama showing the locations of the agencies and the helpers involved in community health.	P
Discussion	13	Discuss and illustrate with pictures and stick-figure drawings the various kinds of community helpers who take care of our health, such as the fire fighter, the police officer, the doctor, the nurse, and the dentist.	P
	14	Collect pictures of ponds, lakes, rivers, and reservoirs and ask the class whether they think it is safe to drink water out of or swim in these places.	P, I
	15	The proper use and maintenance of drinking fountains and lavatories.	P, I
	16	The maintenance of a healthful school environment, including cleanliness, lighting, heating, and ventilation.	P, I
	17	The danger of petting strange animals and the procedures to follow if bitten by one.	P, I
	18	The importance of sanitation, including the disposal of lunch papers and refuse in the school and classroom.	P, I, U
	19	The community rules and regulations concerning garbage and rubbish disposal.	I, U
	20	The relationship of water supply to the sewage disposal system in schools, homes, and rural areas.	I, U
	21	The importance of restaurant sanitation.	I, U
	22	The responsibility of individuals to keep public places clean, such as picnic grounds, parks, campgrounds, and lavatories.	I, U
	23	The effects of water pollution and how local health laws protect against pollution.	I, U
	24	The need for periodic health examinations.	I, U
	25	The use of chemical sprays and dusts in agriculture and the possible dangers involved.	I, U
	26	Ways used by the city to remove and dispose of garbage and trash.	I, U
	27	The effects of radioactive waste dumping near communities.	I, U
Dramatization	28	Prepare and present a play to a parent group on the work of the health department.	I, U
	29	Prepare and present a play to a school assembly that will dramatize community health problems with possible solutions.	I, U
Drawings	30	Make drawings showing the sanitary procedures used in the school cafeteria.	I
Excursion	31	Take an excursion to the lavatories in the school and discuss use and maintenance.	P
	32	Visit a grocery store or food market to observe how perishable foods are stored and how cleanliness is practiced.	P
	33	Take a trip to a dairy to observe the sanitary procedures used in the handling of milk.	I, U
	34	Visit a water purification plant, a sewage disposal plant, or a health department.	I, U

TEACHING TECHNIQUES: COMMUNITY HEALTH—cont'd

		Grades
Excursion—cont'd	35 Visit food markets, restaurants, and other establishments to observe sanitary ways of handling and dispensing food.	I, U
	36 Visit a local hospital.	I, U
Exhibit	37 Display larvae, eggs, pupae, and adult mosquitoes and flies to observe development.	I, U
	38 Display pamphlets, books, and other reading material related to community health.	I, U
Experiment	39 To demonstrate the need for refrigeration in preserving foods, obtain two glasses of milk and cover them. Put one in the refrigerator and leave the other outside at room temperature. Compare the milk in each glass for several days, noting the differences in appearance, texture, and odor.	I, U
Guest speaker	40 Invite the custodian to discuss ways used to protect the health of pupils in school.	I, U
	41 Invite a member of the mosquito abatement office to discuss the control of mosquitoes and flies in the community.	I, U
	42 Invite members of the health department staff such as sanitarians, laboratory technologists, statisticians, and health officers to discuss community health.	I, U
	43 Invite a sanitarian from the local health department to discuss health laws regarding public eating places, public lavatories, and the sale of food in the community.	I, U
	44 Have a food service supervisor discuss rules and regulations regarding the school food program.	U
	45 Have a panel of speakers discuss possible health careers, such as nurses, physicians, dentists, and dietitians.	U
Individual and group reports	46 Write an individual or group letter to the city water department requesting literature on how water is filtered and purified.	I, U
	47 Write a group letter to the health department asking about its role in the health of the community.	I, U
	48 Write a group letter to the local health officer requesting materials that tell how he/she helps to protect the health of the community.	I, U
	49 Pupils prepare a list and conduct a study of the common insects and animals that carry disease and create sanitation problems.	I, U
	50 A pupil committee writes to the mosquito abatement office for information concerning the control of mosquitoes and flies.	I, U
	51 Report on the procedures used to make water safe for drinking in the community.	I, U
	52 Investigate the nature of air pollution and the role of the health department in this problem.	I, U
	53 Pupils write to the World Health Organization, the U.S. Public Health Service, and their state department of public health for information about services and activities.	U

TEACHING TECHNIQUES: COMMUNITY HEALTH—cont'd

		Grades
Individual and group reports—cont'd	54 Consult the local health officer and report on the morbidity and mortality statistics of the community.	U
	55 Pupils report on health heroes in history and their contributions to community health.	U
	56 Investigate ways that the community is protected against disease from people who come from foreign countries by ship and plane.	U
	57 Report on the services rendered to the community by agencies such as the heart and cancer organizations.	U
	58 Pupils write reports on the methods of sewage disposal in the community and the problems related to these procedures.	U
	59 Write reports on ways to purify water and compare them with the procedures used in the community.	U
Interview	60 Pupils interview parents on the major community health problems.	I, U
	61 Interview health officials and obtain information about food poisoning.	I, U
	62 A committee of pupils visits the cafeteria manager to discuss ways used to sanitize dishes, dispose of garbage, and store food.	I, U
	63 A committee of pupils interviews someone from the county or city health department for information about housing laws.	U
Mural	64 Draw a mural showing the location and functions of the various community health helpers.	P, I
Panel	65 Have a panel discussion of the major community health problems and present viewpoints of the nurse, physician, health officer, and others.	U
Posters	66 Make illustrated posters and charts about keeping clean public places, such as parks, lavatories, and campgrounds. Include slogans: "Did you use the garbage can?" "Did you leave the campground clean?"	I, U
	67 Pupils prepare drawings and posters after a trip to the dairy to observe the procedures used in sanitary handling of milk.	I, U
Scrapbooks	68 Prepare scrapbooks containing pictures of and newspaper and magazine articles on community health helpers.	I, U
	69 Make illustrated booklets of the work of the health department or a local hospital or both.	I
Show and tell	70 Have a child tell of a recent visit to a hospital.	P
Role play	71 Children dramatize an unclean classroom or improper sanitation in the cafeteria or a restaurant.	I
Story	72 Write a cooperative story about "Jeremiah Germ" who delights in bad health habits that help him get around the community.	P
Survey	73 A pupil committee surveys school environmental conditions, such as light, heat, and flies, that influence health.	I, U
	74 Have a committee survey the community to determine its "clean-up" need and plan a campaign.	U

TEACHING TECHNIQUES

Consumer Health*

			Grades

Attitude opinionnaire

1 Prepare a series of statements as illustrated below:

Check the appropriate box for each statement below (SA = strongly agree; A = agree; N = neutral; D = disagree; SD = strongly disagree).

	SA	A	N	D	SD
1. A physician is the best person to see when ill.	☐	☐	☐	☐	☐
2. Nurses provide reliable health information.	☐	☐	☐	☐	☐
3. People should treat themselves when ill.	☐	☐	☐	☐	☐
4. Acupuncture helps people with certain illnesses.	☐	☐	☐	☐	☐
5. Special foods and diets help people with arthritis.	☐	☐	☐	☐	☐
6. Books and pamphlets are good places to find out about health.	☐	☐	☐	☐	☐

Grade for item 1: **U**

Bulletin board

2 Display health products advertised in newspapers and magazines for student review and analysis. — I, U

3 Display magazine and newspaper articles related to consumer health that students bring to class. — I, U

4 List local consumer health agencies and organizations and the services they render. Include addresses and telephone numbers. — I, U

Discussion

5 Pupils bring a variety of labels from health products to class for discussion. — I, U

6 Pupils bring advertisements of health products to class for critical analysis. — I, U

7 TV and radio advertisement of health products. — I, U

8 The Pure Food, Drug, and Cosmetic Act. — U

9 Health food fads and fallacies. — U

10 Superstitions and quacks in health. — U

11 Role of the physician, nurse, dentist, and other health practitioners. — P, I, U

12 Use of products in the medicine cabinet at home. — P, I

13 Alternative healing philosophies—acupuncture, faith healing, chiropractic, and others. — U

14 Self-diagnosis and self-medication. — I, U

15 The intelligent health consumer. — P, I, U

16 Reliable sources of health information. — P, I, U

17 Community agencies and organizations to protect the health consumer. — U

18 Food fads—vitamins, wheat germ, yogurt, and others. — I, U

19 Use of aspirin and aspirinlike compounds. — P, I, U

Excursion

20 Visit a Food and Drug Administration laboratory. — I, U

---

*Teacher content information is available in Cornacchia HJ, Barrett S: *Consumer health: a guide to intelligent decisions,* ed 5, St Louis, 1993, Mosby–Year Book.

TEACHING TECHNIQUES: CONSUMER HEALTH—cont'd

		Grades
Exhibit	**21** Display a variety of items that are available in the various health food stores and discuss.	I, U
	22 Display labels from a variety of over-the-counter drugs available in drug stores.	I, U
	23 Have a place in the classroom where pamphlets and publications relating to consumer health are available for pupil use.	I, U
	24 Have the Food and Drug Administration, the Arthritis Foundation, or other organizations display gadgets and items sold by quacks in the community.	U
Guest speaker	**25** Invite the school nurse or a physician to discuss answers to such questions as "How can I choose a competent physician?" "Should I choose my own medication at the drugstore?" "What are the various kinds of specialists who can help me when I am sick and what do they do?"	I, U
	26 Invite a speaker from the Food and Drug Administration to relate how that organization protects the health of the consumer.	I, U
	27 Invite speakers from organizations such as the Federal Food and Drug Administration, the Better Business Bureau, the state Food and Drug Administration, the U.S. Postal Service, the Federal Trade Commission, or the American Medical Association to discuss how they protect the health of the consumer.	I, U
Individual and group reports	**28** Children prepare lists of the health products, or the products that affect health, advertised on radio and TV as well as in newspapers and magazines.	I, U
	29 Pupils collect lists of superstitions, sayings, or customs related to health and health practices.	I, U
	30 Pupils prepare reports on the meaning of the terms *quack* and *nostrum.*	U
	31 Write to the Food and Drug Administration, the Better Business Bureau, the American Medical Association, and other organizations for information and materials about consumer health.	U
	32 Pupils write reports on the different kinds of health specialists found in the community.	U
	33 Pupils prepare individual and group reports on consumer health found in current magazine articles.	U
	34 Compile a list of community sources from which reliable and accurate health information can be obtained.	I, U
	35 Students prepare a list of services rendered by community health agencies and organizations protecting the consumer.	U
	36 Students prepare reports analyzing health publications available for sale.	U

TEACHING TECHNIQUES: CONSUMER HEALTH—cont'd

		Grades

Interview   **37** A committee of pupils interviews a member of the Food and Drug Administration, the Better Business Bureau, the U.S. Postal Service, and other agencies that play a role in consumer health.   U

38 A pupil committee interviews a representative from the advertising department of a local newspaper to learn whether newspapers have criteria for accepting advertising for health products and services.   U

Panel   **39** Have a panel discussion of the question "What are the dangers of self-medication?" Present viewpoints of parents, nurse, and physician.   I, U

40 Have a panel discussion on the question "How should I choose a physician?" Present viewpoints of parents, nurse, and physician.   I, U

Self-test   **41** Prepare a self-test on superstitions, quackery, or health fads.   U

Nutrition facts or fiction?

Place a check mark in the box under the appropriate answer.

	FACT	FICTION	DON'T KNOW
1. Dry cereals are necessary for body energy.	☐	☐	☐
2. Raw eggs are more nutritious than cooked.	☐	☐	☐
3. Eating an egg a day is harmful.	☐	☐	☐
4. Fish and celery are brain food.	☐	☐	☐
5. Frozen orange juice has less nutritive value than fresh.	☐	☐	☐
6. Vegetable juices have magic health-giving qualities.	☐	☐	☐
7. All fruits and vegetables should be eaten raw.	☐	☐	☐
8. It is dangerous to leave food in a can that has been opened.	☐	☐	☐
9. Water is fattening.	☐	☐	☐
10. Drinking ice water causes heart trouble.	☐	☐	☐
11. Wine makes blood.	☐	☐	☐
12. If one vitamin pill a day is good, two or three are better.	☐	☐	☐
13. Meat is fattening.	☐	☐	☐
14. Toast has fewer calories than bread.	☐	☐	☐

Survey   **42** Students ask parents and friends about the kinds and extent of use of over-the-counter drug products purchased.   U

43 Students ask parents and friends about the kinds and extent of use of foods purchased in health food stores.   U

TEACHING TECHNIQUES

Dental Health

		Grades
Bulletin board	**1** Display a collection of magazine pictures about dental health.	P, I
	2 Display illustrated captions on dental health such as the following:	P, I

> I would have been just fine
> If I had kept my place in line
> To the faucet I didn't run
> Broke this tooth and that's no fun.
>
> Here's a tooth so very loose
> As you can see it's not much use.
> 'Cause Tommy refused to look ahead
> And ran into someone else's head.

3 Prepare posters or displays on dental health as illustrated in Figs. 12-10   P ,I ,U
to 12-14.

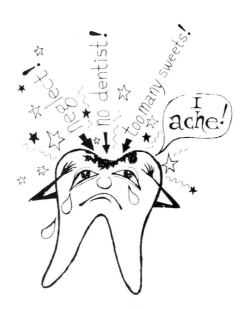

FIG. 12-10

TEACHING TECHNIQUES: DENTAL HEALTH—cont'd

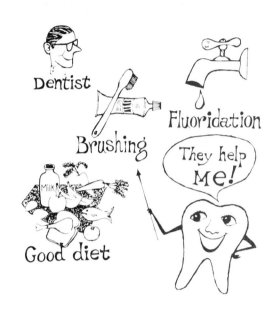

FIG. 12-11

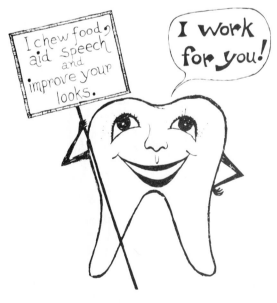

FIG. 12-12

TEACHING TECHNIQUES: DENTAL HEALTH—cont'd

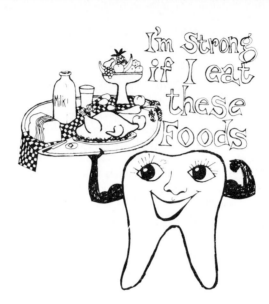

FIG. 12-13

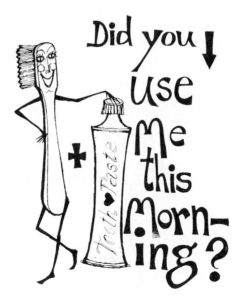

FIG. 12-14

TEACHING TECHNIQUES: DENTAL HEALTH—cont'd

		Grades
	4 Students help the teacher in the preparation of a health chart of practices that contribute to dental health as follows:	P, I

PRACTICES	PRODUCTS NEEDED	SERVICES NEEDED
Brush teeth	Brush	See dentist twice yearly or when problem develops
	Toothpaste	
Floss teeth	Dental floss	

		Grades
Brush-in	**5** Provide toothbrushes and toothpaste to be used in practicing toothbrushing procedures. Use disclosing tablets to determine effectiveness.	P, I
Checklist	**6** Children prepare a daily brushing chart to be taken home and hung in the bathroom to record when their teeth have been brushed.	P, I
	7 Have students complete and discuss "How do I rate?"	I, U

How do I rate?	YES	NO
1. I have had a thorough examination of my teeth in the last 6 months.	☐	☐
2. All dental treatment recommended by my dentist has been completed.	☐	☐
3. I brush my teeth or rinse my mouth with water soon after eating.	☐	☐
4. I understand the importance of having missing teeth replaced.	☐	☐
5. I do not eat sweets between meals	☐	☐
6. I have my teeth cleaned by a dentist or dental hygienist regularly.	☐	☐
7. I know that sugar in candy and soft drinks can lead to tooth decay.	☐	☐
8. My teeth have been treated with a fluoride solution or sealant at the recommended ages.	☐	☐

		Grades
Construction	**8** Children make large construction paper toothbrushes. Each day the child reports the removal of plaque from brushing, the child may hang the brush on the wall-long toothbrush holder.	P
Debate	**9** Have a debate or panel discussion on fluoridation of the water supply.	U
Demonstration	**10** Teacher demonstrates the proper way to brush teeth, and students practice the technique using the flexed fingers of one hand on the cheeks and lips. Distribute toothbrushes and small tubes of toothpaste for all children to take home and use.	
	11 Make tooth powder in class. Students mix the following ingredients in the proportions indicated: 1 teaspoon salt, 2 to 3 teaspoons baking soda, and 1 or 2 drops of oil of peppermint, wintergreen, or cinnamon. Pupils take home some of the mixture to use when brushing teeth.	P, I
	12 Demonstrate proper way to use dental floss and have students practice this skill in class.	I, U

TEACHING TECHNIQUES: DENTAL HEALTH—cont'd

		Grades
Demonstration—cont'd	**13** Demonstrate the proper way to brush teeth using a large toothbrush and a large set of teeth. Children participate in a toothbrush drill using tongue depressors instead of toothbrushes. Pupils also practice rinsing their mouth and swallowing—"swishing and swallowing."	P
	14 Show spoonful amounts of sugar found in candy, soft drinks, and other foods by placing equivalent quantities in plastic bags or other containers. Each container should be labeled and placed on exhibit.	I, U
Discussion	**15** The value of certain foods, such as apples, celery, carrots, and oranges, as tooth cleaners.	P
	16 Display and discuss magazine pictures brought by children showing good and bad foods for teeth using "the happy and sad tooth" chart.	P
	17 The loss of primary teeth (deciduous) as a normal process unless there is tooth decay or an accident.	P
	18 The importance of teeth in speaking after having children pronounce such words as thirsty, thank you, thistle, and sister Susie sitting on a thistle.	P
	19 Show and discuss pictures of people smiling. Illustrate how some of these people would look with missing teeth by blackening a few teeth.	P
	20 The reasons why the dentist is a friend.	P
	21 Have the class discuss how teeth grow by examining a model of the teeth and jaw.	I, U
	22 The types and functions of teeth, using models: incisor—cuts; cuspid—tears; bicuspid—crushes; molar—grinds.	P, I
	23 The qualities and care of a good toothbrush. Draw on blackboard or bring models of toothbrushes to school.	P, I, U
	24 During discussion of teeth have pupils label photocopied diagrams.	I, U
	25 The value of the use of toothpastes or tooth powders.	I, U
	26 Fluoridation.	U
	27 Discuss the decay process using the illustration in Fig. 12-15.	P, I, U
Dramatization	**28** Children set up a dentist's chair and dramatize cleaning teeth and visiting a dentist. A discussion should precede this activity on how to clean teeth and why visits to the dentist are necessary.	P
	29 To show that acid will weaken substances containing calcium (such as tooth enamel), place a whole egg in a bowl of vinegar (acetic acid) for about 24 hours. The eggshell should become soft as the vinegar decalcifies the shell.	P, I, U
	30 Have the class write a play on dental health and present it to a parent group or at a school assembly.	P, I, U
Drawing	**31** Children draw, color, and possibly animate different teeth as well as different parts of teeth.	P, I
Excursion	**32** Visit the community water plant and observe how water is fluoridated.	U

TEACHING TECHNIQUES: DENTAL HEALTH—cont'd

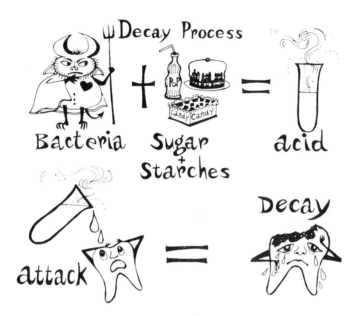

FIG. 12-15

			Grades
Exhibit	**33**	Display pencils, unshelled nuts, buttons, and other hard objects and discuss the dangers to teeth when these items are bitten or chewed.	P, I
	34	Display an explorer and mouth mirror and other implements used by the dentist to examine the teeth and discuss them.	P, I
	35	Build a toothbrush holder and supply each child with a new toothbrush for noon brushing. Be certain that each brush is properly labeled with each child's name on it.	P, I
	36	Display several types of toothbrushes.	I, U
	37	Display booklets, pamphlets, teeth, models, and other items relating to dental health.	I
	38	Display x-ray films and discuss their use in dental care.	I, U
	39	Obtain extracted teeth from a dentist and display to illustrate decayed teeth.	I, U
	40	Display models of orthodontia showing before and after results.	U
	41	Exhibit mouth protectors used in sports such as football and boxing.	U
	42	Show the relative amounts of sugar in different foods, such as candy bars and soft drinks.	U

TEACHING TECHNIQUES: DENTAL HEALTH—cont'd

		Grades
Experience chart	**43** Prepare an experience chart or record listing significant points about dental health, such as:	P

> Teeth are our helpers.
> Teeth must be cleaned.
> Teeth help us to chew.

		Grades
	44 Prepare a chart listing the foods that are good for teeth.	P
Experiment	**45** Observe the progress of decay in two apples by breaking the skin of one and leaving the other intact. Place both apples in a place where they can be seen for a few days and relate to what happens in the dental decay process.	P, I
	46 Have child eat a cracker and with the tongue feel the coating of food on the teeth. Then have each student eat a piece of carrot, celery, or apple and note how much cleaner the teeth feel.	P, I
	47 To show the presence of bacteria in the mouth, sterilize some gelatin (sweetened with sugar) in a pressure cooker for 15 minutes (or heat in oven at 100° to 120° F for 1 hour). Prepare two shallow dishes of the gelatin. Carefully scrape between the teeth and near the gum line to remove food debris (may use a toothpick). Place these scrapings in one dish. Cover both dishes, label, and place in a warm place. After several days fungus growth should appear in the dish exposed to the mouth bacteria, but little or none will be seen in the uncontaminated dish.	I, U
Flannelboard	**48** Compose a story of how a rabbit or other animal took care of its teeth and illustrate the procedures using a flannelboard.	P
	49 Prepare models to compare the parts of a tooth with a hardcooked egg or an apple.	P, I

> *Enamel*—skin of apple or egg shell
> *Dentin*—white of apple or egg white
> *Pulp*—core of apple or egg yolk

		Grades
	50 Discuss appropriate foods for dental health by preparing models for use on the flannelboard and include poor food (candy and soft drinks) models, but do not put sandpaper on the backs of these items. When an attempt is made to place them on the board, they will fall off, indicating poor quality.	P, I, U
	51 Show the parts of the tooth and how decay proceeds by using colored flannel cutouts with black for decay, gray for a filling, pink for the pulp, yellow for the dentin, white for enamel, and red for infection and abscess. Use name tags (enamel, dentin, crown, and others) made of paper with sandpaper backing to identify the flannel parts.	P, I, U
	52 Illustrate the decay process (Fig. 12-15).	P, I, U
	53 Illustrate the progressive stages of dental caries.	P, I, U
Field trip	**54** Students visit a dentist's office.	P, I

TEACHING TECHNIQUES: DENTAL HEALTH—cont'd

		Grades
Flip chart	55 Make a flip chart that shows the importance of retaining all of one's teeth. Show pictures of appetizing foods, such as steak, apples, oranges and celery. Also illustrate types of baby food that would have to be eaten if children did not have teeth.	I, U
Guest speaker	56 Invite a dentist or dental hygienist to class to discuss dental care.	P, I, U
Individual and group reports	57 Children write a brief summary paragraph in answer to the question "What must we do to take care of our teeth?"	P, I, U
	58 Children prepare lists of good dental snacktime foods.	P, I, U
	59 A pupil committee sends a composite letter to the American Dental Association requesting materials on dental health.	I, U
	60 Pupils write reports on the values of x-ray films in dental health.	I, U
	61 Pupils investigate the use of fluoride in preventing tooth decay.	U
	62 Pupils write a group letter to the water commission requesting information about the natural supply of fluoride in the water supply.	U
	63 Students identify foods consumed in 1 day and determine the amount of sugar in each item and total the daily intake. Provide plans for reduction of amount eaten.	I, U
Kit	64 Prepare a plaque control kit containing a toothbrush and flossing material for use at school or at home.	P, I, U
Mural	65 Make a mural in which each child draws a self-portrait and writes a slogan under the picture describing good dental health practices.	I
Poems	66 Create original poems.	P

> We brush the teeth as they grow
> Down from the top and
> Up from below.
> Your teeth look swell
> When you brush them well.
> But your teeth decay
> When you keep the brush away.

Puppets	67 Children participate in puppet shows emphasizing a visit to the dentist, brushing the teeth properly, or eating the proper foods for dental health.	P
Scrapbooks	68 Children prepare scrapbooks of picture cutouts showing good and bad teeth, as well as proper and improper foods for dental health; also drawings of toothbrushes, dental floss, and toothpaste.	P, I
Show and tell	69 Children share a visit to the dentist or the experience of losing a tooth.	P
Songs	70 Create simple toothbrushing or dental health songs.	P

> TUNE: *A Hunting We Will Go*
> A brushing we will go,
> A brushing we will go,
> We'll brush our teeth so white and clean,
> A brushing we will go.

TEACHING TECHNIQUES: DENTAL HEALTH—cont'd

		Grades
Songs —cont'd	TUNE: *Mulberry Bush* This is the way we brush our teeth, Brush our teeth, brush our teeth, This is the way we brush our teeth Right after eating food.	
Stories	71 Have children make up a short story about the care of teeth.	P
Survey	72 Survey the class to determine how many pupils have visited the dentist within the past year.	I, U
	73 Have children keep records of the amount of candy, soft drinks, and other such items consumed and estimate the total amounts of sugar being eaten.	I, U
Tasting party	74 Have a bunny rabbit party in which celery, green peppers, and carrot sticks are served and discuss their importance in helping to clean teeth.	P, I, U
	75 Plan a dental health program for parents and serve nutritious snacktime foods.	P, I, U

TEACHING TECHNIQUES

Disease Control and Prevention (also see HIV/AIDS)

		Grades
Bulletin board	**1** Display a list of good health rules and practices that will protect children from disease.	P
	2 Display illustrations of animals and insects that carry disease.	P, I
	3 Display pictures or drawings showing how to cover the face when coughing or sneezing.	P, I
	4 Prepare posters to illustrate ways to protect others from communicable diseases, such as:	P, I

> Catch that sneeze (use of handkerchief or tissue)
> Cut the apple to share it (rather than taking a bite)
> Use your own comb or towel or washcloth

	5 Display the signs, symptoms, control, and treatment of a particular disease. Different diseases can be featured. Community health organizations often have materials to help with the bulletin board.	U
	6 Prepare pictures of such items as soap, washcloth, toothbrush, comb, and towel. Place caption below reading "We need these to keep clean."	P
	7 Display the hands of all the children in class by tracing them on paper and making cutouts. Place the caption below to read "We wash our hands."	P
Chart	**8** Prepare a chart that lists the ways germs are transmitted from one person to another: talking, sneezing, coughing, dirty hands and objects, carelessness in handling foods, utensils, and dishes.	P, I
	9 Make a "Good health habits" chart to include statements with illustrations of the following:	P

> My hair is combed.
> My face is clean.
> I wash my hands and nails often.
> My clothes are neat and clean.
> My shoes are clean.

Choral speaking	**10** Children participate in choral speaking.	P

My tissue

> See my tissue white as snow,
> I use it when my nose I blow,
> It's not to play with,
> Oh, my, no!!

Construction	**11** Prepare a disease prevention railroad train for bulletin board display using construction paper. The various freight cars should be hauling a comb, toothbrush, handkerchief, washcloth, soap, and other items needed. Each car can be labeled "Comb car," "Toothbrush car," and	P, I

TEACHING TECHNIQUES: DISEASE CONTROL AND PREVENTION—cont'd

		Grades
Construction— cont'd	other appropriate names. The total train might be called "The disease prevention train" or the "Getting ready for school train."	
	12 Construct a TV box and prepare a series of panels on various aspects of cleanliness. Children or teacher could make the panels, which might include soap, comb, wash cloth, children washing, and others. Have a TV show when everything is ready.	P
Demonstration	13 The proper way to blow the nose.	P, I
	14 The way to cover coughs and sneezes.	P, I
	15 The proper way to wash hands.	P, I
	16 The proper use of handkerchief or tissue.	P, I
	17 How to use a paper bag as a sanitary way to discard disposable tissues and other contaminated objects.	P, I, U
	18 Darken the classroom and flash the light from a movie projector on the wall so that the dust particles in the air may be seen. This will show how germs may be spread by the dust to which they attach.	I, U
	19 Have a member of the health department demonstrate different types of disease testing.	I, U
	20 The use of the clinical thermometer in class and its importance in illness.	I, U
	21 Demonstrate how germs may be transmitted by putting fluorescent dye on some coins or other appropriate objects with several pupils handling the items. Have one or two of these pupils wash their hands with soap and water. Using "black light" (ultraviolet) in a darkened room, observe the hands of the children who handled the objects as well as those who washed their hands. If the dye remains on the hands, it will be clearly visible by glowing in the "black light" and thus showing how germs may be spread. The washed hands may or may not fluoresce, depending on the thoroughness of the washing. Ultraviolet light may be damaging if shone directly into the eyes. The nurse may have a Wood's light for use in this demonstration.	I, U
	22 Show pictures of a boy washing hands, a girl washing hands, and hands being washed with soap. Discuss how and when to wash hands. Demonstrate the proper way and follow by having all children practice the proper way to wash hands (Fig. 12-16).	P
	23 Demonstrate the proper ways to wash the hands and face.	P
	24 Make soap in the classroom.	P, I
	25 Show the proper way to clean and file fingernails.	P, I
	26 Have children use a magnifying glass to examine the creases and folds of the skin and the dirt on one hand. After washing the hand have pupils again examine the skin.	I
	27 Examine samples of different kinds of clothing material with magnifying glass. Discuss seasonal appropriateness of each.	I

TEACHING TECHNIQUES: DISEASE CONTROL AND PREVENTION—cont'd

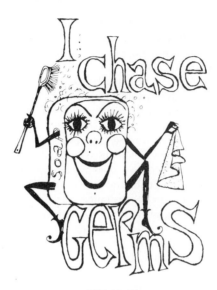

FIG. 12-16

			Grades
Demonstra- tion—cont'd	28	Demonstrate "hidden dirt" on the skin of a child who appears to be clean but has perspired by washing an area of the skin with rubbing alcohol using a piece of cotton. Show the cotton to the class after the demonstration.	I, U
	29	Display two beakers containing warm water in one and cold water in the other with each having a tablespoon of oil and a tablespoon of liquid soap. Stir both beakers and compare the results. Warm water disperses the oil globules more effectively and hence is better for washing.	I, U
	30	Using charts and models, study the structure of the skin and relate this to cleanliness and disease control.	I, U
Discussion	31	Disease control in terms of sleep and rest requirements.	P
	32	Briefly discuss some of the common childhood diseases, their symptoms, prevention, and control.	P
	33	The need for immunizations.	P
	34	Why children should stay at home when they have a fever.	P, I
	35	How to protect ourselves and others from contracting contagious diseases.	P, I
	36	The importance of washing hands before lunch and after using the toilet. Have children practice these habits at the appropriate times.	P, I

TEACHING TECHNIQUES: DISEASE CONTROL AND PREVENTION—cont'd

		Grades
Discussion — cont'd	37 Cleanliness in handling and consuming food; washing of fruits and vegetables before eating and refusing to share bites of food or to eat food that has been dropped on the floor.	P, I
	38 The causes of disease.	P, I
	39 Colds and other contagious diseases in terms of prevention.	P, I
	40 Beneficial and harmful germs. Beneficial germs give cheese its flavor, make bread rise, and turn apple juice to cider. Harmful germs cause disease and illness.	P, I
	41 The importance and significance of poliomyelitis immunization.	P, I, U
	42 The use of disinfectant in the control of disease.	I, U
	43 The methods that help to destroy bacteria: soap and water, pasteurization, sterilization, light, and air.	I, U
	44 Tuberculin test and its meaning.	I, U
	45 Food poisoning and how it may be prevented.	I, U
	46 The heart and heart disease using a model of the heart and a chart of the circulatory system.	U
	47 Weather and seasonal changes that require different kinds of clothing.	P, I
	48 Pictures of appropriate shoes and clothing for work and play, as well as for different kinds of weather.	P, I
	49 The correct disposal of tissues.	P, I
	50 Such questions as "Why should I keep clean?" "What should I do before I eat?"	P, I
	51 Need, frequency, and methods of bathing.	P, I
Dramatization	52 Dramatize a visit to the doctor to be immunized or to obtain treatment for a contagious disease.	P
	53 Getting ready for school using towels, soap, nail file, mirror, nail brush, comb and brush, toothbrush, and tissue.	P
Excursion	54 Visit the school health office and meet the school nurse.	P
Exhibit	55 Display pamphlets and materials on communicable diseases for student use.	I, U
	56 Display samples of clothing for use in different kinds of weather. Have children discuss and select appropriate apparel for the weather indicated by the teacher or by pupils.	P
Experience chart	57 Prepare an experience chart about good health practices in preventing and controlling communicable disease.	P
Experiments	58 To show the existence of germs on the hands, wash with soap and water and place salt on them. Try to rub off the salt until none is visible. By touching the tongue to the hands it can be shown that salt still remains. Wash hands again with soap and water and touch tongue to hands to show that the salt has been removed.	P, I

TEACHING TECHNIQUES: DISEASE CONTROL AND PREVENTION—cont'd

		Grades
Experiments— cont'd	**59** To discover the conditions that may affect the growth of germs, have pupils wet two pieces of cloth and place one in a dark, warm place and the other in sunlight and air for 1 week. The results will show that warmth, moisture, and darkness help molds and bacteria to grow, whereas sunshine prevents this process.	P, I
	60 To discover that hands are germ carriers, have pupils with dirty hands touch a piece of bread and place it in a labeled jar. Have children with freshly scrubbed and dried hands touch another piece of bread and place it in a second labeled jar. After a week or more, the piece of bread that was touched with the dirty hands will have much more mold than that touched with clean hands.	P, I
	61 To discover how germs are spread, push a needle into the moldy part of an orange. Pierce a second orange with the contaminated needle. Clean and sterilize the needle by boiling and pierce a third orange. Label all oranges and observe the changes that occur daily for a week or more. Mold will grow on the contaminated orange.	I, U
	62 To discover the presence of germs, wash, dry, and sterilize (heat directly on an electric plate at medium temperature for 1 hour on each side) two Petri dishes (may use metal lids and glass squares). Prepare a sterile solution by dissolving ½ ounce of plain gelatin in 1¾ cups of water and boil for 1 hour. Pour this substance into the Petri dishes. Cough into one Petri dish and cover. Merely cover the second dish. Place these dishes in a warm dark place and observe them daily for 1 week. Colonies of bacteria will develop in the contaminated dish.	I, U
	63 To discover that sunlight kills bacteria, inoculate two Petri dishes (prepared as previously described) from a dish where bacteria are growing. Place one dish in the open sunlight and the other in a warm, dark place. After one dish has been in the sunlight for several hours, place it in the dark, warm place with the other dish. Examine the two dishes each day for several days.	I, U
	64 Using a magnifying glass, study the molds that have grown on stale bread, fruit, or other material. Bring a microscope to class for each child to view this mold.	I, U
	65 To show the growth of germs, boil some small, peeled potatoes, keeping them firm, and place one in each of four sterile pint jars with lids. Maintain one jar as a control, but contaminate the potatoes in the other three jars by (a) rubbing with dirty hands, (b) rubbing with hands after washing with soap and water, and (c) rubbing with tissue after blowing nose. Put lids on all jars, label, and place in a warm but visible location. Observe daily the growth of bacteria and compare with the control potato.	I, U

TEACHING TECHNIQUES: DISEASE CONTROL AND PREVENTION—cont'd

		Grades
Experiments— cont'd	66 Touch different articles in the classroom with swabs and touch these to Petri dishes containing agar. Incubate the dishes so that the germs will grow. Ask a laboratory technologist from the health department to identify some of the germs.	I, U
	67 To teach the importance of cleanliness, put some dust on a sterile agar Petri dish (may use gelatin if agar not available), cover, and place in a warm, dark place. Use a sterile Petri dish as a control, cover, and place with the first dish. Observe results daily for about 1 week and compare the growth of germs.	I, U
	68 To show how flies spread disease, have one crawl across a sterile agar Petri dish (may use thin layer of gelatin if agar not available), cover, and place in a warm, dark place. Use a sterile Petri dish as a control; cover, and place with the first dish. Observe results daily for about 1 week and compare the growth of germs.	I, U
Finger plays	69 Children participate in finger plays.	P

Here is my little washcloth,	Here is Johnny, ready for bed;
Here is my bar of soap.	Down on the pillow he lays his head.
This is the way I wash my face,	He pulls up the covers over him tight,
Until it's clean, I hope.	This is the way he sleeps all night.
This is the way I brush my teeth,	Morning comes, the sun is bright,
Until they are so white.	Back with a kick the covers fly.
I drink my milk and eat my cereal	He jumps up and gets dressed
So at school I feel just right.	And goes to school to play with the rest.

		Grades
Flannelboard	70 Use paper dolls on a flannelboard to illustrate appropriate clothing for school and different kinds of weather.	P, I
Guest speakers	71 Invite the health officer or nurse to discuss communicable diseases.	P, I, U
	72 Invite guest speakers from the heart, cancer, and lung associations to discuss the nature of chronic diseases.	U
	73 Invite a nurse, dermatologist, or other physician to discuss skin problems or care of the skin.	U
Individual and group reports	74 Children write a brief summary paragraph or two in answer to the question "Why is it necessary to wash our hands and when should this be done?"	P, I
	75 Children write a brief report on "Why I should stay home when I am ill."	I, U
	76 Pupils read about such health heroes as Antonie van Leeuwenhoek, Robert Koch, and Louis Pasteur and write about their contributions to the control of disease.	I, U
	77 Pupils read and write reports about communicable disease transmitted by insects or animals to humans, including methods of control.	I, U
	78 Pupils write to the health department, requesting materials about the control of diseases.	I, U

TEACHING TECHNIQUES: DISEASE CONTROL AND PREVENTION—cont'd

		Grades
Individual and group reports — cont'd	79 Pupils prepare written reports for publication in the school newspaper on tuberculosis, poliomyelitis, colds, and other communicable diseases.	I, U U
	80 Form pupil committees to report on diseases such as tetanus, measles, hepatitis, and chicken pox.	I, U
	81 Pupils read and write about harmful bacteria in drinking water, milk, or food.	I, U
	82 Pupils write reports on TV or radio programs they have seen or heard on the control of diseases.	I, U
Interview	83 A pupil committee interviews health department officials about the prevention and control of disease in the community.	I, U
Mobile	84 Make a mobile showing a toothbrush, comb, washcloth, nail file, and other items needed for cleanliness and disease control.	P
Pantomime	85 Discuss the various procedures a child should follow when getting ready for school. Have children pantomime these procedures and let the class guess the activities being dramatized.	P
Poem	86 Children or teacher or all create poems.	P, I, U

Dirt

Dirt is fine:
　For gardens and roads,
　For worms and toads,
　For puppies to dig—
　And maybe for pigs—
　For cats
　For rats
　For night-flying bats,
　For lambs
　And clams
　And even for dams,
　For slugs and snails,
　But
　　Under my nails,
　Not mine!

If you cough,
Or if you sneeze,
Cover your mouth
With a tissue, please.

Cover your mouth when you sneeze,
'Cause if you don't
Someone might get a disease.

TEACHING TECHNIQUES: DISEASE CONTROL AND PREVENTION—cont'd

		Grades
Poem—cont'd	**The man with the flying sneeze**	

Germs fly through the air with the greatest of ease,
Whenever you cough or whenever you sneeze.
So don't be a goose,
A clean tissue use,
Anytime with a flying sneeze.
    Ah—Chooooooooo————

Good food we should eat,
And get plenty of sleep.
When water is deep,
Away from it keep.
Be on the alert
And don't be a jerk
Anytime with a flying sneeze.

Posters	87 Children make posters about the control and prevention of communicable diseases.	P, I, U
Problem solving	88 Jimmy and his parents are going on a camping trip for a week where there are no modern facilities such as tap water, electricity, or other conveniences. Help Jimmy answer the following questions: How can we keep clean? How can we obtain safe drinking water? What should we do if we get a cut knee? What other things must be done to protect ourselves from diseases?	I, U
Puppets	89 Make two puppets and call them "Healthy Harry" and "Sick Sam." Dramatize children coming to school who feel sick.	P
Quiz	90 Show students a series of pictures and have them tell or write the answers to these questions.	P, I

PICTURES	QUESTIONS
Washing hands	1. When do we do this?
Brushing teeth	2. When do we do this?
Going to bed	3. How much sleep do we need?
Coughing or sneezing	4. What must we do?
Wearing raincoat	5. Why do we need this?

Research	91 Children read and write reports on how disease germs are spread and controlled.	I
	92 Committees prepare oral and written reports on the following diseases: heart, cancer, diabetes, asthma, allergies, and arthritis.	U
Riddle	93 Make up riddles such as "I'm thinking of something we should do after we play and before we eat. What is it?"	P, I
Scrapbooks	94 Prepare scrapbooks of magazine and newspaper articles and pictures relating to communicable diseases.	I
	95 Pupils collect magazine articles, pictures, and other information on chronic diseases and prepare scrapbooks.	U
Self-test	96 Prepare a self-test on the prevention and control of disease.	I, U

TEACHING TECHNIQUES: DISEASE CONTROL AND PREVENTION—cont'd

			Grades
Show and tell	97	Children report experiences about illnesses at home.	P
Role play	98	The school health examination.	P, I
	99	The immunization procedure.	P, I
	100	The procedures for the proper handling of foods.	P, I
	101	The role of the nurse and the physician in the prevention of disease.	P, I
Stories and songs	102	Prepare creative stories and songs about the physician, nurse, and health habits.	P
Survey	103	Survey the nature of illness and the extent of immunizations of the children in class.	I, U

TEACHING TECHNIQUES

Drugs

		Grades
Advertisements	1 Students bring drug advertisements to class for analysis.	U
Brainstorming	2 Have students identify ways they can contribute to the control of drugs in the school and the community.	U
Bulletin board	3 Display magazine and newspaper articles brought to class by pupils.	U
	4 Display illustrations of popular drugs used and abused.	I, U
	5 Display pamphlets and other reading materials and permit students to select items they wish to read or report on.	U
	6 Display of ways to say "no."	I, U
Buzz groups	7 Discussion questions: Why should students not use drugs? Why should marijuana not be legalized? Does "everybody's using drugs" mean everyone should do so?	U
Comparative analysis	8 Have students seriously think about something they like to do above all else—art, music, reading, football—and ask them to jot down in several brief, concise phrases their feelings of what this activity does to and for themselves. Teachers list all the phrases on the chalkboard without reference to the activity. Give students a copy of a list of phrases extracted from drug abusers about their feelings of what drugs do for them. Compare this list with the chalkboard list, which might include:	U

It makes you aware.	It gives you a sense of awe of nature.
My mind is broadened.	It's an intense total experience.
It does something to my perception.	You appreciate your senses better.
I notice differences more.	It puts me in a world by myself.
It increases my potential.	I don't understand why people find
The world is more interesting.	boredom in living.
	I am totally involved in the environment.

	Ask students to identify the similarities and differences in the two lists and give the reasons why. This procedure should encourage a discussion of alternatives to drugs.	
Discussion	9 The kinds of medicines that are used by members of the family such as cough medicine, aspirin, antacids, antihistamines, and others. Also talk about the effects of these drugs on the body: sedation, relief of pain, and relief of symptoms.	I, U
	10 Read current newspaper articles about drugs and have pupils prepare questions that they wish to have answered. List these questions on the blackboard and have pupils determine how to find answers.	U
	11 The importance of taking prescription drugs under parents' and doctors' supervision.	P, I
	12 The factors that put people at risk for early use of drugs.	P, I
	13 Why people use drugs.	U

TEACHING TECHNIQUES: DRUGS—cont'd

			Grades
Discussion—cont'd	14	The physiological effects of drugs such as marijuana, heroin, morphine, barbiturates, amphetamines, volatile chemicals, hallucinogens, and others on the body.	I, U
	15	Sociological factors, including laws of drug use and abuse.	U
	16	Drug usage by students in schools.	U
	17	Poisonous substances in the home.	P, I
	18	Emergency procedures when poisonous substances are ingested.	P, I, U
	19	How young people are introduced to drugs.	I, U
	20	The federal and state regulations concerning the sale and use of drugs.	U
Dramatization	21	A student is urged by friends to ingest an unknown substance.	I, U
Exhibit	22	Display a variety of containers that contain drugs obtainable at drug stores.	U
	23	Display a variety of pamphlets, magazine articles, and other materials for pupil use in writing and preparing reports.	U
Field trip	24	Students attend a court session involving illegal drugs.	U
	25	Students visit and talk with recovering drug abusers.	U
	26	Entire class visits a jail.	U
Guest speaker	27	Invite a member of the sheriff's office, the local police department, or the state narcotics office to discuss narcotic drugs.	U
	28	Invite a physician or pharmacist to come to class to discuss the effects of drugs on the human body.	U
Individual and group reports	29	Vocabulary lists and definitions of such drugs as narcotics, heroin, morphine, marijuana, barbiturates, amphetamines, hallucinogens, volatile substances.	U
	30	Use of drugs by individuals and their effects on the body.	I, U
	31	Oral and written reports on the use of drugs in medicine.	U
	32	Origins of drugs.	U
	33	Federal, state, and local laws about the sale and use of drugs.	U
Music	34	Have students relate rock music, or music in general, to the drug scene.	U
Newspaper articles	35	Students collect articles about drugs for discussion in class.	I, U
Interview	36	A committee of pupils interviews a physician to obtain information about the values, dangers, and abuses of the use of drugs.	U
Panel	37	Have a panel discussion describing the effects of such drugs as aspirin, sleeping pills, and tranquilizers on the human organism.	U
Peer group	38	Upper-grade students prepare presentation for sixth-grade pupils or seventh and eighth graders.	U
Posters	39	Students plan a drug education program for schools using a variety of posters.	U
Pretest	40	Give a pretest to determine the extent of pupils' knowledge about drugs.	U

TEACHING TECHNIQUES: DRUGS—cont'd

		Grades
Problem solving	41 Provide samples of tobacco and alcohol advertising and have students identify the techniques that encourage use.	U
	42 Procedures to be followed to ensure the proper use of medicines.	P, I
	43 If you discovered your brother, sister, or friend using drugs, what would you do? What should you do?	U
	44 What might be the consequences if you are attending a party or are in a car where drugs are being used?	U
Puppets	45 Prepare stick or other types of puppets and dramatize use of medicine in the home.	P
Questions and answers	46 Pupils prepare anonymous questions that they would like answered about drugs.	U
	47 Provide opportunities for students to meet voluntarily in small groups or on a one-to-one basis with a school person who communicates easily with students and is knowledgeable about the drug scene.	U
Reports	48 Have students prepare reports on: my philosophy of life; what I value; peer pressure and drug use; drug laws and minors.	U
Records	49 Play records of rock bands related to drugs. Prepare verses to songs and discuss contents.	U
Role playing	50 Students dramatize a parent giving medicine to a sick child.	P
	51 Students dramatize someone refusing an offer to smoke a marijuana cigarette.	I, U
Scrapbook	52 Pupils make scrapbooks containing drawings, newspaper and magazine articles, and written reports on drugs.	U
Sociodrama	53 Conduct a sociodrama so students can look strong while saying "no" to drug or alcohol use.	U
Student information center	54 Establish a location in school staffed by students where pupils seeking information may go for help.	U
Survey	55 Students attempt to discover the extent of the use of drugs in school.	U
Television	56 Students view a current program about drugs and prepare a report for class.	U

TEACHING TECHNIQUES

Exercise and Body Mechanics*

		Grades
Bulletin board	**1** Display drawings or pictures of proper sitting, standing, and walking posture.	P, I, U
	2 Display charts of the muscles and bones (skeleton) with captions or illustrations showing their relation to exercise, movement, and body mechanics.	P, I, U
	3 Display a series of pictures or drawings of beneficial activities and exercises.	I, U
Debate or panel	**4** Have a debate or panel discussion on the "Soft American." Bring in viewpoints of physicians, parents, and others.	U
Demonstration	**5** Children observe own posture in a full-length mirror.	P, I, U
	6 The correct way to pick up objects.	P, I, U
	7 Correct sitting, standing, and walking posture. Conduct activities in which pupils practice these procedures.	P, I, U
	8 Correct body alignment using a plumb line.	I, U
	9 Have pupils walk attempting to carry a book on their heads after they have assumed the correct posture.	I, U
	10 To show the effect of exercise on pulse rate, have pupils take own pulse while sitting or at rest. Permit them to stand in the aisles and jump up and down about 10 times and again take own pulse rates. Range of pulse rates before and after exercise can be noted on board with individual differences and relationships to exercise discussed.	I, U
	11 Conduct posture parade monthly in which the class votes on the boy or girl demonstrating the best walking posture. Children should determine in advance how they plan to make their selection.	I, U
	12 To show the effect of exercise on breathing and oxygen intake, have children count the number of breaths they normally take per minute using a watch with a sweep second hand. Have pupils stand in the aisles, jump up and down about 10 times, and count the number of breaths needed after exercise.	I, U
	13 Children stand against a wall and try to make their heads, shoulders, hips, and heels touch the wall. Follow this action by having pupils walk away from the wall retaining this position.	P, I, U
Diorama	**14** Prepare a diorama of suitable physical education activities and exercises using pipe cleaners for figures.	I, U
Discussion	**15** The importance and need for exercise in the maintenance and development of physical fitness.	P, I, U
	16 The relationship of muscles and bones to good body mechanics.	P, I, U
	17 The factors that influence posture, such as food, sleep, exercise, and mental attitudes.	I, U
	18 The relationship of exercise and eating to good posture.	I, U

TEACHING TECHNIQUES: EXERCISE AND BODY MECHANICS—cont'd

		Grades
Discussion— cont'd	19 The types of exercise and sports activities that are beneficial.	I, U
	20 The importance of muscular strength in preventing fatigue and in performing daily activities.	I, U
Guest speaker	21 Invite the physical education teacher or supervisor to discuss and demonstrate good body mechanics.	P, I, U
	22 Invite the physical education teacher or supervisor to visit the classroom to discuss "keeping in condition" and its importance in daily living.	I, U
Individual and group reports	23 Pupils write or give oral reports on such topics as "How I exercise each day," and "The sport I like best."	I, U
	24 Pupils prepare written or oral reports on the values of exercise.	I, U
	25 Children prepare written reports about their favorite sports and list the parts of the body that are exercised most in these activities.	I, U
Model	26 Pupils make a posture model (use heavy cardboard) for use in the discussion of body mechanics.	I, U
Mural	27 Make a mural of the variety of kinds of beneficial pupil activities and exercises.	I, U
Music	28 Walk to music, exhibiting good posture.	P, I
Poems, songs, and plays	29 Children create poems, songs, and plays about exercise and its values.	P
Posters	30 Make posters showing the importance of exercise in daily living.	P, I
Scrapbook	31 Make a series of drawings and collect magazine pictures and stories demonstrating proper body mechanics.	P, I
Shadowgram	32 Children make shadowgrams of each other. Using a piece of craft paper as large as a child, with two students holding the paper, have a third pupil stand between the paper and a source of light. A fourth boy or girl outlines the shadow of the third child using a piece of charcoal or crayon. Discuss these drawings individually in terms of good body mechanics.	I, U
Stories	33 Children write illustrated stories of how exercise helps us.	P, I

_____

*Some activities may not be appropriate for physically handicapped children.

TEACHING TECHNIQUES: EXERCISE AND BODY MECHANICS—cont'd

Grades

Survey | **34** Survey the amount of exercise pupils receive by completing the following: | I, U

How much exercise do I get?

Fill in the amount of time in hours or in fraction of hours.

	S	M	T	W	Th	F	S
Riding a bicycle or walking to and from school							
Playing at recesses							
Playing before school, in the morning, and at noon							
Exercising during the physical education class							
Active playing after school and before bedtime							
TOTALS							

Television box | **35** Survey the kinds of activities in which pupils participate. | U
| **36** Make a TV or motion picture box and have children prepare a series of pictures showing the importance of exercise and body mechanics. | P

TEACHING TECHNIQUES

Family Health*

			Grades
Bulletin board	1	Collect pictures of boys and girls of approximately the ages of students in class for a display illustrating differences in size and body build among children of the same age.	I
	2	Show pictures of ways families spend their time in recreation and during holidays.	I
	3	Collect pictures on family life and magazine and newspaper articles about birth and display them.	I, U
	4	Show pictures of happy families and have students describe what makes the families happy.	P
Charts	5	Construct a chart showing varying ages when boys and girls mature.	I
Discussion	6	What can I do to help my family be happy?	P
	7	Ways in which the community helps the family.	P
	8	Differences in growth rates between boys and girls.	I
	9	Inherited characteristics, such as eye and hair color, and curly or straight hair.	I, U
	10	Meaning of "growing up."	I
	11	Anonymous questions prepared by students.	I, U
	12	Living things come from living things.	P
	13	Family rules and family problems.	I, U
	14	Home responsibilities.	I, U
	15	What family members can do to show love, especially at certain times.	P, I
	16	Family customs, traditions, religions, and patterns.	I, U
	17	Care of pets.	P
	18	Nature and functions of the endocrine glands.	I, U
	19	Secondary sex characteristics of boys and girls as they relate to body shape, size, and growth.	I, U
	20	Moral and ethical values and their relation to sexual activities.	U
	21	Different ways of reproduction, asexual and sexual.	I, U
	22	Human reproduction.	I, U
	23	Good sources of information on sex, reproduction, and family living.	I, U
	24	Attraction between sexes.	U
	25	Ways to resolve family conflicts.	P, I
	26	Animal and plant reproduction.	P
	27	Compare the development of human babies before birth with animal babies.	P
	28	Family changes caused by death, divorce, or separation.	P, I
	29	Responsibilities at home, at school, and elsewhere.	P
	30	Freedom and responsibility.	I
	31	Puberty and maturity.	I, U
	32	Love—marriage, children, family.	U

TEACHING TECHNIQUES: FAMILY HEALTH—cont'd

		Grades
Discussion—cont'd	33 Sex drive, birth process, masturbation, behavior on dates, marriage.	U
	34 People, organizations, and agencies that help people with family problems.	U
	35 Steady dating.	U
	36 Determination of personal values.	I, U
Demonstrations	37 Have male and female guinea pigs or hamsters in the classroom. Pregnancy of the female will offer an opportunity to discuss the creation of new life.	P
	38 Hatch chicks from eggs.	P
	39 Observe the growth of seeds in relation to new life.	P
	40 Observe the growth of frog eggs.	P
Display	41 Make available pamphlets and magazine and newspaper articles about sex, reproduction, and values for student optional reading.	I, U
Drawings	42 Illustrate ways in which families have good times together.	P
	43 Children draw their own family groups and list various family patterns.	P
	44 Illustrate pupil's own family or animal families.	P
	45 Depict mother's, father's, or own work.	P
Exhibit and health fair	46 Students prepare bulletin board displays, posters, charts, and other visual materials for display and exhibit these materials at school. Pupils should be available to discuss their projects, provide information requested, and distribute pamphlets.	I, U
Field trip	47 Tour the school building and include a visit to boys' and girls' lavatories. This should lead to a discussion of anatomic differences of boys and girls and correct names of body parts.	P, I, U
	48 Visit a farm and observe the animals.	P
	49 Visit a local museum, hospital, or clinic to view exhibits of a baby before and after birth.	P, I, U
Films	50 Observe films on birth and growth of animals.	P
	51 See and discuss films on human growth, menstruation, and reproduction.	I, U
Guest speakers	52 Invite a physician or nurse to discuss reproduction, childbirth, and other matters.	I, U
	53 Invite ministers, priests, and other religious representatives to discuss moral and ethical values.	I, U
Graph	54 Prepare a graph that shows the heights and weights of class members; compare with national norms.	I
Mural	55 Develop a mural showing animals and human beings caring for babies.	P
Pretest	56 Develop a test relating to puberty, mate selection, reproduction, sex drive, and other matters.	U
Problem solving	57 Develop relevant situations with alternative solutions concerning dating, behavior on dates, selection of marriage partners, sexual relations. Use these as a basis for class discussion.	U

TEACHING TECHNIQUES: FAMILY HEALTH—cont'd

		Grades
Problem solving—cont'd	58 Have children try to provide answers to these questions: How do you grow? What helps you grow? Why do you grow?	I
Individual and group reports	59 Rh factor, sex drive, marriage, dating, and others.	U
	60 Different ethnic, religious, and cultural backgrounds of people.	I, U
	61 What things do I do that make my family happy or unhappy?	P, I
Puppets	62 Prepare a skit to show how parents help us.	P
Question box	63 Provide a box in an appropriate location for students' anonymous questions.	I, U
Role playing	64 Provide skits relating to family roles of mothers and fathers, getting along with brothers and sisters, and helping to care for a new baby.	P
	65 Develop skits depicting manners and etiquette.	P
Scrapbook	66 Include illustrated materials "All about me," with all the items in terms of family, friends, and things that cause different emotional responses.	I
Story	67 Prepare on open-ended story about the family, its activities, and responsibilities of children. Allow pupils to fill in some of the words.	P
	68 Read appropriate stories about families and family relations.	P, I

*Some activities may need teacher sensitivity to ethnic and racial groups and adopted children and the possibility of embarrassment to overweight as well as taller or smaller than average pupils.

TEACHING TECHNIQUES

Growth and Development*

		Grades
Bulletin board	**1** Teacher prepares a series of large drawings that show the progressive stages of the development of a chick embryo into a full-grown chick. Appropriate colors may be necessary to make these illustrations more attractive.	P, I
	2 Children collect pictures showing differences in growth patterns of adults for a bulletin board display: dwarfs and giants, as well as tall and short persons. Discuss these differences as they relate to the pupils themselves.	I, U
	3 Pupils bring to class pictures of well-known, important people and prepare a bulletin board display of these individuals. Discuss the differences in body build.	I, U
	4 Teacher prepares a display showing the relationship of cells, tissues, organs, and systems to the organism as shown in Fig. 12-17.	I, U
Buzz group	**5** Have a buzz group discussion about the meaning of the term *growing up.*	I, U
Demonstration	**6** Put several articles in a bag and observe whether children can identify the articles by merely touching them and not seeing them. This introduces the fact that the nerves send messages to the brain.	I, U

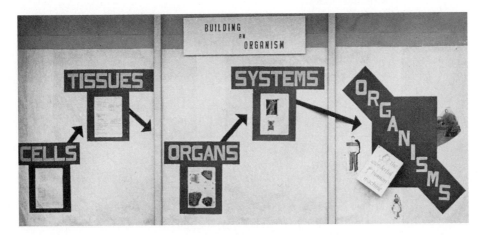

FIG. 12-17 Growth and development bulletin board. (Courtesy Jefferson Union Elementary School District, Daly City, California.)

TEACHING TECHNIQUES: GROWTH DEVELOPMENT—cont'd

		Grades
Demonstration—cont'd	7 Bring an earthworm to class and point out that it has no bones and its only means of locomotion is muscular movement. Mention that without a skeletal system human beings would probably move around like an earthworm. This leads to the concept that each part of the skeleton is shaped for its particular function and that muscles are necessary for locomotion.	I, U
	8 Demonstrate the different rates at which students grow by measuring their heights in the fall and again in the spring.	I, U
	9 Bring a stethoscope to class to demonstrate how a physician uses this instrument.	I, U
	10 Line up pupils in class and have them note the differences in height. Discuss the fact that children do not have the same growth rate, as a result of many factors: heredity, nutrition, and illness.	I, U
	11 Dissect a hog's or cow's heart and identify its parts (see Fig. 12-8, p. 325).	I, U
Discussion	12 Provide an illustrated discussion of the nervous and digestive systems using suitable charts and models.	I, U
	13 Provide an illustrated discussion of the respiratory system using suitable charts and models.	I, U
	14 Provide an illustrated discussion of the heart and the circulatory system using suitable charts and models.	I, U
	15 Provide an illustrated discussion of the muscles of the body using suitable charts and models. Demonstrate how muscles fasten to bones.	I, U
	16 Discuss the nature and function of the skeletal system using suitable charts and models.	I, U
	17 Discuss the endocrine glands and their role in growth and development.	I, U
	18 Discuss and compare the human body with a machine (automobile). Mention the intake of fuel and the conversion to energy.	I, U
	19 Disassemble a model of the human torso and ask pupils to identify the separated parts. Pupils might also try to reassemble the torso at the conclusion of this discussion.	I, U
	20 Provide pupils with diagrams of the nervous, digestive, respiratory, skeletal, and circulatory systems and have them label the parts.	I, U
	21 Discuss growth as an individual matter and show the differential patterns.	I, U
	22 The story of heredity.	I, U
	23 Ask such questions as: How do you know you have a heart? How big is your heart? What is pulse? Can you feel it? How many times does your heart beat, and how many times do you breathe in 1 minute?	I
Display	24 Bones from a variety of animals including human beings; have students try to identify them.	I, U
Dramatization	25 Dramatize a small boy trying to pick a fight with a large boy. Discuss the implications in terms of growth and development.	I, U

TEACHING TECHNIQUES: GROWTH DEVELOPMENT—cont'd

		Grades
Drawings	26 Children draw, color, and label various systems and organs of the human body.	I, U
Exhibit	27 Display pamphlets and other publications on growth and development in the classroom for review by interested children.	P, I, U
	28 Display animal bones obtained from a meat market. Show some cross sections and longitudinal sections of bones.	I, U
Experiment	29 Demonstrate how baby chicks, ducks, or other animals grow when given the proper food. The white rat experiment (see p. 315) also may be used to illustrate the growth process.	P, I
	30 Provide a flannelboard and a box containing cutouts of the bones of the human body. Permit children to try to build the human skeleton on the flannelboard.	I, U
Films	31 Show and discuss films on human growth and menstruation.	I, U
Game	32 Play the game "Who am I?" A child describes the function of a particular organ of the body and pupils try to identify the organ. Another version of this game is to have children mention bones of the body and then have other pupils name bones to which they attach.	I, U
Graph	33 Construct a giraffe out of heavy paper and place measurements on its neck. Have children periodically measure themselves and record these findings on a graph that they have prepared.	P
	34 Have each child prepare a height and weight graph. Children take their measurements once a month and plot their findings. Separate graphs using height and age or weight and age may also be advisable to make and use.	I, U
Guest speaker	35 Invite the school nurse to meet with the girls to discuss menstruation.	I, U
	36 Invite the school nurse to come to class to discuss the process of human reproduction.	I, U
	37 Invite a physician or other qualified person to class to discuss sexual growth and development.	U
Individual and group reports	38 Pupils compile a list of causes of individual differences in growth.	I, U
	39 Pupils find the meaning of the words *heredity* and *environment*.	I, U
	40 Pupils prepare lists of the characteristics they have inherited and acquired.	I, U
Model	41 Children make clay models of different organs of the body after they have seen pictures or drawings of these parts.	I, U
	42 Children make a stethoscope using the material shown in Fig. 12-18. Have pupils hold funnel firmly over the heart and listen to heart sounds. Discussion of structure, function, and related diseases could follow.	I, U
	43 Display plastic models of the heart and other body organs.	I, U

TEACHING TECHNIQUES: GROWTH DEVELOPMENT—cont'd

Grades

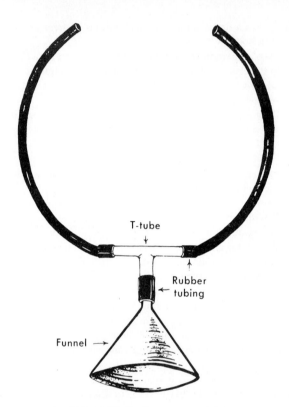

T-tube

Rubber
tubing ←

Funnel →

FIG. 12-18 Stethoscope model.

Problem solv- ing	**44** Encourage pupils to raise questions about growth and development and list these on the blackboard. Have pupils determine ways to find answers to the listed problems.	I, U
	45 Present these or similar questions to pupils for discussion: What does *growing up* mean? How do individuals grow? Do boys and girls grow at the same rate? Why doesn't everyone grow at the same rate? How does one know when growth is taking place? What factors are involved in growth?	I,U
Question box	**46** Provide a question box for pupils' anonymous questions about menstruation, reproduction, and other aspects of growth and development.	I, U
Self-test	**47** Prepare a self-test on the various aspects of growth and development, systems of the body, endocrine glands, and heredity.	I, U

*Teachers must be sensitive to activities that may cause pupil embarrassment.

TEACHING TECHNIQUES

HIV/AIDS

		Grades
Books	**1** Read the book *What's a Virus, Anyway? The Kids' Book About AIDS* (written in both English and Spanish).	P, I
	2 Read the book *Jimmy and His Family* (written in both English and Spanish). Have the children discuss how they might feel if they found out that they had a fatal illness.	P, I
	3 Read *Jimmy and the Eggs Virus*. This book contains a child's first-person description of what it was like to learn that he was HIV positive.	P, I
Bulletin board	**4** Illustrate the ways that HIV/AIDS is spread.	I, U
	5 Have students collect newspaper and magazine stories about HIV/AIDS. Post the stories on a bulletin board. Then use the stories as a basis for discussion.	I, U
	6 Prepare a bulletin board that depicts how the immune system fights disease.	I, U
	7 Prepare a bulletin board emphasizing the importance of not touching other people's blood because of the remote possibility of transmitting HIV.	P, I, U
Brainstorming	**8** In groups of five, have students brainstorm ways that they can avoid the risk of HIV/AIDS.	I, U
Buzz group	**9** Place students into small groups to discuss: "Why do people fear people with HIV/AIDS?" Be prepared to dispel any myths that arise from the groups.	I, U
Chart	**10** Have students graph the incidence and prevalence of HIV/AIDS in the world, the United States, and in their state.	U
Coloring book	**11** Secure copies of *Hey, Do You Know You Can't Get AIDS From . . .* from the Oklahoma Department of Health, AIDS Division. After the students color the pictures, a collage could be made with them.	P
Computer-assisted instruction	**12** *True Stories* available from the Seattle/King County Department of Public Health. It contains nine dramas in which students choose what the characters say and determine how the story proceeds. Complete with teacher's guide.	U
Demonstration	**13** Show how proper handwashing can reduce the spread of germs. Have children put some oil on their hands and rub their hands together. Sprinkle some glitter on their hands. Have some of the children wash their hands with cold water only, some wash their hands with warm water only, and some wash their hands with soap and warm water.	P
	14 Fill a syringe with colored water. Press the plunger to discharge the water. Do not wash the syringe and refill it with fresh water. Again discharge the water and note that some of the color from the first filling has "tinted" the new water. This demonstrates that HIV can be passed through the use of "dirty" needles.	I, U

TEACHING TECHNIQUES: HIV/AIDS—cont'd

			Grades
Discussion	15	How do you think people with HIV/AIDS feel when they know others are talking about them?	I, U
	16	How might students your age help a student your age who has learned he or she is infected with HIV?	I, U
	17	What might a person do to indicate that he or she did not want to use any type of drug because use of needles with drugs could result in the transmission of HIV.	U
	18	Discuss newspaper articles or magazine articles that have appeared about both adults and children who have contracted HIV/AIDS.	U
	19	Discuss how you feel when someone in your family has a serious illness. What might you do to help that person feel even a little better or happier?	P, I
	20	Discuss how you feel when you are ill. Do you like to have people call you or visit you or send you cards? Do you think that people who have HIV/AIDS might feel the same way as you do when you are ill?	P, I
	21	Discuss the rights of the individual who has HIV/AIDS to attend school. Why should students with HIV/AIDS be treated any differently from children with other chronic diseases?	U
Field trip	22	Visit the health department and meet with the infectious disease control personnel. Have them discuss the ways that the health department is dealing with HIV/AIDS and what young people can do to decrease their risk of encountering HIV.	I, U
Game	23	*TLC Game,* available from the Harvard Community Health Plan Foundation. Provides parents and children age 9 years and older with a way to begin family discussions about sex, sensitive topics, and AIDS.	I, U
Guest speaker	24	Invite a physician who deals with HIV/AIDS patients to discuss some of the myths associated with HIV/AIDS and children.	I, U
Poster	25	Have students create a poster that depicts the fact that there are three basic groups of people with HIV/AIDS: those who have AIDS (2% to 5%), those with AIDS-related conditions (5% to 8%), and those who are HIV infected but do not have symptoms.	U
	26	Have students create a poster that shows that it is all right to remain friends with someone who has HIV/AIDS.	I, U
Reports	27	Have students develop a report about how they can decrease their risk of contracting HIV.	U
Scrapbook	28	Collect stories about HIV/AIDS and make a scrapbook. Combine this with discussion of the myths surrounding HIV/AIDS.	I, U

TEACHING TECHNIQUES

Mental Health

		Grades
Bulletin board	**1** Collect and display pictures and drawings of happy children and families, as well as of people showing kindness.	P, I
	2 Display work by each child as often as possible to encourage responsibility in doing his or her best work.	P, I
	3 Display a list of class helpers for a week, eventually giving everyone in class a chance to be a leader.	P, I
	4 Prepare a bulletin board of examples found in newspapers and magazines that show good deeds, good sportsmanship, and other qualities.	P, I, U
	5 Display an illustrated list of the hobbies of the children in class.	P, I, U
	6 Prepare a bulletin board with a variety of illustrated mental health phrases such as "Meet friends halfway," "Be cheerful," and "Control your anger."	I, U
	7 Display pictures of a variety of emotions with the caption: "Emotions with which we live."	P, I
	8 Pupils collect for display magazine and newspaper articles that describe mental health problems of concern to pupils.	U
	9 Prepare the display illustrated in Fig. 12-19 (pp. 380-381). The teacher can prepare questions in first panel and pupils can bring pictures for second panel and also help to obtain definition and lists for third panel.	I, U
Brainstorming	**10** Students prepare lists of problems they consider important and develop plans to resolve them.	I, U
Buzz group	**11** Conduct a buzz group discussion on the character traits a pupil likes or dislikes in a person.	U
	12 Have a buzz group discussion of how boys and girls may become better acquainted.	U
	13 Discuss such questions as: What is reality? Does "everybody's doing it" mean everyone should do it?	U
Checklist	**14** Pupils complete checklists and teacher either holds individual conferences with pupils or anonymously discusses some of the problems in class. Some sample statements on this list might include:	I, U

> I am often embarrassed when I am with others.
> I usually do not know how to act in company.
> I usually feel inferior to my classmates.
> I lack self-confidence.

| Consequences | **15** Students periodically prepare written statements for discussion of the questions that follow regarding any or all of the actions identified or others deemed appropriate:
 Questions—Do you consider the consequences before taking action? Should you? How frequently? Why? What are the possible consequences of your actions? | I, U |

TEACHING TECHNIQUES: MENTAL HEALTH—cont'd

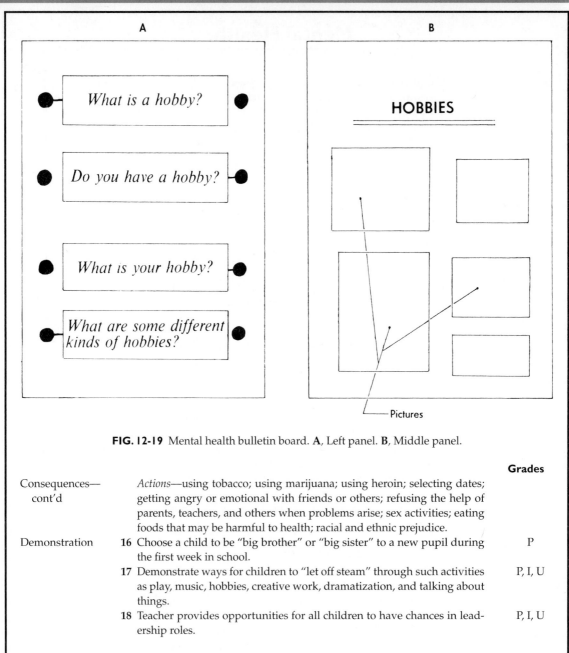

FIG. 12-19 Mental health bulletin board. **A,** Left panel. **B,** Middle panel.

		Grades
Consequences—cont'd	*Actions*—using tobacco; using marijuana; using heroin; selecting dates; getting angry or emotional with friends or others; refusing the help of parents, teachers, and others when problems arise; sex activities; eating foods that may be harmful to health; racial and ethnic prejudice.	
Demonstration	**16** Choose a child to be "big brother" or "big sister" to a new pupil during the first week in school.	P
	17 Demonstrate ways for children to "let off steam" through such activities as play, music, hobbies, creative work, dramatization, and talking about things.	P, I, U
	18 Teacher provides opportunities for all children to have chances in leadership roles.	P, I, U

TEACHING TECHNIQUES: MENTAL HEALTH—cont'd

C

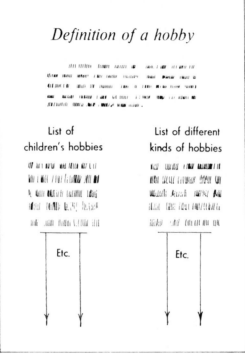

Definition of a hobby

List of
children's hobbies

List of different
kinds of hobbies

Etc.

Etc.

FIG. 12-19—cont'd. C, Right panel.

		Grades
Demonstra- tion—cont'd	19 Teachers provide a warm, friendly atmosphere in the classroom with many centers of interest.	P, I, U
Discussion	20 Children have opportunities to experiment with planning, carry out plans, and evaluate results of a variety of experiences.	P
	21 Talk about how to make friends.	P
	22 Ways to be helpful at home, happy times with the family, and ways to be unselfish about listening to the radio and watching TV.	P
	23 The use of the words *please* and *thank you*.	P
	24 What it feels like when you know someone cares about you.	P, I
	25 Children's feelings and the need for control over such actions as crying easily, temper tantrums, and fighting.	P, I
	26 Behaviors in class and in school in terms of getting along with one another and related problems.	P, I

TEACHING TECHNIQUES: MENTAL HEALTH—cont'd

		Grades
Discussion— cont'd	27 What it means to be a leader and a follower.	P, I
	28 When playing games in physical education, discuss the need to rotate positions to give opportunities for all.	P, I
	29 Discuss what to do when one feels sad, what to do to help others who are unhappy, and ways to behave when something unfortunate happens.	P, I
	30 The need to forgive those who have made mistakes.	P, I
	31 The need for the development of self-responsibility by keeping desk clean, hanging clothes in closet, taking care of pets.	P, I
	32 The quality of friendship.	P, I
	33 How people differ in their abilities to do things.	P, I, U
	34 Ways to cope with and solve problems when they arise. What specific procedures should a pupil follow when faced with a situation for which he/she can find no answer?	I, U
	35 What it means to "put oneself in another person's shoes."	I, U
	36 How people can be considerate of the feelings of others and how to handle hurt feelings.	I, U
	37 Honesty and truthfulness.	I, U
	38 Develop standards for acceptable behavior in the classroom, on the playground, to and from school, on the bus, in the library, on study trips, and at home.	I, U
	39 Children who are embarrassed by physical limitations and what others can do to help these individuals.	I, U
	40 Inadvisability of keeping emotional tensions, worry, and fear bottled up inside. Discuss the need for friends to talk to, hobbies as outlets, being able to face up to problems, and other solutions.	I, U
	41 Have pupils prepare a list of qualities they like in a person as well as those qualities they do not like and post these on the bulletin board or put them in the school newspaper.	I, U
	42 The following personality traits: kindness, helpfulness, reliability, tactfulness, cheerfulness, good sportsmanship, good manners, intelligence, sense of humor, loyalty, and honesty.	I, U
	43 Evaluate ways boys and girls have of gaining acceptance through such means as conforming to clothing fads, using current slang, forming clubs, and participating in school-sponsored social activities, plays, and other projects.	U
	44 Discuss the question "At what age should one start dating?"	U
	45 Habits and ways of behaving that will give parents confidence in allowing boys and girls increasing freedom to make decisions and to participate in activities outside the home.	U
	46 Reactions to other individuals who do not act, look, or believe as you do.	U
	47 The values of people.	U

TEACHING TECHNIQUES: MENTAL HEALTH—cont'd

		Grades
Dramatization	**48** Dramatize the following: thoughtfulness, courtesy, self-reliance, sharing, playing and working together, helping at school, following directions, respecting each other's property, lost and found, self-control, rudeness, good manners, and criticism.	P, I
	49 Dramatize emotional behavior exhibited such as anger, fear, jealousy, sorrow, hate, love, and temper.	P, I
	50 Dramatize such incidents as the following:	P, I, U

> Things that make me happy.
> Things that make others happy.
> Things that make me sad.
> Problems on playground or in classrooms.
> Things I like to do.
> How to make new friends.
> Other kids do things I can't do.
> Others won't play with me.

	51 Dramatize introductions to and conversations with other people in public places, bus, school, dance, party, theater, and street.	U
	52 Dramatize how it feels to be different from others in terms of race, nationality, beliefs, and customs.	U
Drawings	**53** Have children make drawings illustrating: things I love; how I feel when hurt, scared, and angry; when I've wanted something I couldn't get.	P, I
	54 Draw a picture illustrating a way to be helpful to someone.	P, I
	55 Draw pictures of objects or animals that make us afraid or make us feel safe.	P
Emotion box	**56** Prepare an emotion box and have students periodically complete forms in which their names, dates, types of emotion experienced, and the reason for same is identified. Teacher occasionally reviews and uses the material as a basis for class discussion and problem solving without indicating students by name.	I
Exhibit	**57** Display pictures brought to class by children of places they would like to visit or where they would like to live. Discuss the reasons these places have been selected.	I, U
Finger paint	**58** Provide children opportunities to finger paint to help release tensions and to explore creative abilities.	P
Flannelboard	**59** Use the flannelboard to illustrate situations of fair play and good sportsmanship and to create stories about fear, anger, hate, friendship, and others.	P, I
Good-deed box	**60** Prepare a good-deed box and have children deposit in writing good things that they have seen classmates do during the day. At the end of the day the teacher reads these to the class without mentioning names.	P, I
Guest speaker	**61** Invite a psychologist or psychiatrist to discuss the meaning of the term *personality*.	U

TEACHING TECHNIQUES: MENTAL HEALTH—cont'd

		Grades
Individual and group reports	62 Children write brief stories or reports on "How to be a better leader or follower."	P, I
	63 Children write a brief summary paragraph or two in answer to the question "Why should we learn to get along with others?"	P, I
	64 Pupils complete an individual written assignment on the topic "When my feelings were hurt."	I, U
	65 Prepare oral or written pupil reports on good manners and courtesy.	I, U
	66 Write a brief paragraph about good citizenship and draw pictures to illustrate.	I, U
	67 Prepare reports on jealousy, prejudice, anger, and others for the school newspaper.	I, U
	68 Boys and girls make up lists of the qualities they like and dislike in other boys and girls. Discuss the common characteristics found in the lists and their meanings to the pupils.	I, U
	69 Pupils prepare written reports about what they do well and what they would like to improve in themselves.	I, U
	70 Pupils write about and discuss the following: what makes me angry, happy, sad, or afraid; what I wonder about; three persons I love; three wishes; what I would like to change at home or at school; what I like about people; what I like about my friends.	I, U
	71 Pupils write reports about the racial, religious, and other prejudices they have noticed that people have against individuals.	I, U
Murals	72 Make murals, charts, and booklets that emphasize sharing in terms of carrying dishes to the table, going to the store, taking care of pets, making the bed, hanging up clothes, running errands, and putting things away.	P, I
Music	73 Use of various types of music to help calm and relax children to help create a beneficial classroom atmosphere.	P, I
	74 Discuss the meaning of lyrics found in a variety of popular songs.	U
Poems	75 Prepare original poems about feelings.	P
	76 Read poems that have positive mental health in messages.	P, I, U
Problem solving	77 Describe a human relations episode to the class, such as lying, stealing, rudeness, or poor sportsmanship, and have children write or orally discuss how they would solve the problem.	I, U
Puppets	78 Make stick, paper bag, or hand puppets and prepare stories or plays around such themes as fear, anger, and jealousy.	P, I
	79 Construct a shadow box or puppet stage with children working together.	P, I
Questionnaire	80 Students complete short answers to the following:	I, U

Happiness is _____ .
Sadness is _____ .
I am fearful of _____ .
I am angry when _____ .

TEACHING TECHNIQUES: MENTAL HEALTH—cont'd

		Grades
Question box	81 Have a question box in class and encourage children to put in questions concerning worries, fears, and other areas of trouble that they would like discussed.	I, U
Role play	82 Students act out such situations as how to make friends; getting along with others; facing dangers; solving problems.	I, U,
Scrapbook	83 Children prepare a scrapbook or notebook with illustrated writings on "What to do when I get angry," "How to play fairly."	P, I
	84 Prepare a scrapbook of pictures and magazine and newspaper articles that illustrate good sportsmanship.	I
Self-test	85 Have pupils complete the following:	I, U

	YES	NO
Friendliness test		
Do you smile easily?	☐	☐
Are you a good listener?	☐	☐
Are you courteous?	☐	☐
Are you a good sport?	☐	☐
Do you refuse to spread rumors?	☐	☐
Do you have a hobby?	☐	☐
Can you laugh at a joke on yourself?	☐	☐
Are you usually in a good humor?	☐	☐
Can your friends depend on you?	☐	☐
Do you try to talk about what interests other people?	☐	☐

Show and tell	86 Provide time for jokes, funny stories, and riddles.	P
	87 Provide opportunities for all children to show and tell something as often as possible.	P
Sociogram	88 Prepare a sociogram (for teacher's information) to find out if children in the classroom have friends. Have each child list the three children he/she would like to sit near.	P, I
Stories*	89 Read, make up, and discuss stories showing thoughtfulness of individuals to other individuals, about fears, cooperation, sharing, fair play, courtesy, sportsmanship, honesty, truthfulness, courage, friendliness, and other personality traits.	P
	90 Tell and read stories about helping at home, sharing of toys, caring for baby, and family living.	P
	91 Read and discuss stories of famous people who have overcome handicaps and failures, such as Thomas Edison, Helen Keller, and Louis Pasteur.	I, U
	92 Have students write an ending to an unfinished story. Have several of them read their endings aloud and follow with discussion.	P, I
Survey	93 Conduct a survey regarding the qualities or traits that the pupils like in their friends. Have a committee tabulate the results and prepare a chart for display titled "Our best friends."	I, U

*See Appendix D for sample fiction and nonfiction books.

TEACHING TECHNIQUES: MENTAL HEALTH—cont'd

		Grades
Survey—cont'd	**94** Conduct a survey of interests; tabulate, and prepare a series of discussion questions on the findings. Some sample items that could be included are the following:	I, U

> I wish I had better grades.
> I wish I didn't get headaches when I read.
> I wish I didn't get into trouble at school.
> I wish I could change some of my teachers.
> I wish my parents got along better.
> I wish my parents really loved me.
> I wish I could take my friends home.
> I wish my father could spend more time with me.
> I wish I weren't afraid of things.

TV box	**95** Make a TV box with a series of drawings illustrating captions such as the following:	P

> This little girl is too lazy to make her bed.
> Are you a good sport?
> Are you helpful at home and school?
> Do you lose your temper and fight?
> Do you cry easily?
> Are you kind to others?

TEACHING TECHNIQUES

Nutrition

Grades

Bulletin board   **1** Prepare a display of new foods tried by children. Include the food item, a picture or drawing of the food, and the name of the student who had eaten the food.   P

2 From cereal boxes and milk and other cartons construct a food train with an engine and four cars containing the basic four foods. Place food models made from construction paper, clay, paper-mache, or cutouts from magazines in the cars.   P

3 Prepare a bulletin board display depicting a rocket ship and in the pilot's seat insert animated fruits or vegetables. Illustrated caption might read: P, I

> *Mr. Carrot:*   "Fly high with me and grow big and strong."
> *Mr. Milk:*   "I fly high and fast because I give lots of pep and energy."

The captions and food items can be changed periodically.

4 Prepare bulletin board displays, showcase exhibits, dioramas, and others using real foods, food models, attractive pictures, children-made cutouts, and papier-mache models showing: P, I, U

A well-balanced breakfast, lunch, or dinner
Wholesome "snack" foods
Milk products, such as whole milk, skim milk, dried milk, cottage cheese, cream, and butter (indicate their importance)
Foods containing vitamins, minerals, proteins, carbohydrates, and fats
Food sanitation including the preparation, serving, cleanup, washing of utensils, and storage of food
Meals or foods to be served in the school lunchroom
Recent newspaper and magazine articles
The amount of sugar contained in various kinds of candy, soft drinks and foods
A model of a boy and girl with illustrations of the foods they need pinned to them
World food problems

5 Construct a "Breakfast Kid" (Fig. 12-20) out of construction or drawing paper as follows: P, I, U

> *Hat*—bowl of cereal   *Hands*—fruits, eggs, bacon, and bread
> *Head*—an orange   *Arms*—bananas
> *Body*—bottle of milk   *Legs*—bacon strips

6 Assign a group of students the responsibility of locating pictures and newspaper and magazine articles related to nutrition. Students should provide statements or comments below each item.   I, U

TEACHING TECHNIQUES: NUTRITION—cont'd

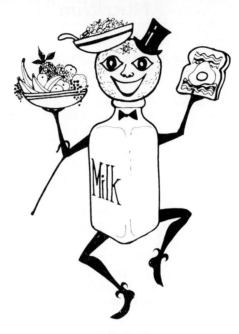

FIG. 12-20

		Grades
Chart	7 Prepare a cooperative chart, or charts, on the kinds of foods (carbohydrates, fats, proteins, minerals, and vitamins) with food pictures to illustrate.	P, I
	8 Cut pictures of foods from magazines and make a basic four classification chart for the classroom.	P, I
	9 Prepare a chart of the food nutrients as follows:	U

Nutrient	What it does	Foods in which found
Proteins		
Vitamins		
Carbohydrates		
Fats		
Minerals		

TEACHING TECHNIQUES: NUTRITION—cont'd

		Grades
Demonstration	**10** Make butter from cream and serve on bread to children in class. Permit each child a chance to shake the jar containing the cream.	P
	11 Make giant paintings of favorite fruits or vegetables on paper bags. Cut holes for the head and arms and have children wear these bags while they tell pupils in other classes what they like about these fruits and vegetables.	P
	12 With the help of parents or teachers, prepare and serve a variety of nutritious breakfasts.	P, I
	13 With parents, plan, prepare, and serve a meal that contains foods from a foreign country.	I, U
	14 Children participate in the planning and preparation of nutritious foods for class or school parties. Avoid the usual cakes, candies, and soft drinks, substituting such items as fruit, fruit juices, popcorn, and nuts.	I, U
	15 Pupil committee tries to improve the attractiveness of the cafeteria through the use of posters, table settings, and flowers.	I, U
	16 Demonstrate ways to test foods for content.	I, U

Starch—Soften, crush, and dissolve foods in water. Place in a test tube with some water and add a drop of iodine (1% solution). If solution turns blue, starch is present.

Fat—Place foods on pieces of paper. Remove foods and place papers on radiator to heat. Fatty foods will leave grease spots.

Protein—Burn foods in direct flame of Bunsen burner. Protein foods (raw, lean meat; cheese; dried beans) will emit odor of burning feathers. May need to burn a feather first so that pupils recognize odor.

Minerals—Burn various foods on a small asbestos or metal plate. High mineral content foods (dried milk, beans, peas, and egg yolk) will leave a gray ash containing one or more minerals such as calcium. Nonmineral foods such as sugar will leave only a small residue of black carbon.

Water—Expose fruits, leafy vegetables, and other foods containing high water content to air and they become shriveled after a while. They may be weighed before and after dehydration to determine the amount of water lost.

		Grades
Discussion	**17** Have children read the cafeteria lunch menu each day and compare this with the balanced food chart found on the bulletin board. On their return from lunch, pupils discuss the meal.	I
	18 Discuss and help plan a school lunch menu.	I, U
	19 Discuss a well-balanced lunch in class and select menus to show foods containing the necessary vitamins and minerals needed for growth. Pupils discuss items purchased in cafeteria and best ways to spend money to obtain proper foods.	I, U
	20 Obesity, weight reducing, and vitamin pills.	U

TEACHING TECHNIQUES: NUTRITION—cont'd

		Grades
	21 The kinds and purposes of foods necessary for growth, as well as the deficiency diseases.	U
	22 Participate as a member of a school health advisory committee to help solve school nutrition problems.	U
Dramatization	23 Dramatize visits to the dairy, grocery store, and food markets by constructing a store having shelves filled with empty food cans, boxes, and other such items. Also play house and dramatize foods eaten for breakfast, lunch, and dinner.	P
	24 Children prepare and participate in plays and radio and TV broadcasts presenting various aspects of nutrition.	P, I, U
Drawings	25 Have children draw pictures of the foods represented below. Enlarge the nine boxes on a full sheet of paper to provide adequate space for each food.	P

Milk	Orange juice	Butter
Bread	Celery	Meat
Eggs	Apple	Carrots

Excursions	26 Visit the dairy, grocery store, and local food markets to observe the availability and storage of different foods.	P
	27 Visit the school lunch room to observe foods being prepared for the noon meal.	P, I
	28 Observe the sanitary methods used in the preparation, serving, and storage of foods in a restaurant or in the school cafeteria.	I, U
	29 Visit milk or food processing plants.	I, U
Exhibit	30 Prepare a display or exhibit of well-balanced breakfasts, lunches, and dinners using real foods or food models.	P, I, U
	31 Have a "Food Fair" during which children display various kinds of foods, adequate lunches, dinners, and breakfasts, and appropriate snack-time foods. Pupils may construct murals, bulletin board displays, write-ups for the newspaper, and invitations to parents.	I, U
	32 Set up a nutrition corner displaying pamphlets, books, magazines, and other materials for pupil reference and use during the nutrition unit.	I, U
Experiment	33 Place grass seed in a sponge, add some water, and watch the sprouts grow.	P, I
	34 Participate in the white rat experiment (see p. 315) to learn the importance of food for life and growth.	P, I
	35 Soak a corn seed in water overnight, remove the bran coat, and then discuss the significance of this outer coat to the white part underneath.	I, U

TEACHING TECHNIQUES: NUTRITION—cont'd

		Grades

Experiment— cont'd

36 Soak a small uncooked chicken bone in vinegar for 3 days. The mineral matter will dissolve and the bone will lose its strength and firmness so that it can be easily bent. This experiment demonstrates the presence of minerals (especially calcium and phosphorus) in bones and points out the importance of minerals in the diet.

I, U

Finger play

37 Prepare finger play, such as:

P

> TUNE: *Mulberry Bush*
> This is the way we drink our milk,
> Drink our milk, drink our milk,
> This is the way we drink our milk,
> Every night and morning.
>
> This is the way it makes us grow,
> Makes us grow, makes us grow.
> This is the way it makes us grow,
> Every single day.

Flannelboard

38 Read the following poem and have children (as many as possible) place the appropriate foods mentioned on the board.

P

Three little pigs and their dinners

> There were three little pigs so happy and gay,
> Said the first little pig, in his house of straw,
> "Now I can eat all the candy I want, hurrah."
> So he filled his tummy with candy and cake,
> 'Till it began to ache and ache.
> "Oh I wish I had listened to Mommy," he said,
> As he rolled over and over in his bed.
>
> The second little pig in his house of twigs,
> Said, "Now I have no Mommy to make me eat figs."
> So he had doughnuts, popsicles, and root beer.
> Soon he yelled loud, "Oh dear! Oh dear!
> My tooth is aching, my tummy's in pain.
> I'll never do that, no never again."
>
> The third little pig, remembering what his Mommy said,
> Had meat, fresh vegetables, milk, and bread.
> He ate oranges and apples, singing their praise,
> As he felt peppy and strong all of his days.
> "I'm always healthy, happy, and strong.
> I get my sleep and nothing goes wrong."
> **MARY STULTZ**

39 Place the following food pictures on a flannelboard and have children prepare three different breakfasts: fruit, whole wheat bread, cocoa, eggs, nuts, bacon, milk, and cereal.

P, I

TEACHING TECHNIQUES: NUTRITION—cont'd

		Grades
Flannelboard—cont'd	40 Have food models available and permit children to show the foods they ate for breakfast, lunch, dinner, and snack time, and also the foods they should eat for breakfast, lunch, dinner, and snack time.	P, I
	41 Use food models to illustrate the basic foods, as well as a balanced breakfast, lunch, and dinner.	I, U
	42 Pictures from magazines are brought to class and children cut out good food items. Pupils paste these foods on cardboard plates and post them.	P
Individual and group reports	43 Pupils prepare lists of foods they like and dislike and make comparisons with the basic food groups.	I, U
	44 Children write a brief summary paragraph or two in answer to the question, "What are the nutritious kinds of foods to eat, and why must we eat them?"	P, I
	45 Serve as a class committee member to meet with the school lunch manager to learn how nutritious lunches are prepared and report findings in an oral or written report to the entire class.	I, U
	46 Pupils write letters of request to various companies for available nutrition materials for use in class.	I, U
	47 Prepare magazine articles regarding school lunch menus, weight reduction, and other important phases of nutrition for publication in the school newspaper.	U
	48 Analyze weight-reducing procedures advertised in newspapers and magazines.	U
	49 Analyze several newspaper or magazine advertisements about foods and food products.	U
	50 Pupils prepare lists of food fallacies and do research to discover why these are considered to be such.	U
	51 Students prepare notebooks of food pictures cut out of newspapers and magazines and grouped according to the basic food groups.	P
	52 Students identify one favorite food and determine the nutrients, caloric value, and contributions to health.	I, U
Mobile	53 Make a food mobile illustrating individual foods found in the basic food groups.	P, I
	54 Teacher prepares a large block (at least 12 inches square) and places pictures of the basic food groups on each side. The block is hung as a mobile during the time that nutrition is being discussed. Manila cardboard also can be used to construct the block because it can be folded and stored more easily.	P, I
Model	55 Prepare food models from clay, sawdust mixtures, cardboard, newspaper clippings, and other materials to be used for exhibit purposes or in the discussion on nutrition.	P, I

TEACHING TECHNIQUES: NUTRITION—cont'd

		Grades
Model—cont'd	**56** Prepare papier-máchê fruits and vegetables using real foods as forms. These items can be used in dramatic play and in the discussion of nutrition.	P, I
Panel	**57** Participate in a panel discussion of the problem "Diet and its relationship to weight control."	U
Poem	**58** Create original poems about nutrition, such as the following:	P

> There was an old woman
> Who lived in a shoe.
> She had so many children
> But she knew what to do.
> She fed them milk, fruit,
> And vegetable greens.
> So they were the best children
> You have ever seen.
>
> Iggildy, piggildy, wiggildy, doo!
> I'm Mrs. Carrot, How do you do!
> I'm lean and crisp.
> I come in a bunch.
> Eat me and see that I'm so good to munch.
> I'm good for teeth.
> I make them chew.
> I make them exercise.
> That's what I do.
> I'm good for eyes to see things, too!
>
> Oodle, doodle, humpty dumpty!
> I'm white and smooth and never lumpy.
> Drinking me keeps you in trim.
> Drink me well 'cause I'm filled to the brim.
> Strong bones and teeth is what I give.
> Drinking me makes you really live!
> My vitamins make skin smooth as silk.
> You should know me,
> I'm Mr. Milk.

Puppets	**59** Make puppets from construction paper and tongue blades (Fig. 12-21). The puppet heads should be about 12 inches high with the following rhymes written on their backs:	P

> *Celery:*   "I'm Mr. Celery
> So much fun to eat
> Serve me at your snacktime
> Then you'll want no sweet."
>
> *Apple:*   "I'm Ms. Apple.
> A juicy, swooshy bite
> Eat me every day
> To keep your teeth just right."

TEACHING TECHNIQUES: NUTRITION—cont'd

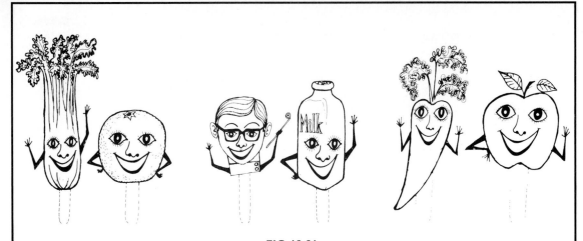

FIG. 12-21

Grades

Puppets—
  cont'd

Orange: "I'm Madam Orange
The sunshine color you see
I protect you from illness
Because I give you vitamin C."

Milk: "I'm your nice, sweet milk
I'll make your bones and teeth grow strong.
Drink and drink and drink some more
Then you'll be healthy your whole life long."

Carrot: "I'm Ms. Carrot
So much fun to eat.
I go crunch, crunch, crunch, crunch
Between your strong, white teeth."

60 Have a puppet show centered around a boy visited by Mr. Candy and   P, I
Ms. Pop, who persuade him to eat these items as snacks instead of oranges and other fruits. Later the fruit (Ms. Orange) and vegetables (Ms.
Carrot and Mr. Celery) come along and persuade the boy to try them as
snack foods.

61 Use puppets or marionettes made in class to dramatize nutrition con-   P, I
cepts, such as drinking milk daily, eating fruits and vegetables, and the
importance of a good breakfast.

Riddle   62 Have children write such riddles as the following: P,I

You find me in the garden,
I'm orange with long green hair,
You might find me on your table
So look for me there.
Who am I?

TEACHING TECHNIQUES: NUTRITION—cont'd

			Grades
Scrapbook	**63**	Locate pictures and information in magazines, newspapers, and pamphlets for making different kinds of sandwiches and preparing lunch boxes more attractively and put them into a booklet to be taken home.	P, I,U
	64	Prepare scrapbooks using pictures from magazines and other sources of such foods as fruits, vegetables, cheese, milk, butter, eggs, meat, fish, and poultry. Also organize these items into nutritious breakfasts, lunches, dinners, and snack foods.	P, I, U
Shadow box	**65**	Make shadow boxes depicting the basic food groups, as well as nutritious breakfasts, lunches, and dinners.	P
Speakers	**66**	Invite such resource people to class as dietitians, school lunch managers, and others to discuss various aspects of nutrition.	U
Stories, songs, and rhymes	**67**	Write stories, songs, rhymes, and plays about nutrition.	P, I
Survey	**68**	Survey the number of children in class who eat breakfast, as well as the nature of the food consumed.	I, U
	69	Survey the number of children purchasing lunches at school and compare this figure with the number who bring their lunches to school.	I, U
	70	Conduct a 1- to 3-day survey of snack foods eaten by pupils.	I, U
	71	Participate in a 3-day diet survey.	I, U
	72	Survey the number of children who eat candy or soft drinks at lunch time, as well as the amounts consumed.	I, U
Tasting party	**73**	Have a bunny party in which children make head bands with paper ears and all eat raw green vegetables and carrots.	P
	74	Participate in the eating of nutritious snack foods by having milk, fruit, fruit juices, nuts, celery, and carrot sticks instead of cake, candy, and soft drinks.	P, I, U
	75	Plan, prepare, and serve nutritious food items for parties and social gatherings at school.	U
Vegetable garden	**76**	Grow such vegetables as lettuce, tomatoes, and carrots to provide knowledge of some of the foods needed for growth and development.	P, I

TEACHING TECHNIQUES

Rest and Sleep

			Grades
Bulletin board	**1**	Display pictures that children bring to class or draw showing sleep, work, play, and relaxation.	P, I
	2	Display humorous illustrations of the basic rules of sleep and rest.	P, I
Chart	**3**	Construct a clock chart that shows children how to budget their time to get adequate amounts of rest, sleep, and exercise.	P, I, U
Demonstration	**4**	Demonstrate a variety of exercises that can help one to relax.	P, I, U
Discussion	**5**	Collect, show, and discuss pictures of animals at sleep and rest.	P
	6	Have children suggest ways to rest and relax and list these on the blackboard: warm bath, lying down, sit with head on desk, listening to music.	P
	7	Importance of sleep and rest and the amount needed.	P, I
	8	Rest, relaxation, and music.	P, I
	9	Children plan the work, play, and rest period for the day.	P, I
	10	Discuss the following questions in class: What happens when we sleep? When did you get up this morning? Did you sleep well? Did you feel rested? What time did you go to bed last night?	P, I
	11	Discuss the best conditions for sleeping and include comments about air, bed, and the room itself.	P, I, U
	12	Discuss the meaning of the terms *relaxation* and *tension*. Demonstrate by having the pupils flex muscles in their bodies and then relax them.	I, U
	13	The causes of fatigue, the signs of fatigue, what to do when fatigued, and the effects of overfatigue.	I, U
	14	Sleep and rest in terms of their value; how one feels and acts when sufficiently rested; and the need for balance between sleep, rest, and exercise.	I, U
	15	Why we tire; how rest affects posture, work, and play; and how anxiety, fear, anger, and eating before bedtime may affect sleep.	I, U
Dramatization	**16**	Children play house and devote part of their play to stressing sleep and rest.	P
	17	Prepare a play emphasizing desirable habits of sleep and rest to be presented in class, to a school assembly, or to a parent group.	I
Drawings	**18**	Draw pictures about sleep, rest, and relaxation.	P, I
Experience chart	**19**	Prepare an experience chart or record of important points about sleep and rest.	P
Experiment	**20**	Tie a weighted string near the tip of the left third finger of a pupil volunteer. Have the pupil raise and lower his/her finger as long as possible. Allow the child to rest for a minute and then repeat the procedure. Try this experiment using different fingers on both hands. The results show that exercise is fatiguing and there is need for rest and relaxation.	P, I, U

TEACHING TECHNIQUES: REST AND SLEEP—cont'd

		Grades
Finger plays	**21** Have children participate in finger plays.	P, I

Rest and listen

I like to rest and listen.
Let me listen while I rest.
My eyes are closed so I can't see.
I'll listen while you count for me.
Sh—whisper, count to ten . . .
Now listen while I rest again.

Time for us to take a rest.
Lock the door up tight (lock lips)
Pull the little window shades (close eyes)
We'll play that it is night.

Let's play rag doll

Let's play rag doll.
Don't make a sound.
Fling your arms and bodies
Loosely around.
Fling your hands!
Fling your feet!
Let your head go free!
Be the raggediest rag doll
You ever did see.

Individual and group reports	**22** Pupils prepare oral and written reports on rest, sleep, fatigue, and relaxation.	I, U
	23 Write a story on the three Rs: rest, relaxation, and recreation.	I, U
Music	**24** Play restful and relaxing music in class.	P, I, U

Brahm's *Lullaby*
Clair de Lune, Debussy
Air from *Suite No. 3 in D Major*, Bach
The Swan from *Carnival of the Animals*, Saint-Saens
The Lake from *Adventures in a Perambulator*, Carpenter
White Peacock, Griffes

Poems	**25** Children listen to, participate in the reading of, and act out poems on sleep, rest, and relaxation.	P, I, U

I am a limp rag doll,
I have no bones,
My feet are flat and still,
My hands are in my lap,
My head is limp,
Now my head rests on my knees
And my hands hang at my sides.

                    SARAH T. BARROWS

TEACHING TECHNIQUES: REST AND SLEEP—cont'd

Poems—cont'd

Grades

Close your eyes, head drops down
Face is smooth, not a frown
Roll to left, head is a ball
Roll to right, now sit tall
Lift your chin, look at me
Deep, deep breath, one, two, three
Big, big smile, hands in lap
Make believe you just had a nap
Now you're rested from your play
Time to work again today.

I went into a circus town
And met a funny Bunny Clown,
He winked his eye, he shook his head,
"This is splendid exercise," he said.
He shook his head, he shook his feet,
He wobbled, bobbled, down the street,
He moved his jaw both up and down
This funny little Bunny Clown.

He played that he was a lazy man
And then sat down like a Raggedy Ann.
His head fell down and his arms fell, too,
And he went to sleep for an hour or two.

The stretching game

Link your thumbs;
Raise your arms
Straight up and past your ears,
Stretch and pull;
Pull and stretch;
Try to touch the sky.
Pull and stretch;
Stretch and pull;
Pull—pull—pull!
Drop your arms, now sigh.

FRANCES C. HUNTER

Poster	26	Make posters or pictures illustrating activities conducive to play, sleep, and relaxation.	P
Puppets	27	Make two puppets and call them "Sleepy Head" and "Wide Awake." Have children dramatize aspects of rest and sleep.	P, I
	28	Make paper-bag puppets and dramatize a problem, such as a boy who wants to stay up past his bedtime to watch TV.	P, I
Scrapbook	29	Prepare scrapbooks of pictures showing restful and relaxing activities.	P, I
Stories	30	Read and create stories about rest, sleep, and relaxation.	P, I

TEACHING TECHNIQUES

Safety

	BICYCLE SAFETY	Grades
Bulletin board	**1** Display children's drawings of bicycle safety.	P, I, U
	2 Display bicycle safety posters and other printed materials available from the American Bicycle Institute and such organizations.	P, I, U
	3 A committee of pupils prepares bulletin board display showing outline of a bicycle labeled with its main parts and the safety rules (Fig. 12-22).	I, U
Chart	**4** Children prepare a chart listing bicycle safety rules, including wearing helmets.	P, I, U
Checklist	**5** Pupils prepare a checklist for use in the inspection of the mechanical safety of bicycles. The assistance of a bicycle repair person may be necessary.	I, U
	6 Organize a bicycle club in school.	I, U
Demonstration	**7** Children demonstrate the following procedures correctly: getting on a bicycle, getting off a bicycle, guiding a bicycle, applying the brake, use of helmets, and stopping and parking the bicycle.	P, I, U
	8 Pupils demonstrate and practice the proper hand signals when riding bicycles.	P, I, U
	9 Demonstrate the mechanical inspection of a safe bicycle in class. It is advisable to bring a bicycle into the room.	P, I, U

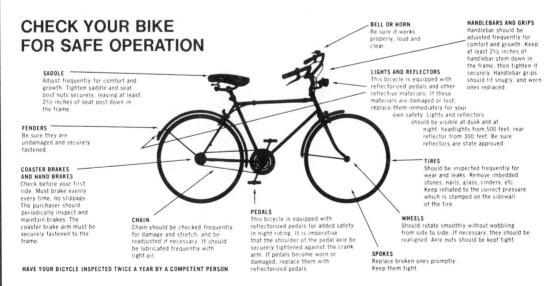

FIG. 12-22 Bicycle safety check. (Courtesy the Bicycle Institute of America, Inc, New York.)

TEACHING TECHNIQUES: SAFETY—cont'd

	BICYCLE SAFETY—cont'd	Grades
Demonstration—cont'd	10 Have a demonstration of minor bicycle repairs. It may be necessary to invite a bicycle repair person to class.	I, U
	11 Conduct a bicycle field day in which pupils participate in a variety of activities that show their ability and skill to ride bicycles safely. Automobile clubs and other organizations in the community often will provide assistance with this program.	I, U
	12 Pupils prepare a demonstration of bicycle safety to be presented to a school assembly.	I, U
Discussion	13 The motor vehicle laws and regulations, in terms of licensing of bicycles, the need to comply with rules, proper hand signals, parking, and others.	P, I, U
	14 Safety factors involved in riding a bicycle to school, including wearing helmets.	P, I, U
	15 Pupils bring newspaper and magazine articles about bicycle safety or accidents to class.	I, U
	16 Pupils discuss the causes of bicycle accidents and how to prevent them. This could lead to a series of unanswered questions and start the problem-solving approach to bicycle safety.	I, U
Dramatization	17 Children dramatize riding a bicycle and demonstrate the necessary safe practices.	P, I, U
Excursion	18 Visit a bicycle repair shop to observe how bicycles are repaired.	I, U
Experience chart	19 Prepare an experience chart or record of bicycle safety rules, including wearing helmets.	P
Guest speaker	20 Invite a police officer to class to discuss bicycle safety traffic rules.	P, I, U
Individual and group reports	21 Prepare oral and written reports on the safest way to ride bicycles to and from school.	I, U
	22 Prepare oral and written reports on bicycle safety.	I, U
	23 Prepare school newspaper articles titled "Bicycle safety tips."	I, U
	24 Write a group letter to the police department or some other organization requesting a speaker to discuss bicycle safety.	I, U
	25 Children prepare a code of safety for bicycle riders. This can be posted on the bulletin board or may be printed in the school newspaper.	I, U
	26 Children write to the Bicycle Institute of America or other organizations for bicycle safety materials.	I, U
	27 Pupils prepare reports on the yearly accidents occurring on bicycles in the nation, state, county, and city.	U
Interview	28 Interview a police officer or some other authority on bicycle safety.	I, U
Scrapbook	29 Prepare a scrapbook containing newspaper and magazine articles, pictures, stories, and other obtainable materials on bicycle safety.	P, I, U
Self-test	30 Prepare a self-test or pretest on bicycle traffic safety.	I, U

TEACHING TECHNIQUES: SAFETY—cont'd

	SAMPLE QUESTIONS	YES	NO	Grades
Self-test— cont'd	1. A bicycle can be ridden on the sidewalk in a business area.	☐	☐	
	2. A bicycle rider should obey all traffic signs, lights and devices.	☐	☐	
	3. Pedestrians do not have the right-of-way in crosswalks.	☐	☐	
	4. You should walk your bicycle across heavily traveled streets.	☐	☐	
	5. Night riding without a light and reflector is unsafe.	☐	☐	
	6. It is safe and proper to carry a passenger on a bicycle.	☐	☐	
	7. Hitching to a moving truck is safe if you are careful.	☐	☐	
	8. It is best to ride three abreast when riding in a group.	☐	☐	
	9. You should give hand signals when turning at all times.	☐	☐	
	10. On a country road you should ride on the left side of the road.	☐	☐	
Survey	**31** Pupils conduct a survey of bicycle traffic violations noted on the way to and from school.			I, U

BUS SAFETY

		Grades
Bulletin board	**1** Display pictures, drawings, slogans, cartoons, and posters about bus safety.	P, I, U
	2 Make a bus out of construction paper and display this along with appropriate captions about bus safety.	P, I, U
Demonstration	**3** With a small tow truck and blocks demonstrate why it is necessary to be seated at all times in the school bus. Show how blocks will fall when a sudden stop is necessary.	P, I
	4 Have children practice bus loading and unloading and discuss safe behavior while riding.	P, I, U
Discussion	**5** The need to cooperate with the bus driver when riding the school bus.	P, I, U
	6 Discuss bus safety with children preparing a list of safe behavior rules.	P, I, U
Dramatization	**7** Arrange chairs in classroom to represent a school bus. Have children act out the right way and the wrong way to get on and off the bus and practice safe bus rules.	P, I
Excursion	**8** Visit a bus and have the driver discuss safe behavior while boarding and riding.	P, I
Experience chart	**9** Prepare an experience chart or record of safe procedures on the bus.	P
Guest speaker	**10** Invite the bus driver to discuss bus safety.	P, I
Mural	**11** Prepare a mural depicting safety on the bus.	P, I
Scrapbook	**12** Construct a scrapbook of pupil drawings about bus safety.	P, I
Songs and poems	**13** Compose songs and poems about bus safety.	P, I

DISASTER SAFETY

		Grades
Bulletin board	**1** Display pictures, drawings, or diagrams of procedures to follow in the event of a flood or tornado.	P, I, U
	2 Prepare an illustrated display of foods suitable for storing for emergency use.	P, I, U

TEACHING TECHNIQUES: SAFETY—cont'd

		DISASTER SAFETY—cont'd	**Grades**
Chart	3	Prepare a wall chart for each classroom showing the floor plans, exits and entrances to the building, and the shortest route to the nearest shelter.	P, I, U
Demonstration	4	Demonstrate the signals in schools that signify alerts and practice identification.	P, I, U
	5	Demonstrate and practice emergency drills for evacuation or seeking cover.	P, I, U
	6	Food pollution through the use of simple fungi and bacteriological experiments.	I, U
	7	How and where to store foods safely at home if an alert occurs.	I, U
	8	How to preserve perishable foods without refrigeration.	I, U
	9	How to properly dispose of polluted food.	I, U
	10	Demonstrate and display an appropriate first-aid kit for emergencies.	I, U
	11	How to preserve and package foods for emergencies.	I, U
	12	First-aid procedures after civil disasters.	I, U
Discussion	13	What children may do (activities) while waiting in a shelter at school until the all-clear signal is sounded.	P, I, U
	14	The procedures to follow if caught outdoors during an alert.	P, I, U
	15	The location of emergency shelters in the school and community.	P, I, U
	16	The meaning of civil defense and why it is necessary.	P, I, U
	17	The problems of emotions, panics, and other behaviors that will occur during disaster.	I, U
	18	First-aid procedures necessary in civil disasters.	I, U
	19	The contamination of food and water and ways to protect these items after floods.	I, U
Dramatization	20	Dramatize proper conduct during disasters.	P, I, U
Exhibit	21	Display pamphlets and other printed materials for pupil reference and use.	I, U
Guest speakers	22	Invite local emergency management officials and Red Cross speakers to discuss aspects of disasters.	I, U
Individual and group reports	23	Have individual or group oral or written reports on plans for the protection of people in the event of disasters.	I, U
	24	Pupils write articles for the local newspaper or school paper on how individuals can protect themselves at home, at school, or when outdoors during a natural disaster.	U
Interview	25	Interview the American Red Cross about the feasibility of community shelters.	
	26	Pupils interview local health officers and medical personnel about the availability of services and hospital facilities in the event of civil disasters.	

TEACHING TECHNIQUES: SAFETY—cont'd

	DISASTER SAFETY—cont'd	**Grades**
Interview—cont'd	27 Pupils interview the health officer or a person from the local emergency management office.	
Survey	28 Survey the school and community to locate the designated shelter areas.	
	FARM SAFETY	
Bulletin board	1 Children obtain pictures or make drawings of tools and machinery found on the farm, such as tractors, cotton pickers, cotton trailers, harvesters, plows, and discs, and place caption "Dangerous equipment" below. Pictures may be obtained from pamphlets available from farm machinery companies or from farm organizations.	P, I, U
Discussion	2 Safe practices when riding on trucks and other farm machinery.	P, I, U
	3 The hazards of insect stings, poisonous sprays, canals, irrigation ditches, tools, and other unsafe places and equipment on the farm.	P, I, U
	4 The hazards of sharp implements such as pitchforks, hoes, saws, and axes used on the farm.	P, I, U
	5 Safety around horses, bulls, and other farm animals.	P, I, U
Experience chart or record	6 Children help prepare an experience chart or record on farm safety rules.	P
Exhibit	7 Display a variety of sharp implements used in farm work and discuss the dangers of their improper use.	P, I, U
Individual and group reports	8 Children prepare oral and written reports on farm safety.	I, U
	FIRE SAFETY	
Bulletin board	1 Prepare an illustrated bulletin board display about fire prevention using construction paper, real clothing materials, or crayons.	P, I, U
	2 Display pictures or news items about fires in the community.	P, I, U
	3 Use pictures and drawings to display the varieties of types of fire extinguishers.	I, U
	4 Display pictures of "drop and roll" and crawling in a smoke-filled room.	P, I, U
	5 Pictorially illustrate the action to be taken when fires occur or smoke appears at home and include escape plan and other procedures.	P, I
Chart	6 Prepare a list of illustrated fire safety rules.	P, I
	7 Make an illustrated chart listing the common causes of fires in the home.	P, I, U
	8 Make an illustrated chart of the fire exits in school.	P, I, U
Demonstration	9 Light two candles and fan one of them to show how moving air causes a flame to burn more vigorously.	P, I,
	10 Sound the fire alarm bell and have children practice responding to it for a fire drill.	P, I, U
	11 The way to report a fire using an alarm box and the telephone.	P, I, U
	12 Ways of putting out fires using a variety of fire extinguishers.	P, I, U
	13 How to put out a fire when someone's clothing is ablaze.	P, I, U

TEACHING TECHNIQUES: SAFETY—cont'd

		FIRE SAFETY—cont'd	**Grades**
Demonstra- tion—cont'd	14	How to use matches safely—use only safety matches and strike match with the cover closed; dispose of burned matches by breaking them and placing in a glass or a metal container.	P, I,U
	15	Drop and roll and crawling low in smoke-filled room procedures.	P, I, U
	16	Demonstrate the making of a fire extinguisher by putting some vinegar in a bottle and adding some baking soda. (Wrap the soda in a tissue before adding it to the vinegar. This will delay the formation of the carbon dioxide gas.) Put a rubber stopper and a pipette in the bottle, turn it upside down, and pour the fluid into a pail or sink.	P, I, U
	17	The combustibility of a variety of materials such as asbestos, glass, paper, water, cotton, cloth, wood, kerosene, and various types of clothing. Also discuss spontaneous combustion.	P, I, U
	18	Place a piece of cardboard against a small light bulb and show the brown spot that occurs. Explain in terms of the fire triangle.	P, I
	19	Teacher lights a candle in class, and pupils watch it burn. A glass is placed over the candle, and children attempt to explain, in terms of the triangle of fire, why the flame was extinguished.	P, I, U
Discussion	20	Fire safety rules and reasons for fire drills.	P, I
	21	Beneficial and hazardous effects of fire.	P, I
	22	Fire hazards on special occasions, such as Christmas, Hannukah, and the Fourth of July.	P, I, U
	23	Discuss and practice fire drills in school.	P, I, U
	24	Discuss these questions: What causes fires? How do fires start? What materials burn? Where should matches be kept? What should you do in case of fire? How should you put out a picnic fire? How can fires be prevented?	P, I, U
	25	The value of the home inspections conducted by firefighters. Introduce common electrical terms, such as wire, plug, socket, bulb, fuse, and fuse box.	I, U
	26	Ways to prevent fires by good housekeeping procedures, proper disposal of rubbish and ashes, safe storage of fuel, correct installation and care of stoves, electric equipment, and furnaces.	I, U
	27	The types of fires and how they may be extinguished.	I, U
	28	Pupils participate as members of the fire-safety patrol to inform other pupils about fire prevention.	I, U
	29	Baby-sitting: responsibilities regarding fire safety.	I, U
	30	Smoke detectors.	P, I, U
	31	Fire escape plans from homes and other buildings.	P, I, U
	32	First-aid procedures for burns.	P, I, U
	33	Hazards and use of electricity and flammable materials.	I, U
	34	Identity and proper storage of flammable liquids.	P, I, U

TEACHING TECHNIQUES: SAFETY—cont'd

	FIRE SAFETY—cont'd	**Grades**
Discussion—cont'd	35 Fires reported in newspapers and magazines in terms of causes and prevention.	I, U
	36 To whom and how to report fires and smoke discovered.	P, I
	37 Combustibility and flammability of various types of clothing and other substances.	I, U
	38 Importance of drop and roll and crawling low procedures.	P, I, U
	39 False alarms.	I, U
	40 Ways to call fire department.	P, I, U
Dramatization	41 Build a fire engine using large blocks, cardboard boxes, and other items. Children participate in dramatic play by having a corner in the classroom as a firehouse. Pupils bring their toy telephones to practice reporting fires.	P
	42 Dramatize the procedures to follow when reporting a fire by telephone.	P, I, U
	43 Dramatize fire safety through sociodramas, puppet shows, and plays.	P, I, U
Drawings	44 Children make drawings of ways to prevent fires, escape from fires, and signal when fire is discovered.	P, I
	45 Draw pictures of wires, plugs, sockets, electric appliances, and other items with descriptions placed below telling of the safe ways to use these items.	I, U
Excursion	46 Visit the firehouse.	P, I, U
	47 Children walk around the school to locate fire hazards or become familiar with the locations of extinguishers, exits, and alarm boxes.	P, I, U
	48 Visit a fireboat.	
Exhibit	49 Invite the fire department to display fire-fighting equipment and its uses.	P, I, U
	50 Display a variety of combustible materials, such as paper, wood, cloth, gasoline, and kerosene.	P, I, U
	51 Display books, magazines, pamphlets, and stories about fire safety for pupil use.	P, I, U
	52 Show pictures and materials of fire hazards, such as overload of electric circuits, trash accumulation, frayed electric wires, and gasoline storage containers.	P, I, U
Experience chart or record	53 Prepare an experience chart or record about fire safety.	P
Experiment	54 Place a lighted candle on a table and let the class watch it burn. Cover the candle with a clear glass so that no air can enter. Have pupils note what happens to the candle—it goes out when the oxygen supply has been used. Relate this to extinguishing fires.	P, I, U

TEACHING TECHNIQUES: SAFETY—cont'd

	FIRE SAFETY—cont'd	**Grades**
Flip chart	**55** Prepare a series of illustrated flip charts for a discussion about fire safety. Include answers to these questions: How is fire helpful? What are the causes of fire? How many fires occur in our community? How can we prevent fires?	P, I, U
Games	**56** Make crossword puzzles, riddles, and other games about fire prevention and fire safety.	P, I, U
Guest speaker	**57** Invite a fire fighter to discuss fire safety.	P, I, U
	58 Invite the fire chief from your local fire department to discuss the junior fire marshall program and to encourage children to participate.	I
	59 Request the local fire department to conduct a demonstration of the types of fire extinguishers and smoke detectors.	U
	60 Invite a member of the National Board of Fire Underwriters Laboratory to discuss the work of this organization in fire safety.	U
Individual and group reports	**61** Write stories about their experiences in fire safety.	P, I
	62 Write to insurance companies and others concerned with fire safety and request materials for display and class reading.	I, U
	63 Prepare oral or written reports on the causes, effects, and prevention of fires.	I, U
	64 Write articles for the school newspaper about fire safety.	I, U
	65 Students prepare reports on baby-sitting and fire safety.	I, U
Inspection	**66** Prepare checklist to search for fire hazards in home or school.	I, U
Map	**67** Prepare a map of your community identifying the locations of fire-houses, hydrants, alarm boxes, and other fire safety features.	I, U
	68 Students prepare home escape-from-fire plans in consultation with parents.	P, I
Models	**69** Construct a fire alarm box, a firehouse, and fire prevention equipment for use in dramatic play.	P
	70 Make fire fighter hats out of construction paper.	P, I
	71 Draw or build a home that is free of fire hazards.	I, U
Mural	**72** Prepare a mural of ways to prevent fires.	P, I
Poems and songs	**73** Create and learn poems, songs, jingles, and stories about fire safety.	P, I
Posters	**74** Conduct a contest for the best school poster on fire safety.	I, U
Scrapbook	**75** Pupils prepare scrapbooks containing pictures, photos, stories, poems, newspaper articles, and written reports about fires and fire prevention.	P, I, U
Self-test	**76** Give the following self-test:	I, U

Circle the correct answers to the right. If you do not know the answer, circle the letter "D."

1. A grease fire may be put out by pouring water on it.	T	F	D
2. One should run to extinguish flames when clothes are on fire.	T	F	D
3. A frayed wire on an electric appliance is a dangerous fire hazard.	T	F	D

TEACHING TECHNIQUES: SAFETY—cont'd

FIRE SAFETY—cont'd **Grades**

4. Fire drills are not necessary at schools.	T F D	
5. It is safe to run a lamp cord under a rug.	T F D	
6. The leading causes of fire are matches and smoking.	T F D	
7. A penny is a good substitute for a blown-out fuse.	T F D	
8. "EXIT" on a door means the door leads to the outside.	T F D	
9. A wood fire may be put out by pouring water on it.	T F D	
10. Gasoline can be stored safely in glass bottles.	T F D	
11. Oily rags can catch fire without a match.	T F D	
12. One should always close the cover of a safety matchbook before striking a match.	T F D	

Show and tell	77	Children tell of their experiences with fire, fire engines, and fire fighters.	P
	78	Children identify names, addresses, and home telephone numbers.	P
Survey	79	Pupils make survey forms to check their homes for fire hazards.	P, I, U
Television box	80	Students make a movie with a title such as "The day Mary's house burned." Pupils draw pictures of the discovery of the fire and what they did.	P
Word lists	81	Prepare a list of new words learned about fire prevention.	P, I, U

FIRST AID

Bulletin board	1	Show pictures and drawings that display first-aid procedures to be followed at school.	P, I, U
Demonstration	2	Display pictures or drawings of poisonous snakes, insects, and plants.	P, I, U
	3	Have nurse or other person demonstrate how to cleanse a wound with soap and water, apply a sterile dressing and bandage, and stop a nosebleed and other bleeding.	P, I, U
	4	Demonstrate the correct procedure for removing foreign objects from the eye.	I, U
	5	Provide for a demonstration of the mouth-to-mouth procedure of rescue breathing.	I, U
Discussion	6	What to do when injured at school, home, or when away from home.	P, I, U
	7	First-aid procedures for sunburn, chapped skin, poison oak or ivy, and insect bites and stings.	P, I, U
	8	Discuss reasons for cleansing wounds and applying sterile dressings and bandages.	P, I, U
	9	First-aid procedures for minor cuts, burns, and bruises.	P, I, U
	10	Dog bites and the necessary first-aid procedures, as well as other action that must be taken.	P, I, U
	11	First-aid procedures for bone fractures.	I, U
	12	The general first-aid procedures when accidents occur.	I, U
Dramatization	13	Children play doctor or nurse attending a child who has been injured.	P
	14	Dramatize the reporting of an accident at school, home, and elsewhere.	P, I
	15	The procedure to follow in an emergency or when someone is injured.	P, I, U

TEACHING TECHNIQUES: SAFETY—cont'd

	FIRST AID—cont'd	Grades
Dramatization—cont'd	16 Dramatize a series of injuries and then permit the class to try to determine the first-aid procedures to be followed: A student is using a penknife at school to whittle on some wood and cuts his/her hand; a student is running his/her hand along a wooden bench that is full of splinters and gets some in his/her hand; a student is tackled playing touch football and falls, striking his/her wrist on the ground.	I, U
Drawings	17 Pupils prepare drawings of first aid being administered to injured children.	P, I
Exhibit	18 Display a variety of poisonous substances or containers that hold such materials.	P, I
	19 Display the contents of a simple first-aid kit. Nurse may be helpful in determining items to be included.	I, U
	20 Display an assortment of materials, such as dressings, bandages, triangular bandages, and splints used in first aid.	I, U
Experience chart or record	21 Construct an experience chart or record that describes what to do when injured at school.	P
Guest speaker	22 Invite the school nurse to come to class to discuss first-aid procedures.	P, I, U
Individual and group reports	23 Children prepare reports on first-aid procedures for snake bites, seizures, frostbite, and fractures.	I, U
	24 Children prepare a letter inviting a member of the Red Cross to come to class to discuss first aid.	I, U
Problem solving	25 Present a series of first-aid problems to individuals or committees and let them try to solve them. Such problems might include: What would you do if a person cut his/her finger while preparing dinner? What would you do if your sister swallowed a poison, such as ammonia? What would you do if a pupil at school fell from the horizontal bar that is 7 feet high?	U
Scrapbook	26 Make scrapbooks containing stories, pictures, magazine articles, and drawings about first aid.	I, U
Self-test	27 Prepare a self-test for use in the discussion on first aid.	I, U
Show and tell	28 Children tell of what they experienced when they were injured.	P
	HOME SAFETY	
Bulletin board	1 Display pictures and magazine and newspaper articles on home accidents and safety.	P, I, U
	2 Pupils construct for display a graph or pie-shaped chart showing the numbers and types of home accidents.	U
Discussion	3 Children's prepared lists of hazardous conditions in and around the home.	P, I
	4 Student-planned "pick-up" day at home to remove hazards.	P, I

TEACHING TECHNIQUES: SAFETY—cont'd

	HOME SAFETY—cont'd	**Grades**
Discussion— cont'd	5 Children's observations of safe and unsafe practices in the home and elsewhere.	P, I
	6 The causes and possible ways to prevent injuries reported in newspaper articles brought to class by students.	I, U
	7 The safe handling of blasting caps and the procedures to follow when they are found.	I, U
	8 How to turn off the electricity and the gas at home.	U
	9 Prepare a list of responsibilities of baby-sitters and discuss the safety problems that sitters may have to handle.	U
Dramatization	10 Children act out such situations as a stranger offering a ride, a cross dog barring the sidewalk, and one child double-daring another to do something reckless. Ask pupils to consider these questions: "What would you do?" and "Would you be acting safely?"	P, I
	11 Dramatize an accident in the home, such as slipping on a scatter rug that has no rubber backing, and discuss how this could have been prevented.	I, U
	12 Prepare a play on home safety for presentation to a parent group or to a school assembly.	I, U
Drawings	13 Following a discussion on safe play areas at home, children draw pictures of where they play at home.	P
	14 Following a unit on home safety, each child draws pictures of what he/she does at home to make it a safer place.	P
Exhibit	15 Children bring some of the dangerous objects found in their back yards for display.	P, I
	16 Children construct a medicine cabinet using cardboard boxes and construction paper and have all items properly labeled.	P, I
	17 Prepare an exhibit of hazardous objects or materials found in the home such as metal toys with sharp edges, sharp knives improperly stored, rugs without rubber backing, and oily rags improperly stored.	P, I, U
	18 Display pamphlets, booklets, and other resource materials on home safety for pupils' use.	I, U
	19 Display poisonous substances found in the home, such as ammonia, disinfectants, drugs, moth balls, and cleaning chemicals.	I, U
Experience chart or record	20 Prepare an experience chart on home safety containing such activities as walking carefully on polished floors, picking up toys when finished with them, and not playing with matches.	P
Flannelboard	21 Prepare home safety stories and use a flannelboard to illustrate them.	P
Guest speaker	22 Invite a representative from the National Safety Council or the local safety council to come to class to discuss home safety.	I, U

TEACHING TECHNIQUES: SAFETY—cont'd

	HOME SAFETY—cont'd	**Grades**
Individual and group reports	23 Pupils use drawings or pictures to illustrate daily activities that will keep themselves safe.	I, U
	24 Collect newspaper articles about accidents in the home and categorize them by types. Committees then do research and write reports about how they could have been prevented.	I, U
Model	25 Pupils construct a cross section of a house out of cardboard or wood and illustrate the possible hazardous places within.	I, U
Mural	26 Make a large cooperative mural of safe play areas in the neighborhood.	P, I
Newspaper	27 Pupils prepare a home safety newspaper to be published periodically containing stories about safety in the home.	I, U
Panel	28 Have a panel discussion on the topic, "Making a safe home."	I, U
Posters	29 Make posters showing how to correct hazardous conditions found in the home, such as not touching radio or electric light cords when bathing, proper position of cooking utensils on stove with handles turned in, and using a stepladder rather than a chair to stand on.	I, U
Scrapbook	30 Children prepare a scrapbook with pictures, stories, and newspaper articles on "Safety at home."	P, I, U
Show and tell	31 Children tell about home injuries.	P
Songs and poems	32 Create home safety songs and poems.	P
Survey	33 Survey the neighborhood and prepare a report on the safe and unsafe places to play.	I, U
	34 Conduct a survey of home hazards using a checklist prepared by children. Discuss how these problems can be changed. Emphasize specific areas such as unlighted, cluttered stairs; unscreened fireplaces; space heaters; electric outlets and wiring; and the proper place to store garden tools, matches, nails, and sewing needles.	I, U
Telephone card	35 Make a card to be hung by the telephone with the number of the fire and police departments, an ambulance, the family physician, the nearest relative, and also the home address.	P, I
Telephone number	36 Children dial home telephone number and give the last name of parent, address, and identity of road and street landmarks.	P, I
	PEDESTRIAN SAFETY	
Bulletin board	1 Prepare a display of student drawings about pedestrian safety.	P, I, U
	2 Develop pedestrian safety slogans for use on the bulletin board such as "Courtesy is safety," "Cross at the crosswalks," and "Wait for the traffic signal before crossing streets."	P, I
	3 Make a series of charts or graphs for display showing the number and kinds of pedestrian injuries.	U
Chart	4 Prepare a chart that lists the pedestrian safety rules.	P, I
Demonstration	5 Demonstrate and practice the proper way to cross streets.	P, I

TEACHING TECHNIQUES: SAFETY—cont'd

	PEDESTRIAN SAFETY—cont'd	**Grades**
Demonstra-tion—cont'd	6 Prepare a table simulating a street corner using small cars, bicycles, police officer, and traffic lights and demonstrate safe pedestrian practices.	P, I
	7 Darken room and have students dressed in various colored clothes walk in front of the room. Be sure to have someone wearing white among these students. Children discuss which colors were more easily seen.	P, I, U
	8 In a darkened room have two lighted flashlights representing auto headlights. Have a student with dark clothes and one with white clothes walk in front of the lights to show the difference in the reflection of light.	P, I, U
Discussion	9 The importance of knowing names, addresses, and telephone numbers.	P
	10 What action to take if a stranger invites you to take a ride in an automobile.	P, I
	11 The school safety patrol and its role in helping children cross streets safely.	P, I
Dramatization	12 Children bring small toy cars, trucks, and buses for use in dramatic play about pedestrian safety.	P
	13 Using a large space in the classroom or on the playground, lay out an intersection with strips of tape or chalk, including crosswalks, and have children cross the street properly. Prepare a number of crossing signal models, such as a traffic light with appropriate color, a walk-wait signal, and a stop sign.	P
Drawings	14 Children make drawings about pedestrian safety.	P, I
	15 Children draw pictures of how they come to school, pointing out safe practices.	P
Excursion	16 Visit the street corner nearest the school to see the traffic signals, the police officer, the yellow crossing lines, and other safety features.	P
Exhibit	17 Display a variety of traffic signs and discuss their meanings for traffic and pedestrian safety.	I, U
Experience chart and record	18 Prepare an experience chart or record of safety pedestrian rules that may include:	P

Red means stop.
Yellow means wait.
Green means go.
Cross at the crosswalks.

Flannelboard	19 Prepare illustrations to tell a story of pedestrian safety with emphasis on the danger of playing or running between parked cars.	P, I
Game	20 Write safety rules on strips of tagboard and cut them in half to form a simple puzzle. Children try to match the cut pieces and locate the correct safety rules.	P, I
Guest speaker	21 Invite a police officer to discuss pedestrian and traffic safety.	P, I, U
	22 Invite a member of the school safety patrol to discuss correct ways to cross streets.	P, I

TEACHING TECHNIQUES: SAFETY—cont'd

	PEDESTRIAN SAFETY—cont'd	**Grades**
Individual and group report	23 Record the number and type of pedestrian injuries listed in local newspapers for a designated period.	I, U
	24 Write letters to the National Safety Council, automobile clubs, and other community organizations requesting material on pedestrian safety for use in class.	I, U
	25 Pupils prepare oral or written reports on the number, kinds, and causes of pedestrian injuries.	U
Interview	26 Pupils interview a traffic police officer and a representative of the automobile club about pedestrian accidents and how to prevent them.	I, U
Map	27 Prepare a large map showing the route each child takes to school and discuss the safest ways to come to school.	P, I
Model	28 Make a traffic signal box with red, green, and yellow lights or signals for use in dramatic play.	P
Poems	29 Children create and learn poems about pedestrian safety, such as the following:	P

> Red says stop,
> Green says go.
> Yellow says wait,
> You'd better go slow.
> When I reach a crossing place,
> To left and right I turn my face.
> I walk, not run, across the street
> And use my head to guide my feet.
>
> Stop, look, and listen
> Before you cross the street.
> Use your eyes, use your ears
> Before you use your feet.

Posters	30 Prepare posters and enter them in the school contest on pedestrian safety.	I, U
Problem solving	31 Have children discuss this problem: "You come to a street corner that you must cross, but there is no signal. How will you get across?"	P, I
Puppets	32 Make puppets and dramatize ways to be a safe pedestrian.	P
Quiz	33 Have children write on a piece of paper the five numbers listed below and place yes or no answers beside the appropriate number to the statements listed.	P

1. We should cross streets at crosswalks.
2. We should cross streets when the traffic light is green.
3. We should look one way when crossing streets.
4. We should always go with the traffic when walking on roadways.
5. We know the yellow light at a crosswalk means wait.

TEACHING TECHNIQUES: SAFETY—cont'd

		Grades
	PEDESTRIAN SAFETY—cont'd	
Riddle	**34** Children make up riddles, such as the following:	P

> It stands near the corner.
> It turns red and green.
> It helps keep us safe.
> What is it?

		Grades
Scrapbook	**35** Make illustrated scrapbooks with pedestrian safety rules, slogans, rhymes, and limericks.	P, I, U
	36 Prepare a scrapbook of pictures and drawings showing safety as a pedestrian.	P, I
Self-test	**37** Pupils take following self-test.	I, U

Do you	YES	NO
1. Cross streets only at intersections or marked crosswalks?	☐	☐
2. Look left and right before crossing streets, making sure that the entire crossing can be made safely?	☐	☐
3. Cross only on green light or "go" signals?	☐	☐
4. Obey directions of safety patrols or officers?	☐	☐
5. Walk on the left side facing traffic if walking on roadway and give way to approaching vehicles?	☐	☐
6. Wear white at night or carry a light?	☐	☐
7. Always get into and out of a vehicle on the side nearest the curb?	☐	☐
8. Give the motorist the right of way where there are no signals?	☐	☐
9. Stay out of streets when playing?	☐	☐
10. Watch for oncoming traffic when catching or leaving a bus?	☐	☐

Score ("yes" answers)

9-10—You may live to a ripe old age.
6-8—You may expect to get hurt before long.
5 or less—Stay in your own yard; you're living on borrowed time.

		Grades
Show and tell	**38** Children tell about pedestrian hazards they have seen.	P
Television	**39** Make a shadow box or TV box and have students prepare a series of drawings about pedestrian safety. Include such illustrations as wearing white at night, crossing at street corners, and waiting for the green light.	P
	RECREATION SAFETY	
Bulletin board	**1** Prepare displays of pictures and drawings of water skiing, hunting, camping, picnicking, fishing, skating, hiking, and vacation safety.	P, I, U
	2 Display posters or drawings showing the correct and incorrect ways to get in and out of rowboats, canoes, and motorboats.	P, I, U
Chart	**3** Pupils prepare and complete charts of summertime safety for reference and use at home during vacation.	I, U

TEACHING TECHNIQUES: SAFETY—cont'd

RECREATION SAFETY—cont'd   **Grades**

Summertime safety

My summer activities:

1. _____
2. _____
3. _____
4. _____

What could hurt me:

1. _____
2. _____
3. _____
4. _____

How to keep safe:

1. _____
2. _____
3. _____
4. _____

		Grades
Demonstration	**4** Have the Red Cross conduct a demonstration of swimming, boating, and beach safety at one of the local swimming pools, lakes, or rivers.	P, I, U
Discussion	**5** Safety on special occasions, such as Halloween and the Fourth of July.	P, I, U
	6 The people who can help when you are injured or lost.	P, I, U
	7 Safety on picnics and outings.	P, I, U
	8 Show pupils pictures of recreational equipment, such as a canoe, skate, sled, ski, baseball bat, and fishhook, and have them tell of a good safety practice when using these items.	P, I, U
	9 Safe and unsafe features of swimming in lakes, rivers, oceans, canals, and other places. Learn how to choose a safe swimming area.	I, U
	10 The laws with which pupils should be familiar when hunting, fishing, and camping.	I, U
	11 Methods of protection while participating in various sports, such as football, baseball, basketball, and skiing.	I, U
	12 Safety in skin and scuba diving.	I, U
	13 Safe hunting procedures.	U

TEACHING TECHNIQUES: SAFETY—cont'd

	RECREATION SAFETY—cont'd	**Grades**
Dramatization	14 Children participate in dramatic play of safe practices while camping or picnicking.	P
	15 Prepare and present a skit on snow safety to an assembly, or a parent group, or broadcast it over the local radio station.	I, U
	16 Pupils write a play ("Comedy of Errors") on how not to go on a camping trip.	I, U
Drawings	17 Make drawings of safe practices while boating, swimming, skiing, playing in the snow or at the beach.	P, I, U
Exhibit	18 Display the items of a "Lost" kit that may be usable when camping or out in the woods, including such things as a single-edge razor blade, fishhooks, fish line and wet flies, pencil and notebook, Band-Aids, soap and disinfectant, compass, sugar lumps, strong string (shoelaces), and matches water-proofed with paraffin. Seal the contents in a can and attach with a belt strap.	P, I, U
	19 Display such hazardous objects as fishhooks, darts, sharp-pointed sticks, and blasting caps.	P, I, U
	20 Display the appropriate clothing to wear in various outdoor activities, such as hiking, camping, hunting, skiing, and boating.	P, I, U
	21 Display the equipment needed for skin and scuba diving and discuss safety features.	I, U
	22 Display safety items that give protection in various sports: football—mouth protectors; baseball—mask; and skiing—safety binders.	I, U
Experience chart or record	23 Make an experience chart or record about safe procedures on vacations, when swimming, and at other times.	P
Game	24 Play the game "Little child lost." The teacher is a police officer and a student is lost. Have children determine what they would do, or should do, if this happens to them.	P
	25 Children collect pictures from magazines and newspapers of safe and unsafe ways of playing. Place all of these in a box and permit each child to select one item and tell whether it is a safe or unsafe procedure.	P, I, U
Guest speaker	26 Invite a member of the Red Cross or the school nurse to discuss first-aid procedures for possible recreation problems, such as sunburn, poisonous plants and insects, and blisters.	P, I, U
	27 Have a forest ranger discuss safe procedures in parks and playgrounds.	P, I, U
	28 Have a representative from the Red Cross or a skin and scuba diving club discuss the safety aspects of this sport.	I, U
	29 Invite guest speakers to discuss safety in activities such as football, basketball, skiing, tennis, and swimming.	I, U
	30 Have a member of the local rifle club demonstrate and discuss safety while hunting or the safe handling of guns.	U

TEACHING TECHNIQUES: SAFETY—cont'd

	RECREATION SAFETY—cont'd	**Grades**
Individual and group reports	31 Pupils prepare oral and written reports on the safety rules when camping, boating, hiking, fishing, swimming, hunting, skiing, and roller or ice skating.	I, U
	32 Pupils write a report of their favorite recreational activities and include the safety rules that should be observed when participating.	I, U
Map	33 Prepare a map showing the safe swimming area in the immediate vicinity and within a comfortable driving distance from the local community.	I, U
Mural	34 Make a mural of safe places and safe ways to play while skiing, boating, swimming, hiking, skating, and others.	P, I, U
Puppet	35 Prepare a puppet show or dramatization of a safe camping or hiking trip.	P, I
Scrapbooks	36 Pupils prepare scrapbooks containing pictures, newspaper and magazine articles, stories, and other items on safety categorized into such areas as fishing, camping, swimming, boating, hunting, skiing, and skating.	I, U

SCHOOL SAFETY

Bulletin board	1 Prepare a display of pictures and drawings showing safety at school.	P, I, U
Cartoon	2 Conduct a school safety cartoon or slogan contest.	I, U
Chart	3 Pupils prepare a chart or graph of the nature, number, and location of accidents that occur in school.	I, U
Demonstration	4 The safe use of tools, blocks, and other equipment.	P, I
	5 The safe way to use stairways, drinking fountains, and school equipment.	P, I
	6 The safe way to use playground apparatus and equipment, such as slides, swings, bats, and tetherballs.	P, I
Discussion	7 School safety helpers, such as the teacher, nurse, custodian, and bus driver.	P
	8 The dangers of throwing sticks, climbing fences, throwing balls improperly, and running in the halls or crowded areas.	P, I
	9 The proper use of fountain pens, scissors, and other implements in class, as well as the proper way to open doors and walk in the corridors.	P, I
	10 Prepare a list of safety rules for the classroom and the playground that may include:	P ,I

> I walk in the halls.
> I use the slides properly.
> I use scissors and pencils carefully.
> I do not push when in line.
> I do not throw rocks or other objects.

	11 What to do when injured at school.	P, I, U
	12 School and playground hazards and accidents.	P, I, U
Dramatization	13 Make puppets and dramatize safety practices at school.	P

TEACHING TECHNIQUES: SAFETY—cont'd

	SCHOOL SAFETY—cont'd	Grades
Dramatization—cont'd	**14** Dramatize safety precautions when playing softball, lining up in the cafeteria, waiting for the bus, and other situations.	P, I, U
Drawings	**15** Make drawings of play areas and equipment and place captions below about school safety.	P, I
Excursion	**16** Walk around the school and locate hazards to safety.	P, I
Exhibit	**17** Children prepare drawings on safety in school, such as keeping feet under tables and desks, not pulling chairs away from others, and the correct way to use the drinking fountain.	P, I
Experience chart or record	**18** Prepare an experience chart or record of safe practices in school.	P
Flannelboard	**19** Make two children out of construction paper (or make drawings) and call them "Safety Sam" and "Silly Billy." Tell a story about school safety including these two characters and use drawings to illustrate their activities.	P, I

Safety Sam:
Waits in line
Stops the swing and gets off
Uses pencils properly

Silly Billy:
Pushes in line
Jumps off the swing
Jabs pencils in his hand

Guest speaker	**20** Invite a physical education teacher or the supervisor of physical education to discuss and demonstrate safety on the playground.	P, I, U
Handbook	**21** A committee of pupils prepares an illustrated handbook of safe practices at school for distribution to all students.	I, U
Individual and group reports	**22** Pupils or pupil committees prepare articles on school safety for the school newspaper.	I, U
	23 Pupils prepare written reports on the causes of school injuries and ways to prevent them.	I, U
Interview	**24** A committee of pupils interviews the school nurse to find out how accidents occur in the school. After reporting their findings in class, they formulate a plan of prevention.	I, U
Map	**25** Prepare a composite map of the neighborhood indicating the location of the traffic lights, stop signs, police officers, and sidewalks. Have students draw the safest way home using colored crayons or yarn. Children may also prepare individual maps to be taken home to parents.	P, I
	26 Draw map of the school grounds and illustrate safe and unsafe places to play.	I, U
	27 Plot locations of hazardous areas on map of school and school grounds.	I, U

TEACHING TECHNIQUES: SAFETY—cont'd

	SCHOOL SAFETY—cont'd	**Grades**
Map—cont'd	28 Teacher prepares map of school showing drinking fountains, bicycle racks, incinerators, and other places. Place on bulletin board and have children mark the hazardous places in school and locate accidents that occur.	P, I
Panel	29 Have panel discussion on "Safety at school."	I, U
Problem solving	30 Discuss solutions to these safety problems:	P, I

A student runs from the cafeteria with an ice cream stick in his/her mouth.
Two groups talking in the corridor meet at a corner.
One student opens a door and bumps two students standing in the corridor.
A student throws his/her bat while playing in a softball game.
A student steps in front of another student who is using the swing.

	31 Form a school safety committee to locate hazardous school areas and plan ways to prevent accidents.	I, U
Questionnaire	32 Prepare a "Do you remember?" questionnaire as a concluding activity to the unit on school safety. Include 15 to 20 questions to be answered verbally by yes or no, such as, "Do I always walk down the halls and stairways properly?"	P, I
Songs and poems	33 Create songs, poems, stories, and drawings about school safety.	P
Survey	34 Children conduct a hazard hunt on school property and safely remove such objects as glass, rocks, wire, tacks, and nails.	P, I
	35 Children are "safety detectives" and locate examples of safety at school.	P, I
	36 Pupils prepare a safety checklist and then survey the school for hazards.	I, U

TEACHING TECHNIQUES

Tobacco

		Grades
Buzz group	**1** Conduct a buzz group discussion on the questions, "Why should people not use tobacco?" "How to say 'no'?"	U
Chart	**2** Pupils prepare charts for bulletin board displays regarding the rise in death rates of major diseases associated with tobacco; comparison of overall death rates of smokers and nonsmokers; location of disorders associated with smoking on an outline figure of the human body; and computation of the cost of smoking one to two packages of cigarettes a day or a week for 1 year and listing of other uses of the same amount of money.	I, U
Debate	**3** Have a debate on the use of tobacco. Try to answer the questions: "Should anyone chew tobacco or smoke? Should tobacco advertising in newspapers and magazines be controlled? How to say 'no'?"	U
Demonstration	**4** Prepare materials as shown in Fig. 12-23. Open and close pinch clamp (acts as siphon—water may need to be replaced several times) to stimulate puffing on cigarette and observe (a) smoke collecting, (b) color of water after shaking flask, and (c) residue on walls of flask. Later discuss relationships to lung tissue in persons who smoke. Place pieces of cotton in glass tube between cigarette and flask without stopping up tube. After smoking several cigarettes (use siphon action previously mentioned), remove cotton and examine. Wipe tar-stained cotton on growing plants and observe results (abnormal growths will appear).	I, U
	5 Blow cigarette smoke through a clean handkerchief or paper tissue with and without inhaling. Observe difference in amount of residue and relate to lung tissue.	I, U
	6 Prepare a smoking machine using materials shown in Fig. 12-24. Insert loosely packed cotton into the tubing and put a cigarette into the open end of tubing. Press firmly on the plastic container to force air out before lighting the cigarette and then proceed with slow and regular pumping action. Later, cotton can be withdrawn from tubing to show the accumulation of tar.	I, U
	7 Prepare a smoking machine using materials shown in Fig. 12-25. Light the cigarette and pump the vacuum so as to draw smoke from cigarette into gallon jar and water until the cigarette is burned completely. Use additional cigarettes until tars can be seen in the water and around the jar. Cotton can be inserted in tubing behind the cigarette and examined later for tars.	
Discussion	**8** The nature of tobacco smoke.	I, U
	9 The physiological effects of tobacco on the human body.	I, U
	10 The relationship of the use of tobacco to lung cancer.	I, U
	11 Analyze the claims of several tobacco advertisements.	I, U

TEACHING TECHNIQUES: TOBACCO—cont'd

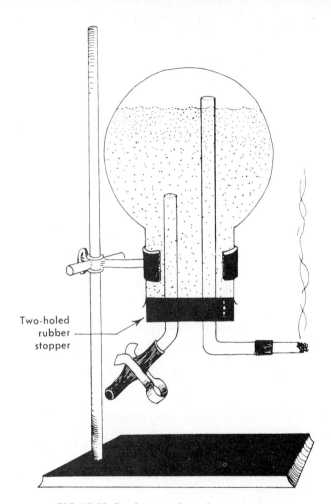

Two-holed
rubber
stopper

FIG. 12-23 Smoking machine demonstration.

			Grades
Discussion—	**12**	Why people smoke.	I, U
cont'd	**13**	Laws related to smoking.	I, U
Dramatization	**14**	Prepare a skit illustrating social pressures used by people to get others to smoke. Follow with a discussion regarding actions pupils should take to handle such situations.	U
Exhibit	**15**	Display magazines, pamphlets, and other materials for student reference and use.	I, U

TEACHING TECHNIQUES: TOBACCO—cont'd

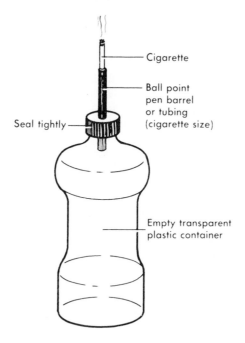

FIG. 12-24 Smoking machine demonstration.

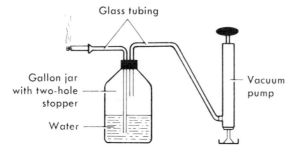

FIG. 12-25 Smoking machine demonstration.

			Grades
Exhibit—cont'd	**16**	Display newspaper and magazine articles on the use of tobacco.	I, U
	17	Display a variety of advertisements found in newspapers and magazines.	I, U
	18	Support the "Great American Smokeout."	I, U
	19	Display a variety of charts and graphs available from the American Cancer Society on the extent and effect of smoking.	U

TEACHING TECHNIQUES: TOBACCO—cont'd

		Grades
Exhibit—cont'd	20 Obtain samples of lungs of smoker and nonsmoker or photographs from the American Cancer Society.	I, U
Experiment	21 Obtain some nicotine and dissolve it in water in a fish bowl. Place a tadpole in the bowl and observe the results.	I, U
Graph	22 Pupils prepare graphs showing the incidence of heart disease, lung cancer, and emphysema among smokers and nonsmokers, as well as the costs of smoking cigarettes yearly.	U
Guest speaker	23 Invite a physician to discuss and answer questions about the effect of tobacco on health.	I, U
Individual and group reports	24 Pupils investigate the laws regarding the sale of tobacco to minors.	U
	25 Pupils prepare oral and written reports on recent magazine articles about tobacco.	I, U
	26 Pupils prepare oral and written reports on emphysema, chronic bronchitis, lung cancer, effectiveness of filter-tipped cigarettes, and number of cigarettes sold.	I, U
	27 Students prepare individual notebooks on tobacco and health, including analysis of advertising, magazine article summaries, research data, and pictures.	I, U
Interview	28 Interview the local health officer for information about the incidence of lung cancer in the community.	U
	29 A committee of children interviews one or more physicians about the effect of tobacco on health.	U
	30 Ask people who smoke and do not smoke for advice on their decision to smoke or not to smoke.	U
Newspaper	31 Prepare articles for the school newspaper as part of an antismoking or an antichewing campaign.	U
Parents	32 Involve parents in an antismoking campaign program with students writing letters against smoking, distributing pamphlets, or inviting them to see a film at school.	I, U
Self-test	33 Conduct a self-test on tobacco.	I, U

What do you know about smoking?

Circle the correct answers to the right. If you do not know the answer, circle the letter "D."

1. Smoking reduces the appetite.	T	F	D
2. Smoking irritates the throat.	T	F	D
3. Inhaling causes a smoker to absorb more nicotine.	T	F	D
4. Smoking may become a habit.	T	F	D
5. Teenagers often start smoking because they want to act like adults.	T	F	D
6. Some people smoke to relieve tension.	T	F	D
7. Smoke from tobacco may be annoying and unpleasant to other persons.	T	F	D

TEACHING TECHNIQUES: TOBACCO—cont'd

	What do you know about smoking? cont'd				**Grades**
Self-test—cont'd	8. Smoking can cause lung cancer.	T	F	D	
	9. Filter-tipped cigarettes prevent the absorption of nicotine into the body.	T	F	D	
	10. The use of tobacco causes a shortness of breath.	T	F	D	
Survey	**34** A committee of pupils conducts an opinion survey of parents, friends, doctors, coaches, and teachers on the use of tobacco by teenagers.				U
	35 Conduct a survey of the tobacco-using habits of pupils in the class. Have pupils post results on the bulletin board in the form of a bar graph.				U

SUMMARY

Methods and techniques of teaching health are important in the instruction program that seeks to develop health practices and attitudes based on scientific information. It is also important for the teacher to use a variety of methods because different approaches will appeal to the particular learning styles of different children. Teachers who are familiar with the variety of activities described in this chapter and are competent in the selection of appropriate activities and content can provide effective health education programs for their students.

Selecting and using good instructional aids for teaching health and evaluation outcomes are closely associated with methods and techniques. The next two chapters deal specifically with instructional aids and evaluation. Teachers should consider all three chapters in planning their programs. Many of the teaching ideas contained in this chapter are a composite of techniques and instructional aids and in some cases also could be used as evaluative techniques.

QUESTIONS FOR DISCUSSION

1. What is the role of the teacher in the learning process in health education?
2. What are the meanings of the terms *method* and *technique?*
3. What factors related to learning must receive teacher consideration?
4. What are the types of methods that contribute to effective health teaching and what are illustrations of each to health education?
5. What are the advantages and disadvantages of the various types of teaching methods that may be used in the health instruction program?
6. What guidelines help the teacher determine the methods of health teaching to be used in the primary, intermediate, and upper grades?
7. What is meant by the term *incidents* or *incidental teaching* in health education? Provide illustrations.
8. What are the limitations and possible problems in the use of incidents in health teaching?
9. How should the textbook be used when teaching health?
10. How can instructional materials be used effectively with methods in health teaching?
11. What are several ways students may be used in peer education programs?
12. What are the relationships between the objectives of health education and the techniques used in teaching?
13. What factors should receive consideration when selecting activities and experiences for health teaching?
14. Why is it important to use a variety of teaching methods when teaching health?
15. What are several activities or experiences suitable for health teaching in the primary, intermediate, and upper grades?
16. What are several health areas in which bulletin boards may be used in health teaching?
17. What are several demonstrations suitable for the primary, intermediate, and upper grades when teaching health?
18. In what grades are the use of buzz groups and self-tests probably most appropriate?
19. What are several experiments suitable for teaching fire safety, dental health, nutrition, and communicable disease control?
20. What are the strengths and weaknesses of cooperative learning?
21. What are some examples of the use of flannelboard in the health instruction program?
22. How can models, charts, and graphs be specifically used in the teaching of health?

SELECTED REFERENCES

Ames EE: Instructional planning for health education. In Cortese P, Middleton K, editors: *The comprehensive school health challenge*, vol 1, Santa Cruz, CA, 1994, ETR Associates.

Centers for Disease Control National AIDS Clearinghouse and National Pediatric HIV Resource Center: *Children and families and HIV/AIDS: educational materials*, Newark, NJ, 1994, National Pediatric HIV Resource Center.

Comprehensive Health Education Foundation: *Here's looking at AIDS and you,* Seattle, WA, 1989, The Foundation.

Cornacchia HJ, Barrett S: *Consumer health: a guide to intelligent decisions,* ed 5, St Louis, 1993, Mosby–Year Book.

Cornacchia HJ, Olsen LK, Nickerson CL: *Health in the elementary school,* ed 8, St Louis, 1991, Mosby–Year Book.

Cornacchia HJ, Smith DE, Bentel DJ: *Drugs in the classroom: a conceptual model for school programs,* ed 2, St Louis, 1978, Mosby–Year Book.

Costa AL, editor: *Developing minds: a resource book for teaching thinking,* Alexandria, VA, 1985, The Association for Supervision and Curriculum Development.

Fassler D, McQueen K: *What's a virus, anyway? The kids' book about AIDS,* Burlington, VT, 1990, Waterfront Books.

Frager AM: Toward improved instruction in hearing health at the elementary school level, *J School Health* 56(5):166-169, 1986.

Gilbert GG, Sawyer RG: *Health education: creating strategies for school and community health,* Boston, 1995, Jones and Bartlett.

Greenberg JS: *Health education: learner-centered instructional strategies,* ed 3, Dubuque, IA, 1995, W. C. Brown Communications.

Harmin M: Value clarity, high morality: let's go for both, *Educ Leadership* 45:(8):23-30, 1988.

Harvard Community Health Plan Foundation: *TLC game,* Wellesley, MA, 1990, Author.

Johnson DW, Johnson RJ: Toward a cooperative effort, *Educ Leadership* 46:(7):80-81, 1989.

Johnson DW, Johnson RJ, Holubec EJ, Roy P: *Circles of learning: cooperation in the classroom,* Alexandria, VA, 1984, The Association for Curriculum Development.

Moody LE, Laurent M: Promoting health through the use of storytelling, *Health Educ* 15(1):8-10, 12, 1984.

National Clearing House for Smoking and Health: *Smoking and health experiments, demonstrations and exhibits,* Washington, DC, 1968, US Department of Health, Education, and Welfare, Public Health Service.

Oklahoma Department of Health, AIDS Division: *Hey, do you know you can't get AIDS from . . . .* Oklahoma City, 1991, Author.

Pollock MB, Middleton K: *School health instruction,* ed 3, St Louis, 1994, Mosby–Year Book.

Sorochan WD, Bender SJ: *Teaching elementary health science,* ed 3, Boston, 1989, Jones and Bartlett.

Raths LE, Harmin M, Simon S: *Values and teaching,* ed 2, Columbus, OH, 1987, Charles E. Merrill.

Sarvela PD, Ritzel DO, Karaffa M, Naseri MK: Applications software packages in the school health program, *Health Educ* 20(3):43-49, 1989.

Seattle/King County Department of Public Health, AIDS Prevention Project: true stories (computer assisted instruction software), Seattle, 1990, Author.

Slavin RE: Cooperative learning and the cooperative school, *Educ Leadership* 45(3):7-13, 1987.

Steinhausen GW: Peer education programs: a look nationally, *Health Educ* 14(7):7-8, 10, 1983.

Talabere LR, Beyrer MK: Health education: perspectives in poetry, *Health Educ* 17(2):15-17, 1986.

Turner SB, Connor MJE: The Brooklyn Center, Minnesota, Student Health Fair: an impetus for learning, *J School Health* 54(9):9-11, 1984.

Wolff MA: According to whom? Helping students analyze contrasting views of reality, *Educ Leadership* 44:(2):36-41, 1986.

Quackenbush M, Villarreal S: *Does AIDS hurt? Educating young children about AIDS,* Santa Cruz, CA, 1992, ETR Associates.

Tasker M: *Jimmy and his family,* Bethesda, MD, 1992, Association for the Care of Children's Health.

Tasker M: *Jimmy and the eggs virus,* Newark, NJ, 1988, National Pediatric HIV Resource Center.

13

Instructional Aids for Health Teaching

KEY CONCEPT

Achievement of favorable health attitudes and health behaviors can be aided through the selection and use of appropriate instructional aids.

If the only tool you have is a hammer, you tend to see every problem as a nail.

ABRAHAM MASLOW

PROBLEMS TO SOLVE

As you prepare to embark on your career as a teacher, you realize that you will need to accumulate many of your own instructional aids for teaching health. Begin to collect instructional aids and prepare a written plan in which you indicate how you have organized the materials for easy storage and retrieval. Include in your plan the types of additional instructional aids you will include in your personal collection, where you will look for them, how you will create them, and how you will ensure that the materials you have or will collect and organize remain up to date.

THE quality and value of health instruction depends largely on the classroom teacher's effective use of appropiate methods, techniques, and strategies and the careful selection of the best available teaching aids. The teacher faces a challenging task in selecting and using instructional aids in health education.

Health instruction must be sensitive to diversity and to the latest and most reliable research and information from the broad spectrum of the biological, social, and physical sciences. Unlike some other areas of the elementary school curriculum, content and concepts in health and safety often change markedly and abruptly with new developments in medicine, public health, dentistry, nutrition, pharmacology, physiology, physical fitness, first aid and emergency care, and many other areas.

Therefore the classroom teacher—involved in a diverse range of subject matter areas—must keep abreast of the significant and applicable contributions of all those fields that bear on personal, family, and community health. To do this, the teacher needs to know where to locate scientifically accurate information and culturally diverse and appealing teaching aids.

Resources and instructional aids are what the teacher makes of them. The best materials may be of little value when used improperly or ineffectively. Before incorporating an instructional aid into classroom activities, the teacher must be familiar with the aid and know how it helps meet the needs of students, the objectives of the program, and the enhancement of the curriculum.

WHAT ARE INSTRUCTIONAL AIDS IN HEALTH EDUCATION?

Instructional aids are any materials or resources used to enhance pupil learning. They are meant to complement effective teaching. Everything in the pupils' environment that contributes in any degree to learning may be considered an aid. Defined in these broad terms, instructional aids include all items that teachers and pupils use, such as bulletin boards, cartoons, charts, pictures and photographs, maps, objects, specimens, models, posters, textbooks, workbooks, programmed instruction guides, newspaper and magazine articles, pamphlets, films, filmstrips, computer software, videotapes, tape recordings, phonograph records, songs, radio and TV programs, slides, transparencies, and exhibits. Pencils, paper, chalk, chalkboards, and so on are also in reality instructional aids, but they will not be discussed in this text.

Aids to learning are used for a variety of purposes, but in general they enhance instruction and serve as (1) sensory experiences that provide greater understanding of abstract thoughts and ideas making them concrete and specific and (2) as important motivational devices.

Bulletin boards are an effective way to present information using cartoons, charts, graphs, maps, posters, and other illustrative materials. Teachers should constantly be alert for potential bulletin board material relating to health and safety; it may appear in newspapers, magazines, pamphlets, and other printed materials. Students can actively participate in locating and preparing suitable material for the bulletin board.

Cartoons relating to a wide range of current problems in child health and safety can be produced by the students or selected from newspapers and magazines. Cartoons often provide the qualities of humor and relevance that can motivate pupils toward improved attitudes and behaviors (Fig. 13-1). Teachers should take care that the cartoon does not contain stereotypes and that the humor does not overshadow the message presented.

Charts, graphs, maps, posters, and *data* (Fig. 13-2) for these visual aids are readily available from numerous sources or can be prepared by students, teachers, or both. They should not be too involved or complicated; they should represent one or a few basic ideas or concepts that can be readily perceived and understood by pupils.

Objects, specimens, and *models* may be animate or inanimate. Hamsters may be used in classroom diet studies. On occasion children may bring a pet to class and talk about caring for its health and

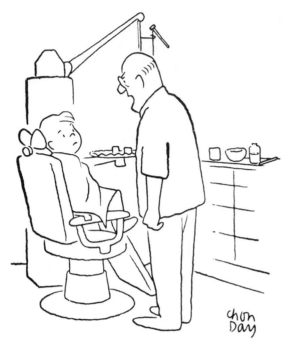

'I don't care if it does run up the light bill . . . brush them!'

FIG. 13-1 (Copyright 1969 by Consumers Union of United States, Inc., Mount Vernon, New York. Reprinted by permission from *Consumer Reports*, March 1969.)

safety. Specimens, such as lung tissue (smoker and nonsmoker) or animal organs, can provide realism in certain learning situations. Anatomic models— a torso, ear, eye, lung, heart, stomach, kidney, head, or brain—can help students better understand the remarkable interrelationships of body organs and systems in maintaining good health.

Textbooks are available and serve as basic reference sources for both pupil and teacher. These aids are discussed in greater detail later in this chapter.

Newspaper items, magazine articles, pamphlets, books, and *other printed material* (Figs. 13-3 and 13-4)—including popular paperbacks and reference books—offer good sources of information for the teacher and students in connection with research projects, class discussion, bulletin board material, and related assignments. Care should be taken to ensure that these sources are up to date and scientifically sound.

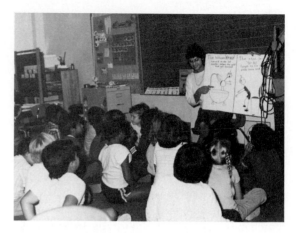

FIG. 13-2 Posters are a good teaching aid.

Poems are generally more effective with younger children. Even with children in the lower grades, the message should be clear and precise, not vague and trite.

Filmstrips, films, videotapes, transparencies, and *slides* are available in many topical areas. Most of these instructional aids are commercially produced, although pupils and teachers can prepare some of their own. See the section on student- and teacher-prepared instructional aids (p. 439) for additional details.

Tape recordings are generally available in two forms: cassette tapes and CDs. The cassette is by far the more popular and easier to handle for use in schools. Tapes are available with prepared audio, or they can be purchased blank. Prepared tapes often accompany some other material, such as a model or filmstrip. Student- and/or teacher-prepared tapes can add much excitement to health learning. Even young students can learn to make their own recordings using a cassette. In addition, the audio portions of radio and TV programs and films can be recorded for use in the classroom. Resource people can be interviewed using tape recordings for enrichment of classroom studies.

Music, phonographs, records, and *songs* appeal to children. Music can aid in relaxation, the lyrics of a catchy tune can assist in conveying health content, and songs can be a fun way of learning, par-

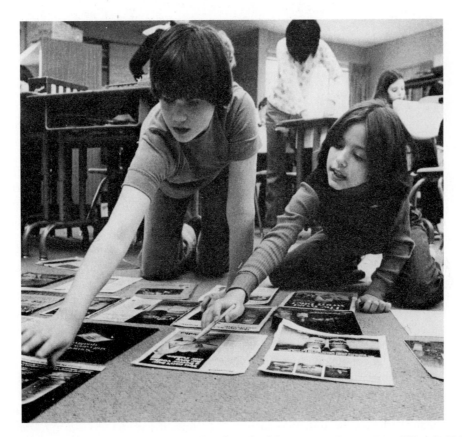

FIG. 13-3 Students use magazine materials to learn health concepts. (Courtesy Mary Wilbert Smith.)

ticularly if students develop their own health-related lyrics to known tunes.

TV and *radio,* both at school and in the home, offer many opportunities for timely and worthwhile health education. Specials on TV and radio often deal with the health and safety problems of children and adults. Problems are usually accurately presented and analyzed by the networks and many local stations. These two all-pervasive media also provide health news items and public service announcements, the latter usually bringing a message from an official or voluntary health agency or a professional society within the health professions.

Even commercials on TV and radio can be used as teaching aids. Students can discuss the questions of the validity and reality of commercials promoting products and services for weight reduction and skin problems, the nutritional value of foods, eye care, toy safety, alcoholic beverages, motor vehicles (including motor-driven cycles, all-terrain vehicles, snowmobiles, and jet skis), and other health-related topics.

Multimedia kits for teaching about specific health topics are now purchased and used by many schools. They generally contain all the material aids a teacher will need to teach some specific health concepts or content. A simple kit might include a set of filmstrips, a record or audiocassette, and a teacher's guide (e.g., American Red Cross text, "Community First Aid & Safety"). More complex kits also include video cassettes, puppets, games, worksheets, posters, and other "hands-on" items. Good kits are extremely helpful

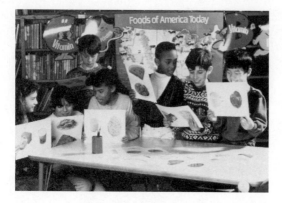

FIG. 13-4 Charts can aid in the study of nutrition. (Courtesy Michigan Department of Education.)

because all the materials needed to teach the unit are located in one place, which saves the teacher much valuable time. Multimedia kits may also be found in computer programs.

Exhibits may be the result of a pupil project or they may be bought, rented, or obtained free from commercial sources, health departments, voluntary health agencies, agricultural extension services, military organizations, and professional—educational, medical, dental, or nursing—societies. Exhibits should be timely and attractive, should offer a clear message, should be culturally diverse and sensitive, and should not be left on display too long. They may serve in three ways: (1) motivation of students, (2) peer education, and (3) parent education.

Computers were first introduced into the classroom in the 1960s and are now readily accepted as classroom teaching aids. Computer-assisted instruction (CAI) is an effective and efficient way to deliver basic factual health information. Computers are particularly useful for presenting a problem to a student as many times as necessary until the problem is solved. The computer also has promise as a tool for providing students with opportunities to use their factual knowledge in problem-solving situations. Another advantage of computer-based instruction is that it frees the teacher from lecturing to the entire class. This time can be used to work with smaller groups of stu-

dents to develop the skills, attitudes, and values that are important components of health education.

Computer-assisted instruction applications generally fall into one of five types. These types include drill and practice, tutorials, demonstrations and simulations, problem-solving applications, and instructional games.

- *Drill and practice:* Involve applications wherein the student is presented with a type of electronic flashcard; the student is presented with a problem, a response is elicited, feedback is provided, and a score is tabulated. These types of application are for relatively low-level learning, such as memorization of facts, terminology, or lists of materials.

- *Tutorials:* Involve somewhat higher level thinking since the student is prompted by the computer based on the responses given to the problems presented. This is quite similar to programmed instruction. Since students may provide different responses to different parts of the problem to be solved, the tutorial program uses a branching technique that allows the student to return to the prior question, request assistance, or review what has already been established. Often graphics or animations are included in tutorial programs.

- *Demonstrations and simulations:* Allow the student to try different approaches without danger to the individual. For example, if certain chemicals were to be mixed in a laboratory situation, an explosion could result. With a CAI application, the use of animation would demonstrate or simulate the explosion, and the student would learn what caused the simulated explosion. These applications require higher level thinking on the part of the student since he or she must remember what created the "problem" in the prior application and not make the same, or similar, mistake again.

- *Problem-solving applications:* Similar to tutorials in that they are generally based within one discipline. For example, if a student is trying to reduce his or her risk of disease, risk tables may be generated based on various decisions the student makes, given certain choices which are presented. This type of program allows the student to apply knowledge previously acquired to new situations, thus aiding in the transfer of learning.

- *Instructional games:* Usually are more than mere entertainment. There are specific rules and there are winners, but there is use of fantasy, drama, and competition. The competition may be against another student, against the computer, or against a character within the program itself. For example, there may be a type of game designed to identify the cause of a disease outbreak within a population, and two or more teams of epidemiologists try to track down the source of the deadly disease. The competition may be to identify the source of the disease and stop it before a total outbreak or just be the first to identify the source of the disease. Instructional games are similar to simulations, but the concept of competition against the computer, the clock, other students, or oneself provides added motivation and entertainment, thus enhancing the learning situation.

With over 2000 new programs being added to the list of more than 12,000 educational software programs currently available, the teacher is faced with a dilemma. The problem is that most of these programs were developed for profit, not for a specific educational purpose. As of 1992, the Association for Supervision and Curriculum Development indicated that only about 136 of the computer-based educational programs available at that time were considered "Only the Best."* Previously, Dorman† had indicated that only about 5% of the programs that were developed each year

could be rated as exemplary. With all of this in mind, how should the teacher evaluate the suitability of computer software? There are many things that must be considered when selecting software. Some of these considerations are applicability to the lesson or unit, program content, hardware compatibility, ease of use by students and teachers, cost, availability of technical support, including instructional manuals, and the amount of time it takes to complete the program. Before the actual purchase of software, the teacher should be familiar with its purpose and applications in the classroom. A guide for the evaluation of computer software programs may be found in Appendix M although considerations for the evaluation of any instructional material, presented in Appendix H should also be considered.

An example of a health-related computer program available is "Grab a Byte," a computer program in nutrition for grades 6, 7, and 8, produced by the Washington State Dairy Council and the Seattle Pacific Science Center. There are three separate programs within this packet:

- *Restaurant:* Students enter their own height, weight, and age into the computer. From an accompanying menu they then choose a variety of foods to create a meal. The computer responds by displaying the nutritional value of the chosen meal based on calories, proteins, vitamins, and so on.
- *Grab a Grape:* Students choose from six nutritional categories to be quizzed at three levels of difficulty. Categories include food facts, weight management, and food and sports, among others.
- *Nutrition Sleuth:* The student becomes "Inspector Good Diet" and is given a clue to solve a nutrition mystery. An incorrect response results in a new clue. The score is displayed as each new nutrition concept is presented.

A major problem with computers in the classroom is nonstandardized equipment. A package programmed for use with certain computer brands often cannot directly be used with others. Teachers must be alert to this problem and select

---

*Association for Supervision and Curriculum Development: *Only the Best,* Reston, VA, 1993, The Association.
†Dorman SM: Evaluating computer software for the health education classroom, *J School Health* 62(1):36, 1992.

software that is compatible with the hardware available within the school. Recent increases in the amount of software available for all major computer systems plus greater compatibility, accompanied by improvement in quality and content, has alleviated the problem.

The computer possibilities for innovative health teaching that will motivate students is extremely exciting. However, since recent research indicates that, when left on their own, boys tend to use computers more often than girls in the school setting, teachers must be alert to scheduling equal computer time for all of the students.

Videodiscs represent perhaps the most recent technology that can be used in the classroom. These discs, although somewhat limited in content at present, represent an interactive mode of learning for the students. If the school has the availability of a videodisc player, videodiscs provide an additional aid that can be used in the classroom. A major advantage of the videodisc is its interactive mode. The student can quickly move from sector to sector within the disc to secure information, which makes the videodisc more facile than videotapes wherein the tape must

be fast forwarded or rewound to specific sections within the tape. At present, videodisc equipment is rather expensive, but, as with computers, the cost most likely will decrease in the future. Evaluation of videodiscs should be based on the same premise as computer software programs (see Appendix M).

HOW SHOULD INSTRUCTIONAL AIDS BE USED?

Teachers should give consideration to certain basic procedures when they use instructional aids if they are to obtain the best results. The following factors must receive consideration: (1) selection of proper aids that meet instructional objectives and enhance instruction, (2) availability of the items, (3) adequate preparation for use, and (4) evaluation (Fig. 13-5).

Guiding Principles

The following suggestions will help guide the teacher in the proper use of instructional aids:

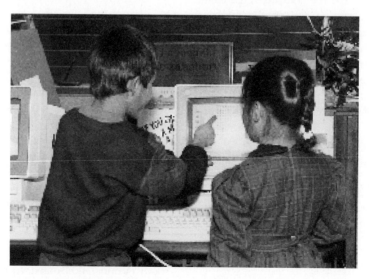

FIG. 13-5 Instructional aids, such as computers, add to learning centers. (Courtesy Austin Independent School District, Austin, Texas.)

- The teacher must clearly know how a particular learning aid fits into a specific situation. Is it relevant to what's being taught? Does it meet the needs of students? Can it be evaluated in terms of its contribution to student learning? Instructional aids should supplement teaching and should be incorporated into the lesson with a proper introduction. They are not meant to do the teaching for the teacher. They should be used to provide greater meaning to the lesson.
- All instructional materials should be previewed by the teacher before use in class. Not previewing materials could result in major problems for the teacher as well as the school.
- Teachers should have aids readily accessible when the lesson starts. If the material is a handout, sufficient copies for all students should be available. It is disconcerting for a class to have to wait for the teacher to locate materials that have been misplaced. When this occurs, continuity and interest in the lesson are often lost.
- If a number of different instructional aids are to be used, it may be advisable to use them one at a time in sequence. More than one item can be displayed at a time when it is necessary to show relationships with graphs or charts. When used in a logical sequence, instructional aids should complement each other.
- Evaluation should take place each time instructional aids are used. Evaluation need not be a cumbersome process. Teacher observations of pupil attention, interest, opinions, and other subjective feedback are often adequate ways of obtaining clues to the effectiveness of a particular learning aid. Questions can be asked to ascertain if students understand the main points represented, if the aids help clarify the relationships to material already introduced, and if the aids help achieve the objectives of the lesson.

Selection of Instructional Aids

The variety of materials in health instruction and the many uses for these materials require careful selection by the teacher. Each type of aid has a particular function; that is, each aid usually can be used to the best advantage with some particular type of presentation. Some examples of this are:

- If an object or its parts are to be named, selected, or manipulated, have the object or a model of it for students to view and use; objects can include items such as actual food, food containers, animal organs, microscopes and slides, bicycles, seat belts, stethoscopes, and sphygmomanometers.
- If an object is inaccessible, perhaps it can be adequately represented by still pictures. A series of still pictures can capture an event. They can be used in station work or on bulletin boards for students to work with in small groups or independently.
- Films, videotapes, computer software, and videodiscs are appropriate when motion and time-space relationships are important, such as when learning about the circulatory and other body systems, environmental concepts, and consumer health issues. These aids are also effective in depicting social interaction and behavioral concepts.

Another important point in the proper selection of any audiovisual aid is its suitability and appropriateness for the age, maturity, ethnicity, family and community background, and experience of the children with whom it is to be used. A teaching aid is most valuable when it meets these criteria. Consequently, if an aid is unsuited to the level of maturity, background, experience, interest, or needs of a particular group, it cannot provide the maximum impact. If an aid is too advanced or difficult for the group, it may be frustrating. If it is below the maturity level of a group, it may stifle interest. Care must also be taken to ensure that the aid is culturally diverse and does not enhance stereotyping of gender roles or ethnicity.

Availability of Instructional Aids

Teachers must plan well in advance of the need for instructional aids to ensure their availability at the time needed. It may take 6 to 8 weeks or longer to reserve films, cassettes, books, or other audiovisual materials from the health resource center, building library, local community health agency, or other source. Planning generally ensures the availability of the desired teaching aids and allows time for preview and examination before classroom use. In addition, should teachers find an item cannot be obtained on the desired date or dates, they have sufficient time to change their teaching schedule, locate substitute materials, or prepare teacher-made aids. Even with good planning, situations will arise wherein the aid does not arrive as planned. Teachers should always have a contingency plan in the event this occurs.

Preparation for Use of Instructional Aids

Adequate preparation by both the teacher and the pupils is necessary for instructional aids to be used effectively. One undesirable tendency in the use of instructional aids is to use them without attempting to ensure that the pupils derive the greatest benefit from their use. An aid should not be used simply because it is available or because the teacher "wants a break." Films and TV have often been used more for entertainment than for their contribution to learning. This does not mean that aids should not be entertaining. It does mean that aids cannot be justified in health education solely on the basis of entertainment value.

With some visual aids (motion pictures, videotapes, slides, and filmstrips), lesson plans and teachers' guides are supplied. In most cases, however, it is necessary for teachers to adapt these lessons or guides based on their knowledge of the students' needs.

Proper preparation by both teacher and pupils helps avoid passive receptivity on the part of the children. The teacher should clearly explain to the students the learning objectives to be derived from using material aids. Thus the learners know what is expected of them, what to examine the

material for, and how the experience relates to their study.

A preplanned question-and-answer period should follow the use of most material aids. This can be done orally or in writing, individually or in groups, and can be led by either the teacher or student(s). Questions similar to the following can help the teacher assess student understanding and perceptions. "What were some of the important things you learned from this videotape?" "How do you think the young girl felt when her dog died?" "How do you think the young boy felt when he learned his family was moving to the city?" "If you were going to make a videotape about this topic, what would you do differently?" "Were there things you didn't understand about the film?" "What were they?"

An important teaching technique is to use the material more than once. For example, a videotape might be introduced and shown to the students. Following a discussion in which students articulate what they observed, heard, and learned, the same film is shown again. Before the second viewing the teacher can suggest certain key points students should look and listen for to clarify discrepancies expressed during the discussion and alert them to detect significant facts that were apparently missed or misunderstood during the first viewing. The second viewing should also be followed by a question-and-answer session or assignment. Also, even during a first showing, a videotape can be paused and an important concept discussed. This is another reason previewing is important; the teacher will know when salient concepts are being introduced and can plan discussions accordingly.

Effective use of instructional aids can improve learning, but aids should not limit the degree of creativity and ingenuity of the teacher or limit student interaction.

Evaluation of Instructional Aids

Instructional aids in health education need to be evaluated to determine (1) their value in the educational process, (2) their contribution to the achievement of instructional goals, and (3) their freedom from racial, ethnic, or gender stereotyping.

Objective evaluation of instructional aids is difficult for the classroom teacher because assessments are complex and time consuming, and reliable and valid instruments are not available. However, subjective measurements can serve as indicators of the value of the aids being used. The following are suggestions for general questions to be asked to determine the effectiveness of instructional aids:

- How well do the materials used contribute to the students' achievement of the objectives?
- Are the materials appealing to the students as evidenced by class interest and attention?
- What changes in the materials are needed to make them more appealing to students and to more effectively achieve the instructional objectives?
- Are arrangements for the use of the materials convenient?
- Is the content accurate?
- Are the materials suitable for grade level, maturity, and experience of students?
- Are there sexual, racial, or other biases in the material?
- Is the material culturally diverse?
- Are the costs reasonable?
- What is the value of the material in terms of effort and time in preparation and expense?

In some cases, the answers to these questions will be all the teacher needs to decide whether or not to use a particular material aid. Other situations may require a more extensive evaluation. Samples of specific evaluation forms for a variety of learning materials including textbooks, films, resource speakers, and others are provided in Chapter 14 and Appendices H and M.

WHERE CAN TEACHERS FIND INSTRUCTIONAL AIDS?

Instructional aids for teaching health may be found within the school building or district, county or regional educational entities including colleges and universities, and organizations outside the school. In schools, the sources include textbooks, libraries/learning resource centers, and individuals. Outside of schools, material may be obtained from health film centers, professional journals, popular magazines, state departments, the federal government, state and national organizations, clearinghouses, professional organizations, various health agencies, and commercial businesses.

Materials Found within the School

School textbooks. Textbooks on health and safety are available for all grade levels in the schools. Many teachers, at some time in their careers, will be confronted with having to make a textbook selection. Several commercial publishers offer series of textbooks that range from grades K-8. Numerous school districts and 22 states* have approved textbook adoption lists that include one or more of the health series to encourage systematic progression of learning, beginning with the primary grades and progressing through the upper elementary grades.

Although the quality of elementary school health textbooks has improved greatly, textbooks still have obvious limitations. First, it is impossible for authors and publishers to keep the contents up to date because of the lag between writing, publishing, and delivering a textbook. The amount of health research and information generated annually is staggering, and it is impossible to incorporate this knowledge into the textbook publishing process in a timely manner.

Second, textbook publishers must give major consideration to including only topics that will be acceptable to screening committees in populous states with statewide textbook adoption lists. Thus topics that might be of great interest to students may be downplayed or omitted for eco-

---

*Mahoney BS, Olsen LK, editors: Statewide textbook adoption. In *Health education: a practical guide for K-12 health education*, Millwood, NY, 1993, Kraus International Publications, pp 301-316.

nomic reasons. Some publishers now offer supplemental booklets on topics considered important but too controversial to include in the text itself.

Finally, the readability of the text will probably be too easy for some students and too difficult for others in the same classroom. Thus some learners may be bored while others are frustrated.

Given these limitations, textbooks can still be a valuable aid in teaching health. They contain much good information in a concise, well-ordered form. Generally, they have been carefully reviewed for accuracy of content, as well as grade-level appropriateness. A good text can serve as the base for an enriched exploration of health topics, but it should be supplemented by appropriate aids as discussed in this chapter. In addition, it can provide an inexperienced teacher of health education with a secure starting point.

There are five major advantages to using a good health textbook:

- It gives an accurate presentation of essential facts.
- It presents an orderly and comprehensible arrangement of the material.
- It furnishes a common core of content for the class.
- It contains such teaching and learning aids as references, questions, summaries, reviews, exercises, pictures, maps, and diagrams.
- It saves time.

Textbook series for elementary schools. The textbook series are generally accompanied by a teacher's manual either bound with the text or as a separate booklet. Some publishers provide free or inexpensive materials for health education, including charts that outline the concepts to be taught at the various grade levels.

Health and safety textbooks for elementary schools can be obtained from the following sources:

- **Scott, Foresman & Co.**
  1900 E. Lake Avenue
  Glenview, IL 60025
  (708) 729-3000
  (800) 554-4411
  Health for Life—K through 8   Copyright 1992

- **Glencoe/McGraw Hill, Inc.**
  936 Eastwind Drive
  Westerville, OH 43081
  (614) 890-1111
  (800) 442-9685
  Health: Focus on You—K through 8   Copyright 1993
  Teen Health—6 through 8   Copyright 1993

- **Harcourt Brace and Company**
  6277 Sea Harbor Drive
  Orlando, FL 32887
  (800) 225-5425
  Being Healthy—K through 8   Copyright 1994

Textbooks frequently contain out-of-date information. An alternative worthy of consideration is the "Great Body Shop" that is available from the Children's Health Market. This is a subscription type program that provides students with take-home materials at a cost of $5 per student per year.

Libraries and learning resource centers. The school library is an excellent first place to look for good teaching aids other than textbooks. In many schools, libraries also serve as learning resource centers where a variety of teaching aids such as filmstrips, flat pictures, small kits, and other materials may be found. In some districts, a separate audiovisual center has been established that may contain instructional health materials. Teachers should develop a close working relationship with the librarians and learning resource center staff.

Fiction and nonfiction books relating to numerous pertinent health topics can be found in the school library. Such books provide a meaningful and appropriate medium for integrating health learning with reading skills. A limited list of health-related library books, categorized by subject area with appropriate grade levels, is found in Appendix D. Annotations are included to illustrate the possibilities of expanding and individualizing the health instruction program through the use of library books.

Encyclopedias and *almanacs* offer an interesting variety of health information that can serve as a valuable resource for integrating and correlating health studies with language skills, mathematics, and research. A sampling of topics contained in these reference materials includes census data, U.S. health expenditures, statistics about the disabled, health costs per capita, information about heart disease including warning signs and risk factors, cardiovascular disease statistical summaries (charts and graphs), suicide rates, and data on fires, accidents, agriculture, air pollution, first aid, nutrition, and many other subjects. Also, most almanacs have a chronology of the year's events, which includes many health-related items. Reference books like these can be valuable, quick, and easy sources of information for students and teachers.

Newspapers often carry special articles by health authorities and science writers and often include daily news items about health and safety. The content is generally accurate but may at times be sensationalized. Newspaper articles can provide current information for bulletin board displays and help pupils develop the ability to critically analyze material.

A major advantage of using the various current materials in health education is that, from an early age, children may be taught to become discriminating and careful in their evaluation of reports that may be sensational, unsubstantiated, or inadequately documented.

Individuals. The *school nurse* can be an invaluable help in locating good teaching aids. Most school nurses are extremely interested in health education and willing to assist the classroom teacher in a supportive and competent manner.

Building principals, district health coordinators, and *curriculum generalists* are additional resource people the teacher can consult to locate appropriate sources of instructional material. Many building principals will also help the teacher find ways to offset the cost of health materials.

One should also check with *other teachers* in the building or district who conduct classes at the same grade level. Most teachers are willing to share not only materials and sources but also teaching/learning activities and teaching ideas.

Materials Located Outside the School Environment

Health film centers. There are many films, videotapes, slide sets, and filmstrips available from a variety of sources outside the school setting. No attempt has been made in this section to identify specific audiovisual aids by title, description, or grade level because distributors continually withdraw old offerings and add new ones to keep lists current. The following list provides the major central sources of these teaching aids. Teachers should check local units for assistance.

- *College and university film libraries* generally have good health and safety films and videotapes and may carry videodiscs. Check with the film librarian or the library nearest to you.
- *Departments of health* at city, county, or state levels usually maintain a health film library. Many of these relate to the health problems of elementary students. Write or call your local or state department of health for a film catalog.
- *Voluntary health agencies* produce and distribute excellent films, videotapes, slide series, and filmstrips. These aids usually deal with those health problems or diseases with which the agency is mainly concerned. Consult your local telephone directory or that of the major city in your state for information about the locations of the leading voluntary agencies. Write or call for a film catalog.
- *Commercial organizations and firms* prepare, distribute, or rent films dealing with health and safety. They also provide catalogs of health films that may be found in the school library or may be obtained by writing directly to the organization. Some organizations such as Blockbuster Video have a selection of videotapes they make available at no charge for use by schools.
- *State departments of education* may maintain a film library. However, as their interest is in both elementary and secondary schools, it is important to check carefully to determine the grade level for which a particular film is designed.

In addition to these centralized general sources, there are many commercial film and videotape distributors. Building librarians and learning resource specialists receive catalogs and other descriptive pamphlets from distributors and producers on a regular basis. Often, films, videotapes, slide sets, and filmstrips can either be rented or purchased.

Professional journals. Health education professional journals (Fig. 13-6) found in many school, college, university, and public libraries, are another source of information about teaching aids. Note that some of the information about aids in these journals is carried in paid advertisements, whereas other aids are examined by authorities and appear in the materials review sections. Professional journals contain many reports and studies of value in the instruction program. They also include information about children's health problems, as well as current content information. Some of these journals include the following:

The Journal of Health Education
The Journal of School Health
Journal of Nutrition Education
American Journal of Public Health
New England Journal of Medicine
Journal of the American Medical Association
Science
Health Values

Scientific American
FDA Consumer
Consumer Reports

Popular magazines. Popular magazines often provide well-written, authoritative articles on new developments in health. These articles must be carefully evaluated for scientific accuracy.

State departments. Local, county, and state health departments often have education sections staffed by individuals willing to help classroom teachers obtain good materials. State departments of education and the state library system may also be contacted for sources of information. The teacher is advised to be specific in making requests.

Federal government. The federal government is a valuable source of free or inexpensive materials. Some telephone directories contain information about federal bookstores and specific regional federal offices. Assistance in obtaining federal publications can usually be obtained from the home office of one's senator/representative. Inquiries and orders can also be made directly by writing the Superintendent of Documents, U.S. Government Printing Office, Washington, D.C., 20402.

State and national organizations. Many national public and private organizations with health improvement goals provide suitable materials for teacher and student use. In some instances the national organizations have state or lo-

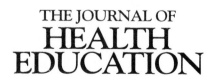
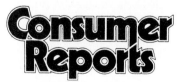

FIG. 13-6 Health source journals.

cal affiliates, such as The American Heart Association, The American Cancer Society, and the March of Dimes Birth Defects Foundation. When a teacher is aware of a state or local affiliate, all requests for material should first be sent to that unit. A list of some of the national organizations that provide free and low-cost health education material is contained in Appendix E.

Clearinghouses. The growth of interest in health is reflected in the number of clearinghouses providing information related to various health topics. A listing of the various clearinghouses is contained in Appendix F.

TEACHER- AND STUDENT-PREPARED INSTRUCTIONAL AIDS

Technological advances have opened the doors for teachers to develop their creativity even further and instill new excitement and meaning into their health instruction programs. Audio and video cassette players, classroom computers, 35-mm and Polaroid cameras, and camcorders are some of the equipment that teachers and pupils can easily operate. This equipment also provides an opportunity for cross-grade teaching with older students working on productions with younger students.

Videotapes and films. Having students role play saying no when offered an alcoholic beverage is a fairly common classroom activity. Recording the role playing on film or videotape brings a whole new dimension to the learning process. Often when students role play in front of the class, they are nervous and do not recall what happened. What they say and do cannot be reflected upon or recalled. Use of a recorder enables pupils to see and hear how they responded. It provides an excellent opportunity to discuss the experience with the pupils, analyze what actually occurred, and explore other effective options.

Pedestrian, bicycle, and motor vehicle passenger safety practices and procedures are often discussed in elementary health lessons. A teacher- or student-made video cassette of actual safety hazards and positive preventive actions in the students' school and community environments can add realism and new meaning to the study.

Films can now be made with relative ease and minimal cost because of technologic advances in the equipment and processing of super 8-mm film and videotape equipment. This provides an opportunity for the elementary school health teacher to develop and maintain an inexpensive film library related specifically to the health curriculum.

Some suggestions for teacher and student films and videotapes include the following:
- Identify the purpose and the objective of the film.
- Limit subject matter to one major idea or concept or a few closely related concepts. The focus should be on the major purpose of the lesson.
- Involve subject matter or techniques that cannot be covered in the normal classroom setting in other ways.
- Develop a storyboard before filming to ensure a logical sequence of action.
- Confine the length of the film to 4 to 6 minutes, although the actual presentation of the film might take longer if the teacher elects to make selective stops during viewing for special emphasis.

Videotaping has many advantages over filming and as most schools have access to the equipment, teachers should be encouraged to use it for enhancing learning in health. Although the following pointers relate specifically to videotaping, many of them are also useful when using 8-mm film.

The video cassette recorder, camera, and monitor are relatively easy pieces of equipment to use, and they are invaluable for providing students fairly immediate feedback of their performance or production. When using this equipment, one should keep in mind the following tips.*

---

*Modified from *Here's looking at you 2000—teacher's guide*, Seattle, 1986, The Comprehensive Health Education Foundation.

- *Know the equipment.* Take time beforehand to become familiar with all of the equipment. Do not waste valuable time during class trying to figure out the various functions of the machinery.
- *Let students adapt.* Have the camera and monitor on when students enter the room. In this way the students can get through the initial shyness, curiosity, and playfulness and be prepared to role play in front of the camera later in the lesson.
- *Do not backlight.* Students will not show up on film well with backlighting, so try to set up the camera with light coming in from the front or side, rather than from a window behind the students.
- *Tape only after practice.* The idea behind videotaping is to make the students look good and enable them to see themselves looking good. Therefore tape only after the student is able to respond appropriately to your cues. It may be that at first a student can master only a memorized sentence, (for example, "What are we going to do there?") rather than an entire sequence of responses. Videotape that sentence and let the student see a successful, albeit limited, performance. Also, shut the monitor off when taping. Watching themselves being taped can prove distracting to students.
- *Play back only successful tapes.* Do not play back mistakes. The class's amusement may be a student's embarrassment.
- *Start with the camera far away, then move in gradually.* The videotape process may intimidate a student, so be as unobtrusive as possible. You can move closer after the class begins to disregard the camera.
- *Keep the camera on target.* There will be times when a student will stand from a sitting position or move from a standing position (for example, when the response calls for the student to leave the situation). Follow the student's face with the camera. Do not get caught focusing on an empty chair or a student's knees.
- *Tape shy students from the side.* There may be some students who cannot get accustomed to the camera; film these students from the side. Similarly, there may be students who positively do not want the class to see them on camera. Approach these students as the class is letting out and offer to show them the tape privately. Use extra reinforcement (for example, [student's name], I think you'll be surprised at how good you look. Why don't you let me show you?).
- *Be mobile.* See if you can obtain a portapack or equipment that will allow you to tape in locations other than the classroom (for example, hallways, playground). Not only will students enjoy the activity more, but they will be more able to transfer learning to situations approximating "real life."

Photographs, pictures, and slides. Photographs, flat pictures (Fig. 13-7), and slides are among the least expensive instructional materials that can be created. Quality pictures can help learning be more interesting and effective. An appropriately selected picture will help a student (1) view more clearly a complex relationship, (2) recall a concrete or specific situation, (3) grasp the appearance of a reality, (4) easily understand an important concept, and (5) come up with questions that will often lead far beyond the immediate purpose of the photographs.

Whether photographs contribute to learning depends on how the teacher structures the learning situation. As in reading, pupils need to have their attention directed to things they can expect to find in photographs. Students must be helped to see rather than merely to look. Carefully planned questions such as the following must be prepared by the teacher: "What do you see in this picture?" "What is the baby trying to reach?" "Is this a safe place to be?" "What do you see that makes you think it is safe?" and "What do you see that makes you think this person is lost?"

The teacher is also responsible for structuring the situation to ensure the attainment of specific outcomes. It is possible to use photographs and get responses ranging from a simple recitation of

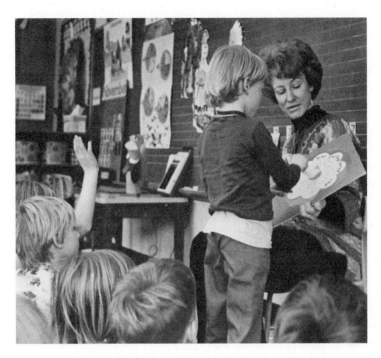

FIG. 13-7 Identification of emotions using "Feelings Wheel." (Courtesy Mary Wilbert Smith.)

facts to complex and creative thinking. Photographs can be mounted on bulletin boards with names or written descriptions covered by flaps of paper. After a student identifies the picture, he/she lifts the flap to check the answer. Students can identify pictures they have not seen before that illustrate the idea or concept under study. They can describe what they see in the photograph along with the application of their own creative thoughts about the concept.

A "home-made" slide presentation with teacher or student narrative is another creative alternative to the presentation of this information.

Teacher-created slides and other materials can be used in testing. A hazardous situation depicted on the screen can be the focus for the questions, "What problems do you see?" "What would you do in this situation?" and "If you saw a younger child here what would you do or what would you tell him or her?"

Flat pictures can either be held up for the entire class to see or mounted on a bulletin board for viewing individually and at greater length by students. They can be placed at a specific class station where students are asked to arrange them in a logical order to show cause-and-effect relationships or changes in sequence. Pictures dealing with the specific topics can be mixed with irrelevant pictures, and students can be challenged to select the pertinent pictures (see Fig. 13-3).

Students may be asked to list appropriate questions about a picture or series of pictures. Photographs can also be used to test students' understanding of relationships and major concepts.

These questions can serve in the selection of photographs appropriate for specific classroom instruction:

- Is the photograph clear and forceful?
- Is the detail clear and large enough for study?
- Is the photograph interesting?
- Does the photograph direct attention to the most significant facts rather than to unimportant details?

- Does the photograph cover information that the students need?

Filmstrips. A filmstrip can be made without expensive photographic equipment from a roll of 35-mm clear movie leader and magic markers or a variety of colored, felt-tipped pens. The leader usually comes in 50-foot rolls and can be purchased at a nominal cost from most photography equipment stores.

A story line, theme, or sequence of events should be developed before the preparation of the filmstrip. Students can then draw or write directly on the leader with the colored markers. Each picture should be about 1 inch by 1 inch in size. A commercially made filmstrip should be available for comparison to ensure that all characters are drawn in the proper direction. (The tops and bottoms of each picture should be adjacent to each other.) The finished product can be shown using a regular 35-mm filmstrip projector.

Puppets. Puppets are excellent teaching aids. There are many types of puppets that children and teachers can make out of inexpensive materials and odds and ends. Paper bag puppets and hand puppets made from old stockings with buttons, yarn, and felt sewn for eyes, mouth, nose, and hair are among the various kinds.

Puppets do not have to be elaborately made for children to enjoy using and identifying with them. With skillful guidance by the teacher, puppets can be used to help students resolve many situations and problems on the playground, deal with feelings of rejection, learn about ways to treat others, deal with someone who cheats or bullies, learn how to say no to pressure from other children, and learn positive ways to express feelings.

SELECTED PROBLEMS WITH INSTRUCTIONAL AIDS
Eliminating Bias in the Selection and Use of Instructional Aids

For years little attention was paid to the hidden messages in many educational materials. Most prominent among these were messages of sexism, ageism, and racism. Although the reasons are complex, girls were generally portrayed as passive and complacent and boys as assertive and adventuresome. Boys became physicians, fire fighters, scientists, and police officers, whereas girls became nurses and mothers. With rare exceptions, senior citizens, African-Americans, Native Americans, Asians, Latinos, Hispanics, and those of other cultures and races either did not exist in these materials or were presented in demeaning ways.

Because of a raised consciousness of these matters, there is no longer any need to tolerate the use of biased materials by any teacher except in a study of bias. The following criteria are listed as illustrative of the kind of considerations the teacher should use to detect bias when reviewing material aids for health instruction.*

- *Check the illustrations.*
    - Look for stereotypes.
    - Look for tokenism.
    - Who's doing what?
- *Check the storyline.*
    - What is the main message?
    - Are one group's standards projected as the ideal?
    - How are problems presented and resolved?
    - Could the story be told if the sex roles were reversed?
- *Examine the lifestyles presented.*
    - Are negative value judgments implied?
    - Do the lifestyles reflect reality?
- *Examine the relationships between people.*
    - Who has the power?
    - Who is portrayed in supporting, subservient roles?
    - How are family relationships depicted?
- *Note the "heroes."*
    - Whose interest is a particular hero really serving?

---

*Modified from *Guidelines for selecting bias-free textbooks and storybooks*, New York, (undated), Council on Interracial Books for Children.

- *Consider the effects on a child's self-image.*
    Are norms established that limit any child's aspirations or self-concept?

    Does the material reinforce or counteract positive associations with the color white and negative associations with the color black?

    Who performs all the brave and heroic deeds?
- *Watch for loaded words.*
    Are there words or phrases that have offensive overtones?

    The generic use of the word *man* was accepted in the past; its use in this way today is outmoded.

Determining Readability of Written Materials

The reading level of a written material indicates the approximate *reading grade level* a student must have attained to be able to read the material successfully. Reading level is an important factor in determining whether written materials are appropriate for the grade levels at which they may be introduced. Within any given elementary school classroom, the wide variance in student reading ability results in pupils being assigned to reading groups according to their skill. Reading specialists sometimes help with this, but the good teacher is able to analyze printed health education materials to determine those items appropriate for students' reading ability in groups or individually.

There are several systems used for determining the readability level of written materials. The Fry Readability Formula (Fig. 13-8, pp. 444-445) is one of the most widely used instruments for measuring readability. Although readability scores arrived at through any procedures must be considered approximations, they are a great asset in analyzing pamphlets, magazine articles, texts, and other written materials.

Factors other than readability level should also be considered by teachers when selecting reading material for students. The appeal of the format and student interest in the topic are major determinants as to whether students will read material. The teacher should also consider nonverbal qualities, such as the use of space, graphs, illustrations, and color when selecting reading material.

Preparing Materials for Students with Low-Level Literacy Skills

Low-level literacy is found in every walk of life, among all races, and at all socioeconomic strata. With few exceptions, it is also found in most elementary school classrooms. Students with low-level literacy skills need special attention and carefully selected or prepared instructional materials.

It is beyond the scope of this text to deal with all the knowledge needed to teach students with low-level literacy skills. However, several basic written and audio materials for students who lack average skills are discussed in this section.

Written materials. Frequently the teacher will have written material that contains the information needed for instruction, but the material may be too difficult for some students to understand. This material should be used as a starting point for preparing a simplified version.

First, decide on the student behavior desired. Identify the information in the original material that is essential to achieve the desired outcome. Organize this information into topics in the sequence needed by students to use the information. Use advance organizers (headings or other clues to alert the readers as to what is coming and to focus them on the intended message). Make the first sentence of each paragraph the topic sentence, and whenever possible make the first word(s) in that sentence the topic (e.g., TV commercials about food can fool you). Be consistent with words (e.g., interchanging "diet" with "meal" may be confusing to these students).

Audiotapes. Audiotaped instruction is especially important for students with low-level literacy skills. However, audiotapes also have literacy levels. The oral language decoding process is similar to that of print decoding in reading. Therefore, professionally prepared English language audio-

GRAPH FOR ESTIMATING READABILITY — EXTENDED

by Edward Fry, Rutgers University Reading Center, New Brunswick, N.J. 08904

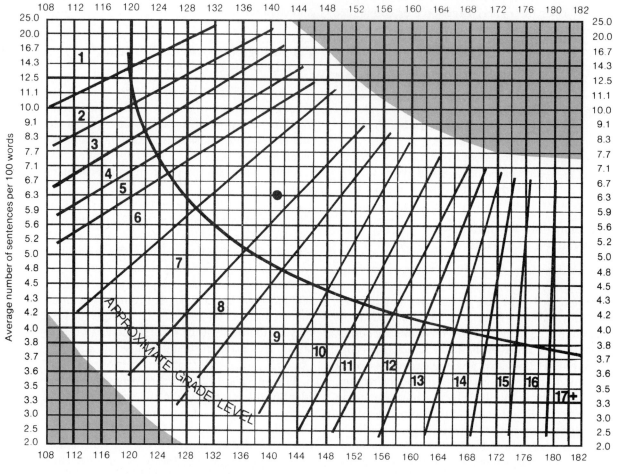

Average number of syllables per 100 words

DIRECTIONS: Randomly select 3 one hundred word passages from a book or an article. Plot average number of syllables and average number of sentences per 100 words on graph to determine the grade level of the material. Choose more passages per book if great variability is observed and conclude that the book has uneven readability. Few books will fall in gray area but when they do grade level scores are invalid.

Count proper nouns, numerals and initializations as words. Count a syllable for each symbol. For example, "1945" is 1 word and 4 syllables and "IRA" is 1 word and 3 syllables.

EXAMPLE:

	SYLLABLES	SENTENCES
1st Hundred Words	124	6.6
2nd Hundred Words	141	5.5
3rd Hundred Words	158	6.8
AVERAGE	141	6.3

READABILITY 7th GRADE (see dot plotted on graph)

For further information and validity data see the Journal of Reading December, 1977.

FIG. 13-8 Fry Readability Graph. (Courtesy Edward Fry, Rutgers University.)

EXPANDED DIRECTIONS FOR WORKING READABILITY GRAPH

1. Randomly select three (3) sample passages and count out exactly 100 words beginning with the beginning of a sentence. Do count proper nouns, initializations, and numerals.

2. Count the number of sentences in the hundred words, estimating length of the fraction of the last sentence to the nearest 1/10th.

3. Count the total number of syllables in the 100-word passage. If you don't have a hand counter available, an easy way is to simply put a mark above every syllable over one in each word, then when you get to the end of the passage, count the number of marks and add 100. Small calculators can also be used as counters by pushing numeral "1", then push the "+" sign for each word or syllable when counting.

4. Enter graph with average sentence length and average number of syllables; plot dot where the two lines intersect. Area where dot is plotted will give you the approximate grade level.

5. If a great deal of variability is found in syllable count or sentence count, putting more samples into the average is desirable.

6. A word is defined as a group of symbols with a space on either side; thus, "Joe," "IRA," "1945," and "&" are each one word.

7. A syllable is defined as a phonetic syllable. Generally, there are as many syllables as vowel sounds. For example, "stopped" is one syllable and "wanted" is two syllables. When counting syllables for numerals and initializations, count one syllable for each symbol. For example, "1945" is 4 syllables and "IRA" is 3 syllables, and "&" is 1 syllable.

FOOTNOTE: This "extended graph" does not outmode or render the earlier (1968) version inoperative or inaccurate; it is an extension.

FIG. 13-8 Fry Readability Graph—cont'd.

tapes may present the same obstacles as written materials for students with limited language skills or for those for whom English is a second language.

One advantage to using teacher-made audiotapes is that they can be tailored for specific topics and outcomes. Furthermore, when students hear their teacher's voice, there is recognition and attentive listening. Also, local language dialects, accents, and references can be used to help make the instruction more relevant. Many copies of the audiotapes can be made for use at listening stations or at home.

The following steps should be followed in the production of teacher-made audiotapes:

- Identify purpose and scope
- List essential points to be covered
- Organize points to be covered in logical sequence
- Determine feedback questions
- Organize instruction into 5-minute segments
- Extemporaneously record or write the script in conversational tone, allowing for minor imperfections
- Pilot test the material with a few students
- Based on pilot test observations, revise if necessary

Other factors to consider. Additional strategies should also be used whenever possible because students with low-level literacy skills are in great need of health information. Link new ideas with already known information using analogies, examples, drawings (simple line drawings work best), pictures, and modeling.

Obtaining regular feedback from students with low-level literacy skills is essential. Be aware that one of the ways such students cope is to agree with whatever is asked of them. If they are asked, "Do you understand?" they answer "Yes." They have learned that a "No" answer is followed by a request to explain what they did not know, and they may not have the vocabulary or fluency to explain what they did not understand. Therefore, instead of asking if they understand, ask them to describe in their own words what they learned. Another useful technique is to have them draw a pic-

ture illustrating the main point of the lesson and then orally explain their picture.

Sponsored Materials

Many groups and individuals offer educational materials for classroom use. Much of this material is good and can be used to supplement, broaden, and enrich the content found in the regular text and reference books. Such material is valuable to the health program in that it can provide students with a variety of points of view on important problems and issues. It also usually represents the special interest of the sponsoring organization; therefore it is referred to as *sponsored material.* The list in Appendix E is illustrative of sources of sponsored material.

An increasing number of noneducational businesses that market products and services, ranging from hamburgers to mouthwash to electrical power, sponsor a variety of promotional materials such as "learning packets," wall posters, "news" broadcasts, computer programs, games, stickers, and the like for school use. Many of these businesses also offer incentive programs that purport to encourage desirable educational behavior on the part of students.

Businesses usually provide their materials to schools free or at nominal cost. These materials are often attractively packaged, easy to use, and focused on current topics. However, business-sponsored materials may be biased. Special care should be taken to review materials provided by a business or business group on topics in which the group has a financial interest. Business-supplied materials about topics such as nutrition, energy, and environmental issues have been especially controversial in the past.

Introduction of sponsored materials into the classroom must be done cautiously. All materials must be carefully evaluated by the teacher with assistance from the grade level team and other personnel such as the nurse and principal. One of the first things a teacher new to a district should learn is the policy and procedures relating to the use of sponsored materials.

The following questions can serve as general guidelines for deciding whether or not to use sponsored materials in the classroom:

- Is the content accurate?
- Is the material helpful in achieving the goals and objectives set up for a particular lesson, unit, or course?
- Can the material be used without obligating the school to an individual or group in any way?
- Is the material free of obtrusive or objectionable advertising?
- Does the material promote or support the point of view of a special interest group? If so, are classroom materials available to present other points of view?
- Is the material culturally sensitive and free of gender, racial, or ethnic stereotyping or bias?

When in doubt as to whether to use sponsored material, teachers should try to view the entire lesson from the perspective of the students. Teachers should determine all the messages the students will receive from the questionable material and the context in which it will be presented. They should also consider the possibilities for modifying the materials. If the content is accurate and important to the lesson, but there is an excess of advertising, the advertising should be physically eliminated.

Games for Health Education

Using games as educational tools is a practice that has met with increased interest. There are many educational games now on the commercial market, and some businesses offer schools free or inexpensive games related to their products. The games most notable among these deal with nutrition. Product-related games must be carefully analyzed by the teacher. Often they teach nothing, or only misconceptions, about health.

Some games promoted as educational aids in reality promote (directly or indirectly) a particular product or brand line. Many games are not adequately field tested or evaluated. Competitive games may encourage winning the game rather than learning. Teachers should critically evaluate any educational health games before trying them with students.

Before deciding to use any specific game for teaching health, the teacher should give consideration to these questions:

- Is the game appropriate for the age group?
- What is the primary function of the game? (What is it to do or represent?)
- How will the game help students reach the objectives of the particular health lesson or unit?
- Is the emphasis of the game on learning or winning?
- What kinds of decisions must the players make? (Pure guesses, chance, logical or evaluative decisions, and so on.)
- Are the anticipated results worth the class time invested?
- Does the game directly or subtly promote a special interest or product?
- What are the potential side effects of the game?

Factors for Effective Use of TV

The teaching effectiveness of instructional TV programs designed for classroom use and programs designed for general viewing is well documented by over 20 years of research. A critical factor in what a child will learn from TV is the presence of a mentor (teacher or parent) who shares the viewing and discusses what is seen with the child. Among the variables that account for successful learning from TV are those listed here.*

Characteristics of effective instructional TV programs. Significant gains in student achievement can take place with TV programs having these characteristics:

- Key concepts are repeated in a variety of ways.

*Modified from *Television in the classroom: what the research says,* Olympia, WA, 1981, State Superintendent of Public Instruction.

- Use is made of animation, novelty, variety, and simple visuals.
- The program entertains and informs.
- A trained communicator is used to present information.
- There are opportunities for students to participate in a learning activity, either in response to information presented in the program or as part of a game presented by the program.
- The length of the program is matched to the attention span of the intended audience.
- The principles of effective audiovisual presentation are followed.

Characteristics of effective instructional TV viewing. Achievement gains from viewing TV occur when teachers do the following:

- Prepare students to receive information to be presented by the TV program
- Provide reinforcing discussions and activities following viewing
- Provide corrective feedback to students in follow-up discussions between students and teachers based on what students reveal they have understood from the program
- Provide students with feedback on their achievement as a result of viewing

The use of TV as an instructional aid also provides an excellent opportunity for parent-teacher cooperation. It provides a convenient and important activity for home and school team teaching. It is the teacher's responsibility to initiate these activities with parents and to provide them with clear guidelines for their involvement.

SUMMARY

Properly selected and applied instructional aids combined with skilled teaching bring excitement and fun to learning about health. The interest of the general population in health has resulted in production of an abundance of information and materials about health-related topics. This abundance of instructional aids has increased the importance of teachers knowing how to select and use health materials wisely and effectively.

Elementary school teachers of health should know the proper and most effective uses of the various forms of instructional aids, where to find them (both within the school and from outside sources), and how to create their own aids when appropriate. Teachers also need to find access to scientifically valid health information through libraries, colleges, and universities; state and federal offices; professional journals; and the mass media.

There are problems associated with many instructional aids. Teachers need to know how to identify and eliminate sexism, racism, and ageism in instructional materials; determine the readability of written materials; and analyze commercial or special-interest messages in sponsored materials. In addition, teachers need to know how to modify existing materials and create special materials for students with low-level literacy skills.

Identification and selection of instructional aids for health teaching is an important responsibility for the elementary school teacher. The school nurse, librarian, learning resource staff, principal, and district health coordinator or curriculum director are key resource people who can help the teacher locate, select, use, and evaluate instructional materials.

QUESTIONS FOR DISCUSSION

1. What are the two main purposes served by instructional aids?
2. Identify some specific kinds of instructional aids and give examples of how they can be used to enhance health teaching.
3. What are the four major factors to consider when using instructional aids? Elaborate on each factor.
4. Explain the statement, "Subjective measurements can serve as indicators of the value of instructional aids."
5. What are the pros and cons concerning the use of textbooks for health instruction?
6. Identify the different kinds of instructional aids for health teaching that can be found in the school library.

7. What sources of instructional aids for health, besides the school library, are available for teachers?

8. What are sponsored materials for health education? How can they be used? Identify any concerns the teacher should be aware of before using sponsored material.

9. Identify and describe the kinds of inexpensive instructional aids that can be made by teachers and students.

10. Describe the major teacher considerations when videotaping students.

11. What are the key considerations for getting the maximum benefit from the use of popular TV as a teaching aid in health instruction?

12. Describe how the classroom teacher can use a variety of materials to teach health to students with low-level literacy skills.

13. How might a teacher modify existing materials so they could be used by students with low-level literacy skills?

SELECTED REFERENCES

Association for the Advancement of Health Education: *Cultural awareness and sensitivity: guidelines for health educators,* Reston, VA, 1994, The Association.

Association for Supervision and Curriculum Development: *Only the best,* Alexandria, VA, 1993, The Association.

Association for Supervision and Curriculum Development: Task Force on Business Involvement in the Schools: guidelines for business involvement in the school, *Ed Leadership* 47:84-87, 1989-1990.

Banks JA: The battle over the canon: cultural diversity and curriculum reform, *Ed Forum* 1:11-13, 1989.

Bullough RV: *Creating instructional materials,* ed 3, Columbus, OH, 1988, Merrill.

Children's books about special children, *Childhood Ed* 57:205-208, 1981.

Dawson ME, Gay G, editors: *Guidelines for avoiding biases and stereotypes in instructional television,* Bloomington, IN, 1978, Agency for Instructional Television.

Deardorff WW: Computerized health education: a comparison with traditional formats, *Health Ed Quart* 13(1):61-72, 1986.

Doak CC, Doak LG, Root JH: *Teaching patients with low literacy skills,* Philadelphia, 1985, Lippincott.

Dorman SM: Evaluating computer software for the health education classroom, *J School Health* 62(1):36, 1992.

Dubois PA, Schubert JG: Do your school policies provide equal access to computers? Are you sure? *Ed Leadership* 43:March, 1986.

Gold RS: *Microcomputer applications in health education,* Dubuque, IA, 1991, WC Brown.

Guidelines for selecting bias-free textbooks and storybooks, New York, (undated), Council on Interracial Books for Children.

Guidelines for the development of instructional materials selection policies, Olympia, WA, revised 1985, Superintendent of Public Instruction.

Jonassen DH: The real case for using authoring systems to develop courseware, *Ed Tech* XXV (2):39-41, 1985.

Lockheed ME, Frakt SB: Sex equity: increasing girls' use of computers, *Computing Teacher* 11(8):16-18, 1984.

Mahoney BS, Olsen LK, editors: *Health education: a practical guide for K-12 health education,* Millwood, NY, 1993, Kraus International Publications.

Martin CE, Stainbrook GL: An analysis checklist for audiovisuals when used as educational resources, *Health Ed* 17(4):31-33, 1986.

Matiella AC, editor: *The multicultural challenge in health education,* Santa Cruz, CA, 1992, ETR Associates.

Moore B: The health information video project, *J School Health* 61(6):265-266, 1991.

Muther C: What every textbook evaluator should know, *Ed Leadership* 42(7):4-8, 1985.

Pahnos M: The continuing challenge of multicultural health education, *J Health Ed* 62(1):24-26, 1992.

Petosa R, Gillespie J: Microcomputers in health education: characteristics of quality instructional software, *J School Health* 54(10):394-396, 1984.

Roberts, Fitzmahan, and Associates: *Here's looking at you, 2000,* Seattle, 1986, Comprehensive Health Education Foundation.

Sager RA: Microcomputer software—the hard part, *Health Ed* 18(3):52-56, 1987.

Standards for evaluation of instructional materials with respect to social content, Sacramento, CA, 1986, California State Department of Education.

Television in the classroom: what the research says . . . , Olympia, WA, 1981, State Superintendent of Public Instruction.

Whiteside MF, Whiteside JA: Microcomputer authoring systems: valuable tools for health education, *Health Ed* 18(6):2-4, 1987-1988.

VI

EVALUATION

14

Evaluating the School Health Program

KEY CONCEPT

Periodic assessment of all facets of the school health program helps ensure that the program is current and is meeting the needs of students and the community at large.

It is a mark of the trained mind never to expect more precision in the treatment of any subject than the nature of that subject permits.

ARISTOTLE

The primary purpose of program evaluation is to collect and analyze information that will assist school leaders and decision makers in making program-related decisions.

DONALD J. IVERSON

PROBLEMS TO SOLVE

How would you proceed to evaluate the school health program? How will you know if your health teaching has been effective? What steps would you follow and what methods would you use? How will you use the results of your evaluation?

Evaluation has always been important to school personnel. Conscientious teachers want and need to know the effect of their teaching on pupils. These understandings are important so that teachers may continually strive to improve. Teachers want to know what they did well and what they did not do so well. In health education evaluation is especially significant in determining the impact of instructional programs on the lives of students. According to Hochbaum,* "The task of health education is to equip people intellectually and emotionally to make sound decisions on matters affecting their health, safety, and welfare." The process used to determine the achievement of this task is referred to as *evaluation.*

School health programs continue to receive little or no evaluation attention. Health education in particular has not received much consideration in this regard. One reason for this neglect has been that authorities have had to concentrate their efforts in gaining acceptance of the need for the establishment of health instruction programs in schools. Also, the evaluation process is more complex in health education than in many other educational areas because of the difficulties faced in trying to determine improvement in students' health behavior. Some pupil health attitudes and practices may be immediately observable, whereas others may not be noted for months or years after the instructional program is completed. These delayed changes may be the result of the additive effects of reinforcing information, new life situations, psychological maturation, or changed environments.

This chapter is designed to provide understanding about evaluation as applied to the total school health program and to offer practical suggestions that teachers may find useful in their classrooms and schools. This coverage is not meant to be all-inclusive because of the complexity of the problem and the limited information available. It includes the four major components of the health program—instruction, services, environment, and coordination—with primary emphasis on instruction.

WHAT IS EVALUATION?

Evaluation is a process of comparing the worth or value of something with a given purpose or objective. This definition contains the three necessary parts of an evaluation: (1) a comparison, (2) a thing or object of interest, and (3) a standard (purpose or objective). The word is often erroneously used synonymously with the term *measurement.* Measurement is the part of evaluation that deals with quantitative results. It is the assignment of numbers to objects, events, or people. It answers the questions: "How much?" "Is there a health instruction curriculum?" "How much time is devoted to health instruction at each grade level?" "How many teaching aids are available?" "How many nurses are employed per 1000 students?" The more important questions that must be answered include, "How good and of what value is the school health program?" "What impact does it have on the lives of elementary schoolchildren?" "How does it help children live in a healthful manner?" "Are all students with health problems identified, and are school programs adjusted to their needs?" "Are teaching materials current and useful?"

Evaluation must be concerned with both quantitative (How much?) and qualitative (How good?) information. Quantitative data refer to such information as the test scores of pupils, the number of nurses employed, and the number of meals served in the school lunch program. Qualitative data provide such understandings as the effectiveness of the program on children in terms of school adjustments and correction of health problems, nurse efficiency, nutritional value of meals in the school lunch or breakfast program, and the extent of behavioral change in pupils.

The technique used to gather information for assessment purposes may provide objective or subjective evidence. Objective data may be obtained through surveys, checklists, inventories, and examinations given before and after pro-

---

*Hochbaum GM: Measurement of effectiveness of health education activities, *Int J Health Ed* 14, 1971.

grams have started, which are then organized and statistically analyzed. Subjective data are derived from the observations and opinions of teachers and others. Regardless of the type of evaluation conducted, it is important that it be appropriate and that the results provide meaningful data from which conclusions can be drawn.

Evaluation is both a process and a product. It is not only a means to an end but an end in itself. It must concern itself with the procedures used to achieve the objectives of the program and with the methods used to reach these goals. For example, the teaching/learning activities and the teaching aids used are interrelated with the pupil behaviors sought by the teacher in the instructional program. These activities are the means to the end (pupil behaviors). If they are inappropriate or ineffective, they may not adequately contribute to the objective of helping pupils live in a healthful manner.

Evaluation is a continuous process. It is not done at the end of a program so that a "grade" can be issued. It involves planned and organized efforts using procedures to gather objective evidence, or it may be day-to-day assessment by teachers to obtain subjective information through observations. Evaluation is an integral part of teaching that is in need of emphasis equal to that for the other phases of the health instruction program. It is needed to identify both strong and weak aspects of the school health program.

WHY EVALUATION IN SCHOOL HEALTH?

Why should the school health program be evaluated?

First, it is sound practice to continually assess the achievement of objectives in the instructional, services, and environmental aspects of the program to ensure that it keeps up with new developments in education and the health services.

Second, there is the responsibility or accountability to measure, evaluate, and report on policies, procedures, and learning outcomes to pupils, parents, school health coordinators, and other concerned persons.

Third, evaluation is an essential part of good teaching. Whereas testing and other evaluative techniques may be overdone in some classes, they are an integral part of the teaching/learning process. Both teacher and pupil can function more efficiently when they are periodically apprised of where they are, where they are going, and how much progress they have made.

Fourth, health services help identify children who are experiencing problems that affect learning, motivation, and discipline. A periodic evaluation of the health services program is essential to ensure that the program is functioning properly and benefiting the maximum number of students on a cost-effective basis.

Fifth, the school environment must be regularly evaluated to be certain teaching effectiveness is maximized and environment-related stress is minimized. An evaluation of the school environment should include the organization of daily activity and the safety of the physical environment.

The *specific uses of evaluation* in school health instruction include the following:

- To use as a diagnostic device. Tests can be given at the beginning of a subject or unit of study for this purpose. Both teacher and pupil benefit from knowing what they know (and, perhaps more importantly, what they do not know), how they feel, and what they

FOR YOUR INFORMATION

Students of all ages who create some of their own [questions for] examinations are forced to reflect upon [and make judgments about] what they have studied. They are forced to ask questions and challenge [their own] answers. They learn how to ask the right questions and how to know good answers from bad, irrelevant from relevant.

Redford Brown
Educ Leadership
47:33, 1989

do with respect to certain health and safety problems.

- To determine progress toward objectives and to appraise the changes in understandings, attitudes, and practices that result from learning experiences in health education. In this way pupil progress may be directly assessed—though it should be kept in mind that important changes in attitude and behavior often may not occur or show for months or years.

- To motivate pupils by stimulating their curiosity about specific health issues. The teacher can then observe the way they react to such problems in thought and practice.

- To identify students who may be in need of special health guidance or counseling.

- To provide data useful in the continual revision of course and curriculum content. Testing affords an objective approach to curriculum improvement in terms of meeting pupil needs.

- To provide a basis for grading. The results of sound tests and portfolios of work provide information for grading and reports of pupils' progress.

- To provide a basis for meaningful parent education and involvement during parent-teacher conferences. Discussing student progress in health studies lends itself to reinforcing parental responsibility for student health and allows the opportunity for the parent to share observed student health attitudes and practices outside of school.

- To provide information useful in program planning. Results of student interest tests and achievement tests can help determine appropriate grade level placement for content and time allotments in the total curriculum.

- To improve instruction by providing feedback about teaching methods and instructional aids.

- To develop good public relations for the health instruction program. Students and parents alike tend to place a higher value on those subjects or courses in which students are tested and assigned a grade. Also, reports of status and progress in specific units of study help communicate the idea that modern health education is significantly more comprehensive and sophisticated than the old "narrow-gauge" hygiene course that was centered around anatomy and physiology.

WHAT SHOULD BE EVALUATED?

The total school health program should be subject to evaluation. This includes the major components of instruction, services, and environment and the coordination of the program. Appendix G contains a good checklist of evaluative criteria for a total program. The suggested evaluation is, to a degree, both quantitative and qualitative.

This section deals primarily with evaluation of the elementary health instruction program, as this is the major purpose of the text. However, attention is also given to health services, environment, and coordination because classroom teachers should be prepared to assist in the evaluation of these components.

School Health Services

On the surface, evaluation of the school health services program may seem to be a rather simple matter of marking yes or no on a checklist. Is the service available or is it not? Checklists for evaluating school health services do help and are a legitimate part of any such assessment. However, they reveal nothing about the quality of service actually available. It is not as important for students, teachers, and parents to know how many nurses are employed or contracted by the district as it is to know how often nurses are available to the school, and how the nurses are contributing to the elementary school health program. Because there are no mandated standards for school health services, one may anticipate a wide divergence in the quantity and quality of programs in local school districts. Appendix G contains one of the better checklists available for evaluating school health services programs.

Checklists for school health services usually include questions relating to health examinations; emergency care; screening tests for vision, hearing, and growth; dental inspections or examinations; immunizations; teacher observation of pupil health; first aid; and follow-up programs. Although a checklist may be useful in describing the scope of services available, it does not help in understanding the teacher's role. Most of the actual services are provided by the nurse or other qualified health professionals. There are, however, four important areas in which teachers have considerable responsibility: (1) observation for health problems, (2) emergency care, (3) follow-up programs, and (4) educational programs that complement some of the health services.

- *Teacher observation* for student health problems is a major responsibility requiring conscientious effort. Few teachers are actually trained to identify children with possible vision, hearing, or postural problems. Lice and ringworm may be easier to spot, but identifying those problems still requires some training and experience. Problems relating to physical, sexual, and mental abuse are often more difficult to observe, as are those concerning drug and alcohol abuse. The teacher should ask, "If observation for health problems is one of my duties, who trains me, or how do I gain the necessary skill?"

- *Emergency care* is a matter all teachers have to face sometime in their career. The situation may involve a simple bruise, a seizure, broken bone, or an appendicitis attack. If the nurse is not in the building all day, is someone else qualified to handle emergency care? Who? Has a clearly written emergency care policy and procedure for district personnel been developed? Has it been approved by appropriate medical and emergency care personnel? Is the teacher expected to give immediate care at the emergency site? If so, will the district provide periodic in-service training for teachers in first aid and emergency skills?

- *Follow-up programs*, in this context, refer to what happens to the child with an identifiable health problem. It may include referral, treatment, and reentry into the school program. It is important that the teacher be kept informed as to the status of the child to plan for a smooth reentry to the classroom. The nurse can help in this situation by carefully instructing the teacher about what to expect from the child and by providing clues for teacher observation to ensure that any signs of remission are noted and quickly reported. Follow-up programs are extremely difficult without the service of a school nurse. Further, many children with chronic conditions (e.g., childhood cancer and leukemia) are now being placed into the regular classroom. The teacher must know how to make adjustments within the classroom so that all children have the best opportunity for optimal learning.

- *Educational programs* should relate to many of the health services provided to children. Basic visual, hearing, and growth and weight screenings offer excellent opportunities to teach about sight, sound, and the body. Too often these opportunities are missed and children go from year to year never knowing what their vision test results were or what having 20/20 vision means. Nor do these children realize that some day they must assume full responsibility for their own health checkups. This is another area in which nurse and teacher should collaborate.

A thoughtful review of the school health services program should lead one to conclude that the nurse is the key element to a good program. An evaluative checklist can show on paper that a program exists; but it is usually the nurse who brings life, depth, and quality to the services. In assessing a school health services program, the key questions to be asked are: "How often is the nurse in the building?" "What is the role of the nurse?" "How much support does he or she receive?" The answers to these key questions will provide a better evaluation of the school health services program than any checklist.

The scope of school health services, including basic policies and procedures, should be *written* and made available to all school employees and parents. This action helps parents gain insight about their role in ensuring that their child or children stay healthy. Teachers must understand their role in relation to student health problems. They should be familiar with what services are available, where and how to make referrals, and the proper procedures to follow.

Healthful School Environment

Many health factors within the school environment are relatively easy to evaluate with a checklist that includes some of these questions: "Is the water supply inspected regularly?" "Does the sewage system function properly and meet state standards?" "Is there an automatic fire alarm system, and is it checked regularly?" "Is playground equipment in good repair, organized for maximum safety, and regularly checked?" "Does the classroom lighting meet acceptable standards?" "Are heat and ventilation systems functioning properly?" "Is the food service safe and sanitary?" Appendix G contains an illustrative instrument that may be used to assess the school environment.

Other factors have a more subtle effect on the school environment. One example is personal space. Students, especially older children, have need for personal space, as well as space for social interaction. Personal space can include a desk for younger students in a self-contained classroom or a locker for older students. It can also include areas such as courtyards where students can find solitude or spend quiet time during breaks or recess. This factor can have a significant impact on the emotional environment of the school and classroom. Noise, color, and odor are other subtle features of a healthy school environment that must receive consideration.

The teacher is the most critical environmental factor in the emotional setting of the school. The emotional climate in the classroom that provides security for children, the opportunity for freedom of student expression, and the fair and just treatment of all students are factors that must constantly be assessed by teachers. Sound teacher health behaviors in regard to rest, nutrition, exercise, and personal health habits are necessary for optimal functioning. Teachers may need to prepare a self-inventory for their own personal use.

Coordination

Coordination refers to the planned interrelation of health instruction, services, and environment. It refers to the consistency with which each of the three components of the health program is performed throughout the district. The degree of coordination of the health program depends not only to a large extent on the size of the district, but also on the implementation and evaluation of each program in each school within the district. If problems are identified, there should be a policy that can be implemented to correct them.

Following are some of the basic questions that should be considered when assessing coordination of the school health program:

- Does the school district have a planned health education program with identified objectives and scope and sequence of instruction for each grade level?
- Are responsibilities for all persons involved in the health program (principals, teachers, school nurses, and others) clearly defined?
- Has the district assigned personnel to provide leadership for the implementation and maintenance of a comprehensive health education program and have the necessary resources been provided?

Additional criteria are listed in Appendix G under "Administration."

EVALUATING THE HEALTH INSTRUCTION PROGRAM

The health instruction program can be assessed in terms of the process used (formative evaluation) and the product (impact on students) (summative evaluation). Each of these categories can in turn be assessed both quantitatively and qualitatively. *Process evaluation* includes assessment of teaching aids and teaching strategies and techniques. It may also cover a variety of other areas, such as adequacy of objectives and content in meeting student needs and interests, the curriculum guide, appropriate grade level for topics, and content and teaching aids. *Product evaluation* refers generally to the effect of the program on students in terms of the extent to which the stated knowledges, attitudes, and practice objectives have been achieved.

Should teachers desire to conduct a brief but limited quantitative assessment of the instructional program, Appendix G contains a section that will be useful. This checklist also includes some qualitative assessment material.

This section of the text limits its coverage of instructional program evaluation to those short-term aspects that are feasible for teacher implementation. These aspects include student achievement and progress, instructional aids, and instructional methods.

Techniques Used in Evaluation

The techniques used in evaluation may also be referred to as instruments, devices, procedures, and strategies. Those that may be appropriate for the teacher to use in the classroom include (1) visual and written procedures, questionnaires, checklists, tests, surveys, anecdotal records, samples of pupils' work (projects, reports), and rating scales and (2) observations of pupils by teachers and parents. The process of evaluation includes self-appraisal, peer and team review, and teacher-based assessment.

Teachers who plan to use paper-and-pencil tests should conduct both pretests and posttests. Without pretests to enable the teacher to make a comparison of learning achievements, there is no way to determine whether the knowledge, attitudes, and practices reflected in posttests existed before the instructional program or whether they can be attributed to the educational activities themselves. The teacher should realize that administering a pretest becomes part of the instruc-

tional program, as it will be a learning experience for the students. Thus student gains on a posttest may be partially a result of the fact that they have taken the pretest.

Primary school-aged students must be tested with great care and consideration. Appropriate sources of information on how well these children are learning and understanding health material may include combinations of the following:

- Systematic observations by teachers, other professionals, and parents.
- Samples of children's work such as drawings, paintings, dictated stories, writing samples, projects, and other activities.
- Test scores if—and only if—appropriate, reliable, and valid tests have been used.

Individual testing procedures are most appropriate for these children. They may have difficulty understanding instructions or using a crayon or pencil to mark the desired responses. Also, children progress at such different rates that it is impossible to maintain a testing speed appropriate for every child. Testing of this nature for primary school-aged students should be in pictorial form (Fig. 14-1).

Evaluating Student Achievement and Progress

How can a teacher know whether pupils have been affected by the health instruction program if no effort is made to determine what they have learned? The need for clear, concise, and measurable cognitive, affective, and action domain objectives must be reemphasized. The taxonomy of objectives by Bloom and others shown in Chapter 11 provides information that will aid in the preparation of these objectives. When written out in this fashion, they give direction to the evaluation process (Fig. 14-2). The teacher should remember, however, that students' abilities at various age levels vary. Therefore it is important to have realistic objectives that students have a realistic chance of attaining.

Measuring health knowledge. Health knowledge is the easiest of objectives to measure. However, teachers will need to determine the type and

A

Mark an X on the picture that shows the health worker who takes your temperature and helps you get ready to see the doctor.

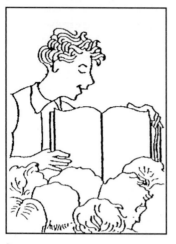 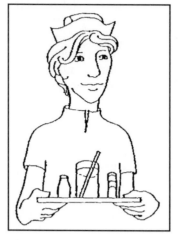 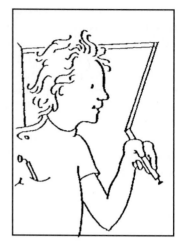

B

Mark an X on the picture that shows the health worker who you go to see when you are ill (sick).

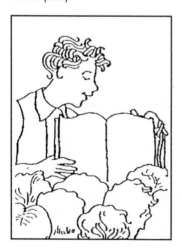 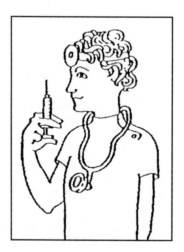 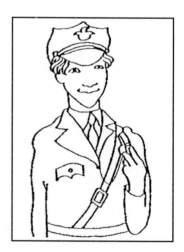

FIG. 14-1 Testing for primary school-aged children may be in pictorial form. (From Pollock MD, Middleton K: *School health instruction,* ed 3, St Louis, 1994, Mosby.)

frequency of devices to use depending on the length of the health instruction program and the amount of time available for evaluation. Teachers can select the strategies that are appropriate for their students from those presented next.

Teacher-prepared paper-and-pencil procedures. Paper-and-pencil procedures are the most universal means of collecting evidence related to health knowledge. They may take the form of tests, self-appraisals, or peer appraisals.

C

Mark an X on the picture that shows where garbage should be kept.

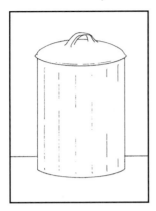 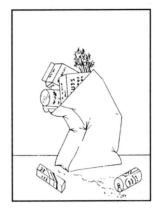 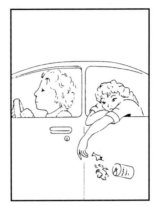

D

Mark an X on the picture that shows what you should drink to help your teeth grow healthy and strong.

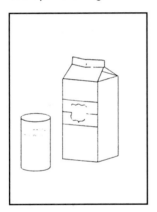 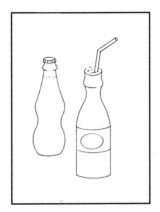 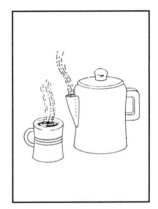

FIG. 14-1,—cont'd. For legend see opposite page.

TESTS. The two kinds of paper-and-pencil tests most often prepared by teachers are the objective test and the written essay or subjective test. Objective test items may be placed in the two broad categories of *recognition* and *recall*. The recognition type of test item requires that the pupil recognize and select the correct answer, which is shown among other, incorrect answers in the test item. The recall type of test item requires that the pupil supply the correct answer, which has been omitted from the test item.

There are several variations of the recognition test item. Some of these include true-false, multiple choice, and matching. In measuring health knowledge, it is recommended that the teacher use a variety of recognition test items rather than rely on one type. The purpose of this is to help offset the limitations involved in the various recognition items.

The true-false test item may have little diagnostic value because a correct response may be merely an indication that the pupil guessed correctly in

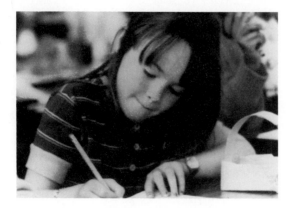

FIG. 14-2 Evaluation should be a learning experience. (Courtesy San Jose Nutrition Project, San Jose, California.)

selecting the answer. When true-false items are used, extreme care should be taken in constructing the false items so they will not leave a fixed false idea with pupils, particularly slow-learning pupils. As a variation, the teacher may ask students to cross out any word or words that make a given statement false and to insert words that will make the statement true. Teachers should use the following criteria when developing or reviewing true-false questions:

- Are statements true or false without additional qualifications?
- Are statements expressed simply and clearly?
- Are items relatively short and restricted to one central idea?
- Are statements ambiguous?
- Do statements contain determiners? False statements—only, never, all, always, none, every, no; true statements—usually, several, sometimes, constantly, often.

The *multiple-choice item*, when carefully prepared, can be thought provoking. It is an excellent way of determining whether pupils have acquired the desired health knowledge and information. In multiple-choice, test items usually have three to five possible responses. Five responses are preferred, because as the number of possible answers is increased the possibility of guessing the correct answer is decreased. Points to consider when developing or reviewing multiple-choice questions include the following:

- Are there three or four distractors with only one answer?
- Are the distractors reasonably plausible?
- Is there grammatical consistency?
- Does the stem contain clues?
- Are choices of answers brief?
- Are ambiguities eliminated?
- Are inclusive options such as "All of the above" or "None of the above" avoided?
- Are words repeated in the distractors that could be included in the stem?
- Are the distractors approximately the same length?
- Are negatively worded item stems avoided?

The matching test item, when properly constructed, can be useful in measuring achievement. The creation of a good matching test begins with clear directions to the student. The directions should indicate the basis for the match or relationship that the test taker should look for between items in the two columns. Directions should also include where and how to indicate an answer and whether a response may be used more than once. Matching test items have the obvious limitation of being the type of items used for the collection of mere factual information. The following five questions can serve as guides in creating or reviewing matching type questions:

- Are lists of comparative items as homogeneous as possible?
- Are some possible responses included that cannot be matched?
- Can questions be easily scored?
- Are lists of responses relatively short?
- Do all the items deal with the same basic topic?

The completion test item requires the pupil to supply the correct answer in the form of a recall or fill-in item. This test item places a premium on rote memorization of health facts. A limitation is that the test item may be such that more than one correct answer can be given. For example, in a recall test such as "Exercise generally shows an increase in _____ development," both "muscular" and "organic" are correct answers, and there may be more. On the other hand, a recall item such as " _____ makes up the greatest part of the body," has only one possible correct answer, which is "water." When there is a possibility of more than one correct answer, the teacher should include all possibilities in the test scoring key.

These three points will help the teacher develop or select good completion-type items:

- Make certain that there is only one correct response.
- Do not put in so many blanks that the question loses meaning.
- Do not permit the syntax of the statement or the length of the blank to give a hint about the answer.

Perhaps the greatest limiting factor among the preceding types of tests is that they all prohibit the students from expressing all their knowledge about the topic. Therefore other types of appraisals are also recommended to provide a well-rounded picture of how well students are progressing in their health education.

ESSAY. *The written or verbal essay* or *subjective test* of health knowledge, although somewhat lacking in objectivity, helps gain evidence of achievement and educative growth that often cannot be measured through the objective test. For example, the teacher can formulate questions in such a way as to provide for better problem-solving situations than are usually possible in straight objective tests. The teacher may ask pupils to write a summary of what has been learned through the study of a certain health unit. If this procedure is undertaken, the teacher should analyze the summaries to determine how closely they are related to the objectives of the unit. In this way the teacher should be able to ascertain to a reasonable degree whether pupils have gained insight into the understanding and concepts that formed the basis for the unit objectives. Caution must be taken so that the focus of the question is not so broad that students do not know how much to write. To realize the optimal benefit from essay-type questions, the following points are suggested:

- Questions should be clearly and carefully constructed.
- Written instructions for answering should be clear and explicit.
- If the question asks students what *they think* about a given topic, there can be no incorrect answers.

SELF-APPRAISALS. Asking pupils to indicate what they have learned by giving them an outline so they can present their comments often provides valuable clues for evaluative information. Students' maintenance of daily journals and logs to note thoughts and new information also may be useful.

PEER APPRAISALS. The technique of having other students assess the learnings of their classmates has advantages if selectively used by teachers. Careful planning is necessary if this technique is to be successful because pupils need to clearly understand the purpose and the procedure. This type of evaluation is particularly useful when conducted in conjunction with cooperative learning strategies.

Oral questioning. When used, oral questioning necessitates that the teacher devise a technique suitable for keeping satisfactory records. Otherwise there will be no documentary evidence of growth when final evaluations and appraisals are made. Some teachers find it desirable and helpful to keep a log in which results of oral questioning can be quickly recorded.

Oral inquiry may be formal or informal. In any event, questions should be such that the teacher can actually determine whether pupils are acquiring and using health knowledge. Because of this, certain types of questions usually should be avoided. For example, questions that require only a yes or no answer may have little value because the pupil will have a 50% chance of guessing the correct answer. On the other hand, questions necessitating critical thinking and judgment can be phrased in ways that enable the teacher to determine evidence of accurate health knowledge. One of the disadvantages that teachers have found in using the oral questioning technique is that it may be difficult to appraise the achievement of all pupils if classes are large. The chief advantage of this means of measurement is that the teacher may obtain a more valid estimate of the individual's learning, especially for those students who experience difficulty with written tests. Oral questioning is particularly suitable for primary children, prereaders, or children who have difficulty reading.

Demonstrations. The measurement of health knowledge through demonstrations can be carried out by either teacher demonstrations or pupil demonstrations. When the teacher demonstrates, the pupils are required to identify those things that are demonstrated. When pupils perform a demonstration, they apply health knowledge, as well as their interest in the topic.

The efficacy of this approach to health knowledge measurement is obvious; it tests pupil knowledge in a lifelike situation, which could be carried over and applied in a practical way, such as helping in the selection of nutritious foods while shopping with the family. Meaningful opportunities that apply new knowledge motivates learning and promotes self-esteem.

Asking pupils to demonstrate certain procedures that were developed in a health unit is a valid way of measuring health knowledge. The chief disadvantage of this technique is the amount of time required. Measurement of health knowledge through pupil demonstration may provide a better indication of educative growth in those pupils who do not express themselves well on written tests.

Pupil projects. Appraisal of learning in terms of health knowledge need not always take the form of testing. For example, the teacher can evaluate notebooks, special projects, and other materials prepared by pupils. This can be done to determine whether pupils have gained insight into certain health concepts necessary for the satisfactory preparation of these materials. Often these works, as well as reports, journals, notes the students have kept, or other examples of written work, are compiled into portfolios. Portfolios provide the teacher with a broad array of the student's achievements, which provides the opportunity to see the assignments as a whole, rather than separately.

Teacher observation. One of the best techniques in health appraisal, teacher observation, can also be a primary measure in the assessment of pupils' progress (Fig. 14-3). Teachers know their pupils. They see them day in and day out. They are in a good position to judge pupil learnings. Because parents also observe their children, communication between teachers and parents is most helpful in evaluating pupil progress.

Standardized tests. Several standardized tests are used to gather information regarding health knowledge. The standardized test is one that has been previously administered to a large number of pupils to establish norms for specific grade levels or combinations of grade levels.

One of the major problems of using standardized tests is that they often lack curricular validity. Because many test items do not relate to the objectives, content, and learning activities of the local school health instruction program, they lack relevance. Careful analysis of standardized tests is

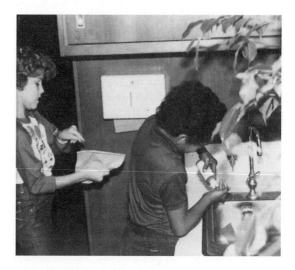

FIG. 14-3 Observation is one way to evaluate health practices. (Courtesy Austin Independent School District, Austin, Texas.)

critical if the teacher plans to use them as the sole means of determining student achievement. Perhaps a better use of standardized tests is using them as a guide for teachers who are developing their own tests.

Appraising health attitudes. Assessment of pupils' attitudes toward health is difficult, and it is almost impossible to obtain objective information. Attitudes are concerned with one's feelings, emotions, beliefs, and values, which are often reflected in behavior. Observations of pupils' actions may provide clues to their feelings and emotions but direct observation may not totally reflect the way students truly feel. Attitudes are elusive and may change with the time of day or the environment or situation. Some pupils may not wish to reveal their true feelings because of their home situations or other conditions. Therefore pupil replies may be unreliable, and the information received from whatever technique used by teachers to assess attitudes should be kept in proper perspective. These data should serve only as indicators of student attitudes. Because attitudes are personal, they should not be "tested" to issue student grades. Rather, attitudes should be assessed to help the teacher gain insight about how students feel about various health topics.

Classroom teachers may use a variety of techniques to assess attitudes. The paper-and-pencil inventory using a Likert-type scale, as shown in Fig. 14-4, is one example. A series of sentence completions on the subject of mental health is another example.

I am happiest when I _____ .
I feel best when people _____ .
What I want most _____ .
I feel important when _____ .
I'd like my friends to _____ .

Other techniques that have been tried with some degree of success include students' completions of unfinished stories about health situations and anonymous pupil self-appraisals of their feelings. Sometimes informal pupil conferences and conversations can reflect health attitudes.

Self-Confidence Survey

Check box to the right of each statement that best indicates how you view yourself.

	No				Yes
	1	2	3	4	5
I am easily upset emotionally	☐	☐	☐	☐	☐
I dislike meeting people	☐	☐	☐	☐	☐
I find criticism hard to take	☐	☐	☐	☐	☐
I have trouble solving problems	☐	☐	☐	☐	☐
I feel inferior most of the time	☐	☐	☐	☐	☐
I will not try anything if it means failure	☐	☐	☐	☐	☐

Perhaps the simplest and most practical strategy is the use of teacher observations. For example, teachers can observe (1) pupils' eating habits in the school cafeteria with regard to food preferences, (2) students freely asking questions informally before and after class about particular health topics covered, and (3) children's behavior on playgrounds during fire drills, and in the interactions with others.

The unreliability of the evidence from the attitude assessment procedures described does not mean they should not be used. Attitudes are closely related to behaviors, and they must be assessed despite the limitations of procedures that only provide indications of pupils' feelings and emotions. It is also important to understand that not all health behaviors are directly observable at school. Objective data may be obtained if teachers keep anecdoctal records of pupils' emotions and comments and periodically analyze them for attitudinal changes. In addition, attitudes can often be validated through conversations with parents and other teachers. A variety of observational resources will provide a much better "picture" of the student than reliance on a single data source.

Assessing health practices. Health practices may be more difficult to assess than attitudes. Most health behaviors are not observable in the classroom because they take place in the home or in the community. Also, many may not emerge for

STUDENT FIRE SAFETY ATTITUDES

Please circle the numbers to the right that best express your feelings about each of the following statements:

	Strongly agree	Agree	Don't care	Disagree	Strongly disagree
1. The stop, drop, and roll procedure should be used when clothes are on fire.	5	4	3	2	1
2. In smoke-filled rooms people should crawl low to get out.	5	4	3	2	1
3. Fire drills at school are important.	5	4	3	2	1
4. Smoke detectors are needed in homes.	5	4	3	2	1
5. Fire and smoke discovered should be promptly reported to fire departments.	5	4	3	2	1
6. Fire fighters are community protectors.	5	4	3	2	1
7. Home escape plans are necessary in case of fire.	5	4	3	2	1
8. Fire burns may be dangerous to people.	5	4	3	2	1
9. Fire inspection of buildings should take place on occasions.	5	4	3	2	1
10. Improper storage of flammable materials is hazardous.	5	4	3	2	1
11. Matches, flammable substances, and electrical appliances should be used safely.	5	4	3	2	1
12. Lightning may cause fires.	5	4	3	2	1
13. Overloaded electrical circuits are hazardous.	5	4	3	2	1
14. Baby-sitter fire safety plans protect individuals.	5	4	3	2	1
15. Electrical equipment that has been tested for fire and safety hazards should be used.	5	4	3	2	1

FIG. 14-4 Student fire safety attitudes.

months or years after pupils have completed their schooling (e.g., selecting a doctor). Therefore most of the information collected may have to be subjective in nature and should come from a variety of sources.

The procedures to use for health practices evaluation include paper-and-pencil or computer software methods, such as questionnaires and checklists, informal conferences and discussions with pupils and parents, and teacher observation. Paper-and-pencil checklists of behavior have limitations because the information received may not be reliable. If students are permitted to complete these forms anonymously, the chances for truthful information are increased.

Informal conferences and discussions with children, parents, and other school personnel may provide indications that pupils are brushing and flossing their teeth, eating nutritious foods, and being safe pedestrians.

In assessing health practices, teachers will have to rely on their own observations as well as the observations and reports of others. Reports may come from nurses, physicians, parents, and school personnel that will provide indications of the extent of behavioral changes or behaviors. Teachers may prepare a parent inventory to be taken home by students before and after a particular health unit. Although this procedure is not completely reliable, it can provide supportive information for teacher observations.

Teacher evaluation of health practices should involve a variety of the strategies presented here to validate the pupil behavior indicators that have been observed. By cross-referencing reports and observation, the teacher can be more confident about the reliability of student behaviors.

Evaluating Health Instruction Material Aids

Instructional material aids generally refer to such items as textbooks, films, cassettes, slides, videotapes, computer software, still pictures, and other things that are helpful in the teaching process. In those instances when they are used for individual instruction, interactive software or self-paced units may in themselves serve as the basic program.

Materials for use in health education should be selected on a systemized basis with thoroughness and awareness of need. Materials should not be selected before the objectives and content of the health education program have been determined.

Health teaching aids should be evaluated on a regular basis, before and after the selection process. Educators should use existing devices for evaluation or create their own. The information collected should be kept on file for reference as needed. Fig. 14-5 illustrates a sample audiovisual evaluation form. Appendix H contains a more detailed instrument that teachers may find more useful. These procedures may be modified to meet specific teacher needs. Teachers also may observe students' reactions to material aids in terms of interest and motivation to obtain a rapid assessment.

Teaching aids should be free of sexual, racial, ethnic, and other biases. Suggestions and criteria for assessing such matters may be found in Chapter 13 and Appendix H.

Resource speakers are considered a type of instructional aid and should be evaluated. Resource speakers should not be selected haphazardly. It is best if the teacher knows the speaker and has heard previous presentations made by her/him. Speakers should be oriented before their presentation and should be evaluated after their presentation. These questions are useful in the assessment process:

- Was the presentation biased or slanted?
- Was the presentation appropriate for the age level addressed?
- Was the presenter well organized?
- What objectives were met by the presentation?
- How did the presenter engage or involve the students?

Students should be asked to respond to the question, "What did you learn from this person?"

Teachers should inform building principals in advance when planning to use an outside resource person. Teachers waive their right of administra-

AUDIOVISUAL EVALUATION FORM

Film   Videotape   Other

Title:

Length:

Year produced:

Production source/publisher: Cost:

Description of content:

Intended audience (age/grade):

Intended teaching purpose(s):

Main ideas and/or skills presented:

Production rating		Encircle	
Photography	Excellent	Good	Poor
Sound	Excellent	Good	Poor
Vocabulary	Excellent	Good	Poor
Acting	Excellent	Good	Poor

Contents rating		
Accurate and authentic	Yes	No
Correlated with curriculum	Yes	No
Presents needed facts	Yes	No
Stimulates pupil activity	Yes	No
Free of racial, ethnic, gender bias	Yes	No

Types of learning   Check
Developing concepts (knowledge)

Values clarification (attitudes)

Critical thinking

Skills/practices

Others

List particular strengths or weaknesses:

FIG. 14-5 Audiovisual evaluation form.

tive support if problems occur with a resource speaker and the principal was not notified *before the event.*

Evaluating Health Instruction Methods

As in other subject areas, the methods teachers use in the classroom are fundamental to the successful achievement of the established objectives in health education. Therefore teachers must continually assess the procedures they use.

One phase of methods evaluation involves the selection of appropriate teaching procedures before instruction starts. Information found in Chapter 12 provides guideline questions that are helpful.

These five rather simple techniques can help in assessing the effectiveness of health instruction methods:

- Teachers observe pupils' reactions and check their own feelings of effectiveness. Experienced teachers know when instruction is going well and when a method or activity is going flat.
- Teachers ask students to respond orally or in writing to these questions:
  "What did you learn today about *(topic)?*"
  "How did you feel when we used *(method/activity)?*"
  "If you were going to teach today's lesson to your friends, how would you do it?"
- Use a tape recorder to capture the dialogue and tone of the class during the lesson. Analyze the tape.
- Videotape the lesson if feasible. Analyze the tape.
- Ask the principal, nurse, coordinator, or another teacher to attend class to evaluate a specific lesson or lessons.

Student Grades in Health Instruction

Pupils and parents alike show great interest in report cards. Pupils generally like to be rated in comparison with their classmates and with their own previous marks. The typical elementary schoolchild expects to get a report on his or her status and progress. Often, the report card provides parents with their only information about what is taught in the school. It can reflect school philosophy and serve as an important medium for communication with the public. Although many elementary schools use the letter system (A-B-C-D-F) for reporting pupil progress and performance, the trend toward more functional and descriptive methods continues.

Many elementary schools today attempt to assess a pupil's progress in light of that pupil's capacities and abilities. Such an approach usually means that a pupil is marked as O for making outstanding progress, S for making satisfactory progress, and U for making unsatisfactory progress. One promising tool for health education is the "Healthy Me Report Card" being developed in Austin, Texas. Students review their progress individually with a classmate and in conferences every 6 weeks. They record progress toward physical, mental, and social objectives with non-letter grade symbols in each classroom as part of a school nurse-led program. The emphasis is on the progress, or educational growth, of each child as an individual. At the elementary school level, progress reports are usually supplemented by parent-teacher conferences. These conferences should bring about a sharing and comparing of knowledge and observation that contributes to a better understanding of the child's performance in school.

The parent-teacher conference should use the report card simply as a point of departure for analyzing the pupil's strengths and needs for improvement. Usually, if parents are objective, they can provide the teacher with significant information about a child's health attitudes and practices in and around the home. Skilled teachers make the most of these all-too-brief conferences.

Principles of grading pupils. There is no single best way to assign grades in health instruction at all grade levels. These are some basic principles teachers can use to assure that grading is fair for all students.

- Grades should reflect *actual class achievement.* Factors such as neatness, spelling, handwriting, and absence do not reflect achievement in health learning and therefore should not be considered as criteria for grading. However, teachers should encourage and strive for quality of performance.

- Grades should be based on a variety of data, including tests, student activities, and student involvement. Having a variety of evaluation activities will provide the teacher with a more valid means of assigning grades than reliance on a single assessment.
- Grades should *not* be used for disciplinary or manipulatory purposes. Such practice detracts from the importance of health learning.
- Students should be well acquainted with the grading method to be used by the teacher.
- Pupils should have access to their grade progress throughout the study of health. They should be provided guidance in ways to improve their standing at any time.

Basis for grading. Teachers should collect sufficient data of student achievement to permit valid judgments to be made. As noted previously, it *is better to use several kinds of indicators of progress rather than one.* Remember, individuals learn in different ways and react to measuring techniques differently. Some students can express themselves and are articulate orally but have little success on written examinations.

Grades should be based on a combination of performances including the following:

- Daily and oral or behavioral indications of learning presentations
- Homework and projects
- Written assignments or graphics
- Examinations and quizzes
- Extra credit opportunities
- Pupil and team self-evaluation

Obviously, some of these activities are too advanced for young children, but many can be modified to provide for a combination of performances. Primary grade students can give simple oral reports. They can use art or print materials to illustrate health learnings, and use new computer programs to "write" simple narratives. They can also role play learning.

Problems in grading. Grades in health education should be based on pupil achievement in terms of knowledge gained, projects and activities completed, and general quality of work performed. Health attitudes and practices, however important in terms of objectives, are virtually impossible to use for grading purposes. Doing so can result in external motivation, untruthfulness, and other problems. Also, determining specific student progress is difficult.

For some pupils, grades become the end purpose of study. These pupils become preoccupied with the process of memorizing subject matter and consider the grade the end result. They do not apply their knowledge to personal decisions that will positively affect their health.

Teachers also can create problems in grading. Some use grades for disciplinary or motivational purposes when other methods fail. Others lack objective, clearly defined criteria for assigning grades. Some teachers tend to grade students with whom they work well higher than the student's achievement warrants. There should be clear communication between the student and teacher about the teacher's grading policy and grading scale. Having open communication about grading will help avert possible problems before they arrive.

Occasionally, personality conflicts between a pupil and teacher can cause the pupil to be penalized when grades are assigned. The problems of discipline and personality conflict must be dealt with as separate issues. Teachers must recognize this potential problem and avoid it.

Many of these problems can be avoided if the teacher is organized, has a well-planned grading system that allows for individual differences, and communicates the proper perspective of grades in the educational process to pupils and parents alike.

WHO EVALUATES?

The answer to the question "Who evaluates?" is based on the answer to the question, "What is to be evaluated?" This chapter deals with evaluating the total school health program. The elementary teacher should not be expected to evaluate the total school health program. This is a major undertaking for which the responsibility should be shared by school administrators, board members, district health or curriculum specialists, teachers, nurses, parents, and in some instances health professionals from the community, local university, and state departments of education.

The teacher is the key person in the evaluation of the instructional program in the classroom. Evaluation of the instructional program includes content, methods, materials, and student progress evaluations. Assistance in this evaluation may come from the principal, nurse, librarian, district health or curriculum specialist, parents, and students.

Effective evaluation is not easy, but it is necessary and can be rewarding. It can result in a teacher feeling like a significant contributor in the development of student, as well as personal, health behavior. Positive community public relations can result when teachers demonstrate pride in their school health programs. More importantly, evaluation enables students to receive improved health instruction and helps them learn to make intelligent decisions about lifestyles that will affect their health.

SUMMARY

Evaluation is a way to determine the worth or value of something. In school health there is need to determine the effectiveness, in terms of process and product, of the total program and its components. These include instruction, services, environment, and coordination.

The teacher has an important role in evaluation. It is limited in terms of the total program, as well as in terms of the services, environment, and coordination aspects. However, the teacher has a major responsibility for determining the impact of the health instruction program on students.

Evaluation of health knowledge objectives can be achieved relatively easily and effectively as long as the instructional objectives are measurable and clearly written. Assessment of health attitudes and practices is more complex and difficult. Teacher observations can be used as indicators of success despite their subjectiveness. These observations should be supplemented by reports from parents and other school personnel. When multiple data sources are used to assess student attitudes and practices, they can be organized to provide objective and fairly reliable information.

The teacher can evaluate student achievement in many ways. The most common means of evaluation is through tests. Teachers would be well advised not to rely on a single source of information for evaluation of student progress. Using a variety of evaluation methods, including tests, student activities, and teacher/parent/school personnel observations, will provide the teacher with a more accurate picture of student progress.

Numerous teaching aids are available for use in health instruction. These aids may include printed, audiovisual, or computer software materials. Guest speakers also may be considered an instructional aid. Regardless of the material aid that is used, each aid should be carefully assessed to ensure that it meets instructional objectives and is appropriate for the grade level, intellectual capacity, and growth and developmental levels of the students. Remember, teaching aids are designed to supplement, not supplant, good health instruction.

Grades are valuable in the health instruction program because they provide student motivation and parent information. They should be based on student achievement. Student attitudes and practices are virtually impossible to grade and therefore should not be a part of the grading system.

QUESTIONS FOR DISCUSSION

1. What is the difference between measurement and evaluation?
2. Why is evaluation important to the school health program?
3. How can parent-teacher-student conferences be used to assess pupil learning in health?
4. What are some key points to consider when selecting instructional aids for health?

5. If you could evaluate only one aspect of the school health services component of the school health program, which one would you select? Why? How might you proceed to evaluate the component that you have selected?

6. Why is it important to have measurable and clearly written health instruction objectives?

7. Explain: Even tests that are purported to be objective, are, in fact, somewhat subjective in nature.

8. What are the specific uses of evaluation in health? Which of these do you consider most important? Explain your response.

9. How are behavioral objectives related to the evaluative procedures and techniques a teacher uses?

10. How can the teacher use standardized tests to evaluate health instruction programs? What are some of the pitfalls of using standardized tests to assess pupil achievement?

11. Can a student's health values be realistically and reliably evaluated? Explain your response.

12. Why should a teacher use multiple sources of data when assessing student attitudes and practices?

13. Why is it important to periodically evaluate teaching methods used in health instruction?

14. Should grades for health be issued to elementary school students? Why or why not? How can progress be summarized?

15. Explain: Evaluation of the school health program is a shared responsibility.

SELECTED REFERENCES

Brown R: Testing and thoughtfulness, *Educ Leadership* 47(4):31-33, 1989.

Christensen PD: An evaluation of quantitative and qualitative assessment techniques on the impact of the SERR curriculum, *J School Health* 55(5):200-204, 1985.

Cleary MJ: Using portfolios to assess student performance in school health education, *J School Health,* 63(9):377-381, 1993.

Contento IR, Kell DG, Keiley MK, Corcoran RD: A formative evaluation of the American Cancer Society "Changing the Course" nutrition education curriculum, *J School Health* 62(9):411-416, 1992.

Dorman S: Evaluating computer software for the health education classroom, *J School Health* 62(1):35-38, 1992.

English J, Sancho A, Lloyd-Kolkin D, Hunter L: *Criteria for comprehensive health education curricula,* Los Alamitos, CA, 1990, Comprehensive Health Education Program, Southwest Regional Laboratory.

Hendricks CM, Peterson F, Windsor R, Poehler D, Young M: Reliability of health knowledge measurement in very young children, *J School Health* 58(1):21-25, 1988.

Iverson DC: Program evaluation versus research: more differences than similarities. In Cortese P, Middleton K, editors: *The comprehensive school health challenge: promoting health through education,* vol 2, Santa Cruz, CA, 1994, ETR Associates.

Kane W: *Step by step to comprehensive school health: the program planning guide,* Santa Cruz, CA, 1993, ETR Associates, Inc.

Maeroff G: Assessing alternative assessment, *Phi Delta Kappan* 73(4):273, 281, 1991.

Mehrens W, Lehmann I: *Using standardized tests in education,* ed 4, New York, 1987, Longman.

Nelson S: *How healthy is your school? Guidelines for evaluating school health promotion,* New York, 1986, National Center for Health Education Press.

Olsen LK, Hambleton R, Simon R, Connell DB, Turner RR, Orenstein D: Development and application of the student test used in the school health education evaluation, *J School Health* 55(8):309-315, 1985.

Robinson J III: Criteria for the selection and use of health education reading materials, *Health Educ* 19(4):31-34, 1988.

Salmon-Cox L: Teachers and standardized tests: what's really happening, *Phi Delta Kappan* 62:631-634, 1981.

Talmage H: Evaluating the curriculum: what, why, and how, *NASSP Bulletin* 57(10):465-468, 1987.

Videto DM: Development of an assessment program. In Mahoney BS, Olsen LK, editors: *Health education teacher resource handbook: a practical guide for K-12 health education,* Millwood, NY, 1993, Kraus International Publications.

VII

APPENDICES

VII

APPENDICES

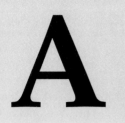

APPENDIX A

HIV Infection/AIDS: Issues for Schools

Supports for Children with HIV Infection in School:
BEST PRACTICES GUIDELINES*

Allen C. Crocker, Alison T. Lavin, Judith S. Palfrey, Stephanie M. Porter, Deirdre M. Shaw, Kenneth S. Weill

CHILDREN with congenital HIV infection are surviving in increasing numbers to reach school age. In the school setting they also join others who have acquired HIV infection, including a significant number of youth now in their teen years. The Maternal and Child Health Bureau, U.S. Dept. of Health and Human Services, requested a review of the circumstances and needs of these children, as well as the challenges experienced by educators and administrators.

The project began with a questionnaire and phone call survey of the nation's largest school districts. Principal information from this survey is reported in two companion publications in the same issue of *Journal of School Health*. Of particular interest was the finding that schools now have partial information only about HIV infection among the student enrollment. The amount of disclosure regarding the diagnosis, or information transfer, is much reduced. Where such knowledge does exist, the maintenance of confidentiality is earnestly pressed. Hence,

generalizations about the number and distribution of students with HIV infection may be difficult for a school or district to make. This greater current anonymity, when present, has some shielding effect regarding possible prejudicial experiences.

In the survey work, and in clinical and personal contact, these children emerged as engaging and valued, and their families as caring and courageous. Society is evolving regarding beliefs and attitudes about pediatric HIV infection; this is true as well for educational and health care professionals. These Guidelines are formulated to be supportive to all of these parties, and to be instructional and protective. We hope that these objectives are achieved. **Duplication and distribution of the BEST PRACTICES GUIDELINES are authorized and encouraged.**

Material on which the Guidelines are based derives from a legal and cultural legacy relating to personal opportunity in the setting of special needs. This setting includes especially the Section 504 amendment of the Rehabilitation Act of 1973, Public Law 94-192, Public Law 99-457, the Americans with Disabilities Act, and precepts of the Centers for Disease Control and Prevention and

*Crocker AC et al: Supports for children with HIV infection in school: best practices guidelines, *J Sch Health* 64(1):32-34, 1994. American School Health Association, Kent, OH.

475

OSHA. The leadership is noted as well of homologous publications from the American Academy of Pediatrics, Child Welfare League of America, American Bar Association, National Association of State Boards of Education, and the American Association of University Affiliated Programs for Persons with Developmental Disabilities. The history of these rules and benchmarks is presented in *HIV Infection and Developmental Disabilities: A Resource for Service Providers.*

In areas where the prevalence of HIV infection is low, or in smaller school districts, it may be appropriate to combine some Advisory Committee and curriculum activities for HIV infection with other school health and education functions. Where higher prevalence creates greater urgency, a richer and more diverse representation would be needed.

I. PREPARATION OF THE SCHOOL SETTING

1. An **advisory committee on HIV-related issues** shall be established for the school district and commissioned by the Superintendent. Membership shall be comprised of health professionals (community physicians, school nurses, and other child and adolescent health workers), parents, teachers, students, persons with HIV infection, attorneys, advocates, and persons representing diversity in the community. At regular meetings, matters shall be discussed concerning HIV that relate to administrative practices, legal and policy questions, educational programs, universal infection control standards, and student welfare. Consultants shall be used as appropriate.

2. The school district shall adopt **policy statements of relevance to students with HIV infection,** in collaboration with the advisory committee. These shall conform with state and federal laws and regulations, and draw on state-of-the-art medical and scientific information from appropriate government sources, model documents from national organizations, research studies, and expert consultation. It may be helpful to use public hearings to gain input into these matters. The policy statements shall then be disseminated to all administrative levels, made available to staff, students, parents, and community leaders, and included in student and parent handbooks. They shall be reviewed at yearly intervals.

3. **Staff education and inservice training** concerning the issues of HIV infection, including transmission, prevention, civil rights, mental health, and death and bereavement, shall be carried out at least annually for all school personnel, including the school board. The program content shall be determined by a multidisciplinary team of appropriate individuals that shall include families of children with HIV infection and also persons with HIV infection. It shall aim to affect staff members' knowledge, feelings, attitudes, behavior, and acceptance of people who are HIV positive. For new employees, this education shall be built into the orientation program, and offered within three months of hire. Teachers responsible for instruction of students regarding HIV infection shall receive specific inservice training.

4. **Universal precautions relating to bloodborne infections,** as adapted for schools, shall be in effect. School clinics and nursing offices shall follow OSHA guidelines for health care facilities. It is the responsibility of the school district to ensure adequate gloves, bleach, sinks, and disposal containers. There shall be systems of quality assurance or monitoring to document compliance with universal precautions in all school settings. These matters shall be featured in the staff education program.

5. The school district shall provide **education relating to the prevention of HIV infection for students in grades K-12,** within the context of a quality comprehensive school health program. Delivered by trained teachers, health educators, and nurses, it shall be developmentally, culturally, and linguistically appropriate. It shall actively promote abstinence as the best protection, and shall also offer explicit information about the use and availability of condoms. Acknowledgement shall be given to the special needs of adolescents regarding emerging sexual orientation. An additional effect of this effort should be to enhance understanding of

the needs of students, staff, and others who are infected with HIV.

II. THE ENROLLMENT PROCESS

6. The parent, guardian, or student shall decide **whether or not to inform the school system** about HIV status or other health conditions. They may support the transfer of this information by another professional or person, including a personal physician or a case manager, but only in the context of strict informed consent procedures. It shall be recognized that disclosure of HIV status often involves revealing related facts, such as medication, parent condition, transmission, and other matters. Under no circumstances shall parents, guardians, or students be required by school personnel to obtain HIV testing or to release information about HIV test results on the student or other family members.

7. Few, if any, personnel in the school or school district shall **receive information about the HIV status** of a student. Determination of those who are to be informed is the prerogative of the parents, guardian, or student, and shall be made in the setting of consideration about special health care or social services that are needed while the student is in school. The terms "need to know" and "right to know" are usually not applicable for school staff, and are best eliminated. Specific release of information by the family as they wish it is obviously acceptable, but such material should then be treated confidentially regarding further dissemination.

8. **Information about a student's HIV status** shall not be included in the educational record, usual school health records, or any other records that are accessible to school staff beyond those the parents, guardian, or student has determined should know. Documentation about specific health care given by school nurses, counselors, clinicians, or other personnel to students with HIV infection shall be put in special health records kept in locked files. If the child changes schools, a plan for the transfer of these records shall be developed with the family and student.

III. ASSURANCE OF APPROPRIATE SERVICES

9. The **design of an individual student's program** shall be based on educational needs and not the status regarding HIV infection. The curriculum and other activities of a student with HIV infection shall be modified only as required per developmental and/or personal health needs. Exclusion or segregation of students solely on the basis of HIV infection is never appropriate.

10. **In-school health services** shall be provided as needed, including special regimens required because of HIV infection, but the origin of these programs shall not be identified at the classroom level. Specific "health care plans" may be formulated by school health personnel for students with symptomatic HIV infection. Notification for families about the presence of other communicable diseases at school (e.g., chicken pox) that place students at risk shall be forwarded universally. Particular notification will be given to families who have informed key school personnel about HIV infection. School nurses, and others with appropriate training, shall participate in counseling for students regarding HIV matters, including the availability of testing. They shall establish quality linkages with youth-serving HIV programs in the community that can provide culturally sensitive, age-appropriate medical, mental health, social, and drug treatment services.

IV. OTHER ELEMENTS

11. School administrators shall provide culturally sensitive information, technical assistance/consultation, and access to resources on HIV issues to the **school's parents and families** through PTAs and other parent organizations. Appropriate issues for discussion include prevention, confidentiality, classroom educational services and related supports, and community resources.

12. Relevant to existing federal and state statutes, teachers, school health professionals, and other qualified employees shall have the **right to employment and confidentiality** regardless of their own HIV status or other health conditions. If they choose to disclose their HIV status to students or other staff this shall not have ramifications regarding employment.

Transmissibility of HIV Infection: What We Know in 1993*

Kenneth McIntosh

WHEN the HIV epidemic began just over a decade ago, it was a mystery where the virus had come from and how it was transmitted. Because HIV infection is a fatal illness, transmissibility remains an area of serious concern. Fortunately, it is not an easy disease to contract, and there are only certain, clearly identifiable ways in which it is transmitted. HIV infection is difficult to contract because of two factors. First, in only a limited number of ways can the virus be passed from one person to another: a) injection of infected blood directly into the blood stream or through the integument, or b) passage of the virus by blood or other infected secretions through mucous membranes. Second, even with the defined mechanisms of transmission, the disease is not passed every time these events occur.

ACCEPTED MODES OF TRANSMISSION

Blood to blood (or blood through skin). Table 1 presents accepted modes of blood and blood product transmission of HIV and estimates risks of an individual contracting HIV through each type of exposure. Extreme rates (greater than 50% risk) are associated with transfusions and transplants where the dose of virus is likely to be high.

Sharing needles and treatment with blood products carry a 5%-10% estimated risk. Risk from a needle stick is low (0.4%) based on actual data. Finally, nonpercutaneous exposure of blood to skin and mucous membranes carries a very low risk. In CDC studies of health care workers, no cases studied prospectively existed where transmission occurred without a break in the skin or a break in some surface.

Transmission from other body fluids. The virus also can be passed between two people who have close enough contact to mix body fluids, often with some contact with the vasculature of the recipient. Work in hospital settings helped clarify which fluids (in addition to blood) can contain HIV in sufficient amounts to pose a threat of infection: semen, vaginal secretions; cerebrospinal fluid; amniotic fluid; synovial fluid; pleural, peritoneal, and pericardial fluids; and others visibly contaminated with blood.

Table 1 also demonstrates how the virus can be transmitted from one individual to another by body fluids. Sexual transmission represents a major mode of transmission. Male-to-male transmission poses a moderate risk (2%-5%). Since semen carries the virus, and since homosexual activity may lead to abraded mucous membranes and perhaps some bleeding, opportunity exists for infection. Male-to-female transmission carries a 0.1% to 2% risk and is substantially higher than female-to-male transmission (Table 2). This difference probably occurs because semen can harbor a larger dose of virus than vaginal secretions do, and because

*McIntosh K: Transmissibility of HIV infection: what we know in 1993, *J Sch Health* 64(1):14-15, 1994. American School Health Association, Kent, OH. Reprinted with permission.

TABLE 1 Accepted Modes of Transmission of HIV

Modes	Estimated risk*
PERCUTANEOUS	
Needle stick from HIV-infected patient	Low (0.4%)
Sharing needles	High
Infected blood product (Factor VIII, before 1981)	High
Infected blood, plasma, platelet transfusion	Extreme
Infected organ transplant	Extreme
MUCOUS MEMBRANE	
Exposure to blood	Very low
GENDER	
Heterosexual	
Male to female	Moderate
Female to male	Low
Homosexual	
Male	Moderate
VERTICAL	
Intrauterine	Very high (10%)
Perinatal	Very high (15%)
Breastfeeding	Very high (?14%)

*Estimated rates (single event): Extreme > 50%; very high 10% to 50%; high 5% to 10%; moderate 2% to 5%; low 0.5% to 2%; very low 0.1% to 0.5%.

the exposed area of mucous membrane is larger in the woman.

Vertical transmission from mother to fetus and newborn carries a high transmission rate. During the intrauterine period the rate probably approaches 10%. With all the bleeding and sharing of fluids during the birth process, it is likely that a 15% risk of transmission exists when the baby passes through the birth canal. While controversial, an analysis of multiple studies from *Lancet* suggests breast feeding by HIV-infected women carries with it as high as a 14% risk of transmission to the breast-fed baby.

TABLE 2 Heterosexual Transmission of HIV

	N	N HIV+	%
Female partners of infected males	307	61	20
Male partners of infected females	72	1	1
Odds ratio 17.5			

From Padian et al. *JAMA*, 366:1664-1667, 1991.

NOT ACCEPTED MODES OF TRANSMISSION

Throughout the AIDS epidemic, periodic fears emerge about how the HIV virus might be spread. Some fears simply involve theories by lay hypotheses. Others derive from case reports in medical journals. Such sporadic infections need substantiation that the secondary instance was caused by the same virus. Lacking such proof, individual reports should be considered "undocumented." Some modes of transmission, while theoretically possible, are now not accepted as real risks. Worldwide experience suggests they are unlikely to represent *bona fide* means of infection. Undocumented concerns include biting; kissing; sports injuries; close contact in school rooms or day care; normal family life; insect bites; contact of healthy intact skin with infected blood; contact with "oozing" nonbloody skin lesions; and contact with urine, feces, saliva, sweat, tears, and other nonbloody body fluids.

CONCLUSION

The real concern for schools involves proper handling of blood in significant amounts. If schools follow the CDC recommendations for Universal Precautions, they can report to school boards, PTAs, teachers, and local news media that they have taken every prudent measure. HIV is hard to spread. Fear of HIV transmission should not stand as a barrier to school admission of children with HIV infection.

APPENDIX

B

Partial Health Units

THE illustrative partial units in this appendix cover a broad approach to pupil health interests and needs. Topical health areas included are community, consumer, dental, disease control (including AIDS), drugs (including alcohol and tobacco), fitness, family, mental, nutrition, safety and first aid, and vision and hearing. This material follows the basic principles identified in Chapter 11.

Teachers can select or modify the material contained herein for use with students when developing health units. Content is presented in outline form to provide the teachers a time-saving format.

More detailed knowledge can be obtained from a variety of sources to ensure current and accurate content (see Chapter 13 and Appendixes D, E, and F). Teaching activities to achieve selected objectives can be chosen from the examples in Chapter 12 or from other sources after the unit framework (teacher scope and sequence) has been constructed from the material in this appendix.

Every effort has been made to present this resource material in a manner that will be useful to teachers regardless of how many times they change grade level teaching assignments.

PARTIAL HEALTH UNITS

Community Health Unit

OUTLINE OF CONTENT

Physiological

Definitions: public health (community health), preventive medicine, preventive health care, immunity, screening tests

Community health problems: communicable diseases (sexually transmitted disease, tuberculosis, upper respiratory infections, hepatitis, measles, German measles, polio, rabies, tetanus, typhoid, mononucleosis, food infections); noncommunicable diseases (heart and circulatory disorders, cancers and leukemias, emphysema and chronic bronchitis, diabetes, arthritis, allergies, ulcers, skin conditions); blindness and other eye defects; dental problems; maternal and child health; mental health; suicide; drug abuse, including alcohol and tobacco; accidents; malnutrition; pollution, accidental pollution

Psychological

Why public health? lack of public understanding of purposes and activities of community health personnel and organizations; improvement of individual, family, and group health; preventive approach, need for group efforts to prevent or correct certain health and accident problems

Social

Public and voluntary health organizations: U.S. Public Health Service; state health department; local health department; World Health Organization; The American Heart Association; The American Cancer Society, Inc.; The American Lung Association; The National Society to Prevent Blindness; The National Association for Mental Health, Inc.; The National Association of Hearing and Speech Agencies; National Clearinghouse for Drug Abuse Information; The Planned Parenthood Federation of America, Inc.; The American Social Health Association; The American National Red Cross; The American Diabetes Association, Inc.; National Sickle Cell Anemia Research Foundation; Muscular Dystrophy Association of America, Inc.; The National Safety Council

Community health programs and activities: prevention and control of diseases (communicable and chronic); infant and maternal deaths; malnutrition; mental illness; drug abuse; accidents; dental and oral defects; hearing problems; blindness and vision disorders; suicide; accidental poisoning; environmental pollution; natural disasters

Public health personnel: increasing need for community health personnel; career opportunities in public health (health educator, public health physician, public health dentist, public health nurse, sanitarian, environmental specialist, safety consultant, mental health counselor, hospital administrator, nurse, and dental hygienist)

Professional societies: medical society, dental society, osteopathic association, optometric association

Spiritual

Values: value of public health in protecting, maintaining, and improving human health

Moral issues: Should citizens contribute money voluntarily to private agencies and through taxes to official organizations for the support of community health programs? Is each individual responsible for the health and safety of others?

Continued.

PARTIAL HEALTH UNITS: COMMUNITY HEALTH UNIT—cont'd

CONCEPTS

Concept	Application of health definition
1 Public health programs protect, maintain, and improve the health of people in a community through group effort.	Social-spiritual
2 As members of the community, children and youths are entitled to public health services and resources.	Social-spiritual
3 Public health agencies and organizations function at the local, state, national, and international level.	Social
4 Community health programs are carried out by official and voluntary organizations.	Social-spiritual
5 All citizens can help improve individual, family, and community health by supporting the work of health departments and health agencies.	Social-spiritual-psychological
6 Public health departments generally are not adequately supported by tax funds.	Social
7 Through careers in the health sciences, many individuals contribute to the health of the community.	Social-spiritual-psychological
8 The school health program is part of the overall community health program.	Social

OBJECTIVES FOR GRADES K TO 3

Domain	Objectives for students	Basic concepts
Cognitive	**1.** Explains the general purpose of public health	1
	2. Identifies several local health agencies	3, 4
	3. Explains why public health services should be available to everyone	1, 2
	4. Lists reasons why people should support community health programs	5, 6
Affective	**1.** Displays interest in learning more about health departments and agencies	3, 4
	2. Asks questions about who pays for community health programs	5, 6
	3. Asks questions about the work of physicians, school nurses, dentists, public health workers, and other people concerned with community health	2, 5, 7
	4. Shows interest in the value of group effort in preventing and solving certain health problems	1, 5
Action	**1.** Cooperates with teachers, school nurses, and others involved in the school health program	2, 5
	2. Assists wherever possible with school or community health efforts	2, 5

OBJECTIVES FOR GRADES 4 TO 6

Domain	Objectives for students	Basic concepts
Cognitive	**1.** Lists the major purposes of health departments	1
	2. Cites examples of public health organizations and agencies	3, 4

PARTIAL HEALTH UNITS: COMMUNITY HEALTH UNIT—cont'd

OBJECTIVES FOR GRADES 4 TO 6—cont'd

Domain	Objectives for students	Basic concepts
Cognitive—cont'd	**3.** Explains chief differences between official and voluntary health agencies	4
	4. Understands the importance of school health and other community programs concerned with child health	2
	5. Explains the need for community support of public health programs	5, 6
	6. Cites examples of health careers	7
	7. Lists health problems that may be prevented or solved by community health programs	1
Affective	**1.** Displays interest in the basic philosophy of public health	1
	2. Asks questions about the different programs and aims of official and voluntary health agencies	3, 4
	3. Accepts the need for community health programs and personnel	1, 2, 5
	4. Appreciates the need for financial and other public support of community health programs	1, 5, 6
	5. Shows interest in and concern for major community health problems	5
	6. Displays interest in career possibilities in public health work	7
Action	**1.** Seeks reliable sources of information regarding community health programs	2, 5
	2. Visits the health department and other local agencies when recommended as part of a community health project	2, 5
	3. Cooperates with school health projects	2, 8

OBJECTIVES FOR GRADES 7 TO 8

Domain	Objectives for students	Basic concepts
Cognitive	**1.** Discusses the importance of public health for all communities	1
	2. Lists reasons why community health programs are especially important for children and youth	2
	3. Explains the nature and functions of health departments at the local, state, national, and international levels	3
	4. Explains differences between official and voluntary agencies with regard to personnel, financing, relative emphasis on services, research, and education	4, 5, 6
	5. Compares the need for the group approach with that of private medical and dental care	1, 7
	6. Cites the reasons for public support for community health programs	5, 6
	7. Identifies major health agencies in the community by purpose, activities, and location	3, 4
	8. Explains the three basic phases of the school health program	8

Continued.

PARTIAL HEALTH UNITS: COMMUNITY HEALTH UNIT—cont'd

OBJECTIVES FOR GRADES 7 TO 8

Domain	Objectives for students	Basic Concepts
Affective	**1.** Appreciates the social values of community health programs	1, 5
	2. Shows interest in the quality of local community health services	2, 5, 6
	3. Asks questions about the most pressing needs in public health at the local, state, national, and world levels	3, 6
	4. Appreciates the purpose of the school health program	8
	5. Offers opinions on the responsibility of government to provide effective public health programs for all citizens	1, 3, 6
	6. Displays interest in differences between official and voluntary health agencies	4, 5
	7. Inquires about public health career opportunities	7
	8. Shows concern for the quality of the school health program	8
Action	**1.** Cooperates whenever possible with special projects of the health department or voluntary agencies	2, 4, 5
	2. Talks with parents about the values of a good community health program	1, 3, 5, 6
	3. Takes part in school health projects	2, 8
	4. Seeks information on needed legislation for the improvement of local, state, and federal public health programs	1, 4, 5, 6
	5. Seeks information on educational requirements and opportunities in one or more public health careers	7

PARTIAL HEALTH UNITS

Consumer Health Unit*

OUTLINE OF CONTENT

Psychological

Definitions: consumer health (economics of health), health products, health services, self-diagnosis, self-medication, prevention, effects of health products, nature of various health examinations, medical care, health insurance

Why consumer health? self-diagnosis and self-medication; advertising inducement; spiraling costs; misinformation and lack of information; vast amount of scientific information; preventive medicine concept

Why do people purchase health products and services? self-diagnosis and self-medication; less expensive treatment; improvement of health status; advertising; the need for help; condition minor in nature; ignorance of hazards; lack of information; religious beliefs; friend or peer recommendations

Why do people go to quacks? lonely; refusal of physician to listen to problems; hopeless case for treatment or cure; mysticism; the desire for pleasant, easy cure; physician's limitation in dealing with problem; psychological problems

Budgeting for health care: estimate of yearly costs of products and services; insurance; emergencies

How to act as an intelligent health consumer: skeptical; critical and analytical of what is read, seen, or heard regardless of source; initiator of investigation; identification of quacks and quackery, fads and frauds, or suspicious of same; knowledge about when to call or visit doctor, dentist, or other health professionals; knowledge about how to select a doctor, dentist, and other health professionals; knowledge of what to expect from a physician, dentist, and other health professionals, and also what is expected by these individuals of patient; application of sound criteria in purchase of health products or services; reading of labels; knowledge of where to seek, how to obtain, and how to seek reliable health information; initiative taken to go to protection agencies and organizations for help

Social

Health products

Arthritis—cures, devices

Athletics and fitness—drugs, vitamins, weight reduction, mechanical aids, spot reducers, vibrator machines, isometric versus isotonic exercises

Cancer—Krebiozen, Laetrile, Hoxsey treatments and cures

Cosmetics—deodorants, hormone creams, and wrinkle removers

Dental—toothpaste, toothbrushes, Water Pik, and others

Drugs—use and misuse, aspirin, over-the-counter, and others

Hearing—hearing aids, mail order of aids

Mechanical—bust developers, rupture devices, silicones, vibrators, seawater

Nutrition—vitamins, food additives, weight control diets, organic and natural foods

Tobacco—smoking cures and filters

Vision—glasses by mail, sunglasses, and contact lenses

Others—cough and cold remedies, laxatives, preparations for hemorrhoids, skin blemish removers, allergic conditions, bad breath, hair restorers, and impotency cures

---

*See also Cornacchia HJ, Barrett S: *Consumer health: a guide to intelligent decisions,* ed 5, St Louis, 1993, Mosby–Year Book.

Continued.

PARTIAL HEALTH UNITS: CONSUMER HEALTH UNIT

OUTLINE OF CONTENT—cont'd

Social—cont'd

Health services

Health examinations—what, when, who does, frequency, and cost

Types of health specialists

    Physicians—general practitioners, internal medicine, pediatrics, or surgery

    Dentists—general practice, orthodontics, oral surgery, and others

    Psychologists—general, clinical, and family counselor

    Also podiatrists, pharmacists, optometrists, osteopaths, and nurses

Hospitals and clinics—types, licensing, standards

Health insurance—types, services, costs

Criteria for selection of health specialists—license to practice, preparation and training, member of local health profession society in good standing, night calls, discussion of fees in advance, opinion of others, hospital affiliation

When to call health specialist—complaint or symptoms too severe to be endured; persistence for more than few days; symptoms' repeated return; accident

Role of business in health products: self-control versus governmental control; psychology of selling; mass communication media; analysis of advertising

Protection of the consumer

Agencies and organizations

    Government—FDA, FTC, U.S. Postal Service, health departments

    Professional—AMA, ADA, American Pharmaceutical Association

    Voluntary—cancer, arthritis, heart, lung, Better Business Bureau

Laws—federal Food, Drug and Cosmetic Act; advertising limitations; labeling of products

Education—formal and informal, sources of information from family, friends, and school

Sources of reliable health information: reputable individuals, such as physicians or dentists; also scientific books, magazines, and publications; questions such as, "What is reputation, training, and experience of authors and sources?" "Is there a profit motive involved in the writing?" "Are the data accurate and up to date?" "What do other sources say about the topic or material?"

Quacks and quackery

Definition—boastful pretender to medical skills; a charlatan; ignorant or dishonest practitioner

Motivational factors—money, power, prestige

Identifying factors—disregard or misinterpretation of scientific evidence; acceptance of money for worthless or questionable treatments, products, or services

Why some quack cures work? spontaneous remission of some diseases, placebo effect, psychosomatic effect of encouragement of patient

Spiritual

Values: differing healing philosophies or cult values—medicine, osteopathy, acupuncture, herbalists, faith healers, Christian Science, Jehovah's Witnesses, and others

What is the effect of differing values on the selection, purchase, and use of health products and services?

Moral issues: Is an ethical code needed in advertising, in the business world? Is an ethical code needed in medicine, dentistry, and the health professions? What should be the relationship between medical practitioners and patients?

PARTIAL HEALTH UNITS: CONSUMER HEALTH UNIT—cont'd

CONCEPTS

Concept	Application of health definition
1 Health products and health services may have beneficial and harmful effects on individuals.	Physiological
2 Self-diagnosis and self-medication and the use of quacks and quackery may be hazardous and costly to individuals.	
3 Individuals purchase and use health products and services for a variety of reasons.	Psychological
4 Wise decisions regarding the selection, purchase, and use of health products and services necessitate individuals acting as "intelligent health consumers."	
5 The use of scientific information is necessary for the effective evaluation, selection, purchase, and use of health products and services.	
6 Appraisal, selection, purchase, and use of health products and services are influenced by past experiences and the environment.	Social
7 There are reliable and unreliable sources of health information.	
8 The community provides a variety of organizations, agencies, and laws to protect the health consumer.	

OBJECTIVES FOR GRADES K TO 3

Domain	Objectives for students	Basic concepts
Cognitive	1. Identifies people who can help promote and protect one's health	8
	2. Identifies people who can help when injured or ill or who prescribe medicines	8
	3. Explains the reasons for caution when taking medicines	1, 2, 4
	4. Lists the reasons adults should help supervise the taking of medicines	1, 4, 8
	5. Concludes that medicines may be necessary at times for health	1, 4, 7
	6. Explains the effect of mass media on the purchase and use of health products	3-6, 8
	7. Identifies a variety of sources of health information	4, 5, 7
Affective	1. Asks questions about the hazards involved in taking medicines without adult supervision	1, 4, 8
	2. Is attentive to the discussion regarding the dangers involved in the consumption of unfamiliar food and liquids	1, 3
	3. Supports the need for medicines when prescribed by physicians	1, 2, 4, 8
	4. Is attentive to discussion about the various people who can help when a person is ill or injured	8
	5. Displays interest in the effect of the mass media on the purchase and use of health products	3-6 8

Continued.

PARTIAL HEALTH UNITS: CONSUMER HEALTH UNIT—cont'd

OBJECTIVES FOR GRADES K TO 3—cont'd

Domain	Objectives for students	Basic concepts
Action (observable)	**1.** Informs parents, teachers, and others when injured or not well	8
	2. Demonstrates skill in analyzing mass media advertising	3, 4, 7, 8
	3. Seeks health information from a variety of sources	4, 5, 7
(nonobservable or delayed)	**4.** Refrains from taking medicine without adult supervision	1, 4, 8
	5. Refrains from consuming unknown foods and liquids	1, 2, 4

OBJECTIVES FOR GRADES 4 TO 6

Domain	Objectives for students	Basic concepts
Cognitive	**1.** List the hazards of self-diagnosis and self-medication	2
	2. Identifies reliable sources of health information	7
	3. Explains factors that affect the reliability of health information	4, 5, 7
	4. Lists the types of mass media that may have an influence on the purchase and use of health products and health services	6
	5. Is able to apply criteria in analyzing labels and advertisement of various kinds	1, 3, 6, 8
	6. Explains the influences of friends and family on the plans to purchase and use health products and health services	6, 8
	7. Identifies a variety of health products that are used in self-treatment and explains problems related to their use	1, 2, 8
	8. Discriminates between reliable and unreliable health information and advertising	7
	9. Cites examples of agencies and organizations that protect the consumer	8
Affective	**1.** Displays interest in the need for reliable sources of health information	5, 7
	2. Asks questions in regard to the hazards of self-diagnosis and self-medication	1, 2
	3. Accepts the need for establishing criteria for use in the selection of health products and health services	4, 5, 7
	4. Is aware of the significance of the influence of religious beliefs, customs, superstitions, fads, and family on consumer health purchasing	3, 6
Action (observable)	**1.** Seeks reliable sources of health information when necessary	5, 7
	2. Seeks appropriate health services personnel when injured or ill	8
	3. Can analyze labels and advertisements using established criteria	3, 4, 8
(nonobservable or delayed)	**4.** Avoids self-diagnosis and self-treatment	2
	5. Uses established criteria when making decisions to purchase and use health products	4, 5, 7

PARTIAL HEALTH UNITS: CONSUMER HEALTH UNIT—cont'd

OBJECTIVES FOR GRADES 7 TO 8

Domain	Objectives for students	Basic concepts
Cognitive	1. Identifies a variety of health products available and explains their effects on individuals	1
	2. Recalls the laws that attempt to protect the health consumer	8
	3. Explains quacks and quackery and their effects on people	1-4
	4. Describes the nature, frequency, cost, and significance of health examinations	2, 4, 8
	5. Identifies the various types of health specialists and services available to help individuals	2, 4, 8
	6. Compares the healing or health treatment philosophies or cults found in society	6, 8
	7. Identifies the criteria to follow to become an "intelligent health consumer"	4
	8. Compares the role of a variety of community organizations and agencies in protecting the health consumer	8
	9. Identifies the reasons why individuals purchase and use a variety of health products and services	3
Affective	1. Accepts the need for reliable sources of health information	4, 5, 7
	2. Displays interest in the need for skepticism in consumer health	4
	3. Supports the need for laws and community organization and agencies to protect the people in consumer health	8
	4. Is supportive of the need to understand quacks and quackery	1, 2, 4, 5, 7
	5. Is attentive to the need for health examinations	1, 8
	6. Listens to the discussion regarding the types of health specialists available	2, 8
	7. Asks questions about the different healing and health treatment philosophies	6
Action (observable)	1. Seeks reliable sources of health information	4, 5, 7
	2. Is skeptical regarding health information from advertising and other sources until it can be verified	4, 5, 7
(nonobservable or delayed)	3. Uses the criteria for an "intelligent health consumer" when considering the purchase or use of health products and health services	4
	4. Seeks the help of community agencies and organizations when information or assistance is needed in regard to health products and health services	8
	5. Refrains from the purchase and use of health products that are detrimental to one's health	1, 2

PARTIAL HEALTH UNITS

Dental Health Unit

OUTLINE OF CONTENT

Physiological

Structure and functions of teeth

Structure—divisions—crown (top), neck, root (base); layers—enamel, dentin, cementum, pulp

Types and numbers of teeth—primary (deciduous), twenty (incisors, cuspids, molars); permanent, thirty-two (eight incisors, four cuspids, eight bicuspids, twelve molars)

Functions—chewing; speech; appearance; primary hold spaces for permanent teeth

Diseases and Disorders

Dental caries—tooth decay

Causes—bacteria plus sugars = acid = decay; pathway—enamel, dentin, pulp; plaque is a gelatin-like substance adhering to teeth where bacteria collect and act on food

Contributing factors—heredity, tooth structure, saliva, bacteria, sugar

Periodontal diseases

  Gingivitis—inflammation of gums; pyorrhea—advanced gingivitis involving gums and bone

  Symptoms—"pink" toothbrush from bleeding gums; red, swollen, tender gums

  Causes—irritation from dental calculus that results from substances secreted by bacteria in plaque; sharp edges of badly decayed teeth, worn-out fillings rubbing on gums; malocclusion, poor nutrition, systemic diseases

  Prevalence—major cause for tooth loss over 35 years

Malocclusion—improper bite; effects—interferes with chewing, speech, and appearance; harder to clean

  Causes—heredity, acquired factors—pressures on teeth including thumb sucking, mouth breathing, tongue twisting, lip sucking, and sleeping habits

Stains—(1) extrinsic—food pigments, tobacco and caffeine, metallic dusts; green stain in children—bacteria, fungi plus inorganic elements (calcium); (2) intrinsic—within tooth structure; caused by pigments in blood; imperfect tooth development

Abscess—infection affecting blood, lymph vessels, and nerves in pulp; caused by neglect of decay

Halitosis—bad breath; caused by poor dental hygiene, carious teeth, unclean mouth, periodontal disease, pyorrhea, infection, possible gastrointestinal problems, and others

Plaque—sticky, almost colorless layer of organized microcolonies of bacteria in a gelatinous substance; clings to teeth, especially near gum line

Calculus—calcified (hardened) plaque, also known as tartar, mineral deposits around gum lines that harden and are removed only by scaling

Nutrition

Need for balanced diet from basic food groups; excess vitamins and minerals (calcium and phosphorus) not generally needed

Good "snack" food—no or minimal sugar and refined sugars: (1) corn chips, popcorn, nuts, cheese, hard boiled eggs, raw fruits and vegetables, unsweetened fruit juices, milk; (2) detergent foods (cleanse teeth and provide exercise), raw vegetables—carrots, celery, green peppers, cauliflower, radishes, raw fruits—apples, oranges

Poor "snack" foods—candy, pastry, cookies, chocolate milk, sweetened beverages, syrups, jellies, and carbohydrate foods that are sticky and cling to teeth

PARTIAL HEALTH UNITS: DENTAL HEALTH UNIT—cont'd

OUTLINE OF CONTENT—cont'd

Psychological

Why oral health? proper tooth functioning necessary for chewing; speech; affects appearance, acceptance and rejection by peers; prevents diseases and disorders

Care of teeth and proper oral hygiene by individuals

Toothbrushing—clean teeth and mouth; eliminate food particles; remove plaque; massage; prevent stains and calculus, when to brush, after eating; if not, "swish and swallow"

Toothbrush—rinse and let dry in sunlight; selection—three to four rows of soft bristles in straight line

Mouthwash—removes excess particles; can do with water; commercial products not effective in removing film, neutralizing acids, curing halitosis, or preventing decay; temporarily freshens and sweetens mouth; may mask disease

Flossing for plaque control with waxed or unwaxed floss between the teeth

Dentifrice—no best kind; possibly one with fluoride

Fluorides—possible use in toothpastes or powders, in tablet form, in bottle water

Periodic dental visits

Proper nutrition

Avoidance of injuries and accidents—follow safe practices; avoid detrimental habits—thumb-sucking, tongue-thrusting, chewing hard objects

Social

Problem: 90% or more of all children and youths need better oral health

Care of teeth

By dentist who examines mouth for diseases and disorders, fills cavities, provide bridges and crowns, applies topical application of fluoride, cleans and polishes teeth, replaces missing teeth, teaches dental hygiene, helps with orthodontia, and uses x-ray films, different types of fillings—silver amalgam, gold, porcelain—mouth mirror and explorer, scaler, drill, and other equipment; when to visit dentist—preferably twice yearly

By community through fluoridation of water supply (1 ppm); sodium fluoride is a chemical that becomes part of the tooth and strengthens it against decay; applied by topical application, in water, and by taking pills; favorable claims—inexpensive; reduces tooth decay significantly; reaches all people; reduces costs of repairs; unfavorable claims—forces people to drink fluoridated water against their will; dangerous to health; type of socialized medicine

Types of dentists—general practice, orthodontia, prosthetics, periodontia, pedodontia, oral surgery, and endodontia

How to select dentist—call local dental society for three names; call reputable hospital and ask chief of dental services for suggestions; see if dentist is member of local dental society; does postgraduate work; attends clinics and does not advertise; ask family dentist in previous community; call nearby dental school; check neighbors who are satisfied with dentist

Effects of mass media including advertising on dental health products and services

Dental health insurance

Cost of products and services for dental care

Continued.

PARTIAL HEALTH UNITS: DENTAL HEALTH UNIT—cont'd

OUTLINE OF CONTENT—cont'd

Spiritual

Values: importance of dental health to self-identity; self-esteem

Moral issue: fluoridation of water supply; responsibility of individual and community (including schools) to help needy students without funds obtain dental health products and services

CONCEPTS

Concept	Application of health definition
1 Positive oral health and oral health neglect have differing effects on individuals.	Physiological
2 Most dental diseases and disorders are preventable and treatable.	
3 Differing motivations influence decisions regarding dental health.	Psychological
4 A variety of environmental factors are important contributing causes of dental diseases and disorders and influence the purchase and use of dental health products and services.	Social
5 The community has a responsibility in the control and prevention of oral health diseases and disorders.	
6 All individuals are affected by dental health neglect.	
7 Community resources are available to assist individuals with oral health problems in varying kinds and amounts.	
8 Dental health is affected by an individual's values.	Spiritual

OBJECTIVES FOR GRADES K TO 3

Domain	Objectives for students	Basic concepts
Cognitive	**1.** Explains ways to clean teeth, as well as when this action should take place	1, 2
	2. Recalls foods that help in promoting dental health	1, 2
	3. Identifies the different teeth and their functions	2
	4. Lists ways to prevent tooth decay or other disorders	1, 2, 4, 7
	5. Explains the proper way to brush teeth	1, 2
	6. States the practices that may be harmful to oral health	4
	7. Identifies the reasons why the dentist or dental hygienist can help individuals	2, 7
	8. Explains the procedures to follow in preparing an inexpensive dentifrice	2
	9. Explains the proper way to floss the teeth	1, 2
Affective	**1.** Displays interest in brushing teeth properly	1, 2
	2. Listens carefully to the ways to prevent tooth decay and other disorders	2, 4

PARTIAL HEALTH UNITS: DENTAL HEALTH UNIT—cont'd

OBJECTIVES FOR GRADES K TO 3—cont'd

Domain	Objectives for students	Basic concepts
	3. Asks questions about teeth and their functions	2
	4. Brings pictures to class, or is attentive to discussion of foods that may be helpful and detrimental to dental health	1, 2, 4
	5. Talks about the need for daily health care	1, 2, 6
	6. Accepts the dentist or dental hygienist as a friend	2, 7
Action	1. "Swishes and swallows" when brushing the teeth is not possible	1, 2
(observable)	2. Prepares an inexpensive dentifrice in the classroom	2
(nonobservable)	3. Eats nutritious foods, including "snack" foods	1, 2
able)	4. Attempts to refrain from harmful dental health practices	2, 8
(nonobservable or	5. Brushes teeth properly after eating when possible	1, 2, 4
able or	6. Attempts to floss teeth once daily	1, 2, 4
delayed)	7. Uses own toothbrush and gives it proper care	1, 2, 4
	8. Visits the dentist periodically	2, 7

OBJECTIVES FOR GRADES 4 TO 6

Domain	Objectives for students	Basic concepts
Cognitive	1. Explains the type, structure, function, growth, and development of teeth	1, 2
	2. Identifies ways in which oral health influences appearance and social relationships	3, 4
	3. Summarizes the procedures to follow for dental health	2, 5, 7
	4. Lists the factors that control and prevent tooth decay	2, 5, 7
	5. Recalls the diseases and disorders that occur from oral health neglect	1, 4, 6
	6. Explains the causes of tooth decay	1, 2, 4
	7. Identifies the reasons for topical application of fluorides to the teeth	1, 2, 6
	8. Recites the services that a dentist can render to an individual	5, 7
	9. Demonstrates the proper way to floss teeth	1, 2
Affective	1. Accepts the responsibility for personal dental health care	1, 3, 6-8
	2. Talks about the need for dental care including periodic dental visits	1, 2, 7, 8
	3. Displays interest in wanting to learn more about the role of nutrition in dental health	1, 2, 4
	4. Listens to discussion about the importance of the individual's oral health	2, 6, 8
	5. Reaches the conclusion that dental health plays a role in the social acceptance and self-esteem of individuals	2, 4, 8
	6. Supports the need for flossing teeth as an important preventive dental health procedure	1, 2, 6

Continued.

PARTIAL HEALTH UNITS: DENTAL HEALTH UNIT—cont'd

OBJECTIVES FOR GRADES 4 TO 6—cont'd

Domain	Objectives for students	Basic concepts
Action	**1.** "Swishes and swallows" when brushing is not possible	2
(observable	**2.** Refrains from using teeth in hazardous ways	1, 2
and non-	**3.** Eats nutritious foods and especially detergent foods	1, 2, 4
observ-	**4.** Limits the consumption of sweets	1, 2, 4
able)		
(nonobserv-	**5.** Attempts to floss teeth daily	1, 2
able or	**6.** Brushes teeth properly after eating when possible	1, 2
delayed)	**7.** Visits the dentist periodically	1, 2, 7
	8. Uses care in the treatment and storage of the toothbrush	2

OBJECTIVES FOR GRADES 7 TO 8

Domain	Objectives for students	Basic concepts
Cognitive	**1.** Compares the claims made for and against fluoridation	3, 5
	2. Compares advertising claims of the product effectiveness on dental health	4
	3. Identifies the community resources available to assist in dental health care	7
	4. Explains the use of x-ray films in the dental care process	1, 2, 7
	5. Lists the importance of teeth to appearance, speech, and digestion	1, 3
	6. Lists the variety of dental specialists and the kinds of services they render	7
	7. Compares the costs of dental services with and without proper dental care	4, 7
	8. Identifies sources of reliable and current scientific dental health information	4, 5, 7
Affective	**1.** Talks about fluoridation of the water supply as a moral issue	7, 8
	2. Displays interest in learning about dental health and its relations to social acceptance and appearance	3
	3. Asks questions regarding the costs of dental services with and without preventive dental care	4, 7
	4. Discusses the place of dental health in an individual's values	8
	5. Is attentive to information presented about the variety of dental specialists and auxiliary dental personnel available in the community	4, 7
	6. Asks questions about the benefits and hazards in the use of x-ray films by dentists	1, 2, 7

PARTIAL HEALTH UNITS: DENTAL HEALTH UNIT—cont'd

OBJECTIVES FOR GRADES 7 TO 8—cont'd

Domain	Objectives for students	Basic concepts
Action (observable and non-observable)	**1.** Is able to differentiate between reliable and unreliable dental health information	4, 7
(nonobservable or delayed)	**2.** Supports community efforts to make dental health services and products available to needy students	6
	3. Is able to make wise decisions regarding personal dental health care	3, 4, 8

PARTIAL HEALTH UNITS

Disease Control Unit

OUTLINE OF CONTENT

Physiological

Definitions: disease, communicable disease, noncommunicable or chronic disease, host (focus), avenue, susceptible, acute, chronic, antigen, antibody, immunity, pathogen, vaccine, serum, antibiotic, resistance, epidemic, transmission, vector

Types

Communicable—respiratory—colds, bronchitis, pneumonia, influenza; tuberculosis, "strep" throat; infectious hepatitis; mononucleosis; skin diseases; sexually transmitted diseases; AIDS; gastrointestinal—food poisoning; childhood—measles, mumps, smallpox, chickenpox, and poliomyelitis

Causes—microorganisms—bacteria (sexually transmissible diseases, tetanus, tuberculosis, "strep" throat); viruses (colds, infectious hepatitis, HIV); fungi (ringworm); protozoa (dysentery, malaria); parasites (worms)

Contributing causes—hereditary; lack of sanitary procedures; individual susceptibility; lack of nutritious food; and exposure

Modes of transmission: air, food, water, direct contact, needle sharing, insects, and animals

Portals of entry—mouth, nose, breaks in skin, and other body openings

Disease process—fever, pain, infection, redness, loss of weight, bleeding, shortness of breath, and other signs and symptoms

Body defenses—skin and mucous membranes; fever; white blood cells; antibodies

Noncommunicable—heart, cancer, allergy, arthritis, diabetes, mental illness, and acne

  Contributing causes—heredity; food; dysfunctioning of body organs; irritations; pressures; and a variety of other environmental factors

Effects—damage, destruction, and altered function of cells, tissues, organs, and systems; illness; disability; death

Prevention and treatment—individual—isolation, health habits; community—control of environment through laws and regulations; immunization; sanitation; water and food controls; drugs and medicines; surgery; radiation; and medical help

Psychological

Effects of diseases and disorders on mental and emotional health: adjustment of self and others; success in social world

  Importance of early diagnosis and treatment

  Individual responsibility in disease control

  Fear of disease, disability, and death

  Disease and death in the family

Social

School and community responsibilities for prevention and control

Control procedures: laws and regulations; sanitary procedures; immunizations; availability of health department services; adequate supply of physicians and hospital and clinic facilities

Sources of help: physicians; health departments; voluntary health agencies

PARTIAL HEALTH UNITS: DISEASE CONTROL UNIT—cont'd

OUTLINE OF CONTENT—cont'd

Spiritual

Values: appreciation of healthy body; differing religious and healing philosophies toward disease

Moral issues: ethics of disease prevention and treatment on the part of individuals and the community; attitudes toward people with disease; appreciation of healing arts; concern for others

CONCEPTS

Concept	Application of health definition
1 Diseases can cause disability, temporary or permanent, and sometimes death.	Physical-social-spiritual
2 Communicable diseases are caused by germs and may be transmitted directly or indirectly from an infected person, or host, to someone who is not immune.	Physical-social
3 For a communicable disease to spread, there must be a host (focus of infection), an avenue or means of transmission, and a susceptible person.	Physical-social
4 Noncommunicable—sometimes called chronic—diseases are caused by hereditary factors, metabolic disorders, aging, diet, stresses, lifestyles, and unknown influences.	Physical-social
5 Elementary school pupils should be routinely immunized against measles, polio, German measles, diphtheria, whooping cough, tetanus, and mumps.	Physical-social
6 Communicable diseases are often spread in elementary schools because of inadequate control measures at home and in school.	Physical-social-spiritual
7 Diseases occur more often among poor children and contribute to lower learning achievement for all elementary pupils.	Social-spiritual
8 Adequate medical care, public health services and personal responsibility are necessary for control of disease in a community	Social-spiritual

OBJECTIVES FOR GRADES K TO 3

Domain	Objectives for students	Basic concepts
Cognitive	1. Tells why it is important to avoid disease	1, 7
	2. Explains the reasons for covering coughs and sneezes in the classroom	2, 3, 6
	3. Lists the ways a communicable disease may be spread	2, 3, 6
	4. Identifies some communicable diseases fairly common among children	2, 3, 6
	5. Tells why it is necessary to be immunized against certain diseases	2, 3, 5
Affective	1. Displays interest in preventing and controlling disease	1, 6
	2. Asks questions about different kinds of diseases	2, 4
	3. Is aware of spread of "catching diseases" among children	2, 3, 5, 6
	4. Accepts the value of immunizations	3, 5
	5. Appreciates the effect of illness on learning	7
Action	1. Covers coughs and sneezes and follows other sanitary practices in school	2, 6
	2. Cooperates in school or community immunization program	5, 6
	3. Remains at home when ill with a communicable disease	6
	4. Talks about reasons why poor people are sick more often than others	7

PARTIAL HEALTH UNITS: DISEASE CONTROL UNIT—cont'd

OBJECTIVES FOR GRADES 4 TO 6

Domain	Objectives for students	Basic concepts
Cognitive	1. Lists the major disease causes of death for all Americans and for children of elementary school age	1
	2. Explains the differences between communicable and chronic diseases	1-4
	3. Cites the differences between a vaccine and a serum	2, 5
	4. Gives reasons for higher rate of disease among poverty groups	4, 7, 8
	5. Lists the communicable diseases against which elementary pupils should be immunized	5
	6. Explains causes, prevention, and medical care for major chronic diseases	1, 4, 8
	7. Identifies ways that AIDS can and cannot be transmitted	2, 3, 8
	8. Identifies way that the AIDS virus damages the immune system	1, 3
Affective	1. Is attentive to information presented on methods for individuals, families, and communities to control diseases	1, 3, 4, 8
	2. Accepts the responsibility for taking steps to avoid spreading disease to others	3, 5
	3. Appreciates the responsibility of parents to have children immunized against certain diseases	5, 6
	4. Supports local, state, and federal efforts to control communicable and chronic diseases	8
	5. Displays interest in government plans for health care of older people and other Americans	1, 7, 8
	6. Accepts responsibility to reduce the risk of getting AIDS	1, 3, 8
Action	1. Follows personal and family practices to prevent disease	1, 6
	2. Seeks medical care when symptoms of illness are present	1, 8
	3. Cooperates with school policy by keeping immunizations up to date and staying home when ill	3, 5, 6, 8
	4. Reports symptoms of illness to parents, teacher, or school nurse	3, 6

OBJECTIVES FOR GRADES 7 TO 8

Domain	Objectives for students	Basic concepts
Cognitive	1. Explains specific causes, preventive measures, and community control of heart diseases, cancers, stroke, and other major diseases	1, 4, 7, 8
	2. Cites differences between communicable and noncommunicable and acute and chronic diseases	1, 2, 4
	3. Lists recent medical and health science advances that have helped control disease	1, 8
	4. Illustrates ways that individuals, families, and communities can help control diseases	1, 6, 8
	5. Identifies signs and symptoms of AIDS and other sexually transmitted diseases	1, 3

PARTIAL HEALTH UNITS: DISEASE CONTROL UNIT—cont'd

OBJECTIVES FOR GRADES 7 TO 8—cont'd

Domain	Objectives for students	Basic concepts
Cognitive—cont'd	6. Identifies reasons that abstinence is the best way for young people to avoid getting AIDS	8
	7. Lists reliable sources of information about AIDS	8
Affective	1. Appreciates the fact that some diseases can be controlled more easily than others	1, 4, 5, 8
	2. Displays interest in plans to provide better medical and hospital care for all Americans	1, 7, 8
	3. Realizes the importance of immunizations for self-protection and the protection of others	3, 5
	4. Appreciates the role of medical science in identifying cures for disease	2, 4, 5, 8
	5. Supports government and other research efforts to improve preventive and control measures for disease	1, 8
	6. Accepts responsibility for having periodic medical checkups	1, 8
	7. Realizes the ways that people's lives change when they get the human immunodeficiency virus (HIV)	1, 8
Action	1. Has regular medical checkups	1, 8
	2. Has all routinely recommended immunizations	3, 5, 6
	3. Participates in personal and family practices to prevent diseases	1, 6
	4. Avoids smoking, drinking, drug use, and other practices that may cause illness	1, 7
	5. Avoids or minimizes physical, chemical, or emotional stresses that may cause disease	1, 4
	6. Uses social skills to avoid contracting HIV	8

PARTIAL HEALTH UNITS

Drug Unit
(Including Alcohol and Tobacco)

OUTLINE OF CONTENT

Pharmacological

Definitions: drug; drug use, misuse, and abuse; addiction; dependency; habituation; tolerance; toxicity; slang terms; tobacco; alcohol; alcoholic beverages; alcoholism

Alcohol synonyms: ethyl alcohol, ethanol

Identification of abused drugs: technical help needed

Classification of drugs:

   Legal and illegal

      Legal—over-the-counter and prescription; alcohol legal for certain age groups, tobacco

      Illegal—marijuana, heroin, cocaine and other drugs; alcohol illegal for certain age groups

   Pharmacological

      Stimulants—amphetamines, tobacco, coffee, cocaine, crack

      Depressants (sedatives-hypnotics)—alcohol, barbiturates, inhalants, marijuana

      Psychedelics—LSD, psilocybin, peyote, STP

      Narcotics—heroin, morphine, opium, codeine, methadone

      Tranquilizers—Thorazine, Compazine, Serpasil

      Over-the-counter—aspirin, ibuprofen, acetaminophen, antihistamines, cough medicines, diet pills, sleeping pills

   Common or trade name (brand) and generic (chemical) identity

Alcoholic beverages: distilled spirits (40% to 50%)—whiskey, brandy, scotch, gin, vodka; wine (12% to 20%); beer (4%)

Tobacco: cigars, cigarettes, pipes, smokeless tobacco

Physiological

The nervous system

Drug effects: dependent on dose response, biologic variability, potency, tolerance, body size

Medical uses: dependent on drug used

Abuse potential: physical and psychological dependence, tolerance

Alcohol

   Short-term effects: intoxication, reaction time slowed, released inhibitions and relaxation at low doses, dulling effects at high doses; also, absorption, metabolism, excretion, brain effects

   Long-term effects: alcoholism, liver malfunction, brain damage

Tobacco

   Short-term effects: stimulation, irritation of mucous membrane, improvement in short-term performance, chronic use affects interchange of O_2, CO, CO_2

   Long-term effects: lung cancer, oral cancer, emphysema, heart disease, and other circulatory disorders

Duration of action: dependent on drug used

Method of administration: pills, capsules, injections, sniffing, liquid, smoking, chewing

PARTIAL HEALTH UNITS: DRUG UNIT (INCLUDING ALCOHOL AND TOBACCO)—cont'd

OUTLINE OF CONTENT—cont'd

Benefits

Alcohol: antiseptic, diet stimulation (small amounts), tonic when prescribed by physicians

Tobacco: stimulation

Psychological

Why people use, misuse, and abuse drugs: curiosity; personal conflicts—insecurity, escape, boredom, rebelliousness: kicks; peer pressure; search for identity-adulthood; rejection of culture including schools; TV; commercial exploitation

Why people don't use: alcohol—religion, no wish to impair physical/mental health, do not like taste, personal convictions against use; tobacco—odor, cost

Characteristics of potential drug abusers: high-risk youths are those with behavioral problems at school with mild conduct disorders; lack of self-confidence; may be self-centered and self-indulgent

Alternatives to drugs: athletics and recreational activities; counseling and group therapy in personal development; improved communications; social service participation; political service activities; intellectual motivation—reading, discussion, creative games; participation in creative art activities; philosophic discussion on ethics, morality, values; spiritual involvement; survival training

Social

Patterns of drug use and abuse: classification of users and abusers

Nature and extent of drug use and abuse: legal and illegal; youth (alcohol—60% to 90%; tobacco—40% to 60%), adults

Factors affecting drug use and abuse:

Conflicts in reality—escape, values

Economics—business and communication media

Social and political climate

Youth lifestyles—counter-culture, youth identity, adolescent revolt

Role of home, school, community: prevention, control, treatment, and rehabilitation

Rehabilitation and treatment: multimodality concept

Crisis intervention

Detoxification

Aftercare

Pharmaceutical—cyclazocine, methadone

Psychiatric—individual counseling in psychiatric hospital

Psychosocial—check for local programs

Religious—Teen Challenge, AA

Courts and the law: laws; enforcement procedures and problems; criminal justice process

Community resources: federal, state, and local government agencies—FTC, FDA, DOE, OSAP, NIAAA, NIDA; private sources; mass media and the business world; education; laws and enforcement; facilities—crisis centers, clinics, hotlines, ongoing groups, self-help groups; drug abuse council or committee

Continued.

PARTIAL HEALTH UNITS: DRUG UNIT (INCLUDING ALCOHOL AND TOBACCO)—cont'd

OUTLINE OF CONTENT—cont'd

Identification of drug abusers

Observations of signs and symptoms

General and specific—change in attendance, discipline, and performance; unusual activity or inactivity; deterioration of personal appearance and health habits; unpredictable outbreaks of temper

Characteristics of potential users

Tell-tale evidence

Peer identification, self-identification, clinical test

Spiritual

Values: developing a value system; self-identity and self-concept

Moral issues: implications of use and abuse of drugs on self, home, and community; drug use by students and adults; commercial interests; the mass media; the sale of drugs; the justice of laws controlling drugs; individual and community responsibilities for drug abusers; the job market for rehabilitated drug abusers or drug abusers in industry

CONCEPTS

Concept	Application of health definition
1 Drugs differ in kind and degree; they have multiple uses with a variety of effects on individuals.	Pharmacological
2 Proper use of drugs may be beneficial to individuals, the family, and the community.	
3 Improper use of drugs may result in health and safety problems to individuals, the family, and the community.	
4 Numerous factors and forces influence the availability, as well as the use and misuse of legal and illegal drugs by individuals and the community.	Psychological-social
5 The individual, the family, and the community have interrelated and reciprocal responsibilities to help control the availability, prevent the misuse and abuse, and assist individuals who become misusers and abusers of drugs in society.	Social
6 The use and misuse of drugs by individuals involve moral principles and issues and are related to one's sense of values, as well as to the humane and just treatment of all people in society.	Spiritual

PARTIAL HEALTH UNITS: DRUG UNIT (INCLUDING ALCOHOL AND TOBACCO)—cont'd

OBJECTIVES FOR GRADES K TO 3

Domain	Objectives for students	Basic concepts
Cognitive	**1.** Identifies drugs commonly used	1
	2. Illustrates ways common drugs are used by individuals	1
	3. Lists beneficial effects of drugs	2
	4. Identifies substances that can be harmful or misused	3
	5. Lists responsible people who can help when medicines are needed	2, 3
	6. Explains why medicines should be taken under supervision of parent as prescribed or recommended by a physician or dentist	4
	7. States conditions under which individuals show lack of responsibility when using medicine	5
	8. Cites ways in which individual shows respect for drugs	5
Affective	**1.** Is aware of differences between alcohol and other drugs and of their usage by individuals	1, 4
	2. Displays interest in learning about the beneficial, as well as harmful, effects of drugs	2, 3
	3. Desires to use drugs in useful and responsible ways	4, 5
	4. Shows interest in discovering people who can help when medicines are needed	5
Action (nonobservable or delayed)	**1.** Takes medicines and drugs only under responsible supervision	3
	2. Refuses to accept substances from strangers	3-5
	3. Refrains from use of drugs, except medicines prescribed and recommended	2, 6

OBJECTIVES FOR GRADES 4 TO 6
(INTRODUCE ALCOHOL/TOBACCO AT THIS LEVEL)

Domain	Objectives for students	Basic concepts
Cognitive	**1.** Identifies varieties of drugs used by individuals	1
	2. Lists reasons for drugs in society	3
	3. Explains medical uses of commonly used drugs	2
	4. Explains physiological effects of some of the commonly used drugs	1
	5. Lists reasons persons react differently to chemicals contained in drugs	1
	6. Cites examples of misuse and abuse of drugs	3, 4
	7. Identifies difficulties or possible problems from misuse and abuse of drugs	3
	8. Explains why misuse and abuse of drugs may start early in life	4
	9. Lists ways society tries to protect individuals from abuse of drugs	4
	10. Identifies ways to protect self against misuse and abuse of drugs	3, 4
	11. Analyzes information about drugs on TV, in newspapers and magazines	4, 5

Continued.

PARTIAL HEALTH UNITS: DRUG UNIT (INCLUDING ALCOHOL AND TOBACCO)—cont'd

OBJECTIVES FOR GRADES 4 TO 6
(INTRODUCE ALCOHOL/TOBACCO AT THIS LEVEL)—cont'd

Domain	Objectives for students	Basic concepts
Affective	**1.** Asks questions about problems involved with misuse or abuse of drugs	3, 5
	2. Seeks further information about community efforts to help people who misuse and abuse drugs	5
	3. Discusses ways to protect self against misuse and abuse of drugs	5, 6
	4. Expresses desire to use drugs responsibly and usefully	2, 6
Action	**1.** Takes medicine and drugs only under responsible supervision	3
(nonobservable or delayed)	**2.** Refrains from use of drugs, except medicines prescribed or recommended, until grown up	3
	3. Refuses to use illegal drugs	3, 6
	4. Starts to develop own practices and habit patterns to protect self against misuse and abuse of drugs	3, 4

OBJECTIVES FOR GRADES 7 TO 8
(INCLUDING ALCOHOL AND TOBACCO)

Domain	Objectives for students	Basic concepts
Cognitive	**1.** Recalls varieties of drugs used by people	1
	2. Describes how medicines can be used to benefit individual	2
	3. Lists variety of individual and social factors that influence misuse and abuse of drugs	4
	4. Interprets role of business and advertising in sale of drugs	4, 5
	5. Identifies differing effects of variety of drugs on the body	1, 4
	6. Compares benefits of smoking, drinking, and using drugs with possible detrimental effects	2, 3
	7. Identifies reasons why people do and do not use, misuse, and abuse drugs	4
	8. Illustrates ways to cope with social and emotional pressures of life other than through use of drugs	4, 5
	9. States procedures used by communities to control availability, sale, and use of drugs	5
	10. Discusses need for development of a value system.	6
Affective	**1.** Shows interest in comparisons of benefits and detrimental effects of alcohol, tobacco, and drugs on individuals and society	2, 3
	2. Gives opinions regarding role of business and advertising in sale and availability of drugs	2, 3, 5
	3. Asks questions about alternatives to drug use	4, 5
	4. Displays interest in developing a value system	6
	5. Is aware and discusses long-term results from frequent and regular misuse and abuse of drugs	4, 5

PARTIAL HEALTH UNITS: DRUG UNIT (INCLUDING ALCOHOL AND TOBACCO)—cont'd

OBJECTIVES FOR GRADES 7 TO 8—cont'd

Domain	Objectives for students	Basic concepts
Action (nonobservable or delayed)	1. Make judgments about drugs and drug users after reviewing all aspects of problem	4-6
		6
	2. Seeks to discover one's own identity and purpose in life	5
	3. Participates in a school-education-information program	4, 5
	4. Seeks help from school personnel in having a drug problem	3-6
	5. Refrains from regular use of drugs that may lead to dependency, disease, or disability	3-6
		3-6
	6. Avoids use of drugs that may affect ability to think clearly and react normally	
	7. Refuses to use illegal drugs	

PARTIAL HEALTH UNITS

Fitness

OUTLINE OF CONTENT

Physiological

Definitions: physical fitness, physiology, physiology of exercise, body mechanics, muscular system, cardiovascular system, strength, speed, endurance, posture, rest, sleep

Exercise

Muscles—types—skeletal (external body control), heart, and smooth (internal organs—blood vessels, glands, others)

Characteristic—contractility when stimulated by nerves

Skeletal muscles:

Structure—attached to bones of body

Locations—back, chest, abdominal wall, arms and legs

Functions—movement of body (exercise), maintenance of posture, production of body heat

Kinds of exercise—many forms; light to heavy, including walking, running, bicycling, hiking, sports, recreational activities

Effects—muscle tone, strength, size and control of skeletal muscles; aid in individual's meeting demands of daily activity; help in creation of reserves for emergencies and safety; aid in cardiovascular, respiratory, and nervous system functioning; improvement of posture, stamina, endurance; relief from tension; fun and pleasure; aid in mental health; control of body weight; one factor involved in heart disease (Fig. B-1)

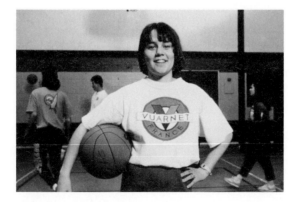

FIG. B-1 Fitness should be promoted. (Courtesy Michigan Department of Education.)

PARTIAL HEALTH UNITS: FITNESS—cont'd

OUTLINE OF CONTENT—cont'd

Rest, relaxation, and sleep

Requirements—need for a balance of work, play, rest, relaxation, and sleep daily; sleep requirements—8 to 10 hours daily for children and adolescents

Fatigue—types—physical, mental, or emotional

Causes—intense or prolonged physical activity; psychologic factors—nervousness, boredom, worry, tensions and stress, emotions, noise; infections and disease conditions

Effects—less attention, drowsy, irritability, lowered resistance to fatigue, less alert to possible hazards—more accident prone, less ability to perform effectively

Procedures for relaxation—sleep, rest, exercise, change of activity, music, art, and other pleasurable activities

Body control

Dependent on proper exercise; practice of bodily movements; adequate rest, relaxation, and sleep; nutrition; and other environmental factors

Poor posture because of lack of, or improper, exercise, rest, and sleep; poor habits of sitting, standing, reclining, or walking; improper nutrition; ill-fitting clothes and shoes

Psychological

Importance of relaxation in helping endure stress

Importance of exercise, rest, and sleep to the individual

Selection of activities to fulfill individual needs

Competition and its psychological effects on children and youth

Games and sports and their provisions for success experiences and self-reliance opportunities

Social

Role of school, home, and community: providing facilities and opportunities for exercise, rest, and relaxation

School curriculum: its inclusion of an education program to help students with postural or exercise problems or to fulfill pupil needs

Social interaction: through games, sport, dance, or other forms of exercise and activity; improvement of teacher-pupil relationships

Spiritual

Values: appreciation of physical fitness, rest, sleep, relaxation, and posture to health and effective living; appreciation of differing attitudes of individuals toward exercise and physical activity

Moral issues: fair play and good sportsmanship in games and sports

Continued.

PARTIAL HEALTH UNITS: FITNESS—cont'd

OUTLINE OF CONTENT—cont'd
CONCEPTS

Concept	Application of health definition
1 Physical fitness is one aspect of total health and requires regular vigorous exercise.	Physical
2 Regular exercise produces good muscle tone and efficient circulation and helps maintain desirable body weight.	Physical-social
3 Everyone needs a balance of exercise and rest for optimal health	Physical-psycho-logical
4 Sports and dance provide opportunities for healthful exercise and pleasant social interaction.	Physical-social-psychological
5 Sound body dynamics improves efficiency and appearance.	Physical-social-psychological

OBJECTIVES FOR GRADES K TO 3

Domain	Objectives for students	Basic concepts
Cognitive	1. Tells why exercise, rest, and relaxation are important for good health	1-4
	2. Identifies ways to relax	3
	3. Recalls pleasant experiences in games or dance activities	4
	4. Identifies the values of good posture and sound body mechanics	5
	5. Explains the importance of rest, relaxation, and sleep to optimal health	3
Affective	1. Appreciates value of exercise, rest, and relaxation in maintaining good health and growth	1, 2
	2. Desires to learn and play games regularly	1, 2, 4
	3. Shows interest in individual and group games and dances	1, 2, 4
	4. Shows interest in using own body most efficiently	5
	5. Is aware of the daily need for rest, relaxation, and sleep	3
Action	1. Takes an active part in games and dances at school and after school	1, 2, 4
	2. Practices good body dynamics in daily activities	5
	3. Sleeps 8 to 10 hours each night and rests occasionally during the day	3
	4. Demonstrates good sportsmanship and a spirit of cooperation in games and dances	4

OBJECTIVES FOR GRADES 4 TO 6

Domain	Objectives for students	Basic concepts
Cognitive	1. Explains physiological reasons for regular, vigorous exercise	1, 2
	2. Understands emotional health values of sports and dance	4
	3. Can demonstrate the basics of functional body movement	5
	4. Lists reasons for adequate rest, relaxation, and sleep	3
	5. Identifies ways to relax at home and school	3

PARTIAL HEALTH UNITS: FITNESS—cont'd

OBJECTIVES FOR GRADES 4 TO 6—cont'd

Domain	Objectives for students	Basic concepts
Affective	1. Appreciates the values of physical fitness as a part of total good health	1, 2, 4
	2. Asks questions about the physiological and mental benefits of exercise	1, 2, 4
	3. Desires to learn more about basic skills, strategy, and rules of sports	4
	4. Is attentive to information on the importance of rest, relaxation, and sleep	3
	5. Appreciates the aesthetic and physiological values of efficient body movement	5
Action	1. Takes an active part in games and dance activities at school	1, 2, 4
	2. Participates in sports after school and on weekends	1, 2, 4
	3. Sleeps 8 to 10 hours each night and rests when fatigued during the day	3
	4. Demonstrates good sportsmanship in sports and dance activities	4
	5. Practices good body dynamics in daily activities	5
	6. Takes time daily to participate in some type of relaxation activity	3

OBJECTIVES FOR GRADES 7 TO 8

Domain	Objectives for students	Basic concepts
Cognitive	1. Explains specific changes in muscular and circulatory systems during exercise	1, 2
	2. Describes mental health values of sports and dance	4
	3. Understands the kinesiology (muscle fuction) of fundamental body movements as in standing, sitting, walking, lifting, pushing, and pulling	5
	4. Cites the physical and mental values of proper sleep, relaxation, and rest	3
	5. Lists health values of regular exercise	1, 2, 4
Affective	1. Believes that physical fitness is one of the values in the good life	1-5
	2. Appreciates the physiological and emotional values of regular exercise	1, 2, 4
	3. Desires to learn more about basic skills, strategy, and rules of sports	4
	4. Appreciates the physical and mental values of adequate rest, relaxation, and sleep	3
	5. Believes that one's appearance and efficiency are enhanced by sound body dynamics	5
Action	1. Participates regularly in sports, dance, or other forms of physical exercise	1, 2, 4
	2. Sleeps 8 to 10 hours each night and rests when fatigued during the day	3
	3. Demonstrates cooperation, leadership, and good sportsmanship in sports or dance activities	4
	4. Maintains desirable muscle development and figure control through exercise	1, 2
	5. Follows principles of sound body dynamics in daily activities	5
	6. Relaxes daily using a satisfactory method	

PARTIAL HEALTH UNITS

Family Health Unit

OUTLINE OF CONTENT

Physiological

Life: purpose and order, a life cycle or pattern of growth, all living things from living things

Characteristics—a beginning, changes, and death; reproduction; need for food, water, air, protection; movement; response to light, sound, cold, pain, danger

Differences—form, structure, functions, life cycle, pattern of growth, dependency and needs, methods of reproduction

Types—plant, animal, and human; plant reproduction—budding, runners, seeds, pollination; animal reproduction—asexually—cell division or fission; sexually—internally with males and females, and externally as in some fish that lay eggs

Human life: human being—unique; rational; decision maker; possessor of freedom, self-awareness, consciousness, and dignity; controller of actions; similarities and differences—heredity, race, size, intellect, ethnic background

Human growth and development

Definitions—"growing," puberty, maturity

Puberty—special growth stage reaching physical adulthood; girls reach this stage 1½ years earlier than boys

Maturity—Growth stage in which the person is more cooperative; has positive sex attitudes; is not easily hurt; is not dominated by moods; is able to meet problems constructively; is able to meet responsibilities; is able to make wise decisions

Cause—action of endocrine glands and their hormones

Results—a variety of physical, emotional, and social changes

Physical—size and shape changes; appearance of secondary sex characteristics; boys—muscle development; hair on face, chest, and pubic areas; seminal emissions; appearance of sex drive; girls—hair under arms and pubic areas; breasts, widening of hips; menstrual cycle; appearance of sex drive

Emotional—physical attraction; fears and emotions with possible moodiness

Social—increase in boy-girl relations; need for friends

Role of heredity—physical characteristics; chromosomes and genes

Human reproduction

Start of life—union of male (sperm) and female (ovum) cells; need for father and mother

Reproductive organs

Male—external—penis, scrotum, testicles; internal—urethra, prostate, seminal vesicles, vas deferens, epididymis

Female—external—labia majora and minora, urethral opening, clitoris, vaginal opening, hymen; internal—vagina, cervix, uterus, oviduct, ovaries, urethra

Other concepts—fertilization, conception, implantation, fetus growth, birth, menstruation, nocturnal emissions, birth control, pubic hair

PARTIAL HEALTH UNITS: FAMILY HEALTH UNIT—cont'd

OUTLINE OF CONTENT—cont'd

Psychological

Understanding self: strengths and weaknesses; personality; worth; ability to succeed, but ability to accept failure; understanding and control of emotions; experience of joy through self-fulfillment; wholesome relations with others; decision making by problem solving process; good use of abilities

Sex drive—normal reaction; perpetuation of population; provides pleasure

Sex behavior in adolescence—interest in one's body and sex normal; questions of sex before marriage; sex deviation—homosexuality, exhibitionism, rape

Factors influencing sex drive—biological makeup; early childhood experiences; parental attitudes; environmental influences

Purpose of family—satisfaction of physical and psychological needs; stability and security important for good mental health; guidance of individuals to adulthood

Social

The family

Nature—size; structure, or composition; culture or ethnic; religion; changes

Types—two parents; one parent; no parents, guardian; stepparents; mixed ethnic

Needs—physical, psychological, and emotional

Functions—different roles because of different types of families and geographical location, but inclusion of sharing and transmission of feelings, ideas, heritage, and income; security by fulfilling needs; aid in education; growth and development; affection, worthy use of leisure time

Role of individual family members—assumption of responsibilities; cooperation in functioning of home; respect of other's rights; consideration; acceptance of differences; trying to understand members; not making unreasonable demands; working together; helping in different ways including financial support; use of constructive ways to solve differences

Family influence on ability of members to make adjustments in society dependent on—cultural background of parents; family dwelling and location; health practices of members; economic status; type of structure; values

Problems and conflicts—parents; siblings; grandparents; money; use of car; discourtesy; failure to assume responsibilities at home, school, or elsewhere; use of drugs; choice and selection of friends; use of time

Boy-girl relations

Development—building of friendships; popularity; qualities boys and girls are seeking

Purpose—sense of belonging; affection; getting along with opposite sex; enjoyment; learning of social behavior

Dating—types; purpose; responsibilities; choosing a date; dating behavior and society's moral code; drinking and drugs

Steady dating—why; advantages and disadvantages; parents' attitudes and reactions

Values of sex in marriage—legal; emotional; social; spiritual

Family planning

Love   *Continued.*

PARTIAL HEALTH UNITS: FAMILY HEALTH UNIT—cont'd

OUTLINE OF CONTENT—cont'd

Spiritual

Values: finding a purpose and meaningfulness in life; a philosophy of life; importance of friendships; interpersonal relationships with adults and peers; influence on personality development; relation to acquisition and use of money

Moral issues: premarital sex; failure to assume home responsibilities; relations with others, including parents

CONCEPTS

Concept	Application of health definition
1 All living things come from living things.	Physiological
2 Individuals in some ways are like all individuals, in some ways like some individuals, and in some ways like no other individual.	
3 The sex drive and reproduction are normal functions of humans.	
4 Maturity is dependent on a variety of physical, social, and emotional factors.	Psychological
5 The family, with its unique features that are subject to change, is the basic unit in American society.	Social
6 Individuals influence and are influenced by the family and its members.	
7 Boy-girl relationships are important preludes to family life and family relations.	
8 Values and moral issues affect attitudes and behaviors regarding the family and sex.	Spiritual

OBJECTIVES FOR GRADES K TO 3

Domain	Objectives for students	Basic concepts
Cognitive	1. Identifies the differences that exist between boys and girls.	2
	2. Concludes the human baby grows and develops inside the mother	1, 2
	3. Recites the correct vocabulary for body parts and body functions	1, 2
	4. Lists the responsibilities to be completed at home and at school	5, 6
	5. Compares how families differ in their composition and functions	5
	6. Recalls that living things come from living things	1
	7. Explains the way parents and family members help individuals	4-6, 8
	8. Identifies the rights of others in need of respect	2, 4-8
	9. Describes the role and responsibilities of family members	5

PARTIAL HEALTH UNITS: FAMILY HEALTH UNIT—cont'd

OBJECTIVE FOR GRADES K TO 3—cont'd

Domain	Objectives for students	Basic concepts
Affective	1. Displays interest in learning about the differences between boys and girls	2
	2. Asks questions about the growth of the baby inside the mother	1, 2
	3. Is interested in wanting to learn the correct vocabulary for body parts and body functions	1, 2
	4. Believes there are responsibilities individuals must give their attention to at school and at home	5, 6
	5. Talks about the differing compositions and functions of families	5, 6
	6. Accepts the conclusion that living things come from living things	1
	7. Believes that parents and family members may be helpful to individuals	4-6, 8
	8. Is supportive of the need to respect the rights of others	2, 5-8
Action (observable) (observable and non-observable)	1. Uses the correct vocabulary for body parts and functions	1, 2 / 5, 6
	2. Assumes responsibilities at school and at home	
	3. Tries to respect the rights of others, including their right to privacy	5, 6

OBJECTIVES FOR GRADES 4 TO 6

Domain	Objectives for students	Basic concepts
Cognitive	1. Identifies the responsibilities that need attention as a family member	5, 6
	2. Lists the rights of others in need of respect	2, 4-8
	3. Is familiar with the terminology used in describing the human reproductive process	1
	4. Summarizes the meaning of puberty and its effect on growth and development	1-4
	5. Explains the responsibilities of all members of a family	5, 6
	6. Recalls that sex is a basic life function	1-4
	7. Identifies the role of heredity in the growth and development of individuals	2-4, 7
	8. Lists the variety of characteristics displayed by the family	5, 6
Affective	1. Believes that it is necessary as a family member to assume home responsibilities	5, 6
	2. Supports the concept that the rights of others must be respected	2, 4-8
	3. Listens to the discussion about puberty and its effect on growth and development	1-4
	4. Displays interest in the responsibilities of all family members	5, 6
	5. Accepts sex as a basic life function	1-3

Continued.

PARTIAL HEALTH UNITS: FAMILY HEALTH UNIT—cont'd

OBJECTIVES FOR GRADES 4 TO 6—cont'd

Domain	Objectives for students	Basic concepts
Affective—cont'd	**6.** Asks questions regarding the role of heredity on the growth and development of individuals	1, 2, 4
	7. Accepts the basic life function of menstruation as an important phenomenon	2, 3
	8. Believes it is necessary to cooperate with other family members to achieve a happy family unit	5, 6
	9. Is aware that families display a variety of characteristics	5
Action (observable and non-observable or delayed)	**1.** Assumes responsibilities at home as a family member	5, 6
	2. Tries to cooperate with family members to achieve a happy family unit	5, 6
	3. Makes efforts to consistently respect the rights of others	2, 4-8
(observable)	**4.** Is able to discuss human reproduction without embarrassment using appropriate terminology	1

OBJECTIVES FOR GRADES 7 TO 8

Domain	Objectives for students	Basic concepts
Cognitive	**1.** Explains the sex drive and its effects on individuals	1-4, 7
	2. Identifies factors that may influence one's sex drive	3, 4, 6-8
	3. Differentiates between physical, emotional, and social maturity	4
	4. Summarizes the human reproductive process from conception through birth	1-3
	5. Concludes that the family is the basic unit of American society and is familiar with its changing roles	5
	6. Identifies the importance of boy-girl relationships and the qualities boys and girls seek in one another	7
	7. Prepares criteria for behavior on dates	3, 4, 7, 8
	8. Compares the advantages and disadvantages of steady dating	7, 8
	9. Discusses sexual behavior in adolescence and before marriage	3-5, 8
	10. Explains the meaning of love	7
	11. Identifies the social, economic, and cultural influences on family life	5, 6, 8
	12. Knows the steps of a problem-solving process to help make decisions about the family and sex behavior	4, 5, 8
	13. Concludes there are moral issues involved in premarital sex	8
	14. Describes the concept and purpose of family planning	3-5, 7, 8
Affective	**1.** Accepts sex as a natural drive and function of individuals that is accompanied by related responsibilities	1-4, 7
	2. Believes that maturity in life is essential for successful living	4

PARTIAL HEALTH UNITS: FAMILY HEALTH UNIT—cont'd

OBJECTIVES FOR GRADES 7 TO 8—cont'd

Domain	Objectives for students	Basic concepts
Affective—cont'd	3. Displays interest in the human reproductive process from conception through birth	1-3
	4. Is sensitive to the acceptance of the family as the basic unit of American society and its changing roles	5
	5. Is aware of the need to develop boy-girl relationships and procedures for building friendships	7
	6. Asks questions regarding the advantages and disadvantages of steady dating	7, 8
	7. Is interested in discussing and preparing criteria for behavior on dates	3, 4, 7, 8
	8. Displays a readiness to want to discuss sexual behavior in adolescence and before marriage	3, 4, 7, 8
	9. Accepts the meaning of love to be more inclusive than physical attraction	7
	10. Is aware of the variety of social, economic, and cultural influences on family life	5, 6
	11. Believes that individuals need to determine the values that help them develop a philosophy of life	8
	12. Is sensitive to the moral issues involved in premarital sex relations, acceptance of responsibilities in the home, and others	3-5, 8
	13. Is aware of the importance of family planning	3-5, 7, 8
Action (observable and non-observable or delayed)	1. Attempts to act as a physically, emotionally, and socially mature individual	4
	2. Tries to become a contributing and effective member of the family	5, 6
	3. Demonstrates the ability to achieve a balance between expression, behavior, and the sex drive	1-4, 7, 8
	4. Develops wholesome relationships with members of the opposite sex	7
	5. Behaves in socially accepted ways with members of the opposite sex	7
(nonobservable or delayed)	6. Attempts to develop values or a value system that will give life meaningfulness	8
	7. Uses the problem-solving process to help make decisions about the family and sex behavior	3, 4, 6

PARTIAL HEALTH UNITS

Mental Health Unit

OUTLINE OF CONTENT

Physiological

Definitions: mental health—adjustment to self and society; faces realities of life; functions effectively
  Mental illness—varying degrees of emotional disturbance; in severe forms—psychoses, neuroses, personality disorders

Growth and development of individual: factors influencing
  Heredity—nervous system and endocrine glands; effect on thinking, feeling, acting
  Environment—economically rich or deprived; stresses and pressure of parents, peers, or teacher; physical atmosphere—housing, climate
  Interrelationship of biological and environmental influences—heredity sets limits; environment determines level of attainment; stress situations may cause biological reactions and anxiety; pleasant environment brings feelings of calmness and tranquility

Psychological

Mentally healthy individual: pursuer of reasonable goals; self-respect; knowledge of being liked and loved; sense of security; ability to think and act rationally; distinguishes between facts and feelings; maintenance of integrity in work and play; ability to work in group; respect for rights of others; faces realities; acceptance of responsibilities

Need of individuals: physical—food, air, water, rest and sleep, housing, clothing, freedom from disease
  Psychological—affection, security, acceptance as an individual, achievement, independence, authority, self-respect, success

Mature personality: a clear self-concept*
  Definition of personality—involving total physical, social, mental, and emotional aspects of individual including interests, size, shape, dress; the way the individual walks, talks, thinks, feels; ability to get along with people
  Understanding of own strengths, weaknesses, and academic, intellectual, and physical potentials
  Understanding of emotions' role in development
    Types—anger, fear, love, hate, jealousy, happiness, prejudice, sorrow, joy
    Effects—helpful or harmful
    Relief from effects by talk with someone, play, work, hobbies
    Influence on personal health—sleep and rest; eating; posture; physical activity
    Control—sense of humor; ability to accept criticism, disappointment, failure, and unhappiness in normal fashion
    Understanding of the physical growth changes taking place

---

*Stenner A.J. and Katzenmeyer W.G. (Self-concept development in young people, *Phi Delta Kappan* December, 1976) reported that children during the early school years who have positive self-concepts are confident of their ability to meet everyday problems and demands and are at ease in their relationships with other people. These children tend to be independent and reliable and are relatively free from anxiety, nervousness, excessive worry, tiredness, and loneliness. They are seldom considered behavior problems. They tend to be above average in reading and mathematics. They view school as a happy, worthwhile place.

PARTIAL HEALTH UNITS: MENTAL HEALTH UNIT—cont'd

OUTLINE OF CONTENT—cont'd

Psychological—cont'd

Ability to make adjustments, develop coping skills

Solving of problems and making decisions after weighing alternatives and consequences about study, work, sex, parent relations, peer relations

Establishment of realistic goals within potentials; achievable to reduce stress

Assumption and carrying out of responsibilities at home, school, and community

Ability to handle stress

Nature—tensions or pressures build attempting to carry out responsibilities, achieve goals, or solve problems resulting in anxieties, fears, worries and other emotional responses; degree dependent on factors involved

Causes—competition, desire to succeed, failure, sibling rivalry, parental expectations, school demands

Values and limits—some individuals work better under slight stress; may be motivational; may interfere with normal response

Relief from—modification of goals; activity change; balance of work and play; assumption of responsibilities; talking it out; taking one thing at a time; working off

Risk taking—positive and negative; includes financial gambles, risks of bodily harm and physical injury, ethical, self-esteem, and social risks

Coping with death and dying, bereavement and grief

Adjustment mechanisms: result from inability to adequately solve problems; individual resorts to other procedures to gain satisfaction, such as rationalization, projection, identification; misuse results in maladjusted behavior

Causes of mental illness: multiplicity of complex environmental factors

Physical and chemical—infections, nutritional deficiencies, accidents, gland deficiencies, alcohol, anemia, physical defects

Psychological—social relations, love and marriage, family conflicts, sibling conflicts, sex adjustments, religious conflicts, parental attitudes and personality, school and peer experiences

Emotional maladjustment or mental illness: mental illness is a matter of degree and kind; for some individuals, mild emotional disturbances; for others, severe mental health problems manifested in a variety of symptomatic behaviors

Death: meaningfulness and relation to birth and life, individuals, animals, and pets; bereavement and grief—stages of grief, need of others, need to be alone, helping others grieve; coping mechanisms—denial, anger, bargaining, depression, acceptance; feelings—perception of death; suicide—causes, signs, and symptoms

Social

Building of satisfying human relations: effective interaction with adults, peers, and opposite sex

Acquisition and retention of friends; sharing possessions and time; development of trust and fair play; respect of people as individuals; willingness to work with people; courteous and considerate; ability to give, as well as to take

Choice of friends: need to establish criteria

Influence of people: rewards; threats; authority; expertness

Warm, safe, and secure home and school climate

Alternative lifestyles   *Continued.*

PARTIAL HEALTH UNITS: MENTAL HEALTH UNIT—cont'd

OUTLINE OF CONTENT—cont'd

Social—cont'd

Successful group functioning involving respect and acceptance of all members; participation of all members; acceptance of responsibilities by each member; need for authority; a must to have constructive ways to resolve differences

Recognition of worth: realization that all individuals have human worths; ability to give consideration to rights of others; value of individual differences including race, religion, or ethnic origin

Community resource available to help with problems: school—nurse, teacher, counselor; home—parents; church—clergy; community—physicians, psychiatrists, organizations and agencies, public health departments

Death: death rituals and funerals—cultural and ethnic differences; communication with terminally ill; costs; suicide—sources of help

Spiritual

Values: the individual needs to attempt to define own values or value system; the individual's acceptance of differing values and value system of others

Moral issue: basic principles to use in the development and retention of relationship with others; recognition that all individuals should receive equal and just treatment regardless of socioeconomic status, religious, cultural, or ethnic backgrounds

CONCEPTS

Concept	Application of health definition
1 Mental health is influenced by biological and environmental factors.	Physiological
2 Each individual is like all others, like some others, and like no others.	
3 Understanding and acceptance of the concept of one's self is important in mental health.	Psychological-spiritual
4 All individuals have dignity and worth.	
5 Individuals should be able to face the realities of life with emotional maturity.	
6 Stress can be both beneficial and detrimental to individuals.	
7 The ability to get along with others is important in mental health.	Social
8 The community has a variety of sources available to help individuals with mental and emotional problems and difficulties.	

OBJECTIVES FOR GRADES K TO 3

Domain	Objectives for students	Basic concepts
Cognitive	1. Explains the reasons why sharing and taking turns are necessary	7
	2. Lists ways to respect the feelings, rights, and property of individuals	4, 7
	3. Lists ways of making and keeping friends	7
	4. Discusses ways emotions may be helpful and harmful and their effects on personal worth	5-7
	5. Recalls possible ways to sublimate or control emotional reactions	1, 3, 5-7

PARTIAL HEALTH UNITS: MENTAL HEALTH UNIT—cont'd

OBJECTIVES FOR GRADES K TO 3—cont'd

Domain	Objectives for students	Basic concepts
Cognitive— cont'd	**6.** Recites ways to assume responsibilities in school and at home	7
	7. Identifies ways to have success and be independent at school	3, 5
	8. Explains ways to prevent hurting someone or causing hard feelings	1, 4, 5, 7
Affective	**9.** Explains life and death in terms of loss of pets and animals	5
	1. Is interested in sharing and taking turns	7
	2. Talks about the feelings, rights, and property of individuals	4, 7
	3. Asks questions regarding ways to prevent hurting people or causing hard feelings	1, 4, 5, 7
	4. Displays interest in wanting and learning how to make and retain friends	7
	5. Supports the need to assume responsibilities in school and at home	7
Action (observable, nonob- servable, or de- layed)	**6.** Realizes that living things must die	5
	1. Participates in sharing and taking turns	7
	2. Experiences success and independence in a variety of ways in school	3, 4
	3. Is able to acquire friends and maintain them	4, 7
	4. Respects the feelings, rights, and property of others	4, 7
	5. Attempts to control emotions	1, 5-7
	6. Is able to express feelings in a mature fashion	1, 5-7
	7. Refrains from behavior that will hurt someone or cause hard feelings	1, 4, 5
	8. Assumes responsibilities expected in **school and at home**	7

OBJECTIVES FOR GRADES 4 TO 6

Domain	Objectives for students	Basic concepts
Cognitive	**1.** Identifies adults who are available to help with problems	8
	2. Lists the rules necessary for classroom behavior	1, 7
	3. Identifies the characteristics in which individuals are alike, different, or unique	1, 2
	4. Identifies goals that are within the possibility of achievement by the individual	3, 5
	5. Describes ways emotions can be controlled	1, 3, 5-7
	6. Explains the reasons for treating all individuals with dignity and respect	4
	7. Discusses the biological and environmental factors affecting mental health	1
	8. Lists situations when stress may occur and discusses helpfulness or harmfulness	1, 6
	9. Illustrates ways to be able to work productively as an individual in small groups	3, 4, 7
	10. Recalls a variety of interesting leisure time activities	1, 3, 8
	11. Identifies ways individuals try to adjust to demands of daily living	5

Continued.

PARTIAL HEALTH UNITS: MENTAL HEALTH UNIT—cont'd

OBJECTIVES FOR GRADES 4 TO 6—cont'd

Domain	Objectives for students	Basic concepts
Cognitive— cont'd	12. Explains the role of the brain, nervous system, and endocrine glands in mental health	7
	13. Explains risk-taking behavior	6
	14. Discusses life and death, meaning and causes	5
Affective	1. Believes a variety of individuals are willing and available to help solve problems	8
	2. Talks about the significance of establishing realistic goals	3, 5
	3. Displays interest in characteristics that identify individuals as alike, different, or unique persons	1, 2
	4. Believes emotions need to be controlled	1, 3, 5-7
	5. Is attentive to the importance of treating all individuals with dignity and respect	4
	6. Asks questions regarding the biological and environmental factors affecting mental health	1
	7. Believes stress situations may be helpful and harmful	1, 6
	8. Displays interest in being able to work productively as an individual and in small groups	3, 4, 7
	9. Enjoys and is interested in participating in a variety of leisure time activities	1, 3, 8
	10. Believes that risk-taking behavior may be hazardous	6
	11. Realizes that grief is part of life	5
Action (observable, nonobservable, or delayed)	1. Participates in the formulation of rules for classroom behavior	1, 7
	2. Seeks help when facing unsolvable problems	8
	3. Attempts to establish realistic goals	3, 5
	4. Treats all individuals with dignity and respect	4
	5. Attempts to control emotions	1, 3, 5, 7
	6. Attempts to avoid or reduce stressful situations	1, 6
	7. Tries to solve problems using scientific principles	5
	8. Is able to work productively as an individual and in groups	3, 4, 7
	9. Participates in a variety of interesting leisure time activities	1, 3, 8

OBJECTIVES FOR GRADES 7 TO 8

Domain	Objectives for students	Basic concepts
Cognitive	1. Describes the values believed to be important to self	3, 4
	2. Explains the interrelationships between biological and environmental influences on mental health	1
	3. Identifies the characteristics of the mentally healthy individual	3, 5
	4. Describes the growth and developmental changes taking place in the individual	1, 2

PARTIAL HEALTH UNITS: MENTAL HEALTH UNIT—cont'd

OBJECTIVES FOR GRADES 7 TO 8—cont'd

Domain	Objectives for students	Basic concepts
Cognitive—cont'd	5. Concludes an individual's personality is comprised of a variety of components and is unique	2
	6. Discusses the procedures necessary and problems faced in attempting to improve relationships with parents and teachers	7
	7. Compares the helpful and harmful aspects of friends and friendships	7
	8. Explains the scientific principles usable in solving problems	5
	9. Interprets the effect of peer pressures on individual behavior	6
	10. Indicates ways stress produced by peer pressures can be handled	6
	11. Identifies the types and symptoms of maladjustive behavior and the community sources and services available	1, 8
	12. Discusses positive and negative aspects of risk-taking behavior	6
	13. Identifies awareness of death and life	5
	14. Lists ways to cope with death of family member or friend	5
	15. Analyzes suicide in terms of causes, signs and symptoms, and sources of help	5
Affective	1. Is attentive to discussion about the interrelationships between biological and environmental influences on mental health	1
	2. Displays interest in the characteristics of the mentally healthy individual	3, 5
	3. Is interested in identifying own personality; characteristics and uniqueness	2, 3
	4. Believes that parent and teacher relationships are important	7
	5. Accepts the fact that friends can be helpful, as well as harmful, to individuals	5, 7
	6. Supports the need to solve problems using scientific principles	5
	7. Listens to the idea that decisions cannot be made without careful consideration	5
	8. Displays interest in learning the effect of peer pressures on behavior	2, 3, 5, 6
	9. Believes that stress created by peers may not always be beneficial	6
	10. Asks questions regarding the types and symptoms of maladjustive behavior and the treatment sources and services available in the community	1, 8
	11. Realizes the positive and negative aspects of risk-taking behavior	6
	12. Asks questions regarding funerals, rituals, and bereavement	5
Action (observable, nonobservable, or delayed)	1. Tries to develop a set of values or a value system	3-5
	2. Attempts to improve the strengths, weaknesses, and potential abilities of the self	7
	3. Endeavors to improve parent and teacher relationships	2, 5, 7
	4. Chooses friends after careful consideration of a variety of factors	
		Continued.

PARTIAL HEALTH UNITS: MENTAL HEALTH UNIT—cont'd

OBJECTIVES FOR GRADES 7 TO 8—cont'd

Domain	Objectives for students	Basic concepts
Action—cont'd (observable, nonobservable, or delayed)	**5.** Solves problems using scientific principles	5
	6. Tries to make decisions after viewing all the alternatives and consequences	5
	7. Attempts not to be unduly influenced by stress created by peers	2, 3, 5, 6
	8. Seeks help when maladjustive symptoms of a persistent nature appear	8
	9. Attempts to help others in time of death of loved ones	5

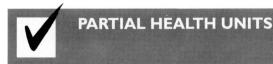

PARTIAL HEALTH UNITS

Nutrition Unit

OUTLINE OF CONTENT

Physiological

Definitions: food, nutrition, calorie

Purposes of food: energy, tissue building, protection and maintenance of bodily functions

Nutrients needed: reasons; good sources of proteins and fats; daily recommended allowances by age, sex, size, activity

Food needed: basic food groups; daily recommended allowances by age, sex, activity

Planning for meals or sample meals: breakfast, lunch, dinner, snacks, camping, picnics, sports, children, elderly, pregnancy, parties

Diet and weight control: desirable weights—age, sex, size; identification of overweight and obesity; food intake; role of exercise; reducing fads and fallacies; sources of help; reliable and unreliable sources of information

Body processing of foods: digestion; absorption; use

Effects on the body: performance—mental, nervous stability, motor, disease; body structure and size—teeth, bones, soft tissues; length of life; energy needs—internal and external body activities

Disorders and diseases: appendicitis, constipation, allergies, diabetes, cancer, food poisoning, heart disease (genetic and environmental risk factors)

Psychological

Food = Power: security; prestige and status; symbol of hospitality and friendship

Effect and outlet for emotions: joy, sorrow, conflict, comfort, fear, worry, anxiety

Motivations for modifying food habits

    Specific—weight reduction; weight control; lower blood pressure; pregnancy; sports; looks and personality; old age

    General—good health; longer life

Social

Eating patterns and preferences: influencing factors including cultural, ethnic, religious, racial, and social customs and traditions—Italian, Mexican, Asian, Native American, black; economic factors; age, sex, size; sensory reactions to food—texture, color, taste, looks; social climate and atmosphere including companionship; education influences—TV, radio, newspapers, magazines, school, family, community, friends, neighbors

Sanitation and safety: home, school, community (restaurants); laws; protective agencies

Preparation, processing, preservation, and storage: procedures—canning, frozen, dehydrated, powdered, refrigerated, pasteurized, irradiated, adulterated

Consumer protection: laws—additives, advertising, safety, adulteration, pasteurization, sanitation, food production, processing; agencies—FDA, FTC, health departments

Fads and fallacies: misconceptions, weight control, natural and organic foods

Selection and purchase of foods: wise economic expenditures

Problems of hunger in society: role in individual and community

Continued.

PARTIAL HEALTH UNITS: NUTRITION UNIT—cont'd

OUTLINE OF CONTENT—cont'd

Spiritual

Values: value of food in human life; importance of food for health of individuals

Moral issues: Does society have the obligation to feed the hungry and the poor? Should the hungry and the poor receive food? How should people treat individuals who are hungry and in need of food?

CONCEPTS

Concept	Application of health definition
1 Foods differ in kind, sources, and nutritive value and serve a variety of purposes for individuals.	Physiological
2 Individuals require the same nutrients but in varying amounts throughout life.	
3 The selection of nutritious foods contained in a balanced diet are necessary for the proper growth, good health, and everyday functioning of the individual.	
4 Lack of nutritious food resulting from a variety of factors may be detrimental to the health of individuals.	
5 Differing motivations influence the types and amounts of food consumed by individuals.	Psychological
6 Cultural, social, economic, and educational factors affect an individual's food selection.	Social
7 Production, processing, storage, preparation, and dispensing of foods influence their nutritional value, safety, and consumption.	
8 Food should be made available to all individuals regardless of their cultural, social, economic, or educational status.	Spiritual

OBJECTIVES FOR GRADES K TO 3

Domain	Objectives for students	Basic concepts
Cognitive	1. Identifies the basic food groups	1-3
	2. Explains the purposes of food and relates to the basic food groups	1, 3
	3. Lists nutritious snack foods	3
	4. Is able to plan simple nutritious breakfasts, lunches, and dinners from the basic food groups	1,3
	5. Recalls the sources of foods from plants and animals	1
	6. Explains the reasons for sanitary practices in the preparing, serving, and eating of foods	7
	7. Identifies the cultural and social differences in foods consumed by people	7
Affective	1. Displays interest in eating a variety of foods	1,3
	2. Raises questions regarding the sources of food from plants and animals	1
	3. Accepts the importance of tasting new and different foods	1,3
	4. Listens to the discussion for socially acceptable behavior at mealtime	5
	5. Talks about cultural and social differences in foods consumed by people	6

PARTIAL HEALTH UNITS: NUTRITION UNIT—cont'd

OBJECTIVES FOR GRADES K TO 3—cont'd

Domain	Objectives for students	Basic concepts
Action (observable)	1. Eats breakfast before attending school or while at school	3
	2. Eats nutritious snack foods	1,3
	3. Acts in a socially acceptable manner at mealtime	1
	4. Follows sanitary practices in the preparing, handling, and eating of foods	7
(nonobservable and delayed)	5. Eats well-balanced meals	1,3
	6. Demonstrates willingness to try and eat a variety of foods, including new ones	1,3
	7. Takes only the amount of food that can be eaten	5

OBJECTIVES FOR GRADES 4 TO 6

Domain	Objectives for students	Basic concepts
Cognitive	1. Recalls the basic food groups	1-3
	2. Identifies the nutrients found in foods, as well as the foods in which they are found	1
	3. Is able to plan nutritious meals with some degree of efficiency	1, 3
	4. Identifies the reasons why individuals need the same nutrients but in varying amounts throughout life	2
	5. Recalls how the body processes foods in terms of digestion, absorption, and use	2, 3
	6. Compares the foods and eating practices of various community, ethnic, religious, racial, and cultural groups of people	6
	7. Explains the relationships of poorly balanced diets and lack of food to diseases and disorders	4
	8. Lists factors that affect choices of foods by individuals	5
	9. Compares the nutritive values of highly advertised foods	1
	10. Identifies reliable sources of nutrition information	6
Affective	1. Displays interest in the selection of nutritious foods	1, 3
	2. Accepts the fact that new and different foods can add interest to eating	1-3
	3. Questions the value of highly advertised foods	1, 3
	4. Raises questions regarding reasons individuals require different types and amounts of food	2
	5. Displays interest in learning more about the relationships of food to disease and disorders	4
	6. Is attentive to discussions regarding the cultural and ethnic patterns and eating practices of individuals	6
	7. Supports the need to locate and use reliable sources of nutrition information	6

Continued.

PARTIAL HEALTH UNITS: NUTRITION UNIT—cont'd

OBJECTIVES FOR GRADES 4 TO 6—cont'd

Domain	Objectives for students	Basic concepts
Action (observable)	**1.** Eats nutritious foods at mealtime and at snacktime	1, 3
	2. Eats breakfast before attending school or while at school	3
	3. Follows sanitary practices in the preparation, serving, storing, and eating of food (Fig. B-2)	7
(nonobservable or delayed)	**4.** Eats a variety of foods and is willing to try new ones	1, 3
	5. Uses reliable sources for nutrition information	6

OBJECTIVES FOR GRADES 7 TO 8

Domain	Objectives for students	Basic concepts
Cognitive	**1.** Explains how it is possible to obtain all the essential nutrients by eating a balanced diet selected from a variety of foods	1, 3
	2. Describes diseases and disorders that may be associated with nutritional practices	4
	3. Lists the dangers to growth, health, and body functioning through the consumption of improper foods or poor eating habits	4
	4. Identifies the differing motivations that bring about changes in food consumption habits, such as sports, weight control, length of life	5
	5. Analyzes TV and other commercials about food and their nutritive value	1, 3, 5, 6

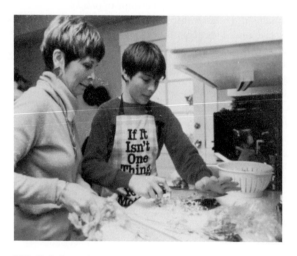

FIG. B-2 Learning to prepare foods. (Courtesy Michigan Department of Education.)

PARTIAL HEALTH UNITS: NUTRITION UNIT—cont'd

OBJECTIVES FOR GRADES 7 TO 8—cont'd

Domain	Objectives for students	Basic concepts
	6. Identifies federal, state, and local agencies and their functions in the control of the purity and quality of foods	8
	7. Explains how weight can be controlled in many individuals through proper diet and exercise	2
	8. Summarizes the current food fads and misconceptions	5, 6
	9. Illustrates the differing effects of food and lack of food on the body	4
	10. Compares the cultural or ethnic food patterns of community groups with the basic food groups	1, 6
	11. Concludes that all people need food and that efforts should be made to ensure that it is available when needed	8
	12. Examines food consumption at breakfast, lunch, dinner, and snacktime and compares with basic food groups	1, 3
	13. Lists reliable sources of nutrition information	6
Affective	1. Displays interest in attempting to help individuals in need of food	8
	2. Accepts the importance of weight control through proper diet and exercise	2
	3. Accepts and understands the cultural and ethnic differences in foods consumed by individuals	6
	4. Asks questions in regard to agencies and their functions that have responsibility for the control of the purity and quality of foods	7
	5. Is attentive to discussions regarding current food fads and misconceptions	5, 6
	6. Displays interest in the differing motivations for food habits	5
	7. Is supportive of the concept that a balanced diet selected from a variety of foods is necessary for proper growth and health	1, 3
	8. Believes that advertising about foods and food products must be carefully analyzed in terms of nutritional value	1, 3, 5, 6
	9. Realizes the role of nutrition as a risk factor in heart disease	4
	10. Accepts the importance of the use of reliable sources of nutrition information	6
Action (observable) (nonobservable or delayed)	1. Eats breakfast before attending school or while at school	3
	2. Eats nutritious foods at mealtime and snacktime	1, 3
	3. Periodically provides assistance by helping needy individuals obtain food	8
	4. Attempts to keep weight and intake of foods under control through the wise selection and consumption of nutritious items	2, 3
	5. Refrains, or attempts to encourage parents to refrain, from purchasing highly advertised foods unless they have been analyzed for nutritional value	1, 3, 5, 6
	6. Reduces intake of foods related to heart disease	4
	7. Uses reliable sources of nutrition information	6

PARTIAL HEALTH UNITS

Safety and First Aid Unit*

OUTLINE OF CONTENT

Physiological

Definitions: injury, sudden illness, hemorrhage, respiration, concussion, fracture, shock, abrasion, laceration, resuscitation, burn classifications, poisons, sprains, strain, contusion, heat stroke and heat exhaustion, defensive driving

Effects of accidents: disability and death

Areas: home; school; community; fire and electric; bicycle; farm; sports and recreation firearms; winter and summer

Psychological

Individual responsibility for safety
Accident proneness
Emotional factors in accidents and emergencies
Alcohol and other drugs in accidents
Emotional effects of accidents and emergencies on first aiders
Emotional influence in shock
Attitude toward mouth-to-mouth resuscitation
Importance of safe practices

Social

Accident costs in money, disability, and death responsibility: safe construction of motor vehicles, highways and information signs, toys, household appliances, farm and ranch equipment, houses and hotels, schools, business and industrial plants, children's clothing, and industrial equipment
Dangerous strangers and dangerous acquaintances
Responsibility for community emergency care programs
Sources of aid in accidents and emergencies

Spiritual

Values: importance of safety and health for all

Moral issues: protection of life and health of others in school, home, and other places; responsibility of individual and community to prevent accidents and provide emergency care

CONCEPTS

Concept	Application of health definition
1 Accident hazards and unsafe conditions exist in all environments.	Physical
2 An individual's safety depends on his or her ability to adjust to his or her environment.	Physical

---

*Also see Chapter 7.

PARTIAL HEALTH UNITS: SAFETY AND FIRST AID UNIT—cont'd

CONCEPTS—cont'd

Concept	Application of health definition
3 Accidents are the leading cause of death and injury among elementary school pupils.	Physical
4 Combinations of factors and forces contribute to the occurrence of accidents.	Psychological-social
5 Individuals, families, and community groups should be prepared to act effectively in the event of injury or sudden illness.	Social
6 Everyone has an obligation to reduce accident hazards in the environment.	Social
7 Safety and emergency care procedures are based on appreciation of the value and quality of life.	Spiritual

OBJECTIVES FOR GRADES K TO 3

Domain	Objectives for students	Basic concepts
Cognitive	**1.** Identifies accident hazards in own immediate environment	1, 2, 6
	2. Explains the reasons for protecting people from accidents	1-3
	3. Lists ways of avoiding accidents	2, 4
	4. Cites examples of disrespect for safety procedures in motor vehicle, home, school, and public activities	4, 6, 7
	5. Explains why first aid is important	5, 7
	6. Identifies ways to care for minor injuries	5, 7
	7. Cites best methods for getting help in emergencies	5, 7
	8. Lists most common kinds of accidents among kindergarten to third-grade pupils	3, 4
Affective	**1.** Asks questions about hazards in the environment	1, 2, 6
	2. Shows interest in the causes of accidents	2, 4, 6
	3. Reacts to class discussion on loss of life and health by accidents	2, 3, 6
	4. Is attentive to information presented on simple first-aid measures and procedures for obtaining expert assistance	5, 7
	5. Displays interest in helping others who may be sick or hurt	5, 7
Action	**1.** Follows safe practices in classroom, lunchroom, hallways, and playground	1-6
	2. Acts in a safe manner enroute to and from school—in bus or car, as pedestrian, or cycling	1-4, 6
	3. Seeks aid from school personnel for injury or sudden illness	5
	4. Helps other pupils when they are hurt or sick	5, 7
	5. Improves safe practices at home and in the immediate environment	1-4, 6
	6. Provides care for minor injuries	5

Continued.

PARTIAL HEALTH UNITS: SAFETY AND FIRST AID UNIT—cont'd

OBJECTIVES FOR GRADES 4 TO 6

Domain	Objectives for students	Basic concepts
Cognitive	1. Identifies the four classes of accidents: motor vehicle, home, public, and occupational	1, 2
	2 Lists new environmental accident hazards resulting from technological advances	1, 2, 4
	3. Explains ways to reduce potential for accidents	1, 2, 4, 6
	4. Tells how mental upsets may help cause accidents	1, 4
	5. Lists the steps in first aid to help someone who has been injured or becomes ill	5, 7
	6. Explains the most common emergency care procedures	5
Affective	1. Asks questions about specific potential causes for various types of accidents	1-4, 6
	2. Shows interest in environmental improvement to remove hazards	1-4, 6
	3. Is aware of the indifference and ignorance of the public with regard to safety	2, 4, 7
	4. Inquires about ways to improve safety conditions in and around the school	1, 3, 6, 7
	5. Expresses desire to become competent in first-aid methods	5, 7
	6. Shows concern for need to improve emergency care programs	5, 7
Action	1. Acts in a safe manner in school and in the community (Fig. B-3)	1-4, 6
	2. Starts to develop habits of helping others in preventing accidents	3, 6, 7
	3. Assists safety patrol or other school personnel when occasion arises	3, 6, 7
	4. Seeks information on underlying causes of accidents	4, 6
	5. Administers first aid for minor injuries	5, 7
	6. Secures information on the community's emergency aid program	5, 7

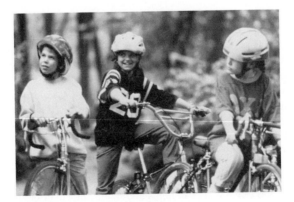

FIG. B-3 Safety is important. (Courtesy Health & Welfare, Canada.)

PARTIAL HEALTH UNITS: SAFETY AND FIRST AID UNIT—cont'd

OBJECTIVES FOR GRADES 7 TO 8

Domain	Objectives for students	Basic concepts
Cognitive	1. Lists deaths and injuries by age groups for the four major classes of accidents	1, 2
	2. Explains the ways in which modern environment can threaten own safety	1, 2, 4, 7
	3. Contrasts of pleasures and dangers of motorcycling, aquatic sports (scuba and skin diving, surfing, and water skiing), snow skiing, and other locally popular sport activities	1, 4, 6
	4. Identifies reliable sources of safety information	1, 3, 6
	5. Identifies safety organizations at the national, state, and local level	1, 6
	6. Explains and illustrates specific major first-aid procedures	5
	7. Lists reasons for needed improvements in community emergency care programs	5, 7
	8. Lists school and community resources that can render assistance in emergencies	5
Affective	1. Displays interest in doing own part to reduce hazards	2, 6
	2. Accepts the need for improving environmental conditions and human behavior	1, 2, 4, 6, 7
	3. Supports the concept that safety is everyone's responsibility	6, 7
	4. Believes that improved safety measures could reduce deaths and injuries among elementary-school-aged children and youth	2, 3, 7
	5. Supports the work of the National Safety Council and other organizations in accident prevention	6, 7
	6. Is aware of the need for better first-aid training for youth and adults	5, 7
	7. Believes that there is an immediate need to improve community programs for emergency care	5, 7
	8. Realizes there are school and community resources that provide assistance in emergencies	5
Action	1. Attempts to act in a consistently safe manner under all conditions	1, 2, 6
	2. Shows leadership in helping others avoid accidents	2, 3, 6
	3. Demonstrates acceptance of the values of safe behavior	2, 7
	4. Seeks solutions to accident problems in a scientific manner	2, 4, 6
	5. Demonstrates leadership in school, home, or community emergency care program	1, 5, 7
	6. Uses school and community resources in emergencies	5-7
	7. Effectively carries out sound first-aid measures if and when an emergency occurs	5, 7

PARTIAL HEALTH UNITS

Safety—Fire Unit*

OUTLINE OF CONTENT

Physiological

Effects

Harmful—3 million fires; 300,000 injuries (50,000 hospitalized); 8,800 deaths; $4 billion property damage yearly

Beneficial—warmth, cook food, manufacture products, scientific research, others

Leading causes of fire: electrical, smoking and matches, heating and cooking equipment, incendiary, children and matches, open flames, flammable liquids, lightning, chimneys and flues, spontaneous ignition

Types of fires: slow-burning, flash, explosion

Classes of fires: combustibles (A); flammable liquids, grease, and oil (B); electrical (C); metals (D)

Fire essentials: heat, fuel, oxygen

Where fires start in homes in rank order: living room, den or family room, basement, kitchen, bedroom, bathroom

Fabric flammability: cotton, linen, and silk burn more easily; tight-weave materials and those treated with flame-resistant substance and also nylon, acrylic, or polyester materials are more difficult to ignite; nylon, and so on, when ignited melts and causes severe burns

Control of fires: remove fuel (turn off electricity, dispose of wood, trash, and so forth), remove heat (cool), remove oxygen (smother)

Psychological

Risk-taking behavior hazards: injuries, deaths, property damage

Prevention behaviors

Before fires occur

   Public places—hotels, theaters, restaurants, and others—identify escape exits and plan for escape; schools—participate in fire drills

   Homes

      Escape plans, periodic inspection of hazards, installation of smoke and flame detectors

      Safety procedures

         General—good housekeeping—trash removal, as well as clutter in basements, attics, and other places; safe storage of flammable materials; remove damaged wires

         Specific

            Matches—close matchbook before striking, extinguish completely, do not play with

            Outside fires—burn trash only when permitted, do not burn unless with adult, do not use flammable liquid to start and rekindle, among others

            Lightning—stay indoors in storms; be away from metal objects, such as wire fences; if outside avoid trees and small sheds, get away from water

            Flammable liquids—do not use for home dry cleaning

---

*National Fire Protection Association in Quincy, MA, developed and launched this fire prevention and safety program in American schools some years ago. To date (1994), there is documented evidence that 298 lives from 118 fires have been saved in the United States as a result of this program.

PARTIAL HEALTH UNITS: SAFETY—FIRE UNIT—cont'd

OUTLINE OF CONTENT—cont'd

Psychological—cont'd

Prevention behaviors—cont'd

Specific—cont'd

Electrical appliances—turn off when not in use, do not use if fuse blown, keep away from objects that can burn, inspect regularly

Electricity—do not overload circuits, remove broken or bare wires, replace blown fuses

Clothing—wear sturdy jeans, tight-fitting jerseys, blouses without frills, jersey pajamas, tight-fitting or short-sleeve clothes

Baby-sitter—know all exits, escape plan, emergency telephone number; do not leave children alone

Holidays—do not use fireworks, use flashlight rather than candles on Halloween, do not use paper decorations, keep Christmas trees moist and in water and turn off lights when not at home or nearby

After fires occur

General—survival, escape, alarm, rescue, first aid

Specific

Home or building—follow escape plan

Report of fire—telephone, alarm box

When trapped—*crawl low* and get out of room, check door before opening and, if hot, fill cracks and signal for help in window with light-colored cloth or use telephone

First aid—burns, asphyxiation, summon medical aid

Clothing—drop to ground and roll

Social

Fire department: sole responsibility to fight fires, services usually available 24 hours daily, telephones readily available

Fire alarm boxes: purpose to summon fire fighters quickly, false alarms delay saving of lives and property

Fire codes, regulations, and laws

Spiritual

Values: importance of fire prevention and safety to prevent injuries and death and protect property

Moral issue: protection of people and property is a responsibility of all individuals

CONCEPTS

Concept	Application of health definition
1 Fire has both beneficial and harmful effects.	Physical
2 Risk-taking behavior is the result of a variety of motivations.	Psychological
3 Individuals, families, and communities can prevent fires, save lives, and prevent injury and loss of property.	Psychological-social
4 Fire fighters are friends and necessary community helpers who render necessary services.	Social

Continued.

PARTIAL HEALTH UNITS: SAFETY—FIRE UNIT—cont'd

CONCEPTS—cont'd

Concept	Application of health definition
5 Fire codes, regulations, and laws are necessary for the protection of individuals and property.	Social
6 Individuals have responsibility to protect their own lives and property, as well as their neighbors'.	Spiritual

OBJECTIVES FOR GRADES K TO 3

Domain	Objectives for students	Basic concepts
Cognitive	1. Identifies the benefits and harmful effects of fire	1-3, 6
	2. Describes the actions to take in a fire drill	3-6
	3. Demonstrates the proper stop, drop, and roll technique when clothes are on fire	3, 6
	4. Describes the crawling low method to exit from a smoke-filled room	3, 6
	5. Lists the procedures to follow when smoke or fire is discovered in a building	3, 6
	6. Explains the reasons for reporting fire and smoke conditions immediately	1, 3, 4, 6
	7. States reason to look for two exits from every building	1, 3, 5, 6
	8. Lists the dangers of playing with or using matches improperly	1-3, 6
	9. Recalls the dangers and safety procedures around heat-producing appliances	1-3, 6
	10. Lists the types of electrical hazards in homes	1, 3, 5, 6
	11. Recites the need for fire-safe holidays	1-3, 6
	12. Recalls the way combustibles can be ignited	1-3, 6
Affective	1. Values fire and smoke drills as necessary for fire safety	3, 5, 6
	2. Values the need for prompt action when smoke or fire is discovered	1, 3, 4, 6
	3. Realizes why fire and smoke conditions should be reported immediately	1, 3, 6
	4. Realizes the importance of identifying and being able to locate two exits at all times	3, 6
	5. Wishes to protect self and others from the hazards of improper use of matches	1-3, 6
	6. Wishes to keep family members fire safe when camping, picnicking, or cooking outdoors	1-3, 5, 6
	7. Recognizes that electrical hazards may result in fire, injury, death, and loss of property	1-3, 6
	8. Believes in identifying and removing fire hazards	1, 3, 4, 6
	9. Supports the need for fire-safe holidays	1-3, 6
	10. Realizes the hazard of inserting objects into electrical outlets	3, 6

PARTIAL HEALTH UNITS: SAFETY—FIRE UNIT—cont'd

OBJECTIVES FOR GRADES K TO 3—cont'd

Domain	Objectives for students	Basic concepts
Action	1. Participates in fire and smoke drills at schools	3, 5, 6
(observable	2. Participates in the planning of a home evacuation plan	3, 4, 6
and	3. Immediately reports fire, heat, or smoke conditions to a responsible adult	3, 4, 6
nonobserv-	4. Refrains from playing with or improperly using matches in home, school, or outdoors	1-3, 6
able)	5. Refrains from playing near stoves, heaters, or fireplaces	1-3, 6
	6. Reports electrical hazards to responsible adults	1, 3, 4, 6
	7. Is able to crawl low to exit from a smoke-filled room	3, 6
	8. Applies cold water to minor burns if no adult is present	3, 6
	9. Seeks help for severe burns	3, 6
	10. Practices and encourages family members to practice fire safety when camping, picnicking, or cooking outdoors	1-3, 5, 6
	11. Practices and encourages fire safety on holidays and special occasions	1, 3, 6

OBJECTIVES FOR GRADES 4 TO 6

Domain	Objectives for students	Basic concepts
Cognitive	1. Describes the actions to take in fire drills	3-6
	2. Demonstrates the proper way to stop, drop, and roll when clothes are on fire	3, 6
	3. Identifies hazardous types of clothing	3, 6
	4. States reason for crawling low in a smoke-filled room	1, 3
	5. Lists procedures to follow when smoke or fire is discovered	1, 3, 4, 6
	6. Describes the purpose of two exits from buildings	3, 4, 6
	7. Identifies the first-aid procedures for burns	3, 6
	8. Explains the procedures for fire safety when serving as a baby-sitter	1, 3, 6
	9. States the reasons for remaining clear of fire fighters while fires are in progress	4
	10. Recites the reasons for refusing to turn in false fire alarms	2, 4
	11. Lists the dangers of playing with or using matches improperly	1-3, 6
	12. Identifies fire safety behavior around lighted stoves, heaters, and small appliances	1-3, 6
	13. Recalls how to store flammable liquids safely	1-3, 5, 6
	14. Explains the ways to extinguish outdoor fires	1, 3, 6
	15. Identifies the types of electrical hazards in homes	3, 6
	16. States the reasons for conducting periodic home hazard inspections	2, 3, 6
	17. Recalls the need to use gasoline in well-ventilated places outside of buildings	2, 3, 6
Affective	1. Values fire and smoke drills for fire safety	3-6
	2. Values the need to use the stop, drop, and roll technique when clothes are on fire	3, 6

Continued.

PARTIAL HEALTH UNITS: SAFETY—FIRE UNIT—cont'd

OBJECTIVES FOR GRADES 4 TO 6—cont'd

Domain	Objectives for students	Basic concepts
Affective— cont'd	3. Realizes the importance for prompt action when smoke or fire is discovered	1-4, 6
	4. Appreciates the importance of locating two exits from buildings	3, 4, 6
	5. Realizes the need for immediate attention to burns	3, 6
	6. Supports the need to refrain from interfering with fire fighters while fires are in progress	4
	7. Believes that false fire alarms are dangerous	4
	8. Wishes to protect self and others from the misuse of matches and lighted objects	1-3, 6
	9. Realizes the hazards of lighted stoves, heaters, and small appliances	1-3, 6
	10. Recognizes the hazards of improperly stored flammable liquids	1-3, 5, 6
	11. Believes in the importance of the use of nonflammable substances inside homes and buildings	1-3, 6
Action (observable) (observable and non-observable)	1. Helps teachers conduct fire drills	3, 6
	2. Helps family in the preparation and the following of a home evacuation plan	3, 6
	3. Immediately reports fire, heat, or smoke observed to a responsible adult after leaving a building	1, 3, 4, 6
	4. Refrains from improperly using matches and helps store them properly	1-3, 6
	5. Practices and encourages others to practice fire safety	1-3, 5, 6
	6. Assists in regular inspection of buildings and grounds	3, 6
(nonobservable)	7. Performs accurately the stop, drop, and roll technique when clothes are on fire	3, 6
	8. Properly performs the crawling procedure to exit a smoke-filled room	1, 3, 6
	9. Establishes an evacuation plan in case of fire in a multistoried building	3, 5, 6
	10. Applies cold water to a minor burn if no adult is present or seeks help with a severe burn	3, 6
	11. Aids fire fighters on arrival regarding location of fire and whether persons are in building	4, 5
	12. Refrains from turning in false fire alarms	4, 5
	13. Helps maintain storage of flammable liquids in proper containers	1-3, 5, 6
	14. Encourages safe smoking habits in buildings, outdoors, and other places	2, 3, 6
	15. Persuades others to use gasoline and other volatile substances in well-ventilated places	1-3, 6

PARTIAL HEALTH UNITS: SAFETY—FIRE UNIT—cont'd

OBJECTIVES FOR GRADES 7 TO 8

Domain	Objectives for students	Basic concepts
Cognitive	1. Identifies reasons for fire drills	3-6
	2. Demonstrates proper technique for stop, drop, and roll technique to use when clothes are on fire	3, 6
	3. Identifies reason to crawl low to exit from smoke-filled room	1, 3, 6
	4. Lists procedures to follow when smoke or fire is discovered	1, 3, 4, 6
	5. Explains reasons for reporting fire and smoke conditions immediately when discovered	1, 3, 4, 6
	6. Demonstrates first aid for use with burn victims	3, 6
	7. Describes procedures to plan a baby-sitter safety plan	3, 6
	8. States the importance of remaining clear of fire fighters while fires are in progress	4
	9. Lists the hazards of false fire alarms	4
	10. Lists the hazards of the improper use of matches	1-3, 6
	11. Recalls the dangers and safety procedures when around cooking, heating, and other heat-producing appliances	1-3, 6
	12. Describes the flammability dangers from volatile substances	1-3, 6
	13. Identifies the safety procedures for use in outdoor fires	1-3, 5, 6
	14. Explains the purposes of fuses and the safe way to replace them	1, 3, 6
	15. Lists procedures used in the regular inspection of buildings for fire hazards	3, 6
	16. Lists the procedures to follow for fire-safe holidays	3, 6
	17. Recalls the need for safe smoking habits in buildings, outdoors, and in automobiles	1, 3, 5, 6
	18. Explains the types, costs, and operation of fire and smoke detectors	3, 5, 6
	19. Describes the significance of the use of the UL label on electrical appliances and equipment	3, 5, 6
	20. States the reason for licensed or certified personnel performing electrical repairs and maintenance	3, 5, 6
Affective	1. Supports the need for fire drills and accepts responsibility for sharing in their conduct	3-6
	2. Values the need to use the stop, drop, and roll technique when clothing is on fire	3, 6
	3. Values the need for prompt action when smoke or fire is discovered	1, 3, 4, 6
	4. Believes it is necessary to help children escape from fire when serving as a baby-sitter	3, 6
	5. Supports the need to refrain from interfering with fire fighters while fires are in progress	4
	6. Believes that false fire alarms should not be turned in	4
	7. Realizes the importance of using matches safely	1-3, 6

Continued.

PARTIAL HEALTH UNITS: SAFETY—FIRE UNIT—cont'd

OBJECTIVES FOR GRADES 7 TO 8—cont'd

Domain	Objectives for students	Basic concepts
Affective—cont'd	**8.** Willingly accepts the responsibility to protect children when around heat-producing equipment	1-3, 6
	9. Recognizes the hazards of improperly used and stored flammable liquids	1-3, 6
	10. Desires to practice fire safety outdoors	2, 3, 5, 6
	11. Realizes the need for fuses and circuit breakers to protect from electrical overloads	3, 5, 6
	12. Values the importance of periodic building inspections for fire hazards	3, 6
	13. Supports the need for fire-safe holidays and special occasions	3, 5, 6
	14. Recognizes the high risk of smoking in bed and the improper disposal of smoking materials	2, 3, 6
	15. Supports the need for fire and smoke detectors	3, 5, 6
	16. Recognizes the need for the repair and maintenance of electrical equipment by licensed or certified personnel	3, 5, 6
Action (observable) (observable and non-observable) (nonobservable)	**1.** Willingly participates in fire and smoke drills at school and assumes responsibility to help conduct same	3-6
	2. Participates in helping family and others develop and follow a home escape plan	3, 6
	3. Prepares fire evacuation plan for use in multistoried building	3, 5, 6
	4. Conducts or assists in periodic building fire safety inspections	3, 6
	5. Performs stop, drop, and roll technique to use when clothes are on fire	3, 6
	6. Performs crawling low procedure to exit from smoke-filled room	3, 6
	7. Immediately reports observed fire, heat, or smoke after leaving a building to responsible adult or fire department	1, 3, 4, 6
	8. Administers first aid for minor burns and shock and seeks medical help for major burns	3, 6
	9. Plans safety procedures with parents when baby-sitting	3, 6
	10. Assists fire fighters regarding location of fires and persons in burning buildings	3, 4, 6
	11. Refrains from turning in false fire alarms	3, 4, 6
	12. Refrains and discourages others from the improper use of matches	1-3, 6
	13. Helps keep children away from heat-producing equipment and appliances	3, 6
	14. Aids in the proper use and storage of flammable liquids	1, 3, 6
	15. Assists with the removal of electrical hazards in the home	3, 6
	16. Encourages safe smoking habits in buildings, outdoors, and automobiles	1, 3, 6
	17. Persuades others to install fire and smoke detectors and to purchase electrical equipment with the UL label	1, 3, 5, 6
	18. Encourages adults to install lightning protection on buildings where appropriate	1, 3, 6

PARTIAL HEALTH UNITS

Vision and Hearing Unit

OUTLINE OF CONTENT

Physiological

Definitions: hyperopia, myopia, astigmatism, amblyopia, glaucoma, color blindness, night blindness, strabismus, conjunctivitis, ophthalmologist, optometrist, optician, otitis media, otitis externa, conduction deafness, nerve deafness

Structure and function of eyes and ears

Eye structure—cornea, iris, lens, retina, optic nerve

Eye function—vision

Ear structure—outer ear, middle ear, inner ear, auditory nerve

Ear function—hearing

Refractive errors; eye diseases and ear disorders

Signs and symptoms of problems (see Appendix I)

Psychological

Emotional problems: caused by strabismus, nearsightedness and farsightedness, partial or complete blindness, partial or complete deafness, learning difficulties

Purposes of testing and care of vision and hearing

Social

Selection of eye specialist

Selection of physician for earache or hearing problem

Choice of glasses, contact lenses, or hearing aid if needed

Periodic eye and ear examinations or screening tests—types, frequency

Spiritual

Values: importance of eye and ear health to self-image

Moral issues: provision of eye and ear care by government funding or private sources; protection of workers' vision and hearing in certain industries; attitudes toward blind and deaf people; responsibility to help blind and deaf persons

CONCEPTS

Concept	Application of health definition
1 Vision and hearing are the two most important senses for life and health.	Physical
2 Visual disorders may cause learning difficulties or psychological problems	Psychological-social
3 Hearing disorders may cause learning difficulties or psychological problems.	Psychological-social
4 During the elementary school years, parents have the primary responsibility for correction of hearing or vision problems in pupils.	Spiritual
5 Prompt professional care can correct or improve most disorders of vision and hearing in their early developmental stages.	Physical

Continued.

PARTIAL HEALTH UNITS: VISION AND HEARING UNIT—cont'd

OBJECTIVES FOR GRADES K TO 3

Domain	Objectives for students	Basic concepts
Cognitive	1. Tells why good eyesight and hearing are important	1
	2. Explains the reasons for having vision and hearing tests	2, 3, 5
	3. Identifies the main parts of the eye and ear	1
	4. Lists ways that good sight and hearing can help learning	2, 3
	5. Discusses factors that may impair vision or hearing	1
	6. Recalls any experiences of visual difficulty or earache	5
Affective	1. Is aware of the importance of good vision and hearing	1
	2. Accepts the need for vision and hearing tests	4, 5
	3. Displays interests in how the eyes and ears function	1
	4. Listens carefully to the ways to protect vision and hearing	1
Action	1. Participates cooperatively when vision or hearing tests are given at school	4, 5
	2. Tells about any personal seeing or hearing difficulty	5

OBJECTIVES FOR GRADES 4 TO 6

Domain	Objectives for students	Basic concepts
Cognitive	1. Explains the basic structure and function of eyes and ears	1
	2. Identifies ways to protect vision and hearing	1, 4, 5
	3. Cites major causes of visual and hearing disorders	1
	4. Illustrates how middle ear infection can cause hearing loss	1
	5. Describes effect of glare on visual acuity and eye fatigue	1
	6. Explains important effects of color blindness and night blindness	1, 2
	7. Explains the importance of regular eye and ear checkups and follow-up for corrections	2, 3, 5
Affective	1. Understands and appreciates the critical value of good vision and hearing	1, 2, 3
	2. Accepts responsibility along with parents for care of eyes and ears	1, 4
	3. Displays interest in the effects of heredity on eye and ear disorders	1, 4, 5
	4. Appreciates the role of parents, teachers, school nurses, and health specialists in the prevention and correction of eye and ear defects	1, 5
	5. Believes that healthy vision and hearing are necessary for a good education	1, 2, 3
Action	1. Takes an active, cooperative part when vision or hearing tests are given at school	5
	2. Protects own eyes and avoids endangering the eyes of others in sports and other physical activities	1

PARTIAL HEALTH UNITS: VISION AND HEARING UNIT—cont'd

OBJECTIVES FOR GRADES 4 TO 6—cont'd

Domain	Objectives for students	Basic concepts
Action— cont'd	3. Reports any personal problem of seeing or hearing to the teacher, school nurse, or other professional person	5
	4. Avoids probing ears with sharp objects, looking directly at sun, or other practices that can be harmful	1
	5. Avoids exposure to excessively loud rock music or other high-decibel noise	1

OBJECTIVES FOR GRADES 7 TO 8

Domain	Objectives for students	Basic concepts
Cognitive	1. Explains major errors of refraction in terms of altered structure and function and professional care	5
	2. Cites causes, prevention, and reasons for professional care of middle ear infection	1, 3, 5
	3. Lists types of environmental noise that can damage hearing	1
	4. Analyzes differences between and among ophthalmologists, optometrists, and opticians	5
	5. Describes possible effects on studying and learning of eye and ear disorders	2, 3
	6. Describes possible emotional effects of eye and ear disorders	2, 3
	7. Compares advantages and disadvantages of glasses and contact lenses	1
	8. Cites dangers of delayed treatment for amblyopia (lazy eye) and glaucoma	1
Affective	1. Understands and appreciates the critical value of good vision and hearing	1, 2, 3
	2. Accepts responsibility for protecting and caring for own eyes and ears	1, 5
	3. Recognizes the responsibility of parents to seek professional care for children with eye or ear problems	1, 4
	4. Discusses the problems of providing medical care for the poor who have eye or ear problems	1, 5
	5. Recognizes and appreciates the growing problem of noise pollution in the environment	1

Continued.

PARTIAL HEALTH UNITS: VISION AND HEARING UNIT—cont'd

OBJECTIVES FOR GRADES 7 TO 8—cont'd

Domain	Objectives for students	Basic concepts
Action	**1.** Takes an active, cooperative part when vision or hearing tests are given	4, 5
	2. Protects own eyes and avoids endangering the eyes of others in sports, laboratory work, and other physical activities	1
	3. Is able to make wise decisions regarding personal eye and ear care	1
	4. Supports school and community efforts to protect and improve eye and ear health	1, 5
	5. Seeks reliable information on eye and ear health	1, 5
	6. Consistently wears glasses or hearing aid if prescribed	1
	7. Avoids exposure to excessively loud rock music or other high-decibel noise	1, 3

C

Education for Health in the School Community Setting
*A Position Paper**

The school is a community in which most individuals spend at least 12 years of their lives, and more if they have the advantages of early childhood programs, college education, and continuing education for adults. The health of our school-aged youth will determine to a great extent the quality of life each will have during the growing and developing years and on throughout the life cycle. Their capacity to function as health-educated adults will in turn help each to realize the fullest potential for self, family, and the various communities of which each individual will be a part.

The American Public Health Association (APHA) believes that health education should be a continuing process, from conception to death, and that such education must be comprehensive, coordinated, and integrated in all community planning for health.

The school as a social structure provides an educational setting in which the total health of the child during the impressionable years is of priority concern. No other community setting even approximates the magnitude of the grades K to 12 school educational enterprise, with an enrollment in 1973-1974 of 45.5 million in nearly 17,000 school

districts comprising more than 115,000 schools with some 2.1 million teachers. This is to say nothing of the administrative, supervisory, and service manpower required to maintain these institutions. In addition, more than 40% of children aged 3 to 5 are enrolled in early childhood education programs. Thus it seems that school should be regarded as a social unit providing a focal point to which health planning for all other community settings should relate.

Schools provide an environment conducive to developing skills and competencies that will help the individual confront and examine a complexity of social and cultural forces, persuasive influences, and ever-expanding options as these affect health behavior. Today's health problems do not lend themselves to yesterday's solutions. Specificity of cause is multiple rather than singular. The individual must assume increasing responsibility for solutions to major public health problems and consequently must be educated to do so.

Education for and about health is not synonymous with information. Education is concerned with behavior—a composite of what an individual knows, senses, and values, and of what one does and practices. Factual data are but temporary assumptions to be used and cast aside as new information emerges. Health facts unrenewed can become a liability rather than an asset. The health-educated citizen is one who possesses resources and abilities that will last throughout a lifetime,

---

*Modified from Governing Council of the American Public Health Association: *Education for health in the school community setting; a position paper*, New Orleans, October 23, 1974, The Council. A "position paper" is defined as a major exposition of the Association's viewpoint on broad issues affecting the public's health.

such as critical thinking, problem-solving, valuing, self-discipline, and self-direction, and that will lead to a sense of responsibility for community and world concerns.

The school curriculum offers an opportunity to view health issues in an integrated context. It is designed to help the learner gain insights about the personal, social, environmental, political, and cultural implications of each issue. Planning for health care delivery, for example, is not simply a matter of providing for manpower, services, and facilities. These things must be considered in concert with housing, employment, transportation, cultural beliefs and values, and the rights and dignity of the persons involved. Nor will nutritional practices be improved substantially by programs based on groupings, labeling, or issuing stamps, because food practices and eating patterns are equally influenced by how, when, where, why, and with whom one eats.

APHA is concerned about the traditional crisis approach to health care. The expense involved in treatment, rehabilitation, recuperation, and restoration to health has sent medical costs soaring. More facilities, services, and manpower to staff the facilities and to provide the services appear to be the nation's leading priorities. The alternative is a redirection of the nation's health goals toward a primary preventive—and constructive—approach to health, through education for every individual.

Because of vested interests, political pressures, mass media sensationalism, and health agency structures with categorical interests, health education programs in schools are compelled to deal with a multitude of separate health issues, with only a few of these given priority at any given time. Too often programs developed to deal with crucial issues are eliminated, although the problems remain because another crisis emerges calling for more new crash programs. A revolving critical issue syndrome has been the result, with the same problems considered crucial a decade or more ago emerging once again. Focusing on selected categorical issues has potential value if time, energy, personnel, and money are available to sustain the emphasis and expand such efforts into an integrated and viable health education framework. A broad concept of healthful living that has consideration for psychosocial dimensions should be the basis for health education.

APHA is encouraged by recent developments in an increasing number of states that attest to recognition of the significance of a comprehensive health education program in grades K to 12. Also encouraging are the exemplary programs being established in many school districts and the expressed intention of the federal government to implement an action plan for "better health through education."

Therefore the American Public Health Association supports the concept of a national commitment to a comprehensive, sequential program of health education for all students in the nation's schools, kindergarten through the twelfth grade. The Association will exert leadership through its sections and affiliates to assure the following for health education:

- Time in the curriculum commensurate with other subject areas.
- Professionally qualified teachers and supervisors of health education.
- Innovative instructional materials and appropriate teaching facilities.
- Increased financial support at the local, state, and national levels to upgrade the quantity and quality of health education.
- A teaching/learning environment in which opportunities for safe and optimal living exist, and one in which a well-organized and complete health service is functioning.

D

A Sample of Health Education Fiction and Nonfiction Books

MORE than 40,000 books specifically written for children are now in print. In addition, approximately 3000 new titles are added each year. This wealth of literature provides the teacher with rich material that can be used in teaching health.

Naturally, the teacher cannot review all of these books; numerous reference compendia are available to teachers that review trade books with health themes. For ease in locating these references, we have listed several that were used in the compilation of the selected list of books contained in this Appendix. The annotations were adapted from a variety of sources. Teachers wishing additional information about any particular book should obtain the book and read it before using it in the classroom. The titles included in the annotated section are likely to be found in an elementary school library and are related to specific areas that could be included in an elementary school health education program.

The list has been organized by topic areas, with books listed alphabetically by authors. Books that deal with diversity are marked with an asterisk (*). Approximations of reading levels are specified using the following code: *P,* primary, *I,* intermediate; and *U,* upper.

GENERAL REFERENCE TEXTS

Azarnoff P: *Health, illness, and disability: a guide to books for children and young adults,* New York, R.R. Bowker, 1983.

> More than 1000 books that deal with health concerns and issues are described.

Bernstein J: *Books to help children cope with separation and loss,* ed 3, New York, R.R. Bowker, 1989.

> Information about bibliotherapy and an annotated list of books about death, divorce, adoption, foster children, and similar topics.

Child Study Children's Book Committee at Bank Street College: *Children's books of the year,* New York, Author.

> An annual listing of more than 500 books that are published in the current year.

Children's Literature Association: *The children's literature association quarterly,* Battle Creek, MI quarterly, Author.

> A quarterly publication that contains book reviews and articles about children's literature. Special sections that deal with plays, poetry, censorship, teaching children's literature, and other related topics are included.

Council on Interracial Books for Children: *Interracial books for children bulletin,* New York, The Council.

> A periodical that contains articles and book reviews that deal with diversity, including ethnic, religious, and gender experiences. A feature is reviews of books that deal with children with disabilities and handicaps.

Lee L, editor: *The elementary school library collection, a guide to books and other media,* ed 19, Williamsport, PA, Bro-Dart Foundation, 1994.

An annotated bibliography of more than 12,000 children's books and other nonprint media arranged in several fashions. A twentieth edition will be available in January 1996 and will include telephone numbers (including 800 numbers), FAX numbers, and E-Mail numbers. Book is available in print, or CD-ROM. The materials included are particularly appropriate for grades K–6.

Lima C: *A to zoo, subject access to children's picture books,* ed 3, New York, R.R. Bowker, 1989.

A listing of over 4000 titles and authors of books designed for preschool through grade 2. They are arranged by subject headings, subject guide, bibliographic guide, title, and illustrator. They are not annotated.

Manna AL, Symons CW: *Children's literature for health awareness,* Metuchen, NJ, The Scarecrow Press, 1992.

A general description of how children's literature can be used in health education. Includes an extensive annotated bibliography of children's books, organized by health topics areas and subdivided by grade and/or reading level and specific subjects.

AGING

Berger, Terry, *Special Friends,* Julian Messner, 1979. (P-I)

A young girl and her neighbor, Aunt Rose, spend many happy days together. The girl tells Aunt Rose about her day and Aunt Rose shares books and cookies. The girl helps Aunt Rose with things she has trouble with because her eyes are bad. Photos enhance this warm story about the love shared between generations. Fiction.

De Paola, Thomas, *Now One Foot, Now the Other,* G.P. Putnam's Sons, 1981. (P)

Bobby, named for his beloved grandfather Bob, learns to deal with his grandfather's stroke. When Bob is hospitalized, Bobby misses him terribly. He thinks about the stories Bob used to tell about teaching Bobby to walk, now one foot, now the other. When Bob finally returns home, he cannot walk, talk, or recognize family members. Bobby is frightened by his grandfather and the strange noises he makes. When

he thinks he sees a tear on Bob's face, Bobby is convinced his grandfather knows him. Together they begin Bob's slow recovery. Now Bobby tells of how he taught Bob to walk, now one foot, now the other. A hopeful and tender look at the aging process and recovery from illness. Fiction.

Farber, Norma, *How Does It Feel To Be Old?* E.P. Dutton, 1979. (P-I)

When a granddaughter questions her grandmother about being old, the grandmother explains. She tells about both the good and the bad. The text rhymes and the illustrations complement the realistic verse. This story may help answer questions children have about aging. Fiction.

Gauch, Patricia. *Grandpa and Me,* Coward, 1972. (I)

Beautifully illustrated portrayal of grandfather and grandson in a vacation setting. Older man is strong, active, and caring. Fiction.

Goffstein, M.B., *Fish for Supper,* Dial, 1976. (P)

Independent older woman catches, cleans, and cooks her own fish in this simple, well-illustrated book for very young children. Fiction.

Guthrie, Donna, *Grandpa Doesn't Know It's Me,* Human Science, 1986. (P-I)

Grandpa suffers from Alzheimer's disease. When it becomes too dangerous for him to live alone, he moves in with Lizzie's family. She describes her fears and the pain of not being recognized. Lizzie's family patiently tries to keep Grandpa active and safe. Coping with any disease can be difficult, and this story can help students learn some positive ways to deal with various situations that may arise with aging. Fiction.

Hein, Lucille, *My Very Special Friend,* Judson, 1974. (I-U)

Sensitive relationship between a young girl and her elderly, yet active and creative, great-grandmother. Fiction.

Hurd, Edith, *I Dance in My Red Pajamas,* Harper & Row, 1982. (P)

Warned by her parents not to be too noisy at her grandparents' house, Jenny knows better. Grandma and Grandpa like nothing better than singing, dancing, and being active with their lively granddaughter. Jenny's special bond with her loving, noisy, and lively grandparents shows that the elderly can still enjoy life. Fiction.

Kirk, Barbara, *Grandpa, Me and Our House in the Tree,* Macmillan, 1978. (I)

After there is a debilitating illness, grandfather and grandson must restructure their formerly physically active relationship. Sensitive portrayal of the needs of both. Fiction.

Lasky, Kathryn, *I Have Four Names for My Grandfather,* Little, Brown, & Co., (P)

Grandfather and grandson are photographed in both active and passive situations. Especially good presentation of communication across generations. Nonfiction.

Maclachlan, Patricia. *Through Grandpa's Eyes,* Harper & Row, 1980. (P)

John loves to visit his blind Grandpa who teaches him how to "see" through touch, sounds, and smell. A tender story with poetic illustrations. Fiction.

Mathis, Sharon Bell, *Hundred Penny Box,* Viking, 1975 (Newberry Honor Book). (I)

When Michael's 100-year-old, Great-Great-Aunt Dew comes to live with them, she brings along an old, beat-up box, with as many pennies as her age in it. He loves to hear the tales she tells about the year she got each penny, while he counts out the pennies. A warm story of the love between old age and youth. Fiction.

Maxer, Norma Fox, *Figure of Speech,* Delacorte, 1973 (I)

Thirteen-year-old Jenny has always found it difficult to relate to anyone in her family except Grandpa. But her parents refer to the 83-year-old man as "failing," and she overhears them say that "everyone passes away," and "his time is coming." That night they find that Grandpa has pinned a note to the bulletin board saying, "I ain't going to pass away. I'm goin' to die. My time ain't going to come. I'll be dead." Jenny and Grandpa share together his attempt to salvage the last shreds of his dignity in a touching and also realistic tale. Fiction.

Whitman, Sally, *A Special Trade,* Harper & Row, 1978. (I-U)

At first an elderly man and a young girl are presented with the man as the initiator—caring, helping, teach-ing. After there is a serious illness, roles changes, but the relationship remains strong and mutual. Fiction.

Williams, Barbara, *Kevin's Grandma,* Dutton, 1975. (P)

Two boys compare grandmothers. One is conventional, yet interesting and self-sufficient. The other is outrageous, delightfully eccentric, and not quite believable. Fiction.

ALCOHOL

Al-Anon, Inc., *What's "Drunk," Mama?,* Al-Anon, 1977. (P-I)

Christy's life is filled with unkept promises and constant worry. She is angry and frightened by her daddy's drinking. Her mama is always crying or mad. Through Al-Anon, her family begins the long process of recovery and learn how to care for themselves. May be a bit simplistic in the way the story portrays the ease of recovery. Fiction.

Dorman, N.B., *Laughter in the Background.* Elsevier/Nelson, 1980. (U)

Following a rape attempt by her alcoholic mother's boyfriend, an obese and slovenly teenager learns to take control of her life. Fiction.

Fitzmahan, Don, *The Roller Coaster,* Comprehensive Health Education Foundation, Seattle, WA, 1986. (I)

This beautifully illustrated book describes the impact an alcoholic mother has on her family. It is a positive story that provides specific ideas on how family members can cope with the problem and maintain their own sense of wellness. Fiction.

Hamilton, Dorothy, *Joel's Other Mother,* Herald, 1984. (U)

The story of a young boy who has an alcoholic mother and how he locates help for her. Fiction.

*Lampman, Evelyn Sibley, *The Potlatch Family,* Atheneum, 1976 (I-U)

A young Native American girl is ashamed of her family, particularly of her alcoholic father. An exploration of how she deals with her feelings. Fiction.

Mazer, Harry, *War on Villa Street,* Delacorte, 1978. (I-U)

Willis Pierce is an eighth-grade boy with an alcoholic father and an overworked mother. A lonely and unhappy boy, repeated threats and beatings by a bully and his gang only increase his frustration. But Willis, while sensitive, is not a quitter. Tutoring a sixteen-year-old retarded boy in athletic skills while daring to compete in track himself, he gains in confidence. This memorable portrait of adolescence is very popular with young readers. Fiction.

Neveille, Emily Cheney, *Garden of Broken Glass*, Delacorte, 1975. (I-U)

Brian, his sister, and their mother who is an alcoholic, fat Martha, Dwayne, and his parents who force him to keep a straight and narrow path . . . these are the friends whose life in a black ghetto is described by a Newberry Prize Winner with perception and understanding. Fiction.

Nickerson, Sara, *Peter Parrot, Private Eye*, Comprehensive Health Education Foundation, 1988. (I-U)

Peter Parrot is a detective working on his first case: to find out about alcohol and its effects on people. He tells readers why some people drink, what alcohol does to their bodies, how people become addicted to alcohol, how to deal with an alcoholic family member, and why children should never drink alcohol. The book concludes with myths and facts about chemical dependency. Fiction.

Seixas, Judith S., *Living with a Parent Who Drinks Too Much*, Greenwillow, 1979. (I-U)

Explains what it is like to live with a parent who drinks too much by describing alcoholism, behavior of alcoholics, and problems the family faces. Suggests ways to cope with medical emergencies for the alcoholic and counseling help for the child. Nonfiction.

Silverstein, Alvin, and Silverstein, Virginia B., *Alcoholism*, Lippincott, 1975. (U)

After learning the medical and historical facts about drinking, the authors hope readers will be able to make an intelligent decision about drinking. In a clear, concise text these reknowned authors discuss all major aspects of alcohol use and abuse, causes and treatment of alcoholism, teenage drinking, and living with an alcoholic parent. Nonfiction.

*Wallin, Luke, *Ceremony of the Panther*, Bradbury, 1987. (U)

A teen is treated for drug and alcohol abuse. How he copes with the treatment and what people are trying to do for him. Fiction.

ANATOMY AND PHYSIOLOGY

Allison, Linda, *Blood and Guts: A Working Guide to Your Own Insides*, Little, Brown, 1976. (I)

A refreshing and fun look at the parts of the human body. They are all described in text and stories, and there are experiments and projects explained to discover how our parts function. Many humorous cartoons illustrate the experiments and descriptions. A real up-tempo book that will appeal to many students. Nonfiction.

Barrett, Judith, *I'm too small, YOU'RE TOO BIG*, Atheneum, 1981. (P)

A 5-year-old boy compares his size to that of his father. He sees the advantages of being big and of being small. He concludes that someday he will be as big as his father or, "maybe even bigger." Not much text, but nice illustrations to make this a good book for young children. Fiction.

Brandreth, Byles, *This Is Your Body*, Sterling, 1979. (U)

Approaches the study of structure and function of the body in an entertaining, yet accurate, manner. The 26 chapters are alphabetically arranged, offering one or more projects to be completed by an individual. Can be used by individual students or as support material in health or anatomy class. Nonfiction.

Brenner, Barbara, *Bodies*, Dutton, 1973. (P)

Everyone has a body and here in vital, vibrant photos showing bodies of many shapes and sizes you can see how one works and what it can do. Nonfiction.

*Cohen, Robert, *The Color of Man*, Random House, 1968. (U)

An exploration of color differences in humans. Nonfiction.

Curtis, Dr. Robert H., *Medical Talk for Beginners*, Messner, 1976. (U)

When new vocabulary pops up, steer older readers to this book. It is an attractively designed dictionary of medical terms from abdomen to x-ray. Nonfiction.

Gleman, Riata Golden, and Buxbaum, Susan Kovacs, *Ouch? All About Cuts and Hurts*, Harcourt, 1977. (P-I)

The volume is organized alphabetically and is a simple introduction to what happens to the body when common injuries occur, such as black-and-blue marks, bumps, cuts, nosebleeds, stitches, and scars, and how the body reacts to repair such damage. Nonfiction.

Gross, Ruth Belov, *Book about Your Skeleton*, Hastings House. In Canada, Sounders of Toronto, 1979 (A Science starter book). (P)

This lucid explanation of the bone structure of the body includes the various functions of bones and the skeleton. Two complete skeletons are shown at the end, labeled with common and scientific names. Nonfiction.

Kaufman, Joe, *How We Are Born, How We Grow, How Our Bodies Work . . . and How We Learn*, Webster, 1975. (I-U)

Contains a treasure lode of information for children of all ages. An attractive, oversized volume designed to give girls and boys a true understanding of their bodies. It answers many questions children might pose. For example: What makes you yawn when you are sleepy? Where do tears come from? Why does your body shiver when you are cold? Colorful illustrations help illuminate human processes such as birth, sight, digestion, dreaming, learning, and memory. Younger students will glean a great deal just by thumbing through the pages; older students can use the text for reference. Nonfiction.

Klein, Aaron E., *You and Your Body; a Book of Experiments to Perform on Yourself*, Doubleday, 1977. (I)

A different approach to the study of human physiology through a series of quick and easy experiments that do not require any complicated equipment. The directions are clear and concise, and the experiments can be performed by individuals, small groups, or an entire class. Nonfiction.

*May, Julian, *Why People are Different Colors*, Holiday House, 1971. (P-I)

An exploration of superficial human differences. Nonfiction.

McGuire, Leslie, *Susan Perl's Human Body Book*, Platt & Munk, 1977. (A Cricket book). (P-I)

Simple, direct answers for a multiplicity of questions about the human body, such as What holds the body up? and What happens to food after it is eaten? are complimented by delightful, whimsical pictures. A different book to share with younger children. Nonfiction.

Showers, Paul, *A Drop of Blood*, Crowell, 1967. (P)

Explains what blood is, how it works for our bodies, and why it is important to us. Nonfiction.

Showers, Paul, *Your Skin and Mine*, Crowell, 1967. (P)

This book encourages readers to make and examine fingerprints. It is also available in Spanish, as *Tu Piel y la Mia*. Nonfiction.

Thompson, Stephanie, *Know Your Human Body*, Rand McNally, 1977. (I-U)

Each chapter consists of only two pages but explains in detail every aspect of the human body, using large, clear diagrams. A quiz with the answers and a page of suggested projects are also included. Nonfiction.

Tully, Mariane, *Facts about the Human Body*, Watts, 1977. (I-U)

Unusual information is offered in this question-and-answer book about various parts of the human body. Authors have used actual questions from students and have responded with direct answers. Unfamiliar words printed in boldface type are all found in the glossary in the back of the book. Nonfiction.

*Whitefield, Phillip, and Whitefield, Ruth, *Why Do Our Bodies Stop Growing?* Viking, 1988. (I-U)

A book presented in question-and-answer format, about how the body works. Nonfiction.

DEATH

Carrick, Carol, *Accident*, Clarion, 1976. (P-I)

Christopher and his dog Badger walk along the road to meet his father and mother, but when a truck comes along, Badger starts to cross the road and is killed. Christopher is grief stricken, and it is only when he and his father search for a stone marker for Badger's grave that he can express his grief. Fiction.

*Dunlop, Beverley, *The Poetry Girl*, Houghton Mifflin, 1989. (I-U)

Story of a family that moves twice, and how the survivors deal with an attempted suicide by the father. Fiction.

Kral, Brian, *Apologies*, Anchorage Press, 1988. (U)

A play about a suicide of a child and the note that was left. The family and friends are left wondering why this could occur. Fiction.

*Krementz, Jill, *How it Feels When a Parent Dies*, Knopf, 1988. (U)

A telling story by two children who report how they coped with the suicide of a parent. Nonfiction.

L'Engle, Madeline. *A Ring of Endless Light*, Farrar, Straus & Giroux, 1980. (I-U)

A young child learns to deal with life and death during a summer with her grandfather who is dying. Fiction.

Mann, Peggy, *There Are Two Kinds of Terrible*, Doubleday, 1977. (P)

Robbie breaks his arm on the last day of school and has to spend summer with a big cast on it. He thinks that is terrible, but then he discovers that there are two kinds of terrible—regular terrible that can happen to anyone and you can get over—and real terrible that has no end. . . . A story of the death of a loved one written with great insight and emotion. Fiction.

Mazer, Norma Fox, *After the Rain*, Morrow, 1987. (U)

A child has to care for her dying grandfather. The book contains information about how she prepares for her grandfather's death. Fiction.

*Miles, Miska, *Annie and the Old One*, Atlantic Monthly, 1971. (P-I)

Annie is a Navajo child who loves to listen to her grandmother's stories. Her grandmother encourages Annie to watch as her mother weaves a rug. Grandmother says when the rug is finished she will "return to Mother Earth." To keep her beloved grandmother from dying, Annie starts to unravel the rug. Grandmother finds her and explains the cycle of life. Annie begins to understand why her grandmother must die, and the reader is shown how the cycle of life continues. Fiction.

Naughton, Jim, *My Brother Stealing Second*, Harper & Row, 1983. (U)

A story about a child's emotional recovery from the death of an older brother by remembering the good times they had. Fiction.

Olsen, Voilet, *Never Brought to Mind*, Atheneum, 1985. (U)

Four months after the death of two of their friends, peers are still experiencing depression and guilt. They must seek understanding and acceptance from others to cope with the loss. Fiction.

*Taha, Karen, *A Gift for Tia Rosa*, Dillon, 1985. (P-I)

Tia Rosa is Carmela's elderly neighbor. Carmela plans to make something special for Tia Rosa as soon as she finishes the scarf she is knitting for her father, but Tia Rosa dies before she finishes the scarf. Carmela learns to pass on to others the love she had for Tia Rosa with the help of her caring and supportive mother. The idea that life and love go on after a death is touchingly portrayed. Fiction.

Townsend, Maryann, and Stern, Ronnie, *Pop's Secret*, Addison-Wesley, 1980 (P)

Mark talks about his grandfather, Pop. He tells about the things he and Pop do together and enjoys looking at photos of Pop as a child. When Pop dies, Mark makes his own family photo album to help him deal with the sadness he feels over losing Pop. This approach to dealing with the loss of a loved one may help students understand the importance of remembering. Fiction.

Varley, Susan, *Badger's Parting Gifts*, Lothrop, 1984. (P)

Badger is aging and wants his friends to be able to accept his impending death. After Badger dies his animal friends express their grief by telling stories of all the things he taught them. As they share stories with one another, they begin to realize that the skills Badger taught are gifts that should be passed on to others. The value of talking with others who care after the death of a loved one is stressed. Fiction.

Zindel, Paul, *A Begonia for Miss Applebaum*, Harper & Row, 1989. (U)

Students find out that a beloved former teacher has a terminal illness. The ways that they deal with the situation are explained in story format. Fiction.

DENTAL HEALTH

De Groat, Diane, *Alligator's Toothache*, Crown, 1977. (P)

Alligator's predicament—a toothache and fear of the dentist—is eventually resolved through trickery and is eloquently portrayed through the three-color pen-and-ink drawings in this wordless book. Fiction.

Doss, Helen, *All the Better to Bite With*, Messner, 1976. (I)

Here is a guided tour of our teeth and mouth, introduced by a discussion of different animal teeth. Parts of the mouth and teeth, causes and prevention of tooth and gum disease, dentist office procedures, and intelligent choice of foods are all discussed in a clear text accompanied by black and white photographs and diagrams. Nonfiction.

Hammond, Winifred G., *Riddle of Teeth*, Coward-McCann, 1971. (I)

Most chapters of this factual book about teeth contain interesting projects for readers to try at home or in school with classmates. The author is very specific in her discussion of formation of teeth, the different kinds of teeth and how they work, the causes of caries and other dental diseases, and the fight to control and prevent the loss of teeth. Children who are preparing for orthodontia can learn much from this book, and it can be used in health classes, by dentists, and for general reading about the care and protection of the teeth and mouth. Nonfiction.

Lesieg, T., *Tooth Book*, Random House, 1981. (P)

In this beginning reader book, rhymed verses and bright, cartoon-style artwork reveal a wealth of dental facts. An excellent fun and educational book for children that conveys good feelings toward dentists and dental health. Fiction.

Pomerantz, Charlotte, *Mango Tooth*, Greenwillow, 1977. (P)

Posy is starting to lose her baby teeth. The first one is loosened by a mango pit, and it earns her a dime. Then she loses the "chicken bone tooth" and the "Turkish tootsie tooth," each providing another dime. But clever Posy nets two dimes on the fourth tooth, an "elephant tooth." Not many people can loosen a tooth on an elephant. Fiction.

Richter, A., and Numeroff, L., *You Can't Put Braces on Spaces*, Greenwillow, 1979. (I-U)

Eleven-year-old Neil has just started to wear braces. Neil's brother describes what Dr. Sherman did and said as he fitted Neil with braces and how his brother said they felt. Line drawings enhance this story, which presents the prospect of wearing braces as a positive event. Fiction.

Ross, Pat, *Molly and the Slow Teeth*, Lee & Shepard, 1980. (P)

Molly is an unhappy second grader because while all her classmates are losing their baby teeth and getting rewards from the Tooth Fairy, she doesn't even have a loose tooth. She tries to fool the Tooth Fairy with a small white pebble, but that doesn't work. Only weeks and weeks of waiting and a hard apple finally put a gaping smile on Molly's face and her name on the class tooth chart. Fiction.

Schaleben-Lewis, Joy, *The Dentist and Me*, Raintree, 1977. (P)

Two children, Adam and Nikki, describe their trips to the dentist. Adam goes for a checkup and Nikki goes to have her cavity filled. These common procedures are described. Emphasis is placed on preventive care. A good introductory book. Fiction.

DISEASES AND HEALTH PROBLEMS

Allen, Majorie, *One, Two, Three—Ah-Choo!*, Coward, 1980. (P)

Wally Springer is allergic to dust, feathers, and his new puppy. When medication and shots do not completely control his allergy, he must give up the puppy for a different pet. Wally learns about all kinds of pets and finally decides on a hermit crab. After a series of humorous events, Wally and his crab win first place at the school pet show because Wally knows so much about hermit crabs. On the way to pick up his trophy he passes the other pets and begins to sneeze. Wally's acceptance of allergies will help others with the same problem. Fiction.

Colmon, Warren, *Understanding and Preventing AIDS*, Children's Press, 1988. (U)

Information intended to warn children about the dangers associated with AIDS. Myths about the disease and how it is spread are dispelled. Nonfiction.

*Brown, Marion Marsh, *Homeward the Arrow's Flight*, Abingdon, 1980. (I-U)

A fictionalized biography of the first woman Native American physician. Fiction.

*Clifford, Eth, *The Wild One*, Houghton Mifflin, 1974. (U)

Biography of Santiago Ramon, a physician who won the Nobel Prize for medicine in 1906. Nonfiction.

Jacobs, Francine, *Breakthrough: The True Story of Penicillin*, Dodd, Mead, 1988. (U)

The true story of the discovery of penicillin by Fleming and how he worked with others for this historic moment. Nonfiction.

Corcoran, Barbara B., *I Am the Universe,* Atheneum, 1986. (I-U)

A story of how a child copes with her mother's cancer as well as other family problems. In dealing with this, she discovers who she really is. Fiction.

*Coerr, Eleanor, *Sadako and the Thousand Paper Cranes,* Putnam, 1977. (I-U)

A compelling story of a Japanese child who is dying of leukemia developed as the result of radiation sickness that resulted from the bombing of Hiroshima. Fiction.

deSaint Phalle, Nicki, *You Can't Catch It Holding Hands,* Lapis Press, 1986. (U)

This book contains information about intravenous drug abuse, homosexuality, safe sex, and AIDS. It is presented in the form of a letter from a mother to her son. Fiction.

Donahue, Parnell, and Capellaor, Helen, *Germs Make Me Sick: a Health Handbook for Kids,* Knopf, 1975. (U)

Describes a wide variety of diseases and their treatment and offers a brief discussion of germs in general. Included are diseases of the gastrointestinal tract (food poisoning, stomach sickness), the respiratory tract (colds, sore throats, sinusitis), germs on the skin (warts, acne, athlete's foot), and viral exanthems (measles, chickenpox). A separate chapter discusses "Some Diseases You Probably Won't Get," such as meningitis, rabies, and rheumatic fever. The final chapter tells about "Getting Well and Staying There." A glossary and index are appended. Nonfiction.

Keller, Holly, *Cromwell's Glasses,* Greenwillow, 1982. (P)

Cromwell, a young rabbit, is teased when he can't see and is teased even more once he gets his new glasses. Cromwell hates his new glasses even more than he hated not being able to see. Finally, Cromwell and his siblings begin to accept his problem when other rabbits at the park make fun of him and Cromwell's sister defends her younger brother. A fun portrayal of common feelings associated with wearing glasses. Fiction.

Kipnis, Lynne, and Adler, Susan, *You Can't Catch Diabetes from a Friend,* Triad, 1979. (P-I)

Four children, (ages 7, 10, 11, and 14) tell their stories about life with diabetes. In each story, a different aspect of coping with this disease is examined. Al-

though three of the children are older than the target audience, the reading level and explanations of the disease are well within grasp of students in grades 1 to 3. These stories provide a quality introduction and explanation of many aspects of living with diabetes. Fiction.

Marion, Barbara, *Eric Needs Stitches,* Addison-Wesley, 1979. (P)

A bicycle accident sends Eric to the emergency room for stitches. His father explains what will happen once they arrive at the hospital, and a nurse reassures him it's okay to cry if it hurts. The photos are realistic and informative. Eric's story will help prepare children for an unexpected trip to the emergency room. Fiction.

Radley, Gail, *CF in His Corner,* Four Winds, 1984. (U)

The story of a young child who must face the fact that his younger brother has cystic fibrosis. Fiction.

Roy, Ron, *Where's Buddy?,* Clarion, 1982. (P-I)

Buddy is 7 years old and has never accepted responsibility for care of his diabetes. When Buddy is left in the care of his older brother, Mike, he disappears. Mike's frantic search for his brother provides suspense. Mike must give Buddy his insulin shot or Buddy could die. The lesson in responsibility and technical information are nicely integrated in this exciting story. Fiction.

Sampson, Fay, *Watch on Patterick Fell,* Greenwillow, 1980. (U)

Patterick Fell is an English plant that stores nuclear waste from around the world. Teenage Roger's father is the director and his mother a distinguished co-worker, and Roger has never questioned the plant's validity until the protests mount, and his younger sister joins them. When an explosion nearly levels the plant, the family rethinks its commitment. A very timely book, but some British attitudes and idioms may need explanation. Fiction.

Silverstein, Virginia B., and Silverstein, DR. Alvin, *Itch, Sniffle and Sneeze: All about Asthma, Hay Fever and Other Allergies,* Four Winds, 1978. (P-I)

If any of your children sneeze every August, get those annoying itchy bumps on their skin when they eat chocolate, or have trouble breathing when they play with a puppy, this book should be passed on to them. The text succinctly tells what allergies are, how the body reacts to them, things people are allergic to, and how to cope with allergies. Nonfiction.

Starkman, Neal, *Z's Gift,* Comprehensive Health Education Foundation, 1988. (I-U)

Z is a young boy whose teacher has AIDS. He knows he can't catch AIDS from Mrs. Brown, but some parents want to take their children out of school because of her. Z decides that it's time people got the facts about AIDS, and he asks his mother to invite his physician to speak to a group of parents. In a touching conversation between the boy and his teacher, readers discover how compassion can be a wondrous gift. Fiction.

Winn, Marie, *The Sick Book: Questions and Answers about Hiccups and Mumps, Sneezes and Bumps, and Other Things That Go Wrong with Us,* Four Winds, 1976. (P-I)

This is an informative volume about common childhood illnesses. Presented in a lively question-and-answer format, the various sections deal with colds and the flu, allergies, chickenpox, mumps, measles, skin troubles, and broken bones. Each ailment is presented so that readers will understand what happens when they are sick. A special section at the end of the book explains how our bodies work when they are healthy. Nonfiction.

DRUGS

Corcoran, Barbara, *The Woman in Your Life,* Atheneum, 1984. (U)

The diary of a girl in prison who was convicted of transporting drugs across the border for a boyfriend. Fiction.

*Dolan, Edward F, Jr., *Drugs in Sports,* Watts, 1986. (U)

The types of drugs used in sports in an attempt to enhance performance. The effects of the drugs on the body and mind are explained. Nonfiction.

Hawley, Richard A., *Think About Drugs and Society,* Walker, 1988. (U)

An exploration of drugs and drug abuse in our culture. The impact of drug use on society is explored. Nonfiction.

Hyde, Margert O., *Know about Drugs,* ed 2, McGraw-Hill, 1979. (I-U)

Along with the basic information about all drugs, the authors include facts about the use and abuse of mar-

ijuana, alcohol, coca and cocaine, cigarettes, PCP (angel dust), inert inhalants, heroin, barbiturates, methaqualone, and a wide variety of tranquilizers, amphetamines, and LSD and other hallucinogens. Nonfiction.

*Liss, Howard, *The Lawrence Taylor Story,* Enslow, 1987. (U)

A story of legendary professional football player Lawrence Taylor; his career and his comeback after drug abuse problems. Nonfiction.

Marr, John S., *The Good Drug and the Bad Drug,* Evans, 1970. (I)

A city doctor has written in simple terms the course of two complete trips of drugs through the body. By means of illustrations, the good drug is shown as it travels toward the infected area in an effort to effect a cure. Having established certain basic concepts, the doctor then describes the harmful effects of a bad drug. A book that lends itself to class discussion. Nonfiction.

Mohun, Jane. *Drugs, Steroids and Sports,* Watts, 1988. (U)

An explanation of steroid abuse and the side effects of the use of steroids. Nonfiction.

Morey, Walt, *Lemon Meringue Dog,* Dutton. In Canada, Clarke, Irwin, 1980. (U)

Chris, age 20, is the junior member of a new Coast Guard narcotic squad that uses dogs to uncover drugs. On their first assignment on a ship, his dog Mike is curiously diverted by a surprise cache of his favorite lemon meringue pies, ruining the drug bust. Demoted, Chris buys Mike, and moonlighting as a night watchman he redeems them both by uncovering a huge and dangerous drug ring. A good action story with a low reading level. Fiction.

*Shreve, Susan, *Nightmare of Geranium Street,* Knopf, 1977. (P)

Elizabeth's family has chosen to stay on in their long-time home in a deteriorating area of Germantown, Pennsylvania. She has become the "Rex" of a club of children. When Amanda comes to live with her Aunt Tess, the club—the Nightmares—become very curious about what happens in their house. Slowly it becomes evident that Tess is involved in a drug ring, as the children observe and become involved in disclosing. They never actually take drugs themselves—

partly because of the strict discipline in Elizabeth's own family. An interesting and valuable picture of inner-city life from a true child's point of view. Fiction.

FAMILY AND RELATIONSHIPS

*Adoff, Arnold, *All the Colors of the Race*, Lothrop, Lee & Shepard 1982. (I-U)

A series of poems that deal with human differences and similarities. Fiction.

Alexander, Martha, *When the New Baby Comes, I'm Moving Out*, Dial, 1979. (P)

When his mother paints his old highchair in preparation for the new baby, Oliver rebels. He plots a variety of plans for revenge. His mother listens patiently to his threats, then points out all the advantages he will have as the big brother. An understanding mother helps Oliver adjust to changes within the family. Fiction.

*Angell, Judie, *One-Way to Ansonia*, Bradbury, 1985. (I)

Historical fiction about an immigrant family and their nonconformity to society to preserve their heritage. Fiction.

*Appiah, Sonia, *Amoko and Efua Bear*, Macmillan, 1989. (P)

A story of a young girl and her relationship with a fantasy friend. Fiction.

*Barrett, Joyce Durham, *Willie's Not the Hugging Kind*, Harper & Row, 1989. (P)

A moving story that deals with the development of feelings. Fiction.

Blaine, Marge, *Terrible Thing That Happened at Our House*, Four Winds, 1975. (P-I)

Two young children dislike the changes in their family life when Mother goes back to work. Everyone has to rush around in the morning; they have to eat in the noisy, smelly school lunchroom, no one has time to listen; and there's no time for stories, games, or trips to the gas station. Things are just too topsy-turvy. Fiction.

Brandenberg, Franz, *Nice New Neighbors*, Greenwillow, 1977. (P)

When Mr. and Mrs. Fieldmouse and their six children move to a new home, the neighborhood children are unfriendly. The resourceful mouse children invent their own play and suddenly they are very popular. All the neighborhood children beg to join in. Fiction.

*Cameron, Ann, *The Stories Julian Tells*, Pantheon, 1981. (P-I)

Six stories of life in a loving family. Fiction.

*Gay, Kathlyn, *The Rainbow Effect: Interracial Families*, Watts, 1987. (U)

The problems of being a child in an interracial family in America. Children tell their own stories. Fiction.

Grant, Jan, *Our New Baby*, Children's, 1980. (P)

A perceptive pediatrician helps a little girl overcome her feelings of jealously toward the arrival of a new baby. Her parents allow her to help with the preparations, and when the new baby comes home and won't stop crying, the little girl sings a song that soothes the infant. She realizes that "Mom and Dad are really going to need my help with the new baby." This story may help parents prepare a child for the arrival of a new baby. Fiction.

Gordon, Shirley, *The Boy Who Wanted a Family*, Harper & Row, 1980. (P-I)

Michael is an orphan who has been living in several foster homes. One day his social worker takes him to meet a woman who might be interested in adopting him. Michael is wary because he has had his hopes crushed before. He meets Miss Graham and finds he likes her. She would like to adopt him, but it will take a year. During that time the two become close, and Michael loses his fear of being rejected. After signing the official papers, Michael begins planning for his future. This story helps the reader to learn about what it is like to be in foster homes and feelings about adoption. Fiction.

*Guy, Rosa, *And I Heard a Bird Sing*, Delacorte, 1987. (U)

How to cope with and understand family problems. Fiction.

Hazen, Barbara Shook, *Tight Times*, Viking. In Canada, Penguin Books Canada. 1979. (P)

A youngster doesn't understand why something called "tight times" keeps him from getting a dog and causes Mommy to go to work and Daddy to lose his job. But in spite of all their problems, when the child brings home a starved kitten, Mommy and Daddy say the new pet can stay. Fiction.

Kosof, Anna, *Incest: Families in Crisis,* Watts, 1985. (U)

An exploration of incest and the importance of reporting this abuse. Fiction.

*Lewin, Hugh, *Jafta's Mother,* Carolrhoda, 1983. (P)

A young African boy, Jafta, describes his mother by comparing her to the things he sees around him. She is like the sun, waking him each morning, and like the earth, strong and brown. She can be stormy as well, but like most storms her anger is soon to blow over. Like the sky, she is always there. A warm, beautiful portrait of a mother's love for her child. Fiction.

Livingstone, Carole, *Why Was I Adopted?* Lyle Stuart, 1978. (I-U)

Presents facts of adoption in clever and appealing text and illustrations. Focuses on reasons for and ways of being adopted and how special adopted children are to parents. Concludes with questions children frequently ask. Nonfiction.

McCord, Jean, *Turkeylegs Thompson,* Atheneum. In Canada, McClelland & Stewart, 1979. (I-U)

Even pugnacious Turkeylegs (really 12-year-old Betty Ann) has a breaking point. Virtually without friends, she helps her single-parent mother care for her whiny little brother and her enchanting little sister. But buffeted by a person exposing himself to her, her little sister's death, and her alcoholic father's return home, she runs away to the hills she loves, but returns home to face her grief and confusion when her young friend Charlie meets her and counsels patience. A bleak, sometimes painful story, with a very believable main character. Fiction.

*Nolan, Madeena Spray, *My Daddy Don't Go to Work,* Carolrhoda Books, 1978. (P)

A young black girl tells about her daddy who goes out every day looking for a job but just can't find a place that needs him. Although her daddy is discouraged, the little girl likes having him home to play ball with her and listen to her after school. Fiction.

Pursell, Margaret Sanford, *Look at Adoption,* Lerner, 1977. (I-U)

Straightforward discussion of adoption, including reasons children are available and steps necessary for adoption. Nonfiction.

Raynor, Dorka, *This Is My Father and Me,* Whitman, 1973. (P-I)

Photographic essay on the relationship between father and child in many different countries. Nonfiction.

Richards, Arlene Kramer, *How to Get It Together When Your Parents Are Coming Apart,* McKay, 1976. (I-U)

Through many representative stories of adolescents, this guide offers suggestions to young people for coping with divorce. Divided into three parts (marriage trouble, during the divorce, and after the divorce), the emphasis is to assuage guilt feelings on the part of the children and to provide specific addresses for finding outside help. Nonfiction.

Stolz, Mary, *Go and Catch a Flying Fish,* Harper & Row. In Canada, Fitzhenry & Whiteside, 1979 (An Ursual Nordstrom book). (P-I)

The seemingly idyllic life of the Reddick family centers on the sea, sun, and sand of Florida's Gulf Coast. Although the three children—13-year-old Taylor and her younger brothers, aged 10 and 4—are aware that something is wrong, no one, not even her husband, Tony, is prepared for Junie's abrupt departure for "time on her own." Fiction.

Tax, Meredith, *Families,* Little, Brown, 1981. (P)

Positive and humorous description of different kinds of families as told by 6-year-old Angie. Includes animals (lions, dogs, chickens, ants) and people (parents, single parent, stepparents, grandparents, two women). Nonfiction.

HANDICAPS

*Anacona, George, and Beth, Mary, *Handtalk Zoo,* Four Winds, 1989. (P-U)

A group of children and a deaf actress visit the zoo. The signs and finger spellings for various familiar animals are demonstrated. Fiction.

Arnold, Katrin, *Anna Joins In,* Abingdon, 1983. (P-I)

Cystic fibrosis is a chronic disease with which young Anna must come to terms. At times she rebels against the restrictions caused by her condition, and at other times she uses it to manipulate those around her. The story helps the reader understand the difficulty of trying to be a normal child while suffering from a chronic disease. Fiction.

Brightman, Alan, *Like Me,* Little, Brown, 1976. (P)

Rhyming text and beautiful photographs explain the concept of mental retardation for the younger reader. Nonfiction.

Carrick, Carol, *Stay Away from Simon!,* Clarion, 1985. (P-I)

Set in the 1830s, this story tells of a brother and sister who have been taught to stay away from Simon, a mentally retarded boy. Their fears and feelings about Simon change when Simon rescues them from a blinding snowstorm on the way home from school. Excellent for helping children understand others who seem different. Fiction.

Charlip, Remy, and Charlip, Mary Beth, *Handtalk: an ABC of Finger Spelling and Sign Language,* Four Winds, 1980 (reprint of edition published by Parents' Magazine Press, 1974). (P)

All ages will enjoy learning about the ways people can talk using their voices: finger spelling (making words letter by letter with the fingers) and signing (using the hands to convey a picture for a word or idea). Full-color pictures show children how it's done. Nonfiction.

Clifton, Lucille, *My Friend Jacob,* Dutton, 1980. (P)

Sam and Jacob are neighbors and the very best of friends. Although 17-year-old Jacob is mentally retarded, 8-year-old Sam learns they can love and help each other. Fiction.

Cohen, Miriam, *See You Tomorrow,* Charles, Greenwillow, 1983. (P)

Charles is a blind student in the first grade. His new classmates accept him but tend to be overprotective. They praise him for even the smallest accomplishments and remind him not to be sad. At recess, the children sneak into a dark basement and become scared. Charles leads them to safety and they develop respect for him. An appropriate book for discussing a disabled person's need for independence and respect. Fiction.

Corcoran, Barbara B., *A Dance to Still Music,* Atheneum, 1974. (U)

The story of a 14-year-old girl who refuses to accept her deafness. Fiction.

Dacquino, V.T., *Kiss The Candy Days Good-bye,* Delacorte, 1983. (I)

This book tells of Jimmy, who is diagnosed as having diabetes. It describes the adjustments that must be made by Jimmy, his family, and friends. Fiction.

Emmert, Michelle, *I'm the Big Sister Now,* Whitman, 1989. (P)

The story of living with a big sister who has cerebral palsy. Written by the younger sister. Fiction.

Froehlich, M.W., *Hide Crawford Quick,* Houghton Mifflin, 1983. (I)

Twelve-year-old Gracie realizes that something is wrong when her brother is born with a limb abnormality. The main plot is the eventual acceptance of this physically handicapped boy by the rest of his family. Fiction.

*Griese, Arnold A., *At the Mouth of the Luckiest River,* Crowell, 1973. (I)

A convincing tale of Talek, an Alaskan Indian boy who becomes a leader among his people despite being crippled. Set in the nineteenth century. Fiction.

Jones, Ron, *The Acorn People,* Abingdon, 1976. (I)

Teachers may wish to read aloud some parts of this story of five severely handicapped children in a boy scout camp with an unprepared counselor. Older children will learn about courage through their own reading. Fiction.

Kamien, Janet, *What If You Couldn't . . . ? A Book About Special Needs,* Scribner's, 1979. (I)

An informational book about handicaps that includes "experiments" that will help children to understand the everyday problems that confront the handicapped. Nonfiction.

Kulkin, Susan, *Thinking Big: The Story of a Young Dwarf,* Lothrop, Lee & Shepart, 1986. (P-I)

Explores a child's experiences with the world as a dwarf. Fiction.

Lasker, Joe, *He's My Brother,* Whitman, 1974. (P)

Jamie is not retarded, but he is a slow learner who often becomes frustrated at school. The other children make fun of him and tease him. There are many things he can't do well, but Jamie is kind and gentle to animals, babies, and young children. He draws well and is also very good on the drums. His parents are patient and understanding. His brother and sister are good to him and make up stories to tell him they love him. Nonfiction.

Levine, Edna S., *Lisa and Her Soundless World,* Human Science Press, 1974. (I)

Eight-year-old Lisa is deaf and attends special schools to learn to use sign language and to lip read, as well as to improve her speech. Fiction.

Litchfield, Ada, *Captain Hook, That's Me,* Walker, 1982. (P-I)

Judy is an active, fun-loving girl who has a hook in place of her left hand. Her usual confidence is shaken when her father tells her the family is moving. She worries about being accepted in a new school. Judy's new class makes her feel welcome and accepted and she no longer worries about belonging. Although Judy's handicap adds to her worries, other students will be able to understand her fears of being accepted in a new environment. The story may help students to be more tolerant toward new students, handicapped or not. Fiction.

Litchfield, Ada, *Words In Our Hands,* Albert Whitman, 1980. (P)

Michael describes in informative and emotional terms life with his deaf parents and two normal sisters. Michael's family adjusts well until they move to a new town. There everyone feels strange and, for the first time, Michael is embarrassed by his parents' deafness. Adjustment is made easier when the family attends a play done in sign language and meets others with similar problems. Pictures of the sign for each letter of the alphabet enhance understanding and interest in this story. Fiction.

Little, Jean, *Mine for Keeps,* Little, Brown, 1962. (I-U)

The story of a child who must face life in the world after spending 5 years in a home for the handicapped. Fiction.

Maclachan, Patricia, *Through Grandpa's Eyes,* Harper & Row, 1980. (P)

A blind grandfather teaches a child to "see" in other ways. Fiction.

Marek, Margot, *Different, Not Dumb,* Franklin Watts, 1985. (P-I)

Mike needs to go to a special teacher to help him read. He doesn't like having to leave his second-grade class

to go for extra help. Mike learns to look at words a new way with the help of his reading teacher. He and his friend Jeff use Mike's new skills to prevent an accident, and both boys become heroes. Concerns about leaving the classroom for extra help may be eased with the use of this book. Fiction.

Payne, Sherry, *A Contest,* Minneapolis, Carolrhoda Books, 1982. (P)

Mike, a student with cerebral palsy, is in a wheelchair, and has attended a special school, finds himself in a regular class. The other kids stare and are scared until the teacher devises games to show off Mike's strengths. Fiction.

Petersen, Palle, *Sally Can't See,* Crowell, 1977 (A John Day Book). (P)

The life of a blind child and how she learns and plays is described in a brief text illustrated with color photographs. Nonfiction.

Robinet, Harriette Gillem, *Ride the Red Cycle,* Houghton, Mifflin, 1980. (I)

Gutsy, crippled Jerome is determined to learn to ride his tricycle, and with the help of his family, he does. Fiction.

Savitz, Harriet May, *Run, Don't Walk,* Watts, 1979. (I)

Two teenagers confined to wheelchairs take some positive actions to prevent being discriminated against because of their handicaps. Fiction.

Shalom, Debra, *Special Kids Make Special Friends,* Bellmore, NY, An Association for Children with Down syndrome, 1984. (P)

This simply written book, aimed at primary and beginning intermediate students, has excellent photographs. It is about children with Down syndrome.

Siegel, Dorothy Schainman, *Winners: Eight Special Young People,* Messner, 1978. (I-U)

Biographical sketches of eight courageous young people, each with a different handicap. These children have not permitted their problems to curtail their activities more than is absolutely necessary. Nonfiction.

Slepian, Jan, *The Alfred Summer,* Macmillan, 1980. (I-U)

Lester could care less that Alfred is slightly retarded. After all, Alfred doesn't mind about Lester's cerebral palsy. Together with two other friends, they are a memorable quartet. Fiction.

Smith, Lucia B., *A Special Kind of Sister,* Holt, 1979. (P)

> Seven-year-old Sarah talks about her feelings for her retarded younger brother Andy. Fiction.

Sullivan, Mary Beth, Brightman, Alan J., and Blatt, Joseph, *Feeling Free,* Addison-Wesley, 1979. (I, U)

> In this spin-off of the television series by the same name, handicapped children talk about their disabilities. A great aid to mainstreaming, the book is directed toward children and adults who are unprepared to interact with the handicapped. Nonfiction.

White, Paul, *Janet at School,* Crowell, 1978, (A John Day Book). (P)

> Janet has spina bifida and cannot move or feel her legs. As children learn about her daily life in this straightforward, caring account, they will grasp the difficulties people with this disease must overcome. Nonfiction.

Wolf, Bernard, *Don't Feel Sorry for Paul,* Lippincott, 1974. (I)

> Born with his hands and feet incompletely formed, Paul is encouraged to be independent all his life. This book shows his progress. Nonfiction.

Wolf, Bernard, *Anna's Silent World,* Lippincott, 1977. (P)

> Abundant black-and-white photographs show Anna at home, in school, at dancing class, and at the New York League for the Hard of Hearing. Hearing aids and the process of learning to speak are explained. Nonfiction.

*Zelonky, Joy, *I Can't Always Hear You,* Raintree, 1980. (P-I)

> Kim has learned to adjust to her hearing loss, but must now learn to adjust to a regular classroom. Both Kim and her classmates learn that being disabled is not reason for cruelty and laughter. During the course of the story, others learn to accept Kim by realizing that each person is different (tall, wearing glasses, wearing braces, adopted, allergic to chocolate, etc.). Illustrations show a variety of ethnic groups in Kim's class. A wonderful way to discuss differences among people. Fiction.

MENTAL AND EMOTIONAL PROBLEMS

*Andrews, Jan, *The Very Last First Time,* Atheneum, 1986. (P)

> *A Journey into Self-Discovery.* Learning how to deal with fears. Fiction.

Bonsail, Crosby, *Who's Afraid of the Dark?* Harper & Row. In Canada, Fitzhenry & Whiteside, 1980. (P)

> A little boy tries to teach his dog Stella to be unafraid of the dark and the night noises, but the readers know it's really the boy who's scared. Fiction.

*Bryan, Ashley, *Lion and the Ostrich Chicks and Other African Folk Tales,* Macmillan, 1986. (P-I)

> A series of amusing tales set in Africa where an underdog triumphs in each case. Fiction.

*Cameron, Ann, *The Most Beautiful Place in the World,* Knopf, 1988. (P)

> A story about a Guatemalan boy who copes with being abandoned and must deal with poverty, but he triumphs over all. Fiction.

Chapman, Carol, *Herbie's Troubles,* E.P. Dutton, 1981. (P)

> Herbie enjoys school until a bully starts to make his life miserable. Herbie reaches the point where he decides not to go to school any more. His friends and family give him advice about how to handle his problem, and each time he goes to school he tries out their advice. Nothing seems to work until Herbie tries his own solution. Herbie once again enjoys going to school. A helpful story for those coping with similar problems. Fiction.

Cohen, Miriam, *So What?,* Greenwillow, 1982. (P)

> Jim is feeling left out and incapable of doing some of the things his classmates can do. He makes several attempts to be part of the group and in the process hurts the feelings of a new girl. She replies, "So what," to his taunts. When Jim fails again, the girl tells him, "so what," that some people are good at different things, and that it shouldn't bother him. Jim is encouraged by this new outlook on life, and the things that used to upset him don't seem to matter so much any more. An interesting approach to solving problems and looking at oneself. Fiction.

Greene, Laura, *I Am Somebody*, Children's Press, In Canada, Regensteiner, 1980. (P-I)

> Story is told in the first person by a not-so-good ball player. Nathan deals with the frustration of not being chosen first, being tagged out at base, and missing an important catch. There is no miraculous ending. Nathan has a collection of feathers that he shares with a friend. He loves to play baseball, but he is better at collecting. Nonfiction.

*Haseley, Dennis, *The Sacred One*, Warne, 1983. (P)

> A story of personal heritage. Explores the world of human differences. Nonfiction.

*Hall, Malcolm, *Friends of Charlie Ant Bear*, Coward-McCann. In Canada, Academic, 1980. (P)

> Charlie Ant Bear is jealous of his best friend Wild Bob Ding, who is liked by everyone in town because of his funny practical jokes. Gloomy Charlie buys a joke book thinking that he too can become popular. All his jokes and tricks backfire, and Charlie is feeling worse than ever, until he and Bob try one final trick that tops them all. Fiction.

*Hill, E. *Evans Corner*, Holt, 1967. (P)

> A young child seeks a quiet space in his crowded home. Fiction.

*Hirschfelder, Arlene, *Happily May I Walk: American Indians and Alaska Natives Today*, Scribner's, 1986, (I-U)

> An informational book about the Indian people of North America and Alaska natives. The central theme is the acceptance of others. Nonfiction.

*Hobby, J., Robin, G., and Rubin, D., *Staying Back*, Triad, 1982. (P-I)

> Seven students from various ethnic and racial backgrounds tell stories of repeating a grade in school. Reasons for the retention are common, but vary. They include illness, parental pressure, learning disabilities, handicaps, and family problems. The everyday fears of childhood are conveyed in this warm and caring story. Fiction.

Hogan, Paula, *Sometimes I Get So Mad*, Raintree, 1980. (P-I)

> Karen learns how to deal with feelings of jealously, ostracism, and anger when she is rejected and hurt by an older girl she admires. Karen takes out her feelings on her little sister, then realizes that it's not her sister's fault the older girl has spurned her. With help from her mother, Karen learns how to express her feelings verbally to the older girl, and when a choice must be made between the little sister and the older girl, Karen happily chooses her sister. Feelings among family members are nicely supported by the illustrations. Fiction.

*Lattimore, Deborah Nourse, *The Flame of Peace*, Harper & Row, 1987. (P-I)

> Learning how to cooperate and develop a positive self-image. Fiction.

Lopshire, Robert, *I Want to Be Somebody New*, Beginner, 1986. (P)

> A large spotted animal is tired of being in the circus and wants to be something new. The animal has the ability to change its spots from place to place and color to color. Using this talent to change into various other creatures, the animal discovers that it really is best to be oneself. Bold color illustrations enhance the text. Simple sentences provide an opportunity for students to expand the sentences with their own thoughts and opinions. Fiction.

*Mohr, Nicholasa, *Going Home*, Dial, 1986. (P)

> A story about coming to terms with one's ethnic heritage. An exploration of cultural and sexual stereotyping. Fiction.

*Naidoo, Beverly, *Journey to Jo'Burg: A South African Story*, Lippincott, 1986. (I-P)

> Set in South Africa, this book contains an explanation of how to deal with human differences. Fiction.

*Nickerson, Sara, *Martin the Cavebine*, Comprehensive Health Education Foundation, 1989. (P-I)

> The furry, little cavebines' fear of the forest prevents them from venturing outside their cave. The whole community, except for Martin, pitches in with the daily chores. They don't understand why Martin spends day after day staring into the forest instead of helping them. When disaster strikes and the cavebines must leave their home, they discover just how important Martin is! Illustrated with colorful, intriguing drawings by an award-winning artist, *Martin the Cavebine* helps young children become more tolerant, and even appreciative, of other's differences. Fiction.

Park, Barbara, *Don't Make Me Smile,* Alfred A. Knopf, 1981. (I)

Charles is having a hard time dealing with his feelings about the divorce of his parents. He tries to handle things on his own, but just can't deal with his mixed emotions. At his father's request, Charles goes to see a psychologist, Dr. Girard. Although at first resentful, Charles lets Dr. Girard help him sort out his feelings and eventually come to terms with his parents' divorce. This story may be useful in opening the door for discussion of divorce and counseling. Fiction.

Prusski, Jeffrey, *Bring Back the Deer,* Harcourt Brace Jovanovich, 1988. (P)

A story of growth and coming of age. Fiction.

*Simon, Norma, *Nobody's Perfect, Not Even My Mother,* Albert Whitman, 1981. (I)

A group of ethnically and racially varied children tell about the things they do well and the things they don't. Some note that even parents and teachers make mistakes and are good at different things. The story concludes, "Everyone's good at some things. But nobody's perfect." Illustrations are very appealing. Very useful in opening discussions about individual talents and abilities. Fiction.

*Soto, Gary, *Baseball in April and Other Stories,* Harcourt, 1990. (I-P)

A series of stories of how contemporary Mexican-American children deal with typical difficulties of growing up. A glossary of Spanish terms is included. Fiction.

*Springer, Nancy, *They're All Named Wildfire,* Atheneum, 1989. (I-P)

An examination of the effects of prejudice and bigotry. Fiction.

Starkman, Neal, *The Riddle,* Comprehensive Health Education Foundation, 1990. (I-U)

When Maria's teacher has her class choose partners to solve a riddle, Maria reluctantly pairs up with Pete, the new kid. As they spend time together to solve the riddle, however, they solve the secret to making a new friend. *The Riddle* shows children the process of making a new friend. As they read about Maria and Pete, they'll discover making friends is easy . . . and fun. Fiction.

Wilhelm, Hans, *Let's Be Friends Again!,* Crown, 1986. (P)

Being an older brother has its ups and downs. When the boy's little sister sets his turtle free, it's the last straw in a terrible day. He thinks he can never forgive her. Humorous illustrations help tell what circumstances cause him to overcome his feelings of anger toward his little sister. Fiction.

NUTRITION

*Anacona, George, *Bananas: From Manolo to Margee,* Houghton Mifflin, 1982. (I-U)

The story of bananas from the perspective of those who grow and produce them, through the production process. Nonfiction.

*Anderson, Joan,. *The First Thanksgiving Feast,* Clarion, 1984. (I-U)

A dramatized account of the first Thanksgiving. Seventeenth-century life in Plymouth, Massachusetts, is recreated. Fiction.

*Bang, Betty, *The Old Woman and the Rice Thief,* Greenwillow, 1978. (P)

The story of how an old woman cleverly catches a thief who has been stealing her rice. Fiction.

Borghese, Anita, *Down to Earth Cookbook,* Revised edition, Scribner's, 1980. (U)

Introduction to natural cooking for intermediate graders. Contains explanations of terms, utensils, ingredients, gives clear directions for all recipes, and introduces the user to unfamiliar foods. Pleasant illustrations enhance the text. Nonfiction.

*Burns, Marilyn, *The Hanukkah Book,* Four Winds, 1981. (I-U)

An explanation of the spirit of Hanukkah and how it is celebrated. Traditional recipes are included and comparisons to the Christian holiday of Christmas are made. Nonfiction.

Cobb, Vicki, *More Science Experiments You Can Eat,* Lippincott, 1979. (U)

Describes food experiments that investigate spoilage, dehydration, ripening, acidity, flavorings, and extracts. In discussing additives, the author relies on the Food and Drug Administration's questionable Generally Regarded As Safe (GRAS) list. Nonfiction.

Cole, W. (compiler), *Poem Stew,* Lippincott, 1981. (PI)

Fifty-seven humorous poems about table manners, overeating and enjoying food. Fiction.

*Goble, Paul, *Iktomi and the Berries,* Orchard Books, 1989. (P-I)

Story of a Sioux Indian trickster who tries to pick berries that are growing in the river, just for himself. Fiction.

*Hughes, Meredith, and Hughes, E. Thomas. *The Great Potato Book,* Macmillan, 1986. (I-U)

A story of the history, uses, and folklore surrounding the potato. Recipes for use of the potato are included. Nonfiction.

Jones, Hettie, *How to Eat Your ABCs; a Book About Vitamins,* Four Winds, 1976. (I-U)

An attractive, neat format and an informal text will be appealing to many middle graders. The history of vitamin research and the roles each vitamin plays and where to get it are included. Nutrition is stressed in problem-solving menu ideas, food charts, and a few easy and yummy recipes. An important topic today in our world of junk food. This book will be of use in nutrition and food units. Nonfiction.

Kolodny, Nancy J., *When Food's a Foe: How to Confront and Conquer Eating Disorders,* Little, Brown, 1987. (U)

The causes and effects of bulimia and anorexia nervosa are presented. Questionnaires, checklists, and exercises that can be used with students are included. Nonfiction.

Perl, Lila, *Eating the Vegetarian Way: Good Food From the Earth,* Morrow, 1980. (U)

An in-depth discussion as to what vegetarianism is and why it has become a new trend in American eating patterns. Final chapter is devoted to recipes that would appeal to boys and girls. Nonfiction.

Phillips, Barbara, *Don't Call Me Fatso,* Raintree, 1980. (P-I)

Rita is overweight and tired of being called "Fatso." She gets help from the school nurse in starting a safe diet and support from her parents, who decide they could also benefit from a change in eating habits. Rita feels frustrated when the weight loss is slow, and occasionally falls off the diet, but with reassurance from her parents she is able to stick to it and even start

exercising—something she doesn't enjoy. The school nurse is very happy when she weighs Rita and finds that even though she has lost only 5 pounds, she has grown 1 inch. The nurse reminds Rita that a growing girl shouldn't lose too much weight. A very sound approach to diet and exercise for children is presented in this story. Fiction.

Pinkwater, D.M., *Slaves of Spiegel: A Major Moscow Story,* Four Winds, 1982. (I-U)

Fat men from the planet Spiegel are ordered to track down the most fattening food. Includes an interplanetary cooking contest. Fiction.

SAFETY

Benson, Kathleen, *Joseph on the Subway Trains,* Addison-Wesley, 1981. (P-I)

Joseph gets separated from his second grade class during a field trip to New York. Lost and alone on the subway, Joseph asks two boys for help and ends up in a dangerous situation. He finally asks a man at a token booth for help. The man calls the transit police, who tell Joseph that people are looking for him. Joseph is eventually reunited with his class. This story will be helpful in introducing the value of knowing where to go for help in a similar situation. Fiction.

Bograd, Larry, *Lost in the Store,* Macmillan, 1981. (P)

Five-year-old Bruno gets lost in a large department store and is frightened until he meets Molly, who is also lost, and they begin to explore the store together. The two get so involved in play that they almost don't hear Molly's name being announced over the loud speaker. Molly goes to her parents and Bruno returns to where he was before he got lost. There he finds his anxious parents waiting for him. On the way out of the store the two children wave goodbye to each other. The fact that the children are not concerned about being lost and don't know how to seek help may prompt discussion of safety procedures. Fiction.

Chlad, Dorothy, *Bicycles Are Fun to Ride,* Children's, 1984. (P-I)

Bicycle care and safety are described by Mark. He tells ways he keeps both his bike and his body in tip-top shape. Emphasis is placed on having fun in a responsible manner. Fiction.

Chlad, Dorothy, *Strangers*, Children's, 1982. (P)

A preschool child, Suzie, tells about strangers. She relates various safety rules about avoiding strangers and what a child should do if approached by a stranger. Suzie defines "stranger" as "anyone you do not know." A simple and easy to understand concept of personal safety rules. Fiction.

Gobbell, Phyllis, and Laster, Jim, *Safe Sally Seat Belt and the Magic Click*, Childrens Press, 1986. (P-I)

A child tells her classmates how she was saved from being hurt during an automobile accident because she was wearing a seat belt. Fiction.

Morris, Judy K., *The Crazies and Sam*, Viking Kestrel, 1983. (I-U)

A story of how a single parent teaches her child how to recognize danger in a large city. Fiction.

Rockwell, Anne, and Rockwell, Harlow, *Out to Sea*, Macmillan, 1980. (P-I)

When Kate and Jeff discover an old boat, they begin to play in it. When the tide comes in and the boat is washed out to sea, their parents notify the Coast Guard. Water safety rules are nicely blended into the telling of the children's rescue. Fiction.

Snyder, Zilpha, *Come on, Patsy*, Atheneum, 1982. (P-I)

Patsy is led into some dangerous situations by a friend who encourages her to break safety rules by saying, "Come on, Patsy." After suffering the negative consequences of following her friend, Patsy finally learns to say no, and her friend can't understand why Patsy turns her back when the friend says, "Come on, Patsy." Fiction.

Stanek, Muriel, *All Alone After School*, Albert Whitman, 1985. (P-I)

Josh's mother is going back to work, and together they make a list of telephone numbers and safety rules. Despite all the preparation, Josh is nervous on the first day alone. As the days wear on, Josh begins to relax and enjoy the responsibility of being alone. An excellent story for those new at coming home to an empty house. Fiction.

Wachter, Oralee, *No More Secrets for Me*, Little, Brown, 1983. (P-I)

In each of four stories, the main character tells how to defend against unwanted touching. Each story includes ways to express feelings or confide in someone who can be trusted. Emphasis is placed on ways to take care of oneself in the event of uncomfortable touching. Fiction.

SEXUALITY

Burn, Helen Jean, *Better Than the Birds, Smarter Than the Bees; No-Nonsense Answers to Honest Questions About Sex and Growing Up*, Abingdon, 1969. (U)

Frank answers are given to honest questions about sex and growing up asked by adolescents. Compiled by one of the members of the Planned Parenthood Association's speaker's bureau, the book provides simple yet complete and satisfying answers to questions relating to the psychological angle of sex, the physiological differences between boys and girls, the "marriage bit," and the "no-no's." The bibliography includes selected references on aspects of sex education, films for use in sex education, and selected fiction on sexual problems. Nonfiction.

*Freeman, Lory, *It's My Body & Mi Cuerpo es Mio*, Parenting Press, 1985. (P)

Hypothetical situations are presented to help children tell the difference between acceptable and nonacceptable touching. Assertiveness skills designed to help children resist touching by others are presented. Fiction.

Hall, Lynn, *The Boy in the Off-White Hat*, Scribner's, 1985. (I)

The damaging effects of sexual abuse on a child is presented. Clues to behaviors exhibited by abused children are included in the story line. Fiction.

*Hall, Lynn, *Danza*, Aladdin, 1989. (I-U)

A young boy learns responsibility and finds himself. An exploration of adolescent sexuality. Fiction.

May, Julian, *New Baby Comes*, Creative Education, 1970. (P)

By means of illustrations and simple text, the growth of a baby is followed until its birth in a hospital and the beginning of its life as a new member of the family. Despite the low reading level, a practical book for the older child. Nonfiction.

*Riordan, James, *The Woman in the Moon and Other Tales of Forgotten Heroines*, Dial, 1985. (I-U)

Oppressed female characters discover their power. Tales featuring females who are bold, strong, and clever. Nonfiction.

Sheffield, Margaret, *Where Do Babies Come From?* Knopf, 1973. (I)

A first sex education book that has the answer to what children really want to know. All of the facts are included in the text using correct terminology. The direct illustrations are soft colored paintings. The book gracefully creates a mood of reverence for life in representing human reproduction. Adopted from a BBC award-winning program. Nonfiction.

*Smith, Rukshana, *Sumitra's Story,* Coward, 1983. (U)

An exploration of the problems of race, changing mores, family, and the role of women as issues for an East Indian girl. Fiction.

Yost, Don, and Plummer, Carol, *Little Bear,* Bridgework Theater, 1981. (I-U)

A play designed to teach children information and skills that they can use to make them less vulnerable to sexual abuse. A curriculum guide is included. Fiction.

SMOKING

Marr, John S., *Breath of Air and Breath of Smoke,* Evans, 1971. (I-U)

The first part of the book contains a detailed description of the respiratory system with many illustrations. Then the processes of inhalation and exhalation are carefully explained again with illustrations. Without critique, the author describes the effect that smoking has on the body. Three-color illustrations are used on every page to enhance the interesting text. Nonfiction.

Sonnett, Sherry, *Smoking,* Watts, 1977. (U)

The history of tobacco and smoking, how it affects people physically, and the diseases it promotes are clearly explained in this slim book. A good book for student reports and classroom units on cancer and health. Nonfiction.

APPENDIX E

Sources of Free and Low-Cost Sponsored Instructional Aids for Health Teaching

Because some organizations move, change policy, or go out of business each year, it is virtually impossible to prepare a list of sources of free and inexpensive materials that will not require revision periodically. Teachers can keep up-to-date with such changes by conferring with the librarian or by requesting that their letters of inquiry be forwarded. Teacher's manuals that accompany many health textbooks also furnish the teacher with selective lists of printed materials, films and filmstrips, and their sources.

The national organizations listed with asterisks have state or regional affiliates or offices. When this is known, the teacher should first request materials or information from the nearest unit.

Abbott Laboratories
Abbott Park, D-383
Abbott Park, IL 60064
(708) 937-6100

Aetna Life and Casualty Companies
Public Relations and Advertising
151 Farmington Avenue RWAC
Hartford, CT 06156
(203) 273-0123

Aims Media
9710 DeSoto Avenue
Chatsworth, CA 91311-4409
(800) 367-2467

Al-Anon Family Group Headquarters, Inc.*
P.O. Box 862
Midtown Station
New York, NY 10018-0862
(212) 302-7240; (800) 344-2666

Allstate
Corporate Relations Department
Allstate Plaza
Northbrook, IL 60062
(708) 402-5000

American Academy of Pediatrics
141 Northwest Point Boulevard
P.O. Box 927
Elk Grove Village, IL 60009-0927
(800) 433-9016

American Alliance for Health, Physical Education,
    Recreation and Dance
1900 Association Drive
Reston, VA 22091
(703) 476-3400

American Automobile Association*
Traffic Safety Department
1000 AAA Drive
Heathrow, FL 32746
(407) 441-4137

American Cancer Society, Inc.*
1599 Clifton Road, NE
Atlanta, GA 30329
(800) ACS-2345

---

*Have state or regional offices.

564

American Chiropractic Association*
1701 Clarendon Boulevard
Arlington, VA 22209
(202) 276-8800; (800) 368-3083

American Dental Association
Bureau of Health Education and Audiovisual Services
211 East Chicago Avenue
Chicago, IL 60611
(312) 440-2500; (800) 621-8099

American Diabetes Association*
1660 Duke Street
Alexandria, VA 22314
(800) 232-3472

American Foundation for the Blind
15 West 16th Street
New York, NY 10011
(212) 620-2000; (800) 232-5463

American Institute of Baking
Communications Department
1213 Bakers Way
Manhattan, KS 66502
(913) 537-4750

American Lung Association*
1740 Broadway
New York, NY 10019
(212) 315-8700

American Medical Association*
535 North Dearborn Street
Chicago, IL 60610
(312) 464-5000

American Optometric Association
Department of Public Information
243 N. Lindbergh Boulevard
St. Louis, MO 63141
(314) 991-4100

American Osteopathic Association
142 E. Ontario Street
Chicago, IL 60611
(312) 280-5800; (800) 621-1773

American National Red Cross*
17th and D Streets NW
Washington, DC 20006
(202) 737-8300

American School Food Service Association
420 Strickland
Glastonbury, CT 06033
(203) 638-4237

American School Health Association
P.O. Box 708
Kent, OH 44240
(216) 678-1601

American Social Health Association
P.O. Box 13827
Research Triangle Park, NC 27709
(919) 361-8422

American Public Health Association
School Health Education and Services Section
1015 Fifteenth Street, NW
Washington, DC 20005
(202) 789-5600

American Public Health Association
Health Education and Health Promotion Section
1015 Fifteenth Street, NW
Washington, DC 20005
(202) 789-5600

American Veterinary Medical Association
930 North Meacham Road
Schaumberg, IL 60196
(708) 605-8070

Arthritis Foundation
1314 Spring Street, NW
Atlanta, GA 30309
(800) 283-7800

Association for the Advancement of Health Education
1900 Association Drive
Reston, VA 22091
(703) 476-3441

Better Vision Institute, Inc.
1800 N. Kent Street
Suite 1210
Rosslyn, VA 22209
(703) 243-1508

Bulimia Anorexia Self-Help (BASH)
6125 Clayton Avenue, Suite 215
St. Louis, MO 63139-3295
(800) BASH-STL (227-4785)

Channing L. Bete Company, Inc.
200 State Road
South Deerfield, MA 01373
(413) 665-7611; (800) 628-7733

Cheesborough-Ponds
Consumer Affairs
33 Benedict Place
Greenwich, CT 06830
(800) 243-5804

Committee for Children
172 20th Avenue
Seattle, WA 98122
(206) 322-5050

Comprehensive Health Education Foundation (CHEF)
22323 Pacific Highway South
Seattle, WA 98190
(206) 824-2907; (800) 323-CHEF

Consumer Information Center
General Services Administration
Pueblo, CO 81009
(719) 948-3334

Coronet/MTI Film & Video
108 Wilmot Road
Deerfield, IL 60015
(800) 621-2131

Council for Exceptional Children
Dept K 10921
1920 Association Drive
Reston VA 22091-1589
(703) 620-3660

Council of Chief State School Officers
HIV/School Health Project
1 Massachusetts NW, Suite 700
Washington, DC 20001
(202) 336-7027

DINE System, Inc
586 N. French Road, Suite 2
Amherst, NY 14228
(716) 688-2492

Division of Adolescent and School Health (DASH)
Center for Prevention of Chronic Diseases
Centers for Disease Control and Prevention
4770 Buford Highway, NE, MS-K32
Atlanta, GA 30341-3724
(404) 488-5314

Education Development Center, Inc.
55 Chapel Street
Newton, MA 02160
(617) 969-7100

Educational Development Corporation
P.O. Box 470663
Tulsa, OK 74747
(800) 475-4522

Educational Resources
1550 Executive Drive
Elgin, IL 60123
(800) 624-2926

Environmental Protection Agency
PM 211-B
401 M Street SW
Washington, DC 20460
(202) 382-2080; 475-7751

Epilepsy Foundation of America
4351 Garden City Drive
Landover, MD 20785
(301) 459-3700; (800) 332-1000

ETR Associates
P.O. Box 1830
Santa Cruz, CA 95061-1830
(800) 321-4407

FDA/Consumer Communications (HFE-88)
5600 Fishers Lane
Rockville, MD 20857
(301) 443-3170

Harcourt Brace
School Department
6277 Sea Harbor Drive
Orlando, FL 32821-9989
(800) Call-HBJ

Health Edco
P.O. Box 21207
Waco, TX 76702-1207
(800) 299-3366, Ext. 295

Healthy Mothers, Healthy Babies Coalition
409 12th Street SW
Washington, DC 20024-2188
(800) 673-8444, Ext. 2458

Hispanic Books Distributors, Inc.
1665 West Grant Road
Tucson, AZ 85745
(800) 634-2124

The Hogg Foundation for Mental Health
University of Texas—Austin
Publication Division
P.O. Box 7998, University Station
Austin, TX 78713-7998
(512) 471-5041

Kellogg Company
P.O. Box 3447
Battle Creek, MI 49016
(616) 961-2000; (800) 962-1413

Krames Communications
1100 Grundy Lane
San Bruno, CA 94066-3030
(800) 333-3032

Kimberly-Clark Corporation
Consumer Services
P.O. Box 2020, Dept. BA
Neenah, WI 54957-2020
(414) 721-2000; (800) 544-1847

March of Dimes*
1275 Mamaraneck Avenue
White Plains, NY 10605
(914) 428-7100

Medic Alert Foundation International
2323 Colorado
Turlock, CA 95381-1009
(800) ID-ALERT (423-5378)

Metropolitan Life Insurance Company
Health and Safety Education Division
One Madison Avenue
New York, NY 10010
(212) 578-2211

Mothers Against Drunk Drivers
P.O. Box 541688
Dallas, TX 75354-1688
(800) 438-6233 (Victim Hotline)

Muscular Dystrophy Association
810 Seventh Avenue
New York, NY 10019
(212) 586-0808

National Association for Hearing and Speech Action
   (NAHSA)
10801 Rockville Pike
Rockville, MD 20852
(301) 897-8682; (800) 638-8255

National Association of School Nurses
P.O. Box 1300
Scarborough, ME 04074
(207) 883-2117

National Association of State Boards of Education
1012 Cameron Street
Alexandria, VA 22314
(703) 684-4000

National Center for Health Education
72 Spring Street, Suite 208
New York, NY 10012-4019
(212) 334-9470

National Clearinghouse for Alcohol and
   Drug Information (NCADI)
P.O. Box 2345
Rockville, MD 20847
(301) 468-2600; (800) 729-6686

National Council on Alcoholism
12 West 21st Street
New York, NY 10010
(212) 206-6770

National Council on Family Relations
3989 Central Avenue NE
Suite 550
Minneapolis, MN 55421
(612) 781-9331

National Dairy Council*
6300 North River Road
Rosemont, IL 60018-4233
(708) 696-1020

National Education Association
1201 16th Street, NW
Washington, DC 20036
(202) 822-7350

National Fire Protection Association
One Batterymarch Park
P.O. Box 9101
Quincy, MA 02269-9101
(617) 770-3000

National Geographic Society
Educational Services
P.O. Box 98019
Washington, DC 20090-8019
(800) 368-2728

National Health Council, Inc.
350 5th Avenue, Suite 1118
New York, NY 10118
(212) 268-8900

National Heart, Lung, and Blood Institute (NHLBI)
Building 32 Room 4A21
9000 Rockville Pike
Bethesda, MD 20892
(301) 496-4236

National Kidney Foundation
30 East 33rd Street
New York, NY 10016
(212) 889-2210; (800) 622-9010

National Institute of Mental Health
Public Inquiries
5600 Fishers Lane
Rockville, MD 20857
(301) 443-4513

National Livestock and Meat Board*
Nutritional Department
444 N. Michigan Avenue
Chicago, IL 60611
(312) 467-5520; (800) 621-7773

National Multiple Sclerosis Society*
205 East 42nd Street
New York, NY 10017
(212) 986-3240; (800) 227-3166

National Safety Council
1121 Springlake Drive
Itasca, IL 60143-3201
(708) 285-1121; (800) 621-7619

National School Boards Association
1680 Duke Street
Alexandria, VA 22314
(703) 838-6756

Office on Smoking and Health
5600 Fishers Lane
Rm 1-16
Park Building
Rockville, MD 20857
(301) 443-1575

Ortho Pharmaceuticals
Route 202 South
Raritan, NJ 08869
(201) 524-0400; (800) 722-7786

Personal Products Company
P.O. Box 529
Gibbstown, NJ 08027
(800) 635-8478

Pharmaceutical Manufacturers' Association
Department NW-601
1100 15th Street NW, Suite 900
Washington, DC 20005
(202) 835-3400

Planned Parenthood Federation of America, Inc.*
Publications Department
810 Seventh Avenue
New York, NY 10019
(212) 541-7800; (800) 829-7732

Positive Promotions
222 Ashland Pl.
Brooklyn, NY 11217
(800) 635-2666

President's Council on Physical Fitness and Sports
701 Pennsylvania Avenue, NW, Suite 250
Washington, DC 20004
(202) 272-3430

Public Health Service
5600 Fishers Lane
Rockville, MD 20857
(301) 443-2403

Rutgers Center of Alcohol Studies
Smithers Hall
Rutgers University
Piscataway, NJ 08854
(201) 932-5528

Sex Information and Education
   Council of the United States
130 W. 42nd Street, Suite 2500
New York, NY 10036
(212) 819-9770

Smith Kline & Beecham
1500 Spring Garden Street
Mailcode E-51
P.O. Box 7929
Philadelphia, PA 19130
(215) 751-4000; (800) 366-8900

Society for Nutrition Education
1736 Franklin Street, Suite 900
Oakland, CA 94612
(415) 444-7133

State Farm Insurance Companies
Public Relations Department
One State Farm Plaza
Bloomington, IL 61710
(309) 766-2311

Sunkist Growers, Inc.
P.O. Box 7888
Van Nuys, CA 91409
(818) 986-4800

Superintendent of Documents
U.S. Government Printing Office
North Capitol & H Streets NW
Washington, DC 20402
(202) 783-3238

Tambrands
Education Division
One Marcus Avenue
Lake Success, NY 11042
(516) 358-8300

The Travelers Film Library
Travelers Insurance Company
One Tower Square
Hartford, CT 06183
(203) 277-0111

United Cerebral Palsy Association, Inc.
7 Penn Plaza, Suite 804
New York, NY 10001
(212) 268-6655

U.S. Department of Education
Comprehensive School Health Education Office
555 New Jersey Avenue, NW
Washington, DC 20208
(202) 628-1556

U.S. Department of Education
Office of Elementary and Secondary Education
400 Maryland Avenue, SW
The Portals Building, Room 4018
Washington, DC 20202
(202) 401-0039

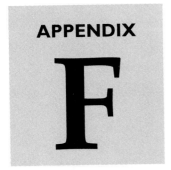

Selected Federal Health Information Clearinghouses and Information Centers

These listings are not meant to be all inclusive. Some of the Clearinghouses and Information Centers will change addresses and telephone numbers. General information about 800 numbers can be secured by calling (800) 555-1212. When writing, request that the letter be forwarded.

AGING

National Resource Center on Health Promotion
  and Aging
1909 K Street NW, 5th Floor
Washington, DC 20049
(202) 728-4476; (800) 729-6686
  Provides access to information and referral services that assist the older American in obtaining services. Distributes Administration on Aging publications.

AIDS

National AIDS Information Clearinghouse
P.O. Box 6003
Rockville, MD 20850
(800) 458-5231
  Responds to the needs of professionals involved in the development and delivery of AIDS programs and distributes single copies of information.

National AIDS Hotline
Atlanta, GA 30333
(800) 342-AIDS
(800) 344-SIDA (Spanish)
(800) AIDS-TTY (Hearing Impaired)
  Provides the most up-to-date information available about the incidence and prevalence of AIDS.

ALCOHOL

National Clearinghouse for Alcohol and Drug Information
P.O. Box 2345
Rockville, MD 20847
(301) 468-2600
(800) SAY-NOTO (729-6686)
  Gathers and disseminates current knowledge on alcohol-related subjects.

ARTHRITIS

Arthritis Information Clearinghouse
P.O. Box 9782
Arlington, VA 22009
(703) 558-8250; (800) 283-7800
  Identifies materials concerned with arthritis and related musculoskeletal diseases and serves as an information exchange for individuals and organizations involved in public, professional, and patient education. Refers personal requests from patients to the Arthritis Foundation.

ASTHMA

Asthma Information Center
National Heart, Lung and Blood Institute
4733 Bethesda Avenue, Suite 530
Bethesda, MD 20814
(301) 951-3260
  Provides educational information about asthma. A
  reading and resource list is available.

BLIND AND PHYSICALLY HANDICAPPED

National Library Service for the Blind and Physically
  Handicapped
Library of Congress
1291 Taylor Street NW
Washington, DC 20542
(202) 707-9287; (800) 424-8567
  Works through local and regional libraries to provide
  free library service to persons unable to read or use
  standard printed materials because of visual or physical impairment. Provides information on blindness
  and physical handicaps on request. A list of participating libraries is available.

CANCER

National Cancer Institute
Office of Cancer Communications
9000 Rockville Pike, Building 31, Room 10A24
Bethesda, MD 20892
(301) 496-5583; (800) 4-CANCER
  Collects information about public, patient, and
  professional cancer education materials and disseminates it to organizations and health care professionals.

Office of Cancer Communication
National Cancer Institute
Cancer Information Service
Bethesda, MD 20014
(301) 496-2351; (800) 638-6694
  Answers requests for cancer information from pa-
  tients and the general public. The National Cancer
  Institute sponsors a toll-free telephone number to
  supply cancer information to the general public.

CHILD ABUSE

National Clearinghouse on Child Abuse and Neglect
P.O. Box 1182
Washington, DC 20013
(703) 385-7565; (800) FYI-3366
  Collects, processes, and disseminates information on
  child abuse and neglect.

CONSUMER INFORMATION

Consumer Information Center
General Services Administration
Pueblo, CO 81009
(719) 948-3334
  Distributes consumer publications on topics such as
  children, food and nutrition, health, exercise, and
  weight control. The *Consumer Information Catalog* is
  available free from the Center and must be used to
  identify publications requested.

DIABETES

National Diabetes Information Clearinghouse (NDIC)
1 Information Way
Bethesda, MD 20892-3560
(301) 654-3327
  Collects and disseminates information on patient education materials and coordinates the development
  of materials and programs for diabetes education.

DIGESTIVE DISEASES

National Digestive Diseases Information Clearinghouse
  (NDDIC)
2 Information Way
Bethesda, MD 20892-3570
(301) 654-3810
  Provides information on digestive diseases to health
  professionals and consumers.

DRUG ABUSE

National Clearinghouse for Alcohol and Drug Information (NCADI)
P.O. Box 2345
Rockville, MD 20857
(301) 468-2600; (800) 729-6686
  Collects and disseminates information on drug
  abuse. Produces informational materials on drugs,
  drug abuse, and prevention.

DRUG EDUCATION

Office for Substance Abuse Prevention
Rockwall II Building, Room 9C03
5600 Fishers Lane
Rockville, MD 20857
(301) 443-0375
(301) 443-0377

Develops, promotes, and distributes prevention materials; provides continuing education training for professionals, and multicultural workshops for professionals, parents, and youth.

ENVIRONMENTAL PROTECTION

Environmental Protection Agency (EPA)
Public Information Center
PM 211-B
401 M Street SW
Washington, DC 20460
(202) 382-2080

Public information materials on such topics as hazardous wastes, the school asbestos project, air and water pollution, pesticides, and drinking water are available. Offers information on the agency and its programs and activities.

FAMILY PLANNING

Family Life Information Exchange
P.O. Box 30436
Bethesda, MD 20814
(301) 907-8198

Collects family planning materials, makes referrals to other information centers, and distributes and produces materials. Primary audience is federally funded family planning clinics.

FAMILY VIOLENCE

Clearinghouse on Family Violence Information
P.O. Box 1182
Washington, DC 20013
(703) 821-2086

Provides information services to those who work to prevent family violence and its victims. Has a library of audiovisual aids and national organizations that can be utilized.

FOOD AND DRUGS

Food and Drug Administration (FDA)
Office for Consumer Communications
5600 Fishers Lane, Room 15B-19 (HFI-40)
Rockville, MD 20857
(301) 443-3220

Answers consumer inquiries for the FDA and serves as a clearinghouse for its consumer publications.

FOOD AND NUTRITION

Food and Nutrition Information Center (FNIC)
10301 Baltimore Boulevard
National Agricultural Library Building, Room 304
Beltsville, MD 20705
(301) 344-3719

Serves the information needs of persons interested in human nutrition, food service management, and food technology. Acquires and lends books, journal articles, and audiovisual materials dealing with these areas of concern.

GENETIC DISEASES

National Clearinghouse for Human Genetic Diseases
805 15th Street NW, Suite 500
Washington, DC 20005
(202) 842-7617

Provides information on human genetics and genetic diseases for both patients and health care workers. Reviews existing curricular materials on genetic education.

HANDICAPPED

Clearinghouse on the Handicapped
Office for Handicapped Individuals
330 C Street
Washington, DC 20202-2524
(202) 732-1244; (800) 999-5599

Responds to inquiries from handicapped individuals and serves as a resource to organizations that supply information to, and about, handicapped individuals.

HEALTH INDEXES

Clearinghouse on Health Indexes
National Center for Health Statistics
Division of Analysis
6525 Belcrest Road, Room 1070
Hyattsville, MD 20782
(301) 436-7035

Provides informational assistance in the development of health measures for health researchers, administrators, and planners.

HEALTH INFORMATION

National Health Information Center (NHIC)
Office of Disease Prevention and Health Promotion
P.O. Box 1133
Washington, DC 20013-1133
(701) 522-2590 (in VA); (800) 336-4797

Helps the public locate health information through identification of health information resources and an inquiry and referral system. Health questions are referred to appropriate health resources that, in turn, respond directly to inquirers.

HEALTH PROMOTION AND EDUCATION

Center for Health Promotion and Education (CHPE)
1300 Clifton Road, Building 14
Atlanta, GA 30333
(404) 501-2222

Provides leadership and program direction for the prevention of disease, disability, premature death, and undesirable and unnecessary health problems through health education. Formerly called the Bureau of Health Education.

HEART HEALTH

National Heart, Lung, and Blood Institute
Education Programs
Information Center
P.O. Box 30105
Bethesda, MD 20824-0105
(301) 951-3260

Serves as a source of information and materials on cholesterol, smoking, asthma, and high blood pressure. Distributes educational materials on request.

HIGH BLOOD PRESSURE

National High Blood Pressure Education Program
Program Information Center
4733 Bethesda Avenue, Suite 530
Bethesda, MD 20814
(301) 951-3260

Provides information on the detection, diagnosis, and management of high blood pressure to consumers and health professionals.

HIGHWAY SAFETY

National Highway Traffic Safety Administration (NHTSA)
U.S. Department of Transportation
400 7th Street SW
Washington, DC 20590
(202) 366-9294; (800) 424-9393

Works to reduce highway traffic deaths and injuries. Publishes a variety of safety information brochures, conducts public information campaigns on vehicle defects and drunken driving, and maintains a toll-free hotline for consumer complaints on auto safety.

HOMELESSNESS

The National Resource Center on Homelessness and Mental Illness
262 Delaware Avenue
Delmar, NY 12054
(800) 444-7415

Provides assistance and information concerning the service and housing needs of homeless mentally ill persons and general information relative to homelessness.

INJURIES

National Injury Information Clearinghouse
5401 Westbard Avenue, Room 625
Washington, DC 20207
(301) 492-6424

Collects and disseminates injury data and information relating to the causes and prevention of death, injury, and illness associated with consumer products. Requests of a general nature are referred to the Consumer Product Safety Commission's Communications Office.

MATERNAL AND CHILD HEALTH

National Center for Health Education in Maternal and
  Child Health
38th and R Streets NW
Washington, DC 20057
(202) 625-8400

Responds to information requests from consumers
and professionals and provides reference and resource materials, including curricula and audiovisuals.

MENTAL HEALTH

National Institute of Mental Health
Public Inquiries Section
5600 Fishers Lane, Room 7C02
Rockville, MD 20857
(301) 443-4513

Acquires and abstracts the world's mental health literature, answers inquiries from the public, and provides computer searches for the scientific and academic communities.

MINORITY HEALTH

Office of Minority Health Resource Center
P.O. Box 37337
Washington, DC 20013-7337
(800) 444-6472

Responds to information requests for information on
minority health. Bilingual staff available.

NUTRITION

Human Nutrition Information Service
Department of Agriculture
6505 Belcrest Road
Hyattsville, MD 20782
(301) 436-7725

Monitors the food and nutrient content of diets of the
American population. Coordinates the review and
publication of the Dietary Guidelines for Americans
and develops information to help Americans put the
guidelines into practice.

PHYSICAL FITNESS

President's Council on Physical Fitness and Sports
701 Pennsylvania Avenue, NW, Suite 250
Washington, DC 22004
(202) 272-3430

Conducts a public service advertising program and
cooperates with governmental and private groups to
promote the development of physical fitness leadership, facilities, and programs. Produces informational materials on exercise, school physical education programs, sports, and physical fitness for youth,
adults, and the elderly.

PRODUCT SAFETY

U.S. Consumer Product Safety Commission (CPSC)
Washington, DC 20207
(800) 638-8326 (in the District of Columbia)
(800) 492-8363 (in Maryland)
(800) 638-8333 (in Alaska, Hawaii, the Virgin Islands,
  and Puerto Rico)
(301) 492-6800; (800) 638-8270 (in all other states)

Evaluates the safety of products sold to the public.
Provides printed materials on different aspects of
consumer product safety on request. Does not answer questions from consumers on drugs, prescriptions, warranties, advertising, repairs, or maintenance.

REHABILITATION

National Rehabilitation Information Center (NARIC)
8455 Colesville Road, Suite 935
Silver Spring, MD 20910
(301) 588-9284

Supplies publications and audiovisual materials on
rehabilitation and assists in locating information on
dates, places, names, addresses, or statistics. The collection includes materials relevant to the rehabilitation of all disability groups.

SMOKING

Office on Smoking and Health
Technical Information Center
Park Building
5600 Fishers Lane, Room 1-16
Rockville, MD 20857
(301) 443-1690

> Offers bibliographic and reference service to researchers and others and publishes and distributes a number of titles in the field of smoking.

SUDDEN INFANT DEATH SYNDROME (SIDS)

National Sudden Infant Death Syndrome Clearinghouse
8201 Greensboro Drive, Suite 600
McLean, VA 22102
(703) 821-8955

> Provides information on SIDS to health professionals and consumers.

Sudden Infant Death Syndrome (SIDS) Alliance
10500 Little Patuxent Parkway, Suite 420
Columbia, MD 21044
(800) 221-SIDS (7437)

> Provides help to families of SIDS babies; offers information to the public; offers referrals for support groups and hospitals.

Criteria for Evaluating the Elementary School Health Program

*California State Department of Education**

CRITERIA for Evaluating the Elementary School Health Program provides school personnel with a tool to use in making an evaluation of the school health program. The results of such an evaluation reveal the strengths and weaknesses of the program. Where weaknesses are revealed, the school health committee may act to bring all the available forces into action for the express purpose of securing strength in the program where weaknesses exist and for planning ways all other phases of the program may be kept strong.

The criteria are organized into four divisions: I—Administration, II—Health instruction, III—Health services, and IV—Healthful school environment. The criteria are expressed in terms of desirable practices presented in the left column. The evaluation should be made by a representative group of the faculty, including administrators, teachers, and health service personnel. The results should express judgments approved by the evaluation committee as a whole.

Provision is made for the quality of each *provi-*

*Modified from *Criteria for evaluating the elementary school health program,* Sacramento, CA, 1977, California State Department of Education.
Note: Although this instrument was developed some time ago, it remains one of the best models available. A 1986 publication by The American School Health Association and other organizations use the criteria with minor modifications.

sion or *practice* stated in the criteria to be judged on a four-point scale: *excellent, good, fair,* or *poor.* If the provision is not made, the practice is not followed; or if the quality is fair or poor, there is space for listing changes needed. At the top of each section, space is provided for recording recommended steps to be taken in relation to the changes needed. Care should be taken to make recommendations that will not have an adverse effect on provisions or practices already judged excellent or good.

SUGGESTED PROCEDURE FOR USING THE CRITERIA FOR EVALUATING THE ELEMENTARY SCHOOL HEALTH PROGRAM

- Determine the membership of study group to evaluate the program.
- Determine the need for consultant help.
- Study thoroughly the criteria and the provisions for making the desired evaluations.
- Determine whether the program meets each criterion.
- If the criterion is met, determine the quality of the provision or practice according to the following scale: *excellent*—near perfection; *good*—satisfactory; *fair*—slightly less than satisfactory; *poor*—unsatisfactory.

- If the criterion is not met—that is, the provision not made or the practice not followed—indicate by a check in the appropriate column.
- Compile a list of the changes needed and determine how the changes can best be secured.
- Set up a priority for accomplishing the changes.

- Develop recommendations for making the needed changes and record in appropriate space at the top of each section.
- Submit the recommendations to the administration for action.

Criteria for Evaluating the Elementary School Health Program

Criteria	Quality of provision or practice					Changes needed
	Excellent (near perfection)	Good (satisfactory)	Fair (slightly less than satisfactory)	Poor (unsatisfactory)	Provision not made or practice not followed	
I. ADMINISTRATION						
A. The policies of the district's governing board provide for a school health program designed to help all pupils achieve the degree of health their potentialities permit through health instruction, health services, a healthful school environment—essentials of the program.	RECOMMENDED STEPS TO BE TAKEN:					
B. A written statement of the school district's point of view regarding the kind and quality of the school health program is available.	RECOMMENDED STEPS TO BE TAKEN:					
C. Responsibility for planning, developing, and administering the district's school health program is delegated by the governing board of the district to the district superintendent of schools.	RECOMMENDED STEPS TO BE TAKEN:					
1. A health committee with a membership that includes school personnel, representatives of community health services, and representatives of the other important segments of the community is assigned advisory responsibilities for the district's school health program.						
D. The principal of the school has outlined the practices that are employed in operating the school health program.	RECOMMENDED STEPS TO BE TAKEN:					
1. A health council or committee with a membership that includes an administrator, teachers, health personnel, and, when possible, counselors, custodians, and school lunch personnel is assigned advisory responsibilities for the school health program.						

I. ADMINISTRATION—cont'd

E. Clerical help, equipment, and supplies, in keeping with the pupil population, are provided for the health services program.

RECOMMENDED STEPS TO BE TAKEN:

F. Health personnel are adequate in number and specialization to provide needed services.

1. School nurses are available in a ratio of 1 nurse for each 1000 to 1400 pupils. (Distances traveled to visit homes and types of terrain should be considered in determining the desired ratio.)

2. Physicians are available for consultation and advice.

3. Dentists are available for consultation and advice.

RECOMMENDED STEPS TO BE TAKEN:

G. The professional library and the school library are well supplied with health materials.

H. Each classroom is supplied with the materials needed for use in health instruction.

1. The classrooms for each grade are supplied with the basic textbooks in health.

2. Each classroom is supplied with health materials, in addition to adopted textbooks, that cover each phase of health.

3. The scope of the materials in each classroom is sufficient to provide for all the pupils, from the slowest to the fastest learner.

RECOMMENDED STEPS TO BE TAKEN:

I. The in-service education program for school personnel provides for health instruction to have the same emphasis as other areas of instruction.

RECOMMENDED STEPS TO BE TAKEN:

J. The in-service education program for school personnel provides for study of the school health services.

RECOMMENDED STEPS TO BE TAKEN:

Continued.

Criteria for Evaluating the Elementary School Health Program—cont'd

Criteria	Quality of provision or practice					Changes needed
	Excellent (near perfection)	Good (satisfactory)	Fair (slightly less than satisfactory)	Poor (unsatisfactory)	Provision not made or practice not followed	
II. HEALTH INSTRUCTION						
A. A course of study for health, a course of study and a teacher's guide, or a combination of study and teacher's guide is provided by the school district or the office of the county superintendent of schools for use in the school.	RECOMMENDED STEPS TO BE TAKEN:					
B. The course of study contains statements of the purposes of health instruction and the objectives to be sought; an outline of the contents that shows both scope and sequence; units of instruction, lists of materials and sources of materials, and recommended means and procedures for evaluating pupils' progress.	RECOMMENDED STEPS TO BE TAKEN:					
1. The scope of the content for the total program includes the following areas:						
a. Consumer health						
b. Mental-emotional health						
c. Drug use and misuse (including alcohol)						
d. Family health (including human sexuality, masculine and feminine qualities, marriage, and family planning)						
e. Oral health, vision, and hearing						
f. Nutrition						
g. Exercise, rest, and posture						
h. Diseases and disorders						
i. Environmental health hazards (including pollution, radiation hazards, accidents, and first aid)						
j. Community health resources						

	RECOMMENDED STEPS TO BE TAKEN:		

II. HEALTH INSTRUCTION—cont'd

2. The basic program of health instruction is developed through the use of units devoted primarily to health.

3. Health instruction is enriched by making it a correlated phase of units in other subjects, such as science, social studies, and homemaking.

4. Pupils' interests and needs are used as motivation for learning.

5. Health instruction is adapted to the pupils' abilities by employing a variety of methods.

6. Instruction is enriched through the use of the up-to-date information that is made available by official and voluntary health agencies and professional associations.

7. Instruction is enriched by the use of up-to-date audiovisual materials, such as films and film strips, charts and pictures, and radio and TV programs.

III. HEALTH SERVICES

A. A health services guide is provided by the school district or by the office of the county superintendent of schools.

B. A health services committee, preferably a subcommittee of the health council or committee, has advisory responsibility for health services.

C. Health services are provided in accordance with the provisions of the guide, provided, however, that the advice of the health services committee is an important consideration in decisions regarding adaptations required to meet special needs of individuals and of the school population.

Continued.

Criteria for Evaluating the Elementary School Health Program—cont'd

Criteria	Quality of provision or practice					Changes needed
	Excellent (near perfection)	Good (satisfactory)	Fair (slightly less than satisfactory)	Poor (unsatisfactory)	Provision not made or practice not followed	
III. HEALTH SERVICES—cont'd						
D. The school health services are of sufficient scope to provide school personnel the information and assistance needed to determine status of, protect, and promote the health of pupils.	RECOMMENDED STEPS TO BE TAKEN:					
1. Guidance and assistance are provided in securing an appraisal of each pupil's health status.						
2. School personnel, pupils, and parents are counseled regarding the results of health appraisals and ways to protect and promote one's health.						
3. Procedures designed to help prevent and control disease are established.						
4. First aid for the injured and emergency care for cases of sudden illness are provided.						
5. School health services are coordinated with those provided by professional health agencies in the community.						
E. School health personnel encourage and guide teacher observation of pupils' health characteristics and accept referrals of pupils whose characteristics are unlike those of the well child.						
F. School personnel inform and advise parents regarding medical examinations their children should have and assist in making provision for the medical examinations as necessary.	RECOMMENDED STEPS TO BE TAKEN:					
1. Parents are advised to have medical examinations for their children before school entrance.						

III. HEALTH SERVICES—cont'd

	RECOMMENDED STEPS TO BE TAKEN:	
2. Provision is made for pupils to have medical examinations as required by existing conditions. (Preferably this provision is made in cooperation with the local medical society.)		
3. Procedures are established for the cumulative health record to follow the pupil from grade to grade and school to school.		
G. School personnel inform parents of the importance of eye examinations for children before school entrance, maintain a vision screening program, and inform and advise parents regarding eye conditions of their children that require the attention of a specialist.	RECOMMENDED STEPS TO BE TAKEN:	
H. School health personnel provide for all pupils to have group hearing tests at regular intervals, individual tests for pupils discovered with hearing difficulties; inform and advise parents regarding their children's need for examinations by ear specialists; and recommend classroom adjustments for children with hearing difficulties.	RECOMMENDED STEPS TO BE TAKEN:	
I. Health services provide for parents to be informed regarding their children's need for regular dental examinations beginning before the children's entrance to school, and for parents of children who have defective dental conditions to be informed regarding the undesirable effects of the conditions and advised regarding essential treatment.	RECOMMENDED STEPS TO BE TAKEN:	
J. Pupils' growth characteristics are observed to determine deviations in growth patterns that merit special attention.	RECOMMENDED STEPS TO BE TAKEN:	

Continued.

Criteria for Evaluating the Elementary School Health Program—cont'd

Criteria	Quality of provision or practice					Changes needed
	Excellent (near perfection)	Good (satisfactory)	Fair (slightly less than satisfactory)	Poor (unsatisfactory)	Provision not made or practice not followed	
III. HEALTH SERVICES—cont'd						
K. Follow-up procedures are taken as necessary—begin when pupils with health difficulties are identified and conclude when the health difficulties have been corrected or their effects minimized.	RECOMMENDED STEPS TO BE TAKEN:					
L. Health counseling and guidance are provided.						
M. Provisions are made for supplying teachers with health information concerning handicapped pupils and for recommending cases for whom home teaching may be necessary.	RECOMMENDED STEPS TO BE TAKEN:					
N. The health services program includes provisions for the prevention and control of communicable diseases.						
1. Parents of preschool children are advised by the school to protect their children as early as possible against communicable diseases for which immunization is available.						
2. School personnel cooperate with representatives of the local health department in planning community immunization programs available to pupils.						
3. The school cooperates with local health agencies in conducting a tuberculosis case-finding program for pupils and school personnel.						

III. HEALTH SERVICES—cont'd

O. The health services program provides emergency service for injury, sudden illness, and disasters.

  1. Updated written policies and procedures for first aid and emergency care are provided to all school personnel.

  2. The policies and procedures pertaining to first aid and emergency care are approved by the local medical society or the health department.

  3. Phone numbers of parents and of physicians to call in emergencies are on file for each pupil.

  4. Parents are notified immediately in instances of serious injury or illness.

  5. Teachers are prepared to render first aid.

  6. First-aid kits are available in each classroom and in the principal's office.

IV. HEALTHFUL SCHOOL ENVIRONMENT

A. The school environment is protected by employing personnel whose health is good, requiring all personnel to have regular health examinations, and providing measures that encourage good health practices.

B. A wholesome emotional climate prevails and essential provisions are made for its maintenance.

  1. The morale of teachers is at a high level.

  2. The following provisions are made for the maintenance of staff morale at a high level.

    a. Leaves of absence without pay are granted for specified purposes.

    b. Sabbatical leaves for study or travel are granted certified personnel in accordance with written policies of the district.

RECOMMENDED STEPS TO BE TAKEN:

RECOMMENDED STEPS TO BE TAKEN:

RECOMMENDED STEPS TO BE TAKEN:

Continued.

Criteria for Evaluating the Elementary School Health Program—cont'd

Criteria	Quality of provision or practice					Changes needed
	Excellent (near perfection)	Good (satisfactory)	Fair (slightly less than satisfactory)	Poor (unsatisfactory)	Provision not made or practice not followed	
IV. HEALTHFUL SCHOOL ENVIRONMENT—cont'd	RECOMMENDED STEPS TO BE TAKEN:					
c. Communication is maintained between the administration and teaching personnel.						
d. A teamwork approach is used in the prevention and solving of staff problems.						
3. The following provisions are employed to create classroom environments that are conducive to learning.						
a. The teachers adapt learning experience to each child's developmental pattern of growth and needs.						
b. The daily program provides for a balance of quiet and active experiences.						
c. Opportunities are provided for each child to release tension by participating in various types of esthetic and physical activities.						
d. Teachers discuss required behavior standards with pupils.						
e. Pupils share responsibility for securing desired classroom behavior.						
f. Discipline and grading procedures are fair and consistent.						
g. The teacher-pupil ratio permits the individualization of instruction to the extent required for maximal learning.						
4. Pupils are given the following types of opportunities to develop as self-directing individuals:						
a. To share responsibility for solving social problems in the school.						

IV. HEALTHFUL SCHOOL ENVIRONMENT—cont'd

RECOMMENDED STEPS TO BE TAKEN:

b. To assume leadership responsibility through participation in classroom and student government activities.

c. To plan and organize school activities under teacher supervision.

5. Teachers are helped by the principal and special school personnel—the school psychologist, counselors, curriculum consultants, and others—to solve problems that arise in their classes.

6. School personnel and parents are encouraged in the following ways to work cooperatively in solving the problems that are causing pupils to make less than maximum use of their abilities.

RECOMMENDED STEPS TO BE TAKEN:

C. The school food services are conducted so that each pupil has opportunity to have a wholesome and nutritionally adequate lunch in an environment that is pleasant and sanitary, and pupils are helped to learn the importance of good eating habits, eating well-balanced meals, and using good table manners.

1. A Type A lunch, a lunch that meets the nutritional standards of a Type A lunch, or both, are served daily.

2. Lunchroom and kitchen facilities are periodically inspected by sanitarians from the local health department.

RECOMMENDED STEPS TO BE TAKEN:

D. The health service unit provides the required space for each type of activity conducted in the unit and is properly equipped with built-in facilities.

E. The school site meets the standards established for schools as set forth by state law.

1. The school is centrally located in the geographic area served.

Continued.

Criteria for Evaluating the Elementary School Health Program—cont'd

Criteria	Quality of provision or practice					Changes needed
	Excellent (near perfection)	Good (satisfactory)	Fair (slightly less than satisfactory)	Poor (unsatisfactory)	Provision not made or practice not followed	
IV. HEALTHFUL SCHOOL ENVIRONMENT—cont'd						
2. The area in which the school is located is relatively free of disturbing noises, noxious odors, and other distractions.	RECOMMENDED STEPS TO BE TAKEN:					
3. Water drains rapidly from outdoor areas.						
F. A planned procedure is followed to detect and correct possible unsafe conditions of buildings, grounds, and equipment.	RECOMMENDED STEPS TO BE TAKEN:					
G. The buildings and play areas are designed to provide for the successful operation of the school program and are kept in good condition.	RECOMMENDED STEPS TO BE TAKEN:					
1. All doors providing exit from buildings are equipped with panic bars.						
2. Ceilings and walls of classrooms and inside corridors are constructed with sound-absorbing materials.						
3. Areas or rooms in which noise-producing activities, such as band practice and playing games, take place are located at points where noises are likely to be least disturbing to classes held in other areas.						
4. The enrollments in classes assigned to rooms are not in excess of the number of pupils for which the rooms were originally planned.						

IV. HEALTHFUL SCHOOL ENVIRONMENT—cont'd

RECOMMENDED STEPS TO BE TAKEN:

H. Essential provisions have been made to secure in each classroom the conditions needed for eye comfort.
1. The lighting in classrooms is soft, even, properly distributed, and sufficiently bright for eye comfort.
2. The colors of the walls, ceilings, and chalkboards are conducive to eye comfort.

RECOMMENDED STEPS TO BE TAKEN:

I. The classrooms and the library are heated or cooled and ventilated as required to provide good working conditions for teachers and pupils.

RECOMMENDED STEPS TO BE TAKEN:

J. Drinking fountains in the building and on the school grounds are sufficient in number, of desirable design, of proper height, conveniently located, and cleaned daily.
1. An adequate number of drinking fountains are available (one for each 75 pupils and at least one on each floor of a multistoried building).
2. The water supply is regularly inspected by health department personnel.

RECOMMENDED STEPS TO BE TAKEN:

K. The handwashing and toilet facilities are sufficient in number and kept clean.
1. The lavatories are readily accessible from classrooms and play areas.
2. Each lavatory contains at least 1 wash basin equipped with hot and cold running water for every 50 pupils using the room.
3. An adequate number of toilets for girls are available (1 for each 30 girls).
4. An adequate number of toilets and urinals are available for boys (1 toilet for each 60 boys, 1 urinal for each 30 boys).
5. A supply of liquid or powdered soap is available near each wash basin.

Continued.

Criteria for Evaluating the Elementary School Health Program—cont'd

Criteria	Quality of provision or practice					Changes needed
	Excellent (near perfection)	Good (satisfactory)	Fair (slightly less than satisfactory)	Poor (unsatisfactory)	Provision not made or practice not followed	
IV. HEALTHFUL SCHOOL ENVIRONMENT—cont'd						
6. The supply of toilet paper and hand towels is replenished each day at specified intervals.	RECOMMENDED STEPS TO BE TAKEN:					
L. Fire prevention equipment is conveniently located and inspected at regular intervals.	RECOMMENDED STEPS TO BE TAKEN:					
1. All school personnel know the location of fire signal switches in the school and of fire alarm boxes near the school.						
2. Fire extinguishers are of a type approved by the local fire department and are inspected at regular intervals by fire officials.						
M. The procedures to be followed in the case of various types of disasters are known by all school personnel and pupils.	RECOMMENDED STEPS TO BE TAKEN:					
1. Written procedures to be followed in times of disaster are displayed in prominent places throughout the school.						
2. School personnel and pupils have practices and know the procedure to be followed in case of a fire, an earthquake, or other disaster.						
3. Fire drills are held monthly.						
4. Drills for disasters other than those that might be caused by fire are held at specified intervals throughout the school year.						

H

General Criteria for Evaluating Health Instructional Materials* and Comparative Text Analysis

The following criteria are to help you evaluate health instructional materials. Indicate your judgment by circling the appropriate number. Each item must be rated. A separate evaluating sheet is necessary for each set of materials considered for recommendation.

NOTE: Comments that would add to this evaluation would be appreciated. Please use last page.

EVALUATED BY _____ DATE _____

COMMITTEE _____ SCHOOL _____

Data for materials evaluated:

Author _____

Title _____

Publisher or producer _____

Copyright date _____ Type of material _____

Grade level of material being evaluated _____

Is this material part of a series?   Yes ☐ Series grade level _____

No ☐

Title of series _____

Cost per item _____

---

*Modified from Handbook I: *Guidelines for the development of instructional materials selection policies*, Olympia, WA, State Office of Public Education.

Summary of Evaluation

	High				Low	M*	NA†
I. Text format	5	4	3	2	1	0	0
II. Audiovisual format considerations	5	4	3	2	1	0	0
III. Organization and overall content	5	4	3	2	1	0	0
IV. Bias content	5	4	3	2	1	0	0
V. Teacher's guide	5	4	3	2	1	0	0
VI. Additional support materials	5	4	3	2	1	0	0
VII. Purchase priority	5	4	3	2	1		

I. TEXT FORMAT	High				Low	M*	NA
1. General appearance	5	4	3	2	1	0	0
2. Size and color practical for classroom use	5	4	3	2	1	0	0
3. Binding: durability and flexibility	5	4	3	2	1	0	0
4. Quality of paper	5	4	3	2	1	0	0
5. Readability of type	5	4	3	2	1	0	0
6. Appeal of page layouts	5	4	3	2	1	0	0
7. Usefulness of chapter headings	5	4	3	2	1	0	0
8. Appropriateness of illustrations	5	4	3	2	1	0	0
9. Usefulness of references, index, bibliography, appendix	5	4	3	2	1	0	0
10. Consistency of format	5	4	3	2	1	0	0

II. AUDIOVISUAL FORMAT AND CONSIDERATIONS	High				Low	M*	NA
1. Sound quality	5	4	3	2	1	0	0
2. Picture quality	5	4	3	2	1	0	0
3. Emotional impact	5	4	3	2	1	0	0
4. Other qualities: vitality, style, imagination	5	4	3	2	1	0	0
5. Authoritative and well-researched, free of propaganda	5	4	3	2	1	0	0
6. Length suitable to audience and content	5	4	3	2	1	0	0
7. Durability	5	4	3	2	1	0	0
8. Usefulness in more than one subject area: write areas here _____	5	4	3	2	1	0	0

_____

_____

III. ORGANIZATION AND OVERALL CONTENT: COVERAGE OF HEALTH AREAS (How comprehensive is the coverage?)	High				Low	M*	NA
1. Anatomy and physiology	5	4	3	2	1	0	0
2. Community health (e.g., noise, chemical, water pollution control; community resources)	5	4	3	2	1	0	0
3. Consumer health (e.g., evaluating health products, use of medicines, components of health examinations, health care delivery system)	5	4	3	2	1	0	0

*Missing; material should have had item but does not.
†Not applicable.

Summary of Evaluation—cont'd

Organization and overall content—cont'd	High				Low	M*	NA
4. Disease prevention (e.g., lifestyle and disease; emotional illness; cancer; cardiovascular disorders; immunizations; diseases of interest to ethnic groups; oral health)	5	4	3	2	1	0	0
5. Adult lifestyle (e.g., changing roles; decisions about sex, marriage, and family; careers)	5	4	3	2	1	0	0
6. Fitness (e.g., benefits of fitness, fitness regimen, grooming and self-concept, fatigue, balanced diets, obesity, ethnic foods)	5	4	3	2	1	0	0
7. Growth and development (e.g., reproduction process, prenatal concerns, tools of inheritance, birth defects, genetic counseling, effects of drugs and nutrition on developing embryo and fetus)	5	4	3	2	1	0	0
8. Mental health (e.g., coping skills, stress, human needs and emotions, self-concept, mental illness, psychological growth and development, stereotyping)	5	4	3	2	1	0	0
9. Safety and first aid	5	4	3	2	1	0	0
10. Smoking, drugs, and alcohol (psychoactive drugs, medical use prescription and over-the-counter drugs)	5	4	3	2	1	0	0
11. Nutrition (e.g., basic necessities; balance; metabolism; changing needs; facts, fads, and fallacies; preparation)	5	4	3	2	1	0	0

IV. BIAS CONTENT	High				Low	M*	NA
1. Presents more than one viewpoint of controversial issues	5	4	3	2	1	0	0
2. Presents accurate facts when generalizations are made	5	4	3	2	1	0	0
3. Includes all socioeconomic levels and settings and all ethnic groups	5	4	3	2	1	0	0
4. Gives balanced treatment of the past and present	5	4	3	2	1	0	0
5. Promotes the diverse character of our nation by:	5	4	3	2	1	0	0
(a) Presenting the positive nature of cultural differences	5	4	3	2	1	0	0
(b) Using languages and models that treat all human beings with respect, dignity, and seriousness	5	4	3	2	1	0	0
(c) Including characters that help students identify positively with their heritage and culture	5	4	3	2	1	0	0
(d) Portraying families realistically (one parent, two parents, several generations)	5	4	3	2	1	0	0
(e) Portraying the handicapped realistically	5	4	3	2	1	0	0

Continued.

Summary of Evaluation—cont'd

	High				Low	M*	NA
6. Includes minorities and women by:	5	4	3	2	1	0	0
(a) Presenting their roles positively but realistically	5	4	3	2	1	0	0
(b) Having their contributions, inventions, or discoveries appear alongside those of white men	5	4	3	2	1	0	0
(c) Depicting them in a variety of occupations and at all levels in a profession	5	4	3	2	1	0	0
(d) Having their work included in materials	5	4	3	2	1	0	0
(e) Presenting information from their perspective	5	4	3	2	1	0	0
(f) Having appropriate illustrations	5	4	3	2	1	0	0

V. TEACHER'S GUIDE FOR TEXTS OR AUDIOVISUAL MATERIALS

	High				Low	M*	NA
1. Easy to use	5	4	3	2	1	0	0
2. Answers provided	5	4	3	2	1	0	0
3. Background information	5	4	3	2	1	0	0
4. Teaching strategies	5	4	3	2	1	0	0
5. Ideas for motivation, follow-up, extension	5	4	3	2	1	0	0
6. Guidelines for evaluation	5	4	3	2	1	0	0
7. Inclusion of script	5	4	3	2	1	0	0
8. Bibliography	5	4	3	2	1	0	0

VI. ADDITIONAL SUPPORT MATERIALS THAT ACCOMPANY TEXT

Please list the materials (e.g., workbooks, tests) and use separate form for each one listed

_____

_____

_____

USE THIS SPACE FOR COMMENTS:

Comparative Text Analysis

The following form, entitled "Comparative Text Analysis," is included as an aid for those who may have the opportunity to review numerous texts in the process of selecting one for local adoption. It can also be used to build a case for replacing old health textbooks. Although the format is designed for facilitating comparison of texts, the items are appropriate for evaluating a single text.

Using the following rating scale, evaluate the material in each area identified.

High............................*Low*	*Missing*	*Not Applicable*
4 3 2 1	0	NA

Fill in *title, publisher,* and *copyright date* for each text.

A. *TECHNICAL QUALITY*
1. General appearance
2. Readability of type
3. Quality of paper and binding
4. Appropriateness of illustrations
5. Format and general organization

B. *EFFECTIVENESS OF MATERIAL*
1. Adapts to individual needs and interests
2. Has appropriate sequential development
3. Provides varied teaching and learning strategies
4. Provides for measuring student achievement
5. Provides management system for tracking student progress
6. Provides clearly organized teacher edition

C. *CONTENT*
1. Consistent with district, program, and course goals
2. Reflects respect for personal worth
3. Aids in building positive attitudes and understandings
4. Depicts cultural diversity
5. Deals effectively with issues and problems
6. Offers accurate and realistic treatment of subject
7. Incorporates balanced viewpoints
8. Makes provision for distinguishing between fact and opinion
9. Stimulates critical thinking

D. *SEX BIAS*
1. Material divides qualities such as leadership, imagination, intelligence, and courage approximately evenly between male and female characters.
2. Females and males are equally represented as central characters in story and illustrative materials.
3. Both men and women are shown performing similar work in related fields.
4. Males and females are shown working together.
5. People are referred to by their own names and roles as often as they are referred to as someone's spouse, parent, or sibling.

Continued.

Comparative Text Analysis—cont'd

High................................Low   Missing   Not Applicable
 4   3   2   1   0   NA

Fill in *title, publisher,* and *copyright date* for each text.

6. Stereotyping language such as "women chatting"/"men discussing" is avoided.
7. Biographical or historical materials include a variety of male and female contributions to society.
8. Both males and females are given credit for discoveries and contributions to social, artistic, and scientific fields.
9. Groups that may include both males and females are referred to in "neutral" language such as people, mail carriers, fire fighters, or legislators.

E. *RACIAL/ETHNIC BIAS*
   1. Materials contain racial/ethnic balance in main characters and in illustrations.
   2. Oversimplifications and generalizations about racial groups are avoided in illustrations and in text material.
   3. Minority characters are shown in a variety of lifestyles in active, decision-making, and leadership roles.
   4. The vocabulary of racism is avoided.
   5. Minority characters are given credit for discoveries and contributions to social, artistic, and scientific fields.

Using the following rating scale, evaluate the material in each area identified.

High................................Low   Missing   Not Applicable
 4   3   2   1   0   NA

Fill in *title, publisher,* and *copyright date* for each text.

SUMMARY INFORMATION
   List total points for each area by Publisher and Title.
A. TECHNICAL QUALITY
B. EFFECTIVENESS OF MATERIAL
C. CONTENT
D. SEX BIAS
E. RACIAL/ETHNIC BIAS

Grand total scores

Additional rationale for selection of these materials: _____
_____
_____

Signs and Symptoms of Health Problems*

Point of observation	Physical signs	Behavior	Complaints
General appearance and behavior	Excessive thinness or overweight; very small or very large in body build for age; pallor; weary expression; poor posture; dark circles under or puffiness of eyes; unusual gait or limp; uncleanliness; lethargic and unresponsive; facial tic	Acts tired or apathetic; is easily irritated; makes frequent trips to toilet; has persistent-nervous habits, such as muscular twitching or biting of nails or lips; fainting, frequent nosebleeds; gets short of breath after mild exertion and climbing stairs; lacks appetite; vomits frequently; has frequent injuries; delayed speech for age	Feels tired; does not want to play; has aches or pains; feels dizzy
Hair and scalp	Stringy, lusterless hair; small bald spots; crusty sores on scalp; nits in hair or live lice on scalp	Scratches head frequently	Head itches
Ears	Discharge from ears; cotton in ear; tired, strained expression long before day is over; watchful, sometimes bewildered expression	Is persistently inattentive; asks to have questions repeated; habitually fails to respond when questioned; mispronounces common words; cocks one ear toward speaker; fails to follow directions	Has earache; has buzzing or ringing in ears; ears feel stuffy; hears noises in head

Continued.

*Basic source: Whaley LF, Wong DL: *Nursing care of infants and children,* ed 4, St Louis, 1991, Mosby–Year Book.

Point of observation	Physical signs	Behavior	Complaints
Eyes	Inflamed or watery eyes; frequent styes; red-rimmed, encrusted, swollen lids; crossed eye; recurring styes; sensitivity to light	Holds book too close to, or too far from, eyes; squints at book or blackboard; persistently rubs or blinks eyes; reads poorly; attempts to brush away blur; tilts head to one side; tends to reverse words or syllables; tends to lose place on page; shuts or covers one eye; unable to see distant things clearly	Headaches; dizziness; nausea; eyes ache, itch, smart, or feel scratchy; cannot see well (blurred or double vision); sensitivity to light
Mouth and teeth	Cavities in teeth; excessive stains; tartar at necks of teeth; malocclusion (uneven bite); irregular teeth; bleeding or inflamed gums; swollen jaw; sores in mouth; cracking of lips at corners of mouth	Acts depressed or resentful if missing teeth or severe malocclusion subjects him or her to teasing or adverse comments from other children; this behavior is especially likely to occur in adolescence	Has toothache; mouth or gums feel sore
Nose and throat (upper respiratory tract)	Frequent or long-continued colds; persistent nasal discharge; persistent mouth breathing; enlarged glands in neck	Is often absent because of a "cold"; constantly clears throat or has frequent coughing spells; is always sniffling or blowing nose; breathes persistently through mouth	Throat feels sore or scratchy; has difficulty in swallowing; nose feels stuffy or sore
Skin	Rashes or inflamed skin areas; scales and crusts; persistent sores, pimples, and blackheads on face; boils; hives; persistent warts; injuries, such as cuts, scratches, bruises, burns, blisters; dry, red, rough skin	Is always scratching; is subject to skin irritations (hives, eczema, puzzling rashes, etc), which suggest sensitivity to one or more substances (allergic manifestations); is easily bruised	Skin itches or burns; is concerned about pimples, blackheads, and other skin conditions that affect personal appearance

Condition	Signs and symptoms	
Allergy	Stuffy and runny nose; sneezing; persistent cough; swollen eyelids; rash; itching; watery and burning eyes; paleness; mouth breathing	Tired and listless, recurrent headaches, recurrent gastrointestinal cramps, vomiting, diarrhea
Cancer	Leukemia: tires easily; irritable, pale (anemic), recurrent and serious infections, prolonged bleeding from injuries	Brain tumors: irritability, fatigability, decreased appetite and activity, intermittent headache

Condition	Signs and symptoms	
Child abuse	Bruises, untreated sores, burns, skin injuries; wears long-sleeved shirts or blouses to hide bruises, cannot sit comfortably; may describe extreme punishment or being photographed nude	Hungry for affection, difficulty relating to others, displays behavioral extremes—timid/fearless, passive/aggressive; undiagnosed learning problems
Child neglect	Unsupervised out of school; kept home to babysit; parent will not get needed health care despite resources	Malnutrition—underweight, fatigue; no breakfast, food, or lunch money
Contagious diseases of childhood	100.4° F temperature taken orally (fever, flushed face, lassitude, malaise); sore or scratchy throat; red, watery eyes; watery nasal discharge	Tight, dry cough; sneezing; headache, earache, or aching in back or legs; nausea or vomiting
Diabetes	Frequent/excess urination, excessive thirst, unusual hunger	Rapid loss of weight, irritability, obvious weakness and fatigue, nausea and vomiting
Diabetic insulin reaction*	Excessive hunger, perspiration, pallor, headache, dizziness, nervousness—trembling, confusion, crying	Irritability, drowsiness, fatigue, blurred vision, poor coordination, abdominal pain or nausea
Epilepsy	Dazed look, loss of consciousness	Tremors of any or all groups of muscles, odd gestures or movements (e.g., chewing or lip-smacking), occasional loss of muscle control (involuntary urination)
Heart problems	Pale, blue lips; short of breath on rest or exertion; undersized, deformed chest	Rapid pulse at rest, clubbed fingers, easily fatigued, undernourished, fainting after exertion or excitement
Hyperactivity (by medical diagnosis)	Easily distracted, impulsiveness, shift from activity to activity, short attention span, difficulty waiting for a turn	Fidgeting, squirms, difficulty remaining seated, difficulty following through task, clumsiness, aggressive behavior, low frustration level, blurts out answers
Lead poisoning	Fatigue, lethargy, stomach pains, constipation, vomiting, anemia, irritability, hearing impairment, learning problems	Headaches, unsteady walking, insomnia, convulsions, loss of coordination, poor appetite or paleness; may be no symptoms
Nutritional deficiencies	General appearance: fatigue slouch or posture; round shoulders or flabby muscles; excessively thin with spindly legs; lack of or finicky appetite; fails to gain weight steadily; excessively fat or poor distribution of fat; strained and worried look; listless; easily fatigued and possibly irritable Hair: dry, coarse, brittle, lacking luster, dull	Eyes: tiny red line (engorged capillaries) extending around or across the cornea and inward toward pupil; dark circles under eyes; inflammation and crusting of lids Teeth and gums: decayed teeth; swollen, bleeding, or spongy gums; or abnormal color Tongue: beefy red and magenta Mouth: scarring, fissuring, or sores on angles of lips Skin: small nodules (like gooseflesh) or scaly and rough Chest, knees, legs and feet: pigeon-breasted, knock-kneed, bow-legged, flatfooted—abnormal bone growth

*Give sugar immediately in form of sugar, fruit juice, carbonated beverages, or candy.

Continued.

Condition	Signs and symptoms	
Posture	Head tilted to side when reading or listening	Shoulders not level: one higher, lower, or forward
	Head tilted forward when sitting, standing or walking	Round shoulders with protruding shoulder blades
	Feet pointed inward or outward; stands with weight on inner ankles (pronated); drags or shuffles feet	One hip higher or more prominent
		Knees pointed inward (knock-kneed), outward or hyperextended (bowlegs)
Rheumatic fever (follows strep infection)	Fever (afternoons), loss in weight; pallor; irritability; flat, nonitchy rash; abdominal pain	Painful swelling in different large joints, poor appetite, unexplained nosebleeds, chorea (aimless movements)
Sexually transmitted diseases	Syphilis (least likely observed): Within 10 to 90 days—small painless sore (chancre) at site where germs entered body	Gonorrhea: Within 3 to 8 days in males—burning sensation on urination, pus from urethra; in females—often no pain until pelvic inflammation, painful urination, vulva soreness
	Chlamydia: Signs may be absent; within 8 to 12 days in males—painful urination, urethral itching or discharge; in females—discharge	HPV (human papillomavirus): genital warts
	Herpes simplex, type II: Blisters on genitalia, sometimes on buttocks and thighs	Nongonococcal urethritis (NGU): pain on urination
Sickle cell anemia	Pain in arms and legs, swelling in joints, loss of appetite	Weakness, pain in abdomen, fever
Social-emotional stress	Overtimidity: withdrawing, crying easily	Excess boasting or showing off
	Overaggressiveness: bullying, quarreling, cruel behavior	Poor sportsmanship
	Excessive daydreaming: persistent inattentiveness	Undue restlessness: hyperactivity, tics, stammering, nail biting
		Frequent accidents or near accidents
	Extreme sensitiveness to criticism: cries easily, temper tantrums	Unusual sex behavior for age
	Failure to advance in school at normal rate despite good physical health and adequate intellectual capacity	Unhappy and depressed
		Gradual deterioration or marked sudden drop in educational achievement
	Stuttering or other speech difficulty or change	Lack of interest or motivation
	Lying, stealing, cheating, truancy	Withdrawal, shyness, self-deprecation
	Resistance to authority: constant complaints of unfairness, "picked on," may engage in vandalism	Demands perfection
		Inconsistent bladder or bowel control
		Constantly seeking attention or popularity
"Strep" throat	Fever, sore throat, swollen neck glands, nausea/vomiting	(Presence of rash is called scarlet fever)

Condition	Signs and symptoms	
Suicidal risk	Sudden shift in quality of work; use of drugs and alcohol; changes in early behavior and learning patterns; extreme fatigue; decreased appetite; inability to concentrate; truancy; gives away prized possessions; "accident-prone"	Psychotic or mental illness—hallucinations; distress signals—"Notice me; I need help; you'll be sorry when I'm dead"; feelings of sadness, hopelessness, loss of interest; isolates self; reacts to stress, usually a loss, by turning aggression inward
Tuberculosis	Persistent cough, blood in sputum, nervousness, lack of energy, easy fatigability, fever Children may have no signs	Loss of weight, chest pain, afternoon fever, pallor, loss of appetite

Other Problems Encountered by Elementary Teachers

Teachers also have self-risk worries about these communicable conditions:

Hepatitis, type A	Young children may have only mild diarrhea; low fever, dark urine, nausea/vomiting, light-color feces, fatigue, jaundice later
Impetigo	Blisters on skin that ooze yellow fluid and crust over
Infectious mononucleosis	High fever, sore throat, swollen glands at back of neck, fatigue
Pediculosis/lice	Small, moving insect(s) on scalp, tiny oval eggs (nits) tightly attached to hair shaft
Tinea/ringworm	Slowly spreading, flat, scaly ring-like skin rash, ring edges may be red and slightly raised; scalp ringworm has slowly spreading balding patches with broken-off hairs
Scabies	Small, raised red or blisterlike bumps that itch intensely, especially at night, usually found in creases of skin

Good Health Characteristics of Children

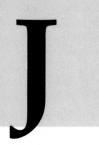

Physical	Social-emotional	Work habits
Endurance: completes a task without undue fatigue	Enthusiastic	Attentive
Enjoys vigorous play	Objective interests: friends, hobbies, games, work, people	Carries a task through to completion
Alert, pleasant	Curious: interested in a variety of things	Ability to concentrate
Looks refreshed in morning	Enters into activities	Persistent in work
Posture expresses confidence, self-worth, sense of security	Happy, cheerful, friendly	Works independently
Muscular coordination and strength	Refrains from quarreling	Orderly in work habits
Hair: clean, groomed	Confident: expects success, learns from mistakes	Shows originality and initiative
Clear skin, clear eyes, clean, neat appearance, inoffensive breath, wholesome appetite	Shares group responsibility	Creative
Body limbs generally symmetrical; no visible differences	Protects others' property	Takes responsibility
Vision: no squinting or unusual posture	Appreciation and understanding for others; respects others	Responds quickly and cheerfully to directions, asks questions if uncertain
Hearing: responds as expected for group; speech sound clear for age and native language; no unusual posture as if straining to hear	Does things for the group, not for self alone	Shares group responsibility
Bladder/bowel: toilet trained, no pain or straining	Shows courage in meeting difficulties	Cooperative with peers; can wait for turn
	Adapts to new situations	Meets deadlines
	Tolerates frustration	Asks for help appropriately
	Has one or more very good friends, able to interact well in small groups	

K

Growth and Development Characteristics

Physical development	Characteristics	Health education content implications
3 TO 5 YEARS OF AGE		
Growth continues at moderately rapid rate	Needs vigorous outdoor activity	Rest and sleep; adequate amounts needed; provide rest periods
Permanent body build evident	Becoming more independent; doing things for self; more self-reliant; can wash and dress self; needs freedom	Dental health: emphasis on food selection and care of teeth
Head and upper body reach adult proportions		Emotional health: needs attention, freedom, and learning to share and get along; provide restraints with love and care; believes death is reversible
Legs and arms lengthening	Needs to learn to get along with others, to share, to take turns	
Bone growth proceeding and cartilage almost completely replaced by bone	Unaware of others' views; thinks, "what's right for me is right for you"	Nutrition: emphasis on adequate diet and amounts of protein, minerals, and vitamins
Girls ahead of boys in skeletal development; usually lighter and shorter than boys	Temper tantrums less likely; may begin to call names, "I don't like you"; much quarreling, hitting, fighting	Sex education: answer questions with simple understandings; recognizes genders; use correct terms and talk about body parts; interested in where babies come from and how they "get in" and "get out"
Primary teeth usually developed	Learns through play; crayons, blocks, large pencils	
Large muscle weight increasing; boys with more muscle tissue than girls; girls more fatty tissue	Language development increases; understands words; can give simple reasons and explanations; can absorb much information; asks questions	Safety: shows concern for school and playground accident prevention
Brain at 90% of adult weight	Asks about word meanings	Exercise: allow for vigorous play involving large muscle activities; small muscle coordination not developed
Motor control; hops and skips; some bedwetting	Can play longer without fatigue	
	Begins to identify own sex; asks why mothers and fathers are different	
	Play includes gender stereotypes	
	Responds when treated as individual	
	Attention hard to hold	

Physical development	Characteristics	Health education content implications
5 TO 7 YEARS OF AGE		
Growth is relatively slow: at age 7 may be 2 to 3 inches and 3 to 6 pounds yearly	On entering school there may be a resumption of earlier tensional behavior; thumbsucking, nail biting, toilet lapses	Mental health:
Large muscles better developed than small ones; improving by age 7	Eager to learn, exuberant, restless; exaggerates, and susceptible to fatigue; dawdling may occur	Wants to get along with peers
Some postural defects may have been established by age of 6	Criticism difficult; thrives on encouragement	Praise, warmth, and patience with independence and encouraging support from adults
Hand-eye coordination is incomplete; 90% are right-handed; small muscle control difficult, especially of fingers and hands	Attention span short but increasing; interested in activity, not results, learns best through active participation	Some responsibilities without pressure of being required to make decisions or meet rigid standards
Eyeballs are still increasing in size; tendency toward farsightedness	Has difficulty making decisions	Help make adjustments in playground; withdrawn child needs encouragement to find place in group
Heart is in a period of rapid growth	Self-assertive; aggressive; wants to be first; becoming self-sufficient; can take care of own toilet needs and dressing; likes to climb and jump; by 7 is apt to be talkative and prone to exaggeration; competition developing	Provide sense of accomplishment for each child; engage in real tasks; needs freedom
Permanent teeth begin to appear; baby teeth begin to be lost		Provide active participation in learning with concrete objects
Susceptible to respiratory infections; childhood diseases such as chickenpox		Exercise and safety: active, boisterous games for large muscles; stress safety
Tires easily	Interest of boys and girls diverging, less play together; gets along best in small groups	Vision care: protect eyes
Teeth: 6-year molars appearing and loss of primary teeth	Able to assume some responsibility concerning right and wrong and simple tasks	Sleep and rest: need 11 or more hours of sleep and possibly daytime naps
	Developing conscience	Dental health: emphasis on tooth care
	Able to compromise if can't get one's way	Disease control: development of personal hygiene; cover coughs, sneezes, keep fingers away from mouth, wash hands, and others
	Careless about others' property; protective of own	Nutrition: concepts of food, eating behavior, and health
	Recognizes others' ideas; believes due to different information	
	Increased ability to organize, generalize, reason	
	Awareness of race and group	
	Enjoys rhythms, active play, fairy tales, comics, TV, myths, dramatic play, and stories	
	Moods fluctuate; quick resistance to bathing	

Physical development	Characteristics	Health education content implications
8 TO 10 YEARS OF AGE		

8 TO 10 YEARS OF AGE

Physical development	Characteristics	Health education content implications
Growth still slow and steady; some children reach plateau preceding growth of preadolescence; differences in individual bone ossification may vary as much as 5 to 6 years; girls' growth spurts at about 10 years	Wants to do well but loses interest if discouraged or pressured; sensitive to criticism	Mental health:
Small muscles developing; manipulative skill increasing	Gangs strong and of one sex only, of short duration and changing membership; response to structured groups and activities	Self-concept; values
Poor posture may develop; presence may indicate chronic infection, fatigue, orthopedic difficulties, emotional distress	Allegiance to peers instead of adult in case of conflict; wants a "best friend"	Needs friends and group membership

Mental health:
- Self-concept; values
- Needs friends and group membership
- Training in skills without pressure
- Wise guidance and channeling of interests rather than domination or overcritical standards
- Praise, encouragement; warmth from adults
- Gains self-confidence by excelling in one thing
- Define responsibility; reasonable explanations; no talking down
- Views death as punishment

Exercise:
- Activities involving use of whole body; sports and games
- Posture development in need of attention

Sleep and rest: 10 to 12 hours of sleep
Nutrition: balanced intake of foods; foods needed daily; wise food choices
Dental health: care of teeth and gums
Disease control: handwashing, nail care, food washing
Safety: accident prevention
Sex education: growth and developmental changes; caring for others; life cycle; gender body parts vocabulary
Grooming: hair washing, clean clothes

Physical development

Growth still slow and steady; some children reach plateau preceding growth of preadolescence; differences in individual bone ossification may vary as much as 5 to 6 years; girls' growth spurts at about 10 years
Small muscles developing; manipulative skill increasing
Poor posture may develop; presence may indicate chronic infection, fatigue, orthopedic difficulties, emotional distress
Hand-eye coordination improved; hands ready for crafts
Eyes:
  Near-sightedness may develop during eighth year
Incisors and lower bicuspids appear; often a period of dental neglect; orthodontia may be necessary
Internal changes in glands and body structure taking place; wide range in beginning of sexual maturity; period of rapid growth comes earlier for girls, it lasts longer in boys:
  Boys: beginning puberty cycle 10 to 13 years; ends 14 to 18½ years
  Girls: appearance of menstruation 10 to 16 years; average 12 years
Lungs and digestive and circulatory systems still developing

Characteristics

Wants to do well but loses interest if discouraged or pressured; sensitive to criticism
Gangs strong and of one sex only, of short duration and changing membership; response to structured groups and activities
Allegiance to peers instead of adult in case of conflict; wants a "best friend"
Capable of prolonged interest; often makes plans and goes ahead on his or her own; increased attention span; realism replacing fantasy
Enjoys conforming to rules of game, testing his or her skill against perfection; can be fairly responsible and dependable
Gaining self-control; conscience becoming strong; awareness of self-energy
Fairly good eater; may neglect vegetables
Decisive, responsible, dependable, reasonable, strong sense of right and wrong; much arguing over fairness of games
Recognizes disagreements with same information; anticipates others' reactions to behaviors but is not able to consider others' viewpoints
Is untidy, deliberately avoids table manners, handwashing, hair combing; protests parents' choice of new clothes; general coolness toward all adults
Is prone to accidents
Health usually good; energetic
Fond of sports and games, collections, comics, adventure stories

Physical development	Characteristics	Health education content implications
11 TO 13 YEARS OF AGE		
A "resting period" followed by a period of rapid growth in height, then weight; usually starts somewhere between 9 and 13 years; girls usually taller and heavier at 11 years than boys	Wide range of individual differences and maturity levels; begins to analyze complex concepts—not future oriented; able to think abstractly, see cause-effect relationships and consequences of actions; considers others' views	Mental health: Self-image; success experiences Warm affection, approval, no nagging or condemnation Increase opportunities for independence Relations with others Sense of belonging and peer group relations—clubs and team sports; needs conflict resolutions without anger
Rapid muscular growth; uneven growth of different parts of body; possible restlessness, listlessness; increased appetite; awkwardness prevalent; posture may be slovenly	Gangs or groups important; prestige is more important than adult approval; gang interest is changing to interest in one or two best friends (girls more than boys)	Values development Individual health and emotional counseling
Secondary sex characteristics beginning to develop; may cause embarrassment; in girls hip and breast development; in boys voice changes	Loves parents but does not show it, cool toward adults; needs affirmation of parents' love	Nutrition: adequate diet importance; amounts and effects of fat, fiber, and cholesterol Rest and sleep: 9 to 11 hours of sleep Exercise: sports and games, both individual and team; satisfaction from risk-taking play
More rest is needed	Strong sense of responsibility about matters thought to be important	Dental health: care of teeth Safety: accident prevention and first aid
Permanent dentition of 28 teeth is completed by 13 to 14 years	Girls mature earlier than boys; girls are taller, heavier	Disease control: acne especially Sex education: Physical and social changes Relationships Sexually transmitted diseases
Resistance to infection may be low	Strong interest in sex, much teasing and antagonism between boy and girl groups; sex consciousness may cause self-consciousness and shyness	Human sexuality is natural Reproductive cycle Pregnancy probability Recognize potential sexual abuse
	Child approaching adolescence often becomes hypercritical, changeable, rebellious, uncooperative; exhibits extremes from independence to childish dependence; may rebel; sensitive to criticism; erratic responses and mood swings	
	Interest in activities to earn money	
	Reading tastes apparent	
	May be overanxious about own health and normalcy; self-conscious about body changes	
	Competition is keen; development of coordination and skills through games	

Joint Statement on School Health by the Secretaries of Education and Health and Human Services

On April 7, 1994, the U.S. Secretaries of Education and Health and Human Services jointly released a historic statement that resulted in the formation of an Interagency Committee on School Health. This committee has been delegated to provide cooperative effort in support of comprehensive school health programs in the United States, especially to achieve the health goals found in the publication, *Healthy People 2000*.

Joint Statement on School Health
by
The Secretaries of Education and Health and Human Services

Health and education are joined in fundamental ways with each other and with the destinies of the Nation's children. Because of our national leadership responsibilities for education and health, we have initiated unprecedented cooperative efforts between our Departments. In support of comprehensive school health programs, we affirm the following:

- **America's children face many compelling educational and health and developmental challenges that affect their lives and their futures.**

  These challenges include poor levels of achievement, unacceptably high drop-out rates; low literacy; violence; drug abuse; preventable injuries; physical and mental illness; developmental disabilities; and sexual activity resulting in sexually transmitted diseases, including HIV, and unintended pregnancy. These facts demand a reassessment of the contributions of education and health programs in safeguarding our children's present lives and preparing them for productive, responsible, and fulfilling futures.

- **To help children meet these challenges, education and health must be linked in partnership.**

  Schools are the only public institutions that touch nearly every young person in this country. Schools have a unique opportunity to affect the lives of children and their families, but they cannot address all of our children's needs alone. Health, education, and human service programs must be integrated, and schools must have the support of public and private health care providers, communities, and families.

- **School health programs support the education process, integrate services for disadvantaged and disabled children, and improve children's health prospects.**

  Through school health programs, children and their families can develop the knowledge, attitudes, beliefs, and behaviors necessary to remain healthy and perform well in school. These learning environments enhance safety, nutrition, and disease prevention, encourage exercise and fitness; support healthy physical, mental, and emotional development, promote abstinence and prevent sexual behaviors that result in HIV infection, other sexually transmitted diseases, and unintended teenage pregnancy; discourage use of illegal drugs, alcohol, and tobacco; and help young people develop problem-solving and decision-making skills.

- **Reforms in health care and in education offer opportunities to forge the partnerships needed for our children in the 1990s.**

  The benefits of integrated health and education services can be achieved by working together to create a "seamless" network of services, both through the school setting and through linkages with other community resources.

- **GOALS 2000 and HEALTHY PEOPLE 2000 provide complementary visions that, together, can support our joint efforts in pursuit of a healthier, better educated nation for the next century.**

  GOALS 2000 challenges us to ensure that all children arrive at school ready to learn; to increase the high school graduation rate; to achieve basic subject matter competencies; to achieve universal adult literacy; and to ensure that school environments are safe, disciplined, and drug free. HEALTHY PEOPLE 2000 challenges us to increase the span of healthy life for the American people, to reduce and finally to eliminate health disparities among population groups, and to ensure access to services for all Americans.

In support of GOALS 2000 and HEALTHY PEOPLE 2000, we have established the Interagency Committee on School Health co-chaired by the Assistant Secretary for Elementary and Secondary Education and the Assistant Secretary for Health, and we have convened the National Coordinating Committee on School Health to bring together representatives of major national education and health organizations to work with us.

We call upon professionals in the fields of education and health and concerned citizens across the Nation to join with us in a renewed effort and a reaffirmation of our mutual responsibility to our Nation's children.

Richard W. Riley
Secretary of Education

Donna E. Shalala
Secretary of Health and Human Services

Issued April 7, 1994.

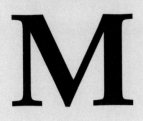

APPENDIX

M General Criteria for Assessing Health Instruction Software

The criteria presented below were developed to help you assess health instruction software. You should respond to each of the items in the form. A separate form should be completed for each piece of software that is assessed. Any comments relative to the software should be included with the form.

EVALUATED BY _____   DATE _____

COMMITTEE _____   SCHOOL _____

Program Title: _____

Author/Distributor: _____

Version: _____   Prior Version: _____   Copyright: _____

Grade Level: _____   Cost: _____   License: _____

Is program compatible with existing hardware: _____

Additional hardware requirements:

    Color Monitor: _____   Printer Type: _____

    Mouse: _____   Memory: _____

    Hard Drive: _____   DOS Version: _____

    RAM Needed: _____   Modem Req: Yes: ___ No: ___

    Floppy Drives: _____

Audience: Elementary: ___   Intermediate: ___   Upper: ___

Computer Skill Level: Novice: ___   Intermed: ___   Advanced: ___

Setting: Individual: ___   Pairs: ___   Small Group: ___

    Classroom: ___   Lab: ___

Technical Information: Graphics: ___   Color: ___   Music: ___

    Time Display: ___   Pull Down Menu: ___Windows: ___

    Student Scores Stored: ___   Score Display: ___

    Class Scores Maintained: ___   Score Display: ___

    Help Screen Available: _____

    Graphics Quality: _____

    Data Save and Reentry at Point of Save: _____

    Teacher Can Personalize: _____

    Ease of Teacher Alteration: _____

Health Content Area: _____

Content Overview: _____

_____

_____

_____

_____

Instructional Objectives:

1. _____

2. _____

3. _____

4. _____

5. _____

Content:

     Accuracy: Good: ___   Fair: ___   Poor: ___   Inaccurate: ___

     Stereotypes: None: ___   Specify: _____

     Bias: None: ___   Specify: _____

     Meets Needs Of: Students: ___   Teacher: ___   Course: ___

Ease of Use: Easy: ___   Intermediate: ___   Difficult: ___

Instructions Provided: _____

_____

Instructional Assessment:

     Personalization Included: _____   Positive Feedback: _____

     Practice Provided: _____   Branching OK: _____

     Examples Provided: _____   Pre-Test: _____

     Post-Test: _____   Rank Indicated: _____

Output:

     Individual Student Data: _____

     Classroom Data: _____

Documentation:

     Teacher: _____   Specific Instructions Provided: _____

     Student: _____   Specific Instructions Provided: _____

     Helpline listed: Local: (_____)_____   Distance: (_____)_____

     Data Interpretation Examples Provided: _____

     Instructional Suggestions Offered: _____

     Time Framework: _____

     Integration Plan Included: _____

Review Comments: _____

_____

_____

_____

_____

_____

_____

Index